The Atlas of
Emergency
Medicine

The Atlas of Emergency Medicine

THIRD EDITION

Editors

Kevin J. Knoop, MD, MS

Director, Professional Education, Naval Medical Center, Portsmouth, Virginia
Assistant Professor of Military and Emergency Medicine,
Uniformed Services University of the Health Sciences,
Bethesda, Maryland

Lawrence B. Stack, MD

Associate Professor of Emergency Medicine,
Vanderbilt University, Nashville, Tennessee

Alan B. Storrow, MD

Vice Chairman for Research and Academic Affairs
Associate Professor of Emergency Medicine,
Vanderbilt University, Nashville, Tennessee

R. Jason Thurman, MD

Assistant Professor of Emergency Medicine
Associate Director, Residency Program, Department of Emergency Medicine,
Vanderbilt University, Nashville, Tennessee

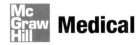 **Medical**

New York   Chicago   San Francisco   Lisbon   London   Madrid   Mexico City

Milan   New Delhi   San Juan   Seoul   Singapore   Sydney   Toronto

The Atlas of Emergency Medicine, Third Edition

The views expressed in this work are those of the individual authors and do not reflect the official policy or position of the Departments of the Navy, Army or Air Force, the Department of Defense, or the U.S. Government.

1 2 3 4 5 6 7 8 9 0   CTP/CTP   14 13 12 11 10 9

ISBN 978-0-07-149618-6
MHID 0-07-149618-1

This book was set in Times Roman by International Typesetting and Composition.
The editors were Anne M. Sydor and Cindy Yoo.
The production supervisor was Sherri Souffrance.
Project management was provided by Rajni Pisharody, International Typesetting and Composition.
The designer was Janice Bielawa; the cover art director was Margaret Webster-Shapiro; the cover designer was Tom Lau.
China Translation & Printing Services, Ltd. was printer and binder.

This book is printed on acid-free paper.

Library of Congress Cataloging-in-Publication Data

Atlas of emergency medicine / editors, Kevin J. Knoop . . . [et al.].—3rd ed.
    p. ; cm.
  Includes bibliographical references and index.
  ISBN 978-0-07-149618-6 (alk. paper)
  1. Emergency medicine–Atlases.   I. Knoop, Kevin J.
  [DNLM: 1. Emergency Medicine–methods–Atlases.   2. Critical Care–methods–Atlases.
3. Emergencies–Atlases.   WB 17 A8817 2009]
RC86.7.A85   2009
616.02'5—dc22
                                                      2009014108

McGraw-Hill books are available at special quantity discounts to use as premiums and sales promotions, or for use in corporate training programs. To contact a representative please e-mail us at bulksales@mcgraw-hill.com.

To Mimi and Stephen, for your warm hearts and clear minds. You make me extremely proud to be your father.

To Mary Jo, still my high school sweetheart! For your tenacity in pursuing your goals, and for your endless support, love and friendship.

To our patients, who trust us in their care and allow their illness or injury to be used to help others.

KJK

To the patients who have allowed us to photograph their physical examination findings—I pray for Gods blessings on you for allowing others to learn from your illness and injuries for the benefit of caring for other patients.

LBS

To my mother, Ruth Ann Storrow, in deep gratitude for your steadfast love, support, and guidance.

ABS

To my wonderful wife, Lauren, whose abundance of patience, love, and encouragement enrich every moment.

To our children, Kate and Ben, who bring joy into every day.

To all those who have generously provided mentoring, especially Drs. Knoop, Stack, and Storrow, whose vision and tireless effort produced the first two editions of this book: I am deeply honored and humbled to have had the opportunity to work alongside them.

RJT

CONTENTS

Part 1 REGIONAL ANATOMY 1

Chapter 1
HEAD AND FACIAL TRAUMA 3

David W. Munter ▪ Timothy D. McGuirk

Chapter 2
OPHTHALMOLOGIC CONDITIONS 25

Marc E. Levsky ▪ Paul DeFlorio

Chapter 3
FUNDUSCOPIC FINDINGS 57

David Effron ▪ Beverly C. Forcier ▪ Richard E. Wyszynski

Chapter 4
OPHTHALMIC TRAUMA 77

Dallas E. Peak ▪ Christopher S. Weaver ▪ Kevin J. Knoop

Chapter 8
UROLOGIC CONDITIONS 189
Jeffery D. Bondesson

Chapter 9
SEXUALLY TRANSMITTED INFECTIONS AND ANORECTAL CONDITIONS 209
Diane M. Birnbaumer ◼ Lynn K. Flowers

Sexually Transmitted Infections 210

Chapter 10
GYNECOLOGIC AND OBSTETRIC CONDITIONS 233
Robert G. Buckley ◼ Kevin J. Knoop

Gynecologic Conditions 234

Obstetric Conditions 249

Part 2 SPECIALTY AREAS 403

Chapter 14
PEDIATRIC CONDITIONS 405

Matthew R. Mittiga ▪ Javier A. Gonzalez del Rey
▪ Richard M. Ruddy

Chapter 15
CHILD ABUSE   457

Robert A. Shapiro ▪ Charles J. Schubert
▪ Kathi L. Makoroff ▪ Megan L. McGraw

Chapter 16
ENVIRONMENTAL CONDITIONS   487

Ken Zafren ▪ R. Jason Thurman ▪ Ian D. Jones

Chapter 17
TOXICOLOGICAL CONDITIONS   533

Saralyn R. Williams ▪ Matthew D. Sztajnkrycer
▪ R. Jason Thurman

Chapter 22
AIRWAY PROCEDURES 689

Steven J. White ■ Richard M. Levitan ■ Lawrence B. Stack

Chapter 23
ECG ABNORMALITIES 733

James V. Ritchie ■ Michael L. Juliano ■ R. Jason Thurman

Part 1: ST-T Abnormalities 734

Part 2: Conduction Disturbances 747

Part 3: Rhythm Disturbances 757

Part 4: Structural Abnormalities 768

J. Michael Ballester, MD
Assistant Professor and Director, Fourth Year Medical
   Student Clerkship
Wright State University
Boonshoft School of Medicine
Dayton, Ohio
Chapter 20

Sean P. Barbabella, DO
LCDR, MC, USN
Associate Residency Director
Emergency Medicine
Naval Medical Center Portsmouth
Portsmouth, Virginia
Chapter 5

Diane M. Birnbaumer, MD
Professor of Clinical Medicine
Emergency Medicine
David Geffen School of Medicine at UCLA
Westwood, California
Chapters 9 and 25

Jeffery D. Bondesson, MD
Attending Physician
Emergency Department
Kaiser San Diego Medical Center
San Diego, California
Chapter 8

Robert G. Buckley, MD, MPH, FACEP
CAPT, MC, USN
Director for Branch Clinics
Staff Physician
Emergency Medicine
Naval Medical Center San Diego
San Diego, California
Chapter 10

Stephen W. Corbett, MD, PhD
Professor
Department of Emergency Medicine
Loma Linda University Medical Center
Loam Linda, California
Chapter 7

Paul DeFlorio, MD
MAJ, MC, USAF
Adjunct Assistant Professor
Military and Emergency Medicine
Uniformed Services University of the Health Sciences
Bethesda, Maryland
Chapter 2

David Effron, MD, FACEP
Assistant Professor
Emergency Medicine
Case Western Reserve University, Metro Health Medical Center
Cleveland, Ohio
Chapter 3

Francisco J. Fernandez, MD, MS
Clinical Instructor
Emergency Medicine
University of Cincinnati College of Medicine
Cincinnati, Ohio
Chapter 5

Lynn K. Flowers, MD, MHA, FACEP
Physician Partner
Emergency Medicine
Apollo MD
Atlanta, Georgia
Chapter 9

Beverly C. Forcier, MD
Ophthalmology
Cleveland Heights, Ohio
Chapter 3

Javier A. Gonzalez del Rey, MD, Med
Professor of Clinical Pediatrics
Department of Pediatrics
University of Cincinnati College of Medicine
Cincinnati Children's Hospital Medical Center
Cincinnati, Ohio
Chapter 14

Brent E. Gottesman, MD
Clinical Instructor
Emergency Department
University Hospital
Cincinnati, Ohio
Chapter 6

Jason Gukhool, MD, RDMS
Director of Emergency Ultrasound
Greater Houston Emergency Physicians
Houston, Texas
Chapter 24

J. Matthew Hardin, MD
Chief Resident, Division of Dermatology
Vanderbilt University
Nashville, Tennessee
Chapter 13

Meg Jack, MD
Assistant Professor of Emergency Medicine
Vanderbilt University
Nashville, Tennessee
Chapter 21

Edward C. Jauch, MD, MS, FAHA, FACEP
Associate Professor
Division of Emergency Medicine & Department of
   Neurosciences
Medical University of South Carolina
Charleston, South Carolina
Chapter 6

Ian D. Jones, MD
Assistant Professor of Emergency Medicine
Medical Director Adult Emergency Department
Vanderbilt University
Nashville, Tennessee
Chapter 16

Michael L. Juliano, MD
LCDR, MC, USN
Attending Physician
Department of Emergency Medicine
Naval Medical Center Portsmouth
Portsmouth, Virginia
Chapters 18 and 23

Kevin J. Knoop, MD, MS
CAPT, MC, USN
Director, Professional Education
Naval Medical Center Portsmouth
Portsmouth, Virginia
Assistant Professor of Military and Emergency Medicine,
    Uniformed Services
University of the Health Sciences
Bethesda, Maryland
Chapters 4, 5, 7, 10

Stephen J. Leech, MD, RDMS
Assistant Clinical Professor
Departments of Emergency Medicine
University of Central Florida School of Medicine
Florida State University School of Medicine
Orlando, Florida
Chapter 24

Richard M. Levitan, MD
Attending Physician
Emergency Medicine Department
Director of Airway Training Center
Albert Einstein Medical Center
Philadelphia, Pennsylvania
Chapter 22

Marc E. Levsky, MD, RDMS
Attending Physician
Division of Emergency Medicine
Seton Medical Center
Daly City, California
Chapter 2

Kathi L. Makoroff, MD
Assistant Professor
Department of Pediatrics
University of Cincinnati College of Medicine
Cincinnati, Ohio
Chapter 15

Megan L. McGraw, MD
Assistant Professor of Clinical Pediatrics
Department of Pediatrics, Division of Child and Family Advocacy
The Ohio State University College of Medicine/Nationwide
    Children's Hospital
Columbus, Ohio
Chapter 15

Timothy D. McGuirk, DO, FACEP
Attending Physician
Emerency Medicine Department
Naval Medical Center Portsmouth
Portsmouth, Virginia
Chapter 1

Matthew R. Mittiga, MD
Assistant Professor of Clinical Pediatrics
Department of Pediatrics
University of Cincinnati College of Medicine
Cincinnati Children's Hospital Medical Center
Cincinnati, Ohio
Chapter 14

Roderick Morrison, MD
Emergency Medicine Resident
Wright State University
Boonshoft School of Medicine
Dayton, Ohio
Chapter 20

David W. Munter, MD, MBA
Assistant Clinical Professor
Department of Emergency Medicine
Eastern Virginia Medical School
Norfolk, Virginia
Chapter 1

Chan W. Park, MD
LCDR, MC, USN
Attending Physician
Department of Emergency Medicine
Naval Medical Center
Portsmouth, Virginia
Chapter 18

Dallas E. Peak, MD, FACEP
Assistant Professor of Clinical Emergency Medicine
Department of Emergency Medicine
Indiana University School of Medicine
Indianapolis, Indiana
Chapter 4

Neha P. Raukar, MD, MS
Assistant Professor
Emergency Medicine
Brown University
Providence, Rhode Island
Chapter 11

George J. Raukar, MD
Orthopaedic Surgery
Coastal Orthopaedics
Fall River, Massachusetts
Chapter 11

James V. Ritchie, MD
CAPT, MC, USN
Assistant Professor
Military and Emergency Medicine
Uniformed Services University of the Health Sciences
Bethesda, Maryland
Chapter 23

Richard M. Ruddy, MD
Professor of Clinical Pediatrics
Department of Emergency Medicine
University of Cincinnati College of Medicine
Director, Division of Emergency Medicine
Children's Hospital Medical Center
Cincinnati, Ohio
Chapter 14

Daniel L. Savitt, MD
Associate Professor
Emergency Medicine and Internal Medicine
Brown University
Providence, Rhode Island
Chapters 11 and 12

Charles J. Schubert, MD
Professor of Clinical Pediatrics
Department of Pediatrics
University of Cincinnati
Cincinnati, Ohio
Chapter 15

Robert A. Shapiro, MD
Professor of Clinical Pediatrics
Department of Pediatrics
Univerisity of Cincinnati College of Medicine
Cincinnati, Ohio
Chapter 15

Paul R. Sierzenski, MD, RDMS, FAAEM, FACEP
Director, Emergency, Trauma & Critical Care Ultrasound
Director, Emergency Ultrasound Fellowship
Emergency Medicine
Christiana Care Health System
Newark, Delaware
Chapter 19

William S. Smock, MD, MS
Professor
Emergency Medicine
University of Louisville School of Medicine
Louisville, Kentucky
Chapter 19

Lawrence B. Stack, MD, FACEP
Associate Professor of Emergency Medicine
Vanderbilt University
Nashville, Tennessee
Chapters 7, 19, 22

Alan B. Storrow, MD, FACEP
Vice Chairman for Research and Academic Affairs
Associate Professor of Emergency Medicine
Vanderbilt University
Nashville, Tennessee

Selim Suner, MD, MS, FACEP
Associate Professor
Emergency Medicine, Surgery and Engineering
Brown University
Providence, Rhode Island
Chapter 12

Matthew D. Sztajnkrycer, MD, PhD
Associate Professor
Emergency Medicine
Mayo Clinic
Rochester, Minnesota
Chapter 17

R. Jason Thurman, MD, FAAEM
Assistant Professor of Emergency
Associate Director, Residency Program
Department of Emergency Medicine
Nashville, Tennessee
Chapters 16, 17, 23

Robert J. Tubbs, MD
Assistant Professor
Department of Emergency Medicine
Alpert Medical School of Brown University
Providence, Rhode Island
Chapter 12

Christopher S. Weaver, MD
Associate Professor
Emergency Medicine
Indiana University School of Medicine
Indianapolis, Indiana
Chapter 4

Steven J. White, MD, FACEP, FAAP
Assistant Professor of Emergency Medicine and Pediatrics
Vanderbilt University
Nashville, Tennessee
Chapter 22

Saralyn R. Williams, MD, FACMT, FACEP
Associate Professor of Clinical Medicine
Departments of Medicine and Emergency Medicine
Vanderbilt University
Nashville, Tennessee
Chapter 17

Dana Woodhall, MD
Resident Physician
Department of Emergency Medicine
Vanderbilt University
Nashville, Tennessee
Chapter 18

Seth W. Wright, MD, MPH
Associate Professor of Emergency Medicine
Vanderbilt University
Nashville, Tennessee
Chapter 21

Richard E. Wyszynski, MD, FACS
Staff Physician
Lorain Institute
Cleveland Clinic Foundaton
Cleveland, Ohio
Chapter 3

Ken Zafren, FAAEM, FACEP, FAWM
Clinical Assistant Professor
Division of Emergency Medicine
Stanford University Medical Center
Palo Alto, California
Chapter 16

Edward S. Amrhein, DDS

CAPT, DC, USN
Head, Dental Department
Director, Oral & Maxillofacial Surgery Residency
Naval Medical Center
Portsmouth, Virginia

Thomas Babcock, MD

Longview Emergency Medicine Associates
Good Shepherd Medical Center
Longview, Texas

Matthew Backer Jr., MD

RADM, MC, USNR (RET)
Attending Physician
Department of Obstetrics and Gynecology
Naval Medical Center
San Diego, California

John D. Baker, MD

Chief of Ophthalmology
Children's Hospital of Michigan
Clinical Professor of Ophthalmology
Wayne State University School of Medicine
Detroit, Michigan

Raymond C. Baker, MD

Professor of Pediatrics
University of Cincinnati College of Medicine
Pediatrician, Division of Pediatrics
Children's Hospital Medical Center
Cincinnati, Ohio

William Barsan, MD

Professor and Chair
Department of Emergency Medicine
University of Michigan
Ann Arbor, Michigan

Keith F. Batts, MD

Department Head
Emergency Medicine Department
Naval Hospital
Bremerton, Washington

Judith C. Bausher, MD

Associate Professor of Pediatrics and Emergency Medicine
University of Cincinnati College of Medicine
Attending Physician, Division of Emergency Medicine
Children's Hospital Medical Center
Cincinnati, Ohio

William Beck, CRA

Clinic Photographer, Florida Eye Clinic
Altamonte Springs, Florida

Debbie Bennes, BS, MLT, ASCP

Mayo Clinic
Rochester, Minnesota

Marion Berg, MD

Assistant Professor of Emergency Medicine
Department of Emergency Medicine
Vanderbilt University Medical Center
Nashville, Tennessee

Frank Birinyi, MD, FACEP

Clinical Assistant Professor of Emergency Medicine
The Ohio State University
Attending Physician
Mount Carmel Medical Center
Mount Carmel East Hospital
Columbus, Ohio

Allison Bollinger, MD

Resident
Department of Emergency Medicine, Vanderbilt University
Nashville, Tennessee

Jeffery D. Bondesson, MD

Attending Physician
Kaiser Permanente Medical Center
San Diego, California

Thomas Bottoni, MD

Staff Emergency Physician
Naval Medical Center
Portsmouth, Virginia

Robert Brandt Jr., MD

Clinical Professor
Department of Family Practice
Boonshoft School of Medicine
Wright State University
Dayton, Ohio

James Paul Brewer, MD

Resident
Department of Emergency Medicine
Vanderbilt University School of Medicine
Nashville, Tennessee

Robert G. Buckley, MD, MPH, FACEP

CAPT, MC, USN
Director for Branch Clinics
Staff Physician
Emergency Medicine
Naval Medical Center San Diego
San Diego, California

Steven D. Burdette, MD, FACP

Associate Professor
Department of Internal Medicine
Boonshoft School of Medicine
Wright State University
Dayton, Ohio

Sean P. Bush, MD, FACEP
Staff Emergency Physician and Envenomation Consultant
Associate Professor of Emergency Medicine
Loma Linda University Medical Center and School of Medicine
Loma Linda, California

William E. Cappaert, MD
Department of Emergency Medicine
MetroHealth Medical Center
2500 MetroHealth Drive
Cleveland, Ohio

Marguerite M. Caré, MD
Assistant Professor of Clinical Radiology
Cincinnati Children's Hospital Medical Center
University of Cincinnati College of Medicine
Cincinnati, Ohio

Mary Jo Chandler, PA-C
Suffolk, Virginia

Richard A. Chole, MD, PhD
Lindburg Professor and Head
Department of Otolaryngology
Washington University School of Medicine
St. Louis, Missouri

Judy Christensen
Medical Illustrator
Graphics Division
Staff Education and Training
Naval Medical Center
San Diego, California

Jason Chu, MD
Assistant Professor of Clinical Medicine
Columbia University College of Physicians and Surgeons
St. Luke's-Roosevelt Hospital Center
New York, New York

Walter Clair, MD
Assistant Professor
Vanderbilt Heart and Vascular Institute
Vanderbilt University School of Medicine
Nashville, Tennessee

Richard A. Clinchy III, PhD, NREMT-P
American College of Prehospital Medicine
Ft. Walton Beach, Florida

Timothy A. Coakley, MD, FAAEM
CDR MC USN DMO
Deputy Force Surgeon
Navy Expeditionary Combat Command NO2M
Norfolk, Virginia

Stephen W. Corbett, MD, PhD
Department of Emergency Medicine
Loma Linda University Medical Center
Loma Linda, California

Robin T. Cotton, MD
Professor
Department of Otolaryngology and Maxillofacial Surgery
Children's Hospital Medical Center
Cincinnati, Ohio

Barbara R. Craig, MD
CAPT, MC, USN
Medical Consultant for Child Abuse and Neglect
National Naval Medical Center
Bethesda, Maryland

James Dahle, MD
MAJ, USAF, MC
Attending Physician
Naval Medical Center
Portsmouth, Virginia
Riverside Emergency Physicians
Newport News, Virginia

Sheila Dawling, PhD
Associate Professor
Vanderbilt University Medical Center
Nashville, Tennessee

Mohamud Daya, MD
Oregon Health and Sciences University
Portland, Oregon

Herbert L. DuPont, MD
Chief, Internal Medicine Service
St. Luke's Episcopal Hospital
Houston, Texas

Lee E. Edstrom, MD
Surgeon in Chief
Division of Plastic Surgery
Rhode Island Hospital
Assistant Professor of Surgery
Brown University
Providence, Rhode Island

David Effron, MD, FACEP
Department of Emergency Medicine
Metro Health Medical Center
Cleveland, Ohio

Mark Eich, MD
Staff Physician
Naval Hospital
Jacksonville, Florida

Edward M. Eitzen, Jr., MD, MPH
Chief, Preventive Medicine Department
US Army Medical Research Institute of Infectious Diseases
Fort Detrick, Maryland

James P. Elrod, MD, PHD
Staff Hemopathologist
St. Thomas Hospital
Nashville, Tennessee

John Fildes, MD, FACS
Attending Surgeon
Division of Trauma
Department of Surgery
Cook County Hospital
Chicago, Illinois

Jeffrey Finkelstein, MD, FACEP
Chief, Division of Acute Care
Chairman, Department of Emergency Medicine
Wilford Hall Medical Center
Attending Physician
Joint Military Medical Centers
Emergency Medicine Residency
San Antonio, Texas

Andreas Fischer, RN
San Diego, CA

Beverly C. Forcier, MD
Department of Emergency Medicine
Metro Health Medical Center
Cleveland, Ohio

Luanne Freer, MD, FACEP, FAWM
Medical Director, Yellowstone National Park
Yellowstone, Wyoming

Sara-Jo Gahm, MD
Resident
Department of Emergency Medicine
Medical College of Pennsylvania
Philadelphia, Pennsylvania
Geisinger Medical Center
Department of Emergency Medicine
Danville, Pennsylvania

W. Brian Gibler, MD
Professor and Chair
Department of Emergency Medicine
University of Cincinnati College of Medicine
Cincinnati, Ohio

Jeffrey S. Gibson, MD
LCDR, MC, USNR
Staff Physician
Emergency Medicine Department
Naval Medical Center
Jacksonville, Florida

Javier A. Gonzalez Del Rey, MD, FAAP
Assistant Professor of Clinical Pediatrics and Emergency Medicine
University of Cincinnati College of Medicine
Attending Physician, Division of Emergency Medicine
Children's Hospital Medical Center
Cincinnati, Ohio

Rob Greidanus, MD
Peace Country Health Region
Alberta, Canada

Ralph A. Gruppo, MD
Professor of Pediatrics
University of Cincinnati College of Medicine
Director, Hemophilia Treatment Center
Children's Hospital Medical Center
Cincinnati, Ohio

Peter Hackett, MD, FACEP
The Institute for Altitude Medicine
Telluride, Colorado

Murray Hamlet, DVM
Former Director of Research
Army Research Institute of Environmental Medicine
Natick, Massachusetts

H. Hunter Handsfield, MD
Professor of Medicine
University of Washington
Director, STD Control Program
Seattle-King County Department of Public Health
Seattle, Washington

J. Matthew Hardin, MD
Chief Resident, Division of Dermatology
Division of Dermatology
Vanderbilt University Medical Center
Nashville, Tennessee

Carson Harris, MD
Regions Hospital/Health Partners Institute of Medical Education
St. Paul, Minnesota

Geoffrey E. Hayden, MD
Clinical Assistant Professor
Vanderbilt University Medical Center
Department of Emergency Medicine
Nashville, Tennessee

Ben Heavrin, MD
Chief Resident and Instructor
Department of Emergency Medicine
Vanderbilt University School of Medicine
Nashville, Tennessee

Thomas R. Hedges III, MD
Director, Neuro-Ophthalmology Service
Co-Director, Electrophysiology Service
New England Eye Center
Boston, Massachusetts

Lawrence E. Heiskell, MD, FACEP, FAAFP
Department of Emergency Medicine
Naval Hospital Twentynine Palms
Twentynine Palms, California

Robert W. Hickey, MD
Associate Professor of Pediatrics
Children's Hospital of Pittsburgh of UPMC
Pittsburgh, Pennsylvania

Briana Hill, MD
Chairman
Department of Dermatology
Naval Medical Center
Portsmouth, Virginia

Stephen Holt, MD
San Antonio, Texas

Meg Jack, MD
Assistant Professor
Emergency Medicine
Vanderbilt Medical Center
Nashville, Tennessee

Jennifer Jagoe, MD
LT, MC, USNR
Resident
Department of Obstetrics and Gynecology
Naval Medical Center
San Diego, California

Timothy Jahn, MD
LCDR, MC, USNR
Attending Physician
Department of Emergency Medicine
Naval Hospital
Great Lakes, Illinois

Thea James, MD
Department of Emergency Medicine
Boston Medical Center
Boston University School of Medicine
Boston, Massachusetts

Edward C. Jauch, MD, MS
Assistant Professor
Department of Emergency Medicine
University of Cincinnati Medical Center
Cincinnati, Ohio

Katie L. Johnson, MD
Resident
Department of Emergency Medicine
Vanderbilt University Medical Center
Nashville, Tennessee

Ian D. Jones, MD
Assistant Professor of Emergency Medicine
Director of Emergency Department Operations
Vanderbilt University Medical Center
Nashville, Tennessee

Michael L. Juliano, MD
Staff Emergency Physician
Department of Emergency Medicine
Naval Medical Center Portsmouth
Portsmouth, Virginia

Arthur M. Kahn, MD, FACS
Assistant Professor of Surgery
UCLA School of Medicine
Attending Surgeon
Cedars-Sinai Medical Center
Los Angeles, California

David Kaplan, MD
Staff Attending Physician
Department of Emergency Medicine
The Miriam Hospital
Providence, Rhode Island

Lee Kaplan, MD
Chief of Dermatology
VA Medical Center, San Diego, California
Associate Clinical Professor of Medicine and Dermatology
University of California
San Diego, California

Tomisaku Kawasaki, MD
Director
Japan Kawasaki Disease Research Center
Tokyo, Japan

Rudy Kink, MD
Pediatric Emergency Medicine Fellow
LeBonheur Children's Medical Center
Memphis, Tennessee

Kevin J. Knoop, MD, MS, FACEP
CAPT, MC, USN
Director, Professional Education
Naval Medical Center
Portsmouth, Virginia

Stephen Knoop
Chesapeake, Virginia

Matthew Kopp, MD
Assistant Professor of Emergency Medicine
UEMF Compliance Director
Department of Emergency Medicine
The Warren Alpert Medical School
Brown University
Providence, Rhode Island

Paul J. Kovalchik, MD, FACS
Colorectal Surgeon
Chesapeake, Virginia

David P. Kretzschmar, DDS, MS
Chief, Department of Oral and Maxillofacial Surgery
2nd Medical Group
Barksdale AFB, Louisiana
Assistant Professor
Department of Surgery
Louisiana State University Medical Center
New Orleans, Louisiana

James L. Kretzschmar, DDS, MS
LTCOL, USAF
OIC Flight Dental Clinic
Holloman AFB, New Mexico

Jeffery Kuhn, MD
CAPT, MC, USN (RET)
Department of Otolaryngology—Head and Neck Surgery
Naval Medical Center
Portsmouth, Virginia

Douglas R. Landry, MD
Staff Physician
Bayside Hospital
Virginia Beach, Virginia

Hillary J. Larkin, PA-C
Director, Medical Sexual Assault Services
Department of Emergency Medicine
Alameda Sexual Assault Response Team
Highland General Hospital
Oakland, California

Lorenz F. Lassen, MD
CAPT, MC, USN
Assistant Professor of Otolaryngology—Head and Neck Surgery
Eastern Virginia Medical School
Service Line Leader
Reparative Services
Naval Medical Center
Portsmouth, Virginia

Laurie Lawrence, MD
Assistant Professor
Vanderbilt University Medical Center
Nashville, Tennessee

Louis Lavopa, MD
Staff Physician
Emergency Medicine Department
Naval Hospital
Agana, Guam

Stephen J. Leech, MD, RDMS
Assistant Clinical Professor
Departments of Emergency Medicine
University of Central Florida School of Medicine, Florida State
  University School of Medicine
Orlando, Florida

William Leninger, MD
LT, MC, USNR
Resident
Department of Obstetrics and Gynecology
Naval Medical Center
San Diego, California

Richard C. Levy, MD
Professor Emeritus of Emergency Medicine
Department of Emergency Medicine
University of Cincinnati
Cincinnati, Ohio

Anne W. Lucky, MD
Volunteer Professor of Dermatology and Pediatrics
University of Cincinnati College of Medicine
Director, Dermatology Clinic
Children's Hospital Medical Center
Cincinnati, Ohio

Binh Ly, MD
Associate Clinical Professor
University of California, San Diego
San Diego, California

C. Bruce MacDonald, MD
Assistant Professor, Department of Otolaryngology
Boston University School of Medicine
Boston, Massachusetts

Mark L. Madenwald, MD
LT, MC, USNR
Chief Resident
Emergency Medicine Department
Naval Medical Center
Portsmouth, Virginia

Kathi L. Makoroff, MD
Assistant Professor
Department of Pediatrics
University of Cincinnati College of Medicine
Cincinnati, Ohio

William K. Mallon, MD, FACEP
Associate Director of Residency Training
Assistant Professor of Medicine
University of Southern California School of Medicine
Los Angeles, California

Scott Manning, MD
Professor and Chief of Pediatric Otolaryngology
University of Washington, Seattle Children's Hospital
Seattle, Washington

Robin Marshall, MD
Emergency Medicine Attending
Naval Medical Center
Portsmouth, Virginia

Thomas F. Mauger, MD
Associate Professor of Ophthalmology
Department of Ophthalmology
William H. Havener Eye Center
The Ohio State University
Columbus, Ohio

Ian T. McClure, MD
Staff Emergency Physician
Sutter General Hospital
Sacramento, California

Megan L. McGraw, MD
Insuring the Children Child Abuse Fellow
Cincinnati Children's Hospital Medical Center
Cincinnati, Ohio

Timothy D. McGuirk, DO, FACEP
CAPT, MC, USN
Department Head
Emergency Medicine Hospital
Okinawa, Japan

Patrick H. McKenna, MD, FACS, FAAP
Assistant Clinical Professor of Urology and Pediatrics
University of Connecticut Health Center
Hartford, Connecticut

Kathy McCue, MD
Staff Emergency Physician
Alaska Native Medical Center
Anchorage, Alaska

Jared McKinney, MD
Assistant Professor
Department of Emergency Medicine
Vanderbilt University Medical Center
Assistant Emergency Medical Services Director
Nashville Fire Department
Nashville, Tennessee

Jeff McKinzie, MD
Assistant Professor
Assistant Professor Pediatrics
Director, Division of International Medicine
Department of Emergency Medicine, Vanderbilt University
Nashville, Tennessee

John Meade, MD
CEO, Statdoc Consulting, Inc.
Gulf Breeze, Florida

Vineet Mehan, MD
Attending Physician,
Greater Washington Plastic Surgery Associates, LLC
Annandale, Virginia

Aurora Mendez, RN
Sexual Assault Response Team Coordinator
Villavu Community Hospital
San Diego, California

James Mensching, DO
Operational Medical Director
Emergency Medical Department
Naval Medical Center
Portsmouth, Virginia

Mark Meredith, MD
Assistant Professor
Department of Emergency Medicine and Pediatrics
Clinical Director Pediatric Emergency Medical Services
Vanderbilt University Medical Center
Assistant EMS Medical Director for Pediatric Care
Nashville Fire Department
Nashville, Tennessee

Benjamin Milligan, MD
Providence, Rhode Island

Sherman Minton, MD
Professor Emeritus
Department of Microbiology and Immunology
Indiana University School of Medicine
Indianapolis, Indiana

Matthew R. Mittiga, MD
Assistant Professor of Clinical Pediatrics
Department of Pediatrics
University of Cincinnati College of Medicine
Cincinnati Children's Hospital Medical Center
Cincinnati, Ohio

Margaret P. Mueller, MD
Department of Emergency Medicine
Rhode Island Hospital and Brown University
Providence, Rhode Island

David W. Munter, MD, MBA
Assistant Clinical Professor
Department of Emergency Medicine
Eastern Virginia Medical School
Norfolk, Virginia

Douglas Nilson, MD
Senior Resident
Brown University
Rhode Island Hospital
Residency Program in Emergency Medicine
Providence, Rhode Island

Daniel Noltkamper, MD
Assistant Chairman
Department of Emergency Medicine
Naval Hospital
Camp Lejeune, North Carolina

Jason T. Nomura, MD
Associate Director of Emergency Ultrasound,
 Department of Emergency Medicine
Associate Director Emergency Ultrasound Fellowship,
 Department of Emergency Medicine
Clinical Faculty, Department of Internal Medicine
Christiana Care Health System
Newark, Delaware

James Nordlund, MD
Professor of Dermatology
Department of Dermatology
University of Cincinnati
Cincinnati, Ohio

Michael J. Nowicki, MD
CDR, MC, USN
Division of Pediatric Gastroenterology
Department of Pediatrics
Naval Medical Center
Portsmouth, Virginia

John O'Boyle, MD
CAPT, MC, USN
Director, Professional Education
Naval Medical Center
Portsmouth, Virginia

Alan E. Oestreich, MD
Professor of Radiology and Pediatrics
University of Cincinnati College of Medicine
Chief, Section of Diagnostic Radiology
Staff Radiologist
Children's Hospital Medical Center
Cincinnati, Ohio

Edward C. Oldfield III, MD
Professor of Medicine
Director, Infectious Diseases Division
Eastern Virginia School of Medicine
Norfolk, Virginia

Sheryl Olson, RN, BSN, CCRN
Flight Nurse
Wilderness Medicine Instructor
WildernessWise
Manitou Springs, Colorado

Gerald O'Malley, DO
LCDR, MC, USNR
Research Coordinator
Naval Medical Center
Portsmouth, Virginia

James O'Malley, MD
Providence Alaska Regional Medical Center
Anchorage, Alaska

John Omara, MD
Department of Cardiology
Dartmouth-Hitchcock Medical Center
Lebanon, New Hampshire

Jared M. Orrock, MD
Department of Laboratory Medicine and Pathology
Mayo Clinic
Rochester, Minnesota

Edward J. Otten, MD
Professor of Emergency Medicine and Pediatrics
Director, Division of Toxicology
University of Cincinnati College of Medicine
Cincinnati, Ohio

James Palma, MD
LCDR, MC, USN
Ultrasound Fellow
Palmetto Health Richland
Columbia, South Carolina

James Palombaro, MD
LCDR, MC, USNR
Attending Physician
Department of Obstetrics and Gynecology
Naval Medical Center
San Diego, California

Lauri Paolinette, PA-C
Sexual Assault Examiner
Department of Emergency Medicine
Alameda Sexual Assault Response Team
Highland General Hospital
Oakland, California

Chan W. Park, MD
Attending Physician
Department of Emergency Medicine
Naval Medical Center Portsmouth
Norfolk, Virginia

Dallas E. Peak, MD, FACEP
Assistant Professor of Clinical Emergency Medicine
Department of Emergency Medicine
Indiana University School of Medicine
Indianapolis, Indiana

Michael P. Poirier, MD
Assistant Professor of Pediatrics
Eastern Virginia Medical School
Division of Pediatric Emergency Medicine
Children's Hospital of the King's Daughters
Norfolk, Virginia

Francisco Bravo Puccio, MD
Universidad Peruana
Cayetano Heredia, Lima

Mark Ralston, MD, MPH
CAPT, MC, USNR
Director
Children's Emergency Unit
Department of Emergency Medicine
Naval Medical Center
Portsmouth, Virginia

Michael Redman, PA-C
Staff, Emergency Medicine
Fort Leonard Wood Army Community Hospital
Fort Leonard Wood, Missouri

William H. Richardson III, MD
Palmetto Health Richland
Columbia, South Carolina

Sue Rist, FNP
CAPT, NC, USN (RET)
Naval Training Center
San Diego, California

James V. Ritchie, MD
CAPT, MC, USN
Assistant Professor
Military and Emergency Medicine
Uniformed Services University of the Health Sciences
Bethesda, Maryland

Michael Ritter, MD
Laguna Beach, California

Harold Rivera, HM1, USN
Optician
Department of Ophthalmology
Naval Medical Center
Portsmouth, Virginia

Gregory K. Robbins, MD MPH
Instructor in Medicine
Massachusetts General Hospital
Partners AIDS Center
Harvard Medical School
Boston, Massachusetts

Karen Rogers, MD
Resident
Vanderbilt University Medical Center
Nashville, Tennessee

Donald L. Rucknagel, MD, PHD
Professor of Pediatrics and Internal Medicine
University of Cincinnati College of Medicine
Comprehensive Sickle Cell Center
Children's Hospital Medical Center
Cincinnati, Ohio

Richard M. Ruddy, MD, FAAP
Professor of Clinical Pediatrics
Department of Emergency Medicine
University of Cincinnati College of Medicine
Director, Division of Emergency Medicine
Children's Hospital Medical Center
Cincinnati, Ohio

Stephan E. Russ, MD
Assistant Professor of Emergency Medicine
Department of Emergency Medicine
Vanderbilt University Medical Center
Nashville, Tennessee

Brad Russell, MD
Emergency Physician
Nashville, Tennessee

Warren K. Russell, MD
LCDR, MC, USNR
Head, Emergency Medicine Department
Naval Hospital
Roosevelt Roads, Puerto Rico

Sally A. Santen, MD
Associate Professor
Department of Emergency Medicine
Emory University
Atlanta, Georgia

Katrina C. Santos, HM3, USN
Ocular Technician
Department of Ophthalmology
Naval Medical Center
Portsmouth, Virginia

Daniel L. Savitt, MD
Attending Physician and Residency Director
Department of Emergency Medicine
Rhode Island Hospital
Associate Professor of Medicine
Brown University
Providence, Rhode Island

Robert Schnarrs, MD
Staff Physician
Department of Plastic Surgery
Sentara Norfolk General Hospital
Norfolk, Virginia

Charles J. Schubert, MD
Assistant Professor of Pediatrics and Emergency Medicine
University of Cincinnati College of Medicine
Attending Physician, Division of Emergency Medicine
Children's Hospital Medical Center
Cincinnati, Ohio

Gary Schwartz, MD
Assistant Professor
Department of Emergency Medicine
Vanderbilt University Medical Center
Nashville, Tennessee

Robert A. Shapiro, MD
Medical Director, Mayerson Center for Safe and Healthy Children
Children's Hospital Medical Center
Cincinnati, Ohio

Virender K. Sharma, MD
Fellow
Division of Digestive Disease and Nutrition
University of South Carolina School of Medicine
Columbia, South Carolina

Rees W. Sheppard, MD, FACS
Assistant Director of Pediatric Ophthalmology
Children's Hospital Medical Center
Volunteer Associate Professor
University of Cincinnati College of Medicine
Cincinnati, Ohio

Anita P. Sheth, MD
Volunteer Assistant Professor
Co-Director, Division of Pediatric Dermatology
Cincinnati Children's Hospital Medical Center
University of Cincinnati College of Medicine
Cincinnati, Ohio

Ellen Sierzenski, RDCS
Newark, Delaware

Paul R. Sierzenski, MD, RDMS, FAAEM
Director of Emergency Medicine Ultrasound
Department of Emergency Medicine
Christiana Care Health System
Newark, Delaware
President, Emergency Ultrasound Consultants, LLC
Bear, Delaware

Arun D. Singh, MD
Director
Department of Ophthalmic Oncology
Cole Eye Institute, Cleveland Clinic
Cleveland, Ohio

Kenneth Skahan, MD
Assistant Professor
Division of Infectious Diseases
University of Cincinnati
Cincinnati, Ohio

Stuart Skinner, MD
Division of Infectious Diseases, University of Saskatchewan
Saskatchewan, Canada

Clay B. Smith, MD
Assistant Professor
Departments of Emergency Medicine, Pediatrics
  and Internal Medicine
Vanderbilt University Medical Center
Nashville, Tennessee

Hannah F. Smitherman, MD
Fort Worth, Texas

William S. Smock, MD
Associate Professor and Director
Clinical Forensic Medicine Fellowship
Department of Emergency Medicine
University of Louisville, School of Medicine
Louisville, Kentucky

Shannon B. Snyder, MD
Assistant Professor
Department of Emergency Medicine
Vanderbilt University Medical Center
Nashville, Tennessee

Aaron Sobol, MD
Medical Director
Laurel Ridge Eyecare
Uniontown, Pennsylvania

Lawrence B. Stack, MD, FACEP
Associate Professor
Department of Emergency Medicine
Vanderbilt University Medical Center
Nashville, Tennessee

Philip E. Stack, MD
Western Carolina Gastroenterology Associates
Sylva, North Carolina

Emily R. Stack
Brentwood, Tennessee

James F. Steiner, DDS
Professor of Pediatrics
University of Cincinnati College of Medicine
Pediatric Dentistry
Children's Hospital Medical Center
Cincinnati, Ohio

Alan B. Storrow, MD, FACEP

Associate Professor of Emergency Medicine Clinical
    Research Director
University of Cincinnati College of Medicine
Cincinnati, Ohio

Richard Strait, MD

Assistant Professor of Clinical Pediatrics
Children's Hospital Medical Center
University of Cincinnati
Cincinnati, Ohio

Selim Suner, MD, MS, FACEP

Assistant Professor of Surgery (Emergency Medicine)
Brown University School of Medicine
Department of Emergency Medicine
Rhode Island Hospital
Providence, Rhode Island

Matthew D. Sztajnkrycer, MD, PhD

Associate Professor
Emergency Medicine
Mayo Clinic
Rochester, Minnesota

Gary Tanner, MD

CDR, MC, USN
Chairman, Department of Ophthalmology
Naval Medical Center
Portsmouth, Virginia

Martin Terry, PhD

Assistant Professor of Biology
Department of Biology
Sul Ross State University
Alpine, Texas

R. Jason Thurman, MD, FAAEM

Assistant Professor of Emergency Medicine
Associate Director, Residency Program
Patient Safety Officer
Department of Emergency Medicine
Associate Medical Director, VU Stroke Center
Vanderbilt University Medical Center
Nashville, Tennessee

Robert Trieff, MD (Deceased)

LCDR, MC, USN
Emergency Medicine Resident
Naval Medical Center
Portsmouth, Virginia

Alexander T. Trott, MD

Professor of Emergency Medicine
University of Cincinnati College of Medicine
Cincinnati, Ohio

Robert J. Tubbs, MD

Assistant Professor
Department of Emergency Medicine
Alpert Medical School of Brown University
Providence, Rhode Island

George Turiansky, MD

Dermatology Service
Walter Reed Army Medical Center
Washington, D.C.

Janice E. Underwood, RDMS

Advanced Health Education Center, Inc.
Houston, Texas

Andrew H. Urbach, MD

Professor of Pediatrics
University of Pittsburgh School of Medicine
Medical Director for Clinical Excellence and Service
Children's Hospital of Pittsburgh of UPMC
Pittsburgh, Pennsylvania

Lynn Utecht, MD

Chairman
Department of Dermatology
Naval Hospital
Rota, Spain

Gerald Van Houdt, MD

CDR, MC, USN
Resident
Department of Emergency Medicine
Naval Medical Center
San Diego, California

Cathleen M. Vossler, MD

Resident
Department of Emergency Medicine
Rhode Island Hospital and Brown University
Providence, Rhode Island

Arden H. Wander, MD

Professor of Clinical Ophthalmology
University of Cincinnati
Cincinnati, Ohio

Steven J. White, MD, FACEP, FAAP

Assistant Professor
Emergency Medicine and Pediatrics
Vanderbilt University Medical Center
Nashville, Tennessee

Saralyn R. Williams, MD, FACMT, FACEP

Associate Professor of Clinical Medicine
Department of Medicine and Department of Emergency Medicine
Vanderbilt University
Nashville, Tennessee

Alex Wilson
Nova Scotia Museum of Natural History
Halifax, Nova Scotia, Canada

John Worrell, MD
Professor of Radiology
Department of Radiology
Vanderbilt University Medical Center
Nashville, Tennessee

Seth W. Wright, MD, MPH
Associate Professor
Emergency Medicine
Vanderbilt University
Nashville, Tennessee

Richard E. Wyszynski, MD, FACS
Department of Emergency Medicine
Metrohealth Medical Center
Cleveland, Ohio

Scott W. Zackowski, MD
Director, Medical Services
Naval Hospital
Naples, Italy

Ken Zafren, FAAEM, FACEP, FAWM
Clinical Assistant Professor
Division of Emergency Medicine
Stanford University Medical Center
Palo Alto, California

Kevin E. Zawacki, MD
Cardiologist
Division of Cardiology
Naval Medical Center
Portsmouth, Virginia

Richard Zienowicz, MD
Attending Physician
Division of Plastic Surgery
Assistant Professor of Surgery
Brown University
Providence, Rhode Island

Regional Anatomy

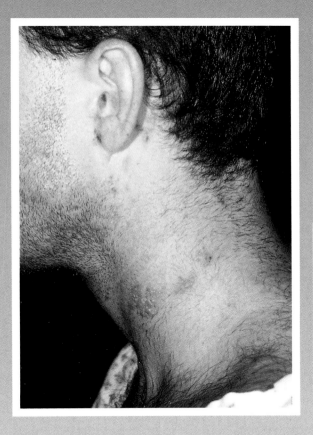

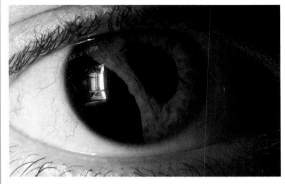

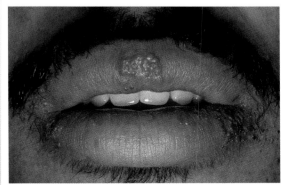

Chapter 1

HEAD AND FACIAL TRAUMA

David W. Munter
Timothy D. McGuirk

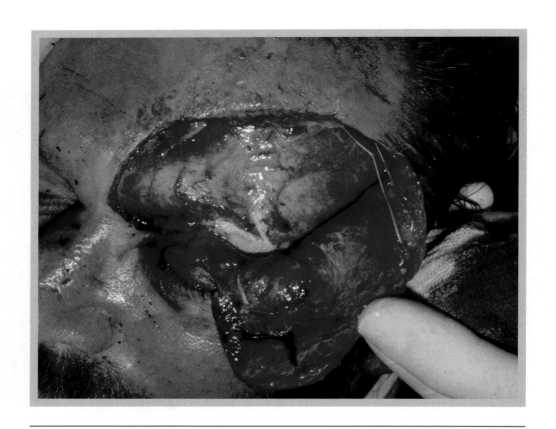

Clinical Summary

The skull base comprises the floors of the anterior, middle, and posterior cranial fossae. Trauma resulting in fractures to the basilar area typically does not have localizing symptoms. Indirect signs of the injury may include visible evidence of bleeding from the fracture into surrounding soft tissue, such as a Battle sign or "raccoon eyes." Bleeding into other structures such as hemotympanum and blood in the sphenoid sinus, evident as an air-fluid level on CT, may also be seen. Cerebrospinal fluid (CSF) leaks may also be evident and noted as clear or pink rhinorrhea. If CSF is present, a dextrose stick test may be positive. The fluid can be placed on filter paper and a "halo" or double ring may be seen.

Emergency Department Treatment and Disposition

The mainstay of management is to identify underlying brain injury, which is best accomplished by computed tomography (CT). CT is also the best diagnostic tool for identifying the fracture site, but fractures may not always be evident. Evidence of open communication, such as a CSF leak, mandates neurosurgical consultation and admission. Otherwise, the decision for admission is based on the patient's clinical condition, other associated injuries, and evidence of underlying brain injury, as seen on CT. The use of antibiotics in the presence of a CSF leak is controversial because of the possibility of selecting resistant organisms.

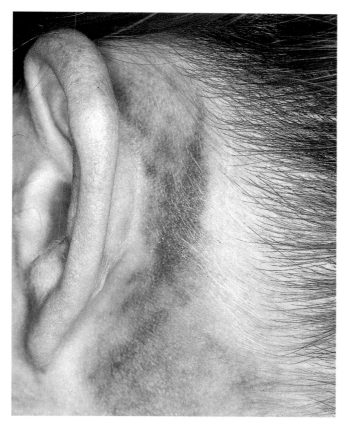

FIGURE 1.1 ■ Battle Sign. Ecchymosis in the postauricular area develops when the fracture line communicates with the mastoid air cells, resulting in accumulation of blood in the cutaneous tissue. This patient sustained injuries several days prior to presentation. (Photo contributor: Frank Birinyi, MD.)

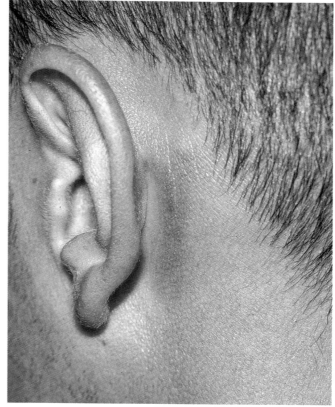

FIGURE 1.2 ■ Battle Sign. A subtle Battle sign is seen in this patient with head trauma. This sign may take hours to develop fully. (Photo contributor: Lawrence B. Stack, MD.)

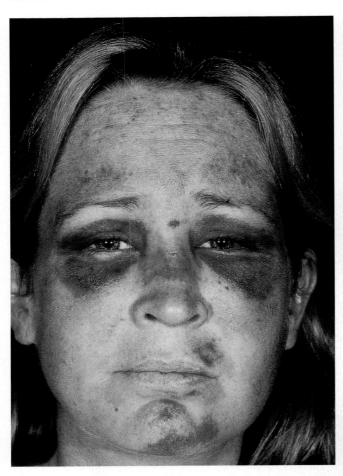

FIGURE 1.3 ■ Raccoon Eyes. Ecchymosis in the periorbital area, resulting from bleeding from a fracture site in the anterior portion of the skull base. This finding may also be caused by facial fractures. (Photo contributor: Frank Birinyi, MD.)

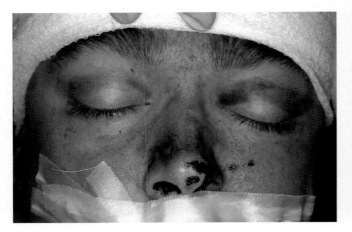

FIGURE 1.4 ■ Early Racoon Eyes. Subtle periorbital ecchymosis manifests 1 hour after a blast injury. (Photo contributor: Kevin J. Knoop, MD, MS.)

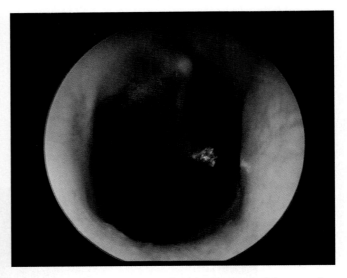

FIGURE 1.5 ■ Hemotympanum. Seen in a basilar skull fracture when the fracture line communicates with the auditory canal, resulting in bleeding into the middle ear. Blood can be seen behind the tympanic membrane. (Photo contributor: Richard A. Chole, MD, PhD.)

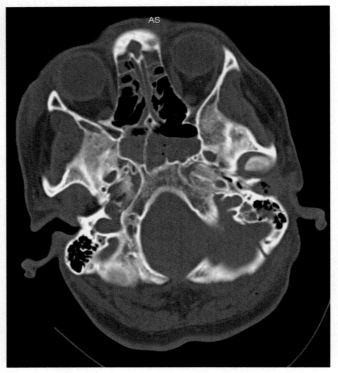

FIGURE 1.6 ■ CT of Basilar Skull Fracture. Bone window demonstrates a fracture of the left sphenoid sinus and an air-fluid level. (Photo contributor: Jared McKinney, MD.)

Pearls

1. The clinical manifestations of basilar skull fracture may take 6 to 12 hours to fully develop.
2. Since plain films are unhelpful, there should be a low threshold for head CT in any patient with head trauma, loss of consciousness, change in mental status, severe headache, visual changes, or nausea or vomiting.
3. The use of filter paper or a dextrose stick test to determine if CSF is present in rhinorrhea is not 100% reliable.
4. Fracture of the temporal bone could result in temporary conductive hearing loss caused by disruption of the ossicular chain.

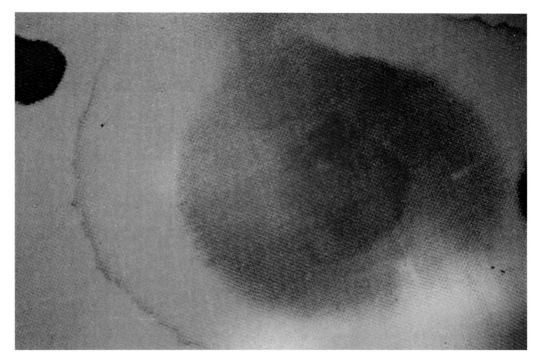

FIGURE 1.7 ■ Cerebrospinal Fluid Leak. This example, obtained from the nose, can be difficult to distinguish from blood or mucus. The distinctive double-ring sign, seen here, comprises blood (*inner ring*) and CSF (*outer ring*). The reliability of this test has been questioned. (Photo contributor: David W. Munter, MD.)

Clinical Summary

Depressed skull fractures typically occur when a significant force is applied over a small area. They are classified as open if the skin above them is lacerated and bone is exposed to the environment, and closed if the overlying skin is intact. Bleeding, abrasions, contusions, and hematomas may accompany the fracture. The patient's mental status varies depending on the associated brain injury. Evidence of other injuries such as a basilar fracture, facial fractures, or cervical spinal injuries may also be present.

Emergency Department Treatment and Disposition

Every laceration to the scalp should be explored and palpated to exclude a depressed fracture. CT is the best radiological study to identify a depressed skull fracture and underlying brain injury. Depressed skull fractures require immediate neurosurgical consultation. Open fractures require antibiotics and tetanus prophylaxis as indicated. The decision to observe or operate immediately is made by the neurosurgeon.

Pearls

1. Explore and palpate all scalp injuries, including lacerations, for evidence of fractures or depression. Fragments depressed more than 3 to 5 mm below the inner table are more likely to penetrate the dura and injure the cortex.
2. Children with depressed skull fractures are more likely to develop epilepsy.
3. Nonaccidental trauma should be suspected in children below 2 years of age with depressed skull fractures.
4. All patients with head injuries must be evaluated for possible cervical spine injuries.

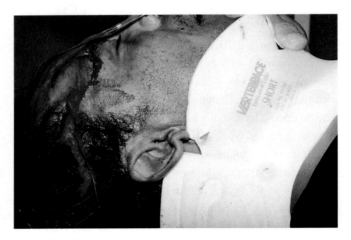

FIGURE 1.8 ■ Depressed Skull Fracture. A scalp laceration overlying a depressed skull fracture. All scalp lacerations should undergo sterile exploration for skull fracture. (Photo contributor: David W. Munter, MD.)

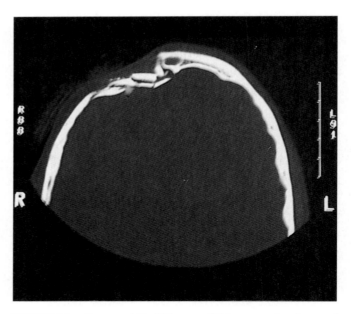

FIGURE 1.9 ■ Depressed Skull Fracture. CT demonstrating depressed skull fracture. (Photo contributor: David W. Munter, MD.)

Clinical Summary

Clinically significant nasal fractures are almost always evident on examination, with deformity, swelling, and ecchymosis present. Injuries may occur to surrounding bony structures, including the orbit, frontal sinus, or cribriform plate. Epistaxis may be caused by a septal or turbinate laceration, but can also be seen with fractures of surrounding bones, including the cribriform plate. Septal hematoma is a rare complication that, if untreated, may result in necrosis of the septal cartilage and a resultant "saddle-nose" deformity. A frontonasoethmoid fracture has nasal or frontal crepitus and may have associated telecanthus or obstruction of the nasolacrimal duct.

Emergency Department Treatment and Disposition

Management decisions for isolated nasal injury rarely require diagnostic radiographic studies. Obvious deformities are referred within 7 days for reduction, after the swelling has subsided. Nasal injuries without deformity need only conservative therapy with an analgesic and a nasal decongestant. Septal hematomas must be immediately drained, with packing placed to prevent reaccumulation. In some cases, epistaxis may not be controlled by pressure alone and may require nasal packing. Lacerations overlying a simple nasal fracture should be vigorously irrigated and primarily closed with the patient placed on antibiotic coverage. Complex nasal lacerations with underlying fractures should be closed by a facial trauma consultant. Nasal fractures with mild angulation and without displacement may be reduced in the emergency department by manipulating the nose with the examiner's thumbs into the correct alignment.

Pearls

1. All patients with facial trauma should be examined for a septal hematoma.
2. Marked isolated traumatic nasal deformity should be reduced in the emergency department by an experienced provider or a facial trauma consultant.
3. Every patient discharged with nasal packing should be placed on antistaphylococcal antibiotics and referred to ENT in 2 to 3 days.
4. Consider cribriform plate fractures in patients with clear rhinorrhea after nasal injury.

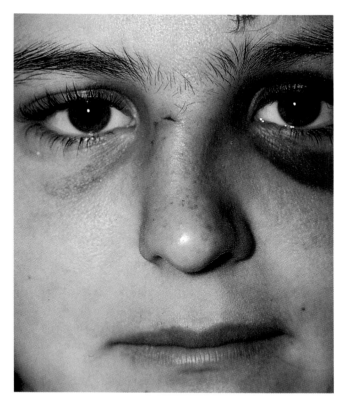

FIGURE 1.10 ■ Nasal Fracture. Deformity is evident on examination. Note periorbital ecchymosis suggesting additional facial fractures (or injuries). Suspicion for nonnasal facial fractures should guide the decision for obtaining diagnostic imaging. (Photo contributor: David W. Munter, MD.)

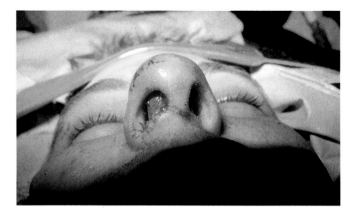

FIGURE 1.11A ■ Septal Hematoma. A bilateral, grapelike mass on the nasal septum. If untreated, this can result in septal necrosis and a saddle-nose deformity. Incision, drainage, and packing are indicated. (Photo contributor: Lawrence B. Stack, MD.)

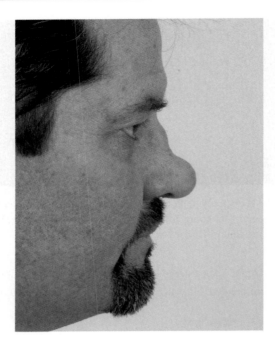

FIGURE 1.11B ■ Saddle Nose Deformity. Nasal septal necrosis resulting in saddle nose deformity is seen here. (Photo contributor: David Effron, MD.)

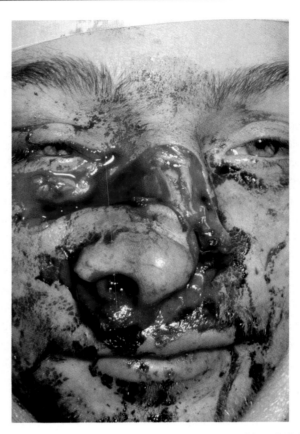

FIGURE 1.13 ■ Open Nasal Fracture. Lacerations with underlying fracture that require multilayered closure should be repaired by a facial trauma surgeon. (Photo contributor: Lawrence B. Stack, MD.)

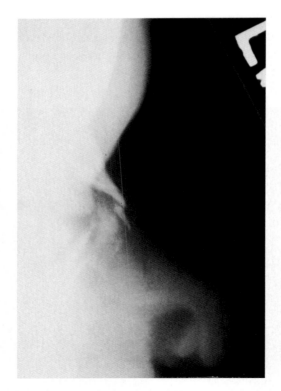

FIGURE 1.12 ■ Nondisplaced Nasal Fracture. Radiograph of a fracture of the nasal spine, for which no treatment other than ice and analgesics is needed. (Photo contributor: Lorenz F. Lassen, MD.)

Clinical Summary

The zygoma is composed of the zygomatic arch and the body. The arch forms the inferior and lateral orbit, and the body forms the malar eminence of the face. Direct blows to the arch can result in isolated arch fractures. These present clinically with pain on opening the mouth secondary to the insertion of the temporalis muscle at the arch or impingement on the coronoid process. A *tripod fracture* consists of fractures through three structures: the frontozygomatic suture; the maxillary process of the zygoma including the inferior orbital floor, inferior orbital rim, and lateral wall of the maxillary sinus; and the zygomatic arch. Clinically, patients present with a flattened malar eminence and edema and ecchymosis to the area, with a palpable step-off on examination. Injury to the infraorbital nerve may result in infraorbital hypesthesia, and gaze disturbances may result from entrapment of orbital contents. Subcutaneous emphysema may be caused by a fracture of the antral wall at the zygomatic buttress.

Emergency Department Treatment and Disposition

Facial CT will accurately demonstrate zygoma injuries. Simple zygomatic arch or minimally displaced tripod fractures without eye injury can be treated with ice and analgesics and referred for delayed operative repair within 7 days. Tripod fractures or those with eye injuries should be urgently evaluated by a facial

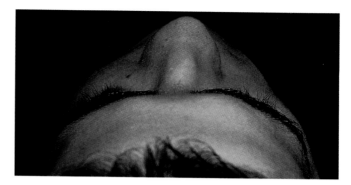

FIGURE 1.15 ■ Zygomatic Fracture. Patient with blunt trauma to the zygoma. Flattening of the right malar eminence is evident. (Photo contributor: Edward S. Amrhein, DDS.)

trauma surgeon. Decongestants and broad-spectrum antibiotics are recommended since the fracture crosses into the maxillary sinus.

Pearls

1. Tripod fractures are frequently associated with ocular injuries. A thorough eye examination should be performed on all patients with a tripod fracture.
2. Infraorbital hypesthesia suggests orbital floor injury extending into the infraorbital foramen and impingement of the infraorbital nerve.

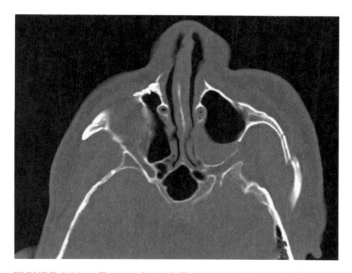

FIGURE 1.14 ■ Zygomatic Arch Fracture. Axial cut of a facial CT which reveals a minimally depressed zygomatic arch fracture. (Photo contributor: Lawrence B. Stack, MD.)

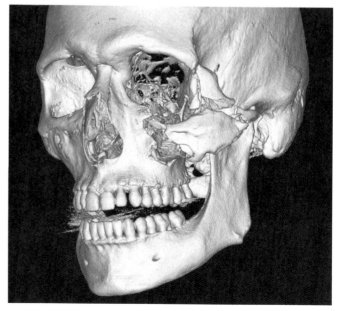

FIGURE 1.16 ■ Tripod Fracture. The fracture lines involved in a tripod fracture are demonstrated in this three-dimensional CT reconstruction. (Photo contributor: David Effron, MD.)

Clinical Summary

All LeFort facial fractures involve the maxilla. Clinically, the patient has facial injuries, swelling, and ecchymosis. LeFort I fractures are those involving an area under the nasal fossa. LeFort II fractures involve a pyramidal area including the maxilla, nasal bones, and medial orbits. LeFort III fractures, sometimes described as craniofacial dissociation, involve the maxilla, zygoma, nasal and ethmoid bones, and the bones of the base of the skull. Airway compromise may be associated with LeFort II and III fractures. LeFort II and III fractures can be difficult to distinguish clinically. Physical examination is sometimes helpful in distinguishing the three. The examiner places fingers on the bridge of the nose and tries to move the central maxillary incisors anteriorly with the other hand. If only the maxilla moves, a LeFort I is present; movement of the maxilla and nose indicates a LeFort II; and movement of the entire midface and zygoma indicates a LeFort III. Because of the extent of LeFort II and III fractures, they may be associated with cribriform plate fractures and CSF rhinorrhea.

Emergency Department Treatment and Disposition

Maxillofacial CT should be obtained if a LeFort injury is suspected. Management of LeFort I fractures may involve only dental splinting and oral surgery consultation, but management of LeFort II and III fractures normally requires admission because of associated injuries as well as need for operative repair. Epistaxis may be difficult to control in LeFort II and III fractures, in rare cases requiring intraoperative arterial ligation.

Pearls

1. Attention should be focused on immediate airway management, since the massive edema associated with LeFort II and III fractures may quickly lead to airway compromise.
2. Nasotracheal intubation should be avoided because of the possibility of intracranial tube placement.
3. LeFort fractures are associated with cervical spine injury, intracranial injury, and CSF leak.

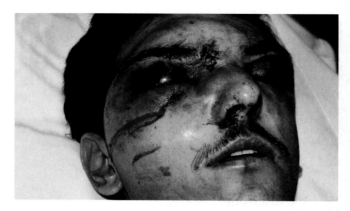

FIGURE 1.18 ■ LeFort Facial Fractures. Clinical photograph of patient with blunt facial trauma. Note the ecchymosis and edema. This patient sustained a LeFort II fracture on one side and a LeFort III on the other, and associated intracranial hemorrhages. (Photo contributor: Stephen W. Corbett, MD.)

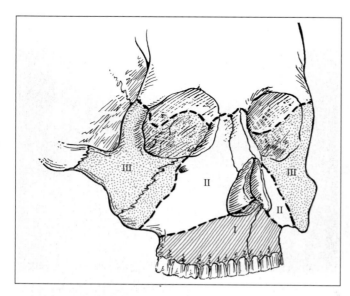

FIGURE 1.17 ■ LeFort Fractures. Illustration of the fracture lines of LeFort I (alveolar), LeFort II (zygomatic maxillary complex), and LeFort III (cranial facial dysostosis) fractures.

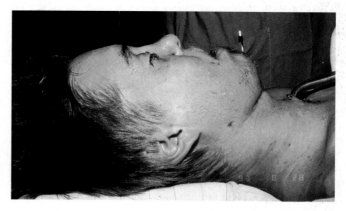

FIGURE 1.19 ■ LeFort Facial Fractures. Clinical photograph of patient with blunt facial trauma. This patient demonstrates the classic "dish face" deformity (depressed midface) associated with bilateral LeFort III fractures. (Photo contributor: Robert Schnarrs, MD.)

Clinical Summary

Orbital floor fractures are seen from two distinct mechanisms. The first is a true "blowout" fracture, where all energy is transmitted to the globe. The spherical globe is stronger than the thin orbital floor, and the force is transmitted to the thin orbital floor or medially through the ethmoid bones, with the resultant fracture. Fists or small balls are the typical causative agents. This mechanism of injury is more likely to cause entrapment and globe injury. The second mechanism of injury occurs when the energy from the blow is transmitted to the infraorbital rim, causing a buckling of the orbital floor. Entrapment and globe injury are less likely with this mechanism of injury. Patients with orbital floor fractures have periorbital ecchymosis, lid edema, and infraorbital numbness from injury to the infraorbital nerve but may sustain globe injuries as well, including chemosis, subconjunctival hemorrhage, corneal abrasion, hyphema, enophthalmos, proptosis, iridoplegia, dislocated lens, retinal tear, retinal detachment, and ruptured globe. If the inferior rectus muscle is extruded into the fracture, it may become entrapped; upward gaze is then limited, with resultant diplopia.

Emergency Department Treatment and Disposition

Orbital CT scan should be performed in all patients with a suspected orbital floor fracture or entrapment. Patients without eye injury or entrapment may be treated conservatively with ice and analgesics and referred for follow-up in 3 days. Patients with blood in the maxillary sinus are usually treated with antibiotics. Patients with a true "blowout" fracture should be seen by ophthalmology, since up to 30% of these patients sustain a globe injury. Patients with entrapment should undergo consultation on a same-day basis.

Pearls

1. Enophthalmos, limited upward gaze, diplopia with upward gaze, or infraorbital anesthesia from entrapment or injury to the infraorbital nerve should heighten suspicion of an orbital floor fracture.
2. Compare the pupillary level on the affected side with the unaffected side, since it may be lower from prolapse of the orbital contents into the maxillary sinus.

Subtle abnormalities may be appreciated as an asymmetric corneal light reflex (Hirschberg reflex).

3. Periorbital swelling after the patient blows his or her nose (from subcutaneous emphysema) or air bubbles emanating from the tear duct suggest orbital wall injury.

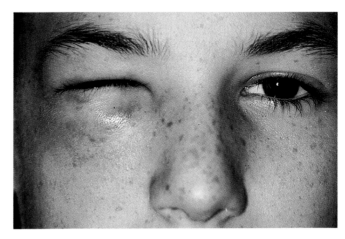

FIGURE 1.20 ■ Orbital Ecchymosis. Sustained from blunt trauma to the globe and the inferior orbital rim. This patient presents with subtle signs only (ecchymosis and swelling with no entrapment or eye injury). This patient demonstrates that orbital floor fractures can present with subtle physical findings. (Photo contributor: Kevin J. Knoop, MD, MS.)

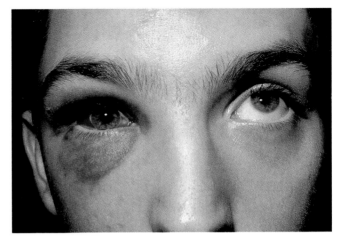

FIGURE 1.21 ■ Inferior Rectus Entrapment. The inferior rectus muscle is entrapped within the orbital floor fracture. When the patient tries to look upward, the affected eye has limited upward gaze and diplopia. (Photo contributor: Lawrence B. Stack, MD.)

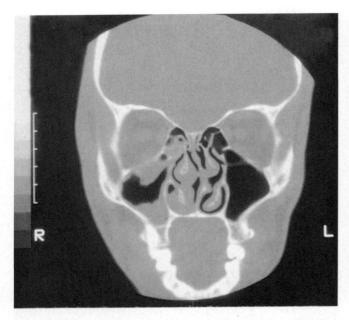

FIGURE 1.22 ■ Orbital Floor Fracture with Entrapment. CT of the patient in Fig. 1.20 demonstrating the entrapped muscle extruding into the maxillary sinus. (Photo contributor: Lawrence B. Stack, MD.)

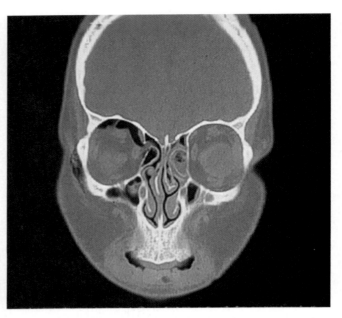

FIGURE 1.24 ■ CT of Medial Wall Orbital Fracture. CT Coronal view of the patient in Fig. 23. Subcutaneous emphysema and orbital air is seen. An opening between the orbit and ethmoid air cells can be seen. (Photo contributor: Lawrence B. Stack, MD.)

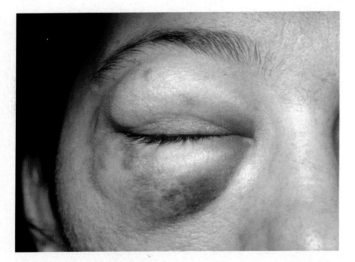

FIGURE 1.23 ■ Medial Wall Orbital Fracture. Periorbital ecchymosis and swelling is seen in this patient with a medial wall orbital fracture. The patient blew her nose after the injury and the swelling became more prominent. (Photo contributor: Lawrence B. Stack, MD.)

Clinical Summary

Blunt trauma, mandibular pain, malocclusion, and inability to fully open the mouth, are clinical features of mandibular fractures. A step-off in the dental line or ecchymosis or hematoma to the floor of the mouth is often present. Mandibular fractures may be open to the oral cavity, as manifested by gingival lacerations. Dental trauma may be seen. Other clinical features include inferior alveolar or mental nerve paresthesias, loose or missing teeth, dysphagia, trismus, or ecchymosis of the floor of the mouth (considered pathognomonic). Multiple mandibular fractures are present in more than 50% of cases because of the ringlike structure of the mandible. Mandibular fractures are often classified as favorable or unfavorable. Those fractures displaced by the masseter muscle are unfavorable and inevitably require fixation, whereas fractures that are not displaced by traction are favorable and in some cases will not require fixation. Injuries creating unstable mandibular fractures may create airway obstruction because the support for the tongue is lost. Mandibular fractures are also classified based on the anatomic location of the fracture. Dislocation of the mandibular condyles may also result from blunt trauma and will always have associated malocclusion, typified by an inability to close the mouth.

Emergency Department Treatment and Disposition

The dental panoramic view followed by plain films (antero-posterior [AP], bilateral oblique, and Townes views to evaluate the condyles) are the best imaging studies to detect mandibular fracture. CT is best utilized for the evaluation of fractures of the mandibular condyles. Nondisplaced fractures can be treated with analgesics, soft diet, and referral to oral surgery in 2 days. Displaced fractures, open fractures, and fractures with associated dental trauma require immediate consultation. All mandibular fractures should be treated with antibiotics effective against anaerobic oral flora (clindamycin, amoxicillin clavulanate) and tetanus prophylaxis given if needed. The Barton bandage has been suggested to immobilize the jaw in the emergency department.

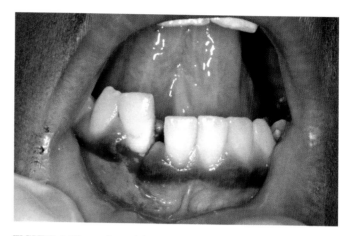

FIGURE 1.25 ■ Open Mandibular Fracture. An open fracture is suggested by the misaligned teeth and gingival disruption. (Photo contributor: Lawrence B. Stack, MD.)

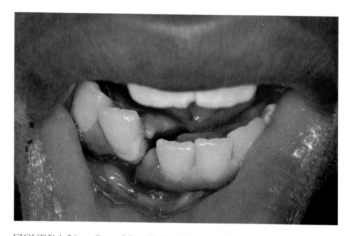

FIGURE 1.26 ■ Open Mandibular Fracture. Same patient as Fig. 1.25 demonstrating marked lingual gingival disruption. (Photo contributor: Lawrence B. Stack, MD.)

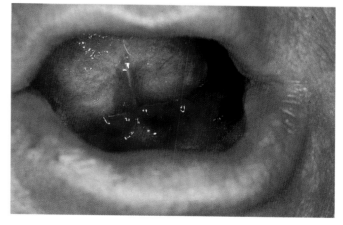

FIGURE 1.27 ■ Sublingual Hemorrhage. Hemorrhage or ecchymosis in the sublingual area is pathognomonic for mandibular fracture. (Photo contributor: Lawrence B. Stack, MD.)

Pearls

1. The most sensitive sign of a mandibular fracture is malocclusion.
2. A nonfractured mandible should be able to hold a tongue blade between the molars tightly enough to break it off. There should be no pain in attempting to rotate the tongue blade between the molars.
3. Bilateral parasymphyseal fractures may cause acute airway obstruction in the supine patient. This is relieved by pulling the subluxed mandible and soft tissue forward and by elevating the patient to a sitting position, if appropriate.

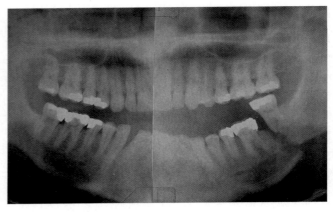

FIGURE 1.29 ▪ Unfavorable Mandibular Fracture. Dental panoramic view demonstrating a mandibular fracture with obvious misalignment due to the distracting forces of the masseter muscle. (Photo contributor: Edward S. Amrhein, DDS.)

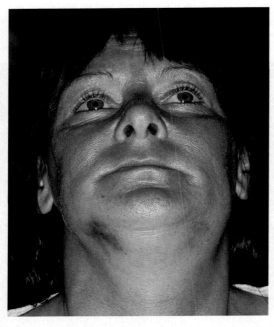

FIGURE 1.28 ▪ Bilateral Mandibular Fracture. The diagnosis is suggested by the bilateral ecchymosis seen in this patient. (Photo contributor: Lawrence B. Stack, MD.)

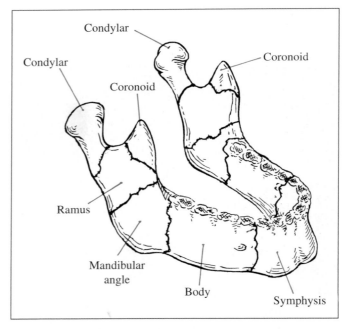

FIGURE 1.30 ▪ Classification of Mandibular Fractures. Classification based on anatomic location of the fracture.

Clinical Summary

Blunt external ear trauma may cause a contusion or hematoma of the pinna which, if untreated, may result in cartilage necrosis and chronic scarring or further cartilage formation and permanent deformity or "cauliflower ear." Open injuries include lacerations (with and without cartilage exposure) and avulsions.

Emergency Department Treatment and Disposition

Pinna hematomas must undergo incision and drainage or large needle aspiration using sterile technique, followed by a pressure dressing to prevent reaccumulation of the hematoma. This procedure may need to be repeated several times; hence, after emergency department drainage, the patient is treated with antistaphylococcal antibiotics and referred to ENT or plastic

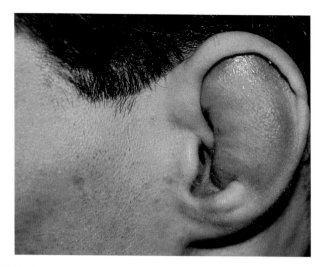

FIGURE 1.32 ■ Pinna Hematoma. A hematoma has developed, characterized by swelling, discoloration, ecchymosis, and fluctuance. Immediate incision and drainage or aspiration is indicated, followed by an ear compression dressing. (Photo contributor: C. Bruce MacDonald, MD.)

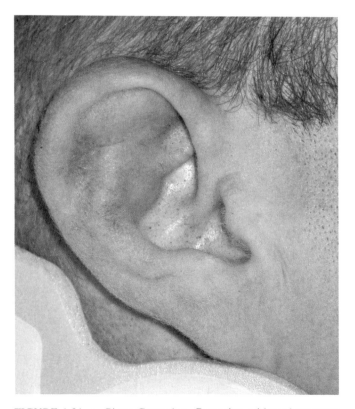

FIGURE 1.31 ■ Pinna Contusion. Contusion without hematoma is present. Reevaluation in 24 hours is recommended to ensure a drainable hematoma has not formed. (Photo contributor: Lawrence B. Stack, MD.)

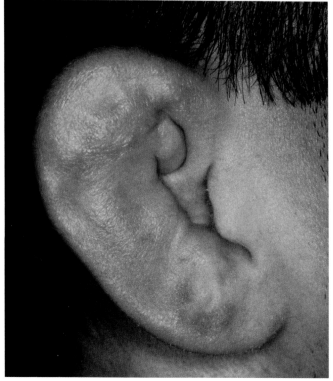

FIGURE 1.33 ■ Cauliflower Ear. Repeated trauma to the pinna or undrained hematomas can result in cartilage necrosis and subsequent deforming scar formation. (Photo contributor: Timothy D. McGuirk, DO.)

surgery for follow-up in 24 hours. Lacerations must be carefully examined for cartilage involvement; if this is present, copious irrigation, closure, and postrepair oral antibiotics covering skin flora are indicated. Simple skin lacerations may be repaired primarily with nonabsorbable 6-0 sutures. The dressing after laceration repair is just as important as the primary repair. If a compression dressing is not placed, hematoma formation can occur. Complex lacerations or avulsions normally require ENT or plastic surgery consultation.

Pearls

1. Pinna hematomas may take hours to develop. Patients with blunt ear trauma require careful discharge instructions, with a follow-up within 24 hours to check for hematoma development.

2. Failure to adequately drain a hematoma, reaccumulation of the hematoma owing to a faulty pressure dressing or inadequate follow-up increases the risk of infection of the pinna (perichondritis) or of a disfiguring cauliflower ear.

3. Copiously irrigate injuries with lacerated cartilage, which can usually be managed by primary closure of the overlying skin. Direct closure of the cartilage is rarely necessary and is indicated only for proper alignment, which helps lessen later distortion. Use a minimal number of absorbable 5-0 or 6-0 sutures through the perichondrium.

4. Lacerations to the lateral aspect of the pinna should be minimally debrided because of the lack of tissue at this site to cover the exposed cartilage.

5. In the case of an avulsion injury, the avulsed part should be cleansed, wrapped in saline-moistened gauze, placed in a sterile container, and then placed on ice to await reimplantation by ENT.

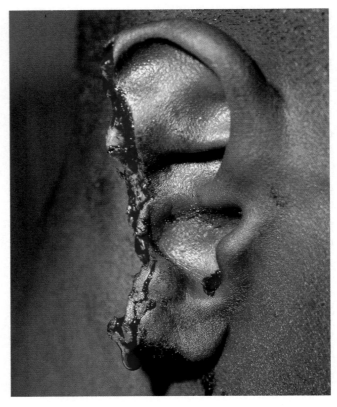

FIGURE 1.34 ■ Complete Avulsion of Partial Pinna. This ear injury, sustained in a fight, resulted when the pinna was bitten off. Plastic repair is needed. The avulsed part was wrapped in sterile gauze soaked with saline and placed in a sterile container on ice. (Photo contributor: David W. Munter, MD.)

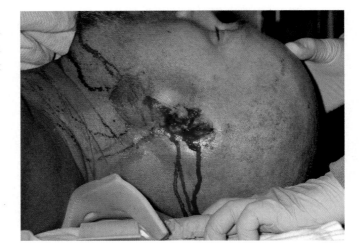

FIGURE 1.35 ■ Complete Avulsion of Entire Pinna. This injury occurred as a result of a motor vehicle crash. The pinna was not found. (Photo contributor: Ian T. McClure, MD.)

Clinical Summary

Blunt trauma to the frontal area may result in a depressed frontal sinus fracture. There frequently is an overlying laceration. Isolated frontal fractures normally do not have the associated features of massive blunt facial trauma as seen in LeFort II and III fractures. Careful nasal speculum examination may reveal blood or CSF leak high in the nasal cavity. Posterior table involvement can lead to mucopyocele or epidural empyema as late sequelae. Involvement of the posterior wall of the frontal sinus may occur and result in brain injury or dural tear. Frontal fractures may be part of a complex of facial fractures, as seen in frontonasoethmoid fractures, but generally more extensive facial trauma is required.

Emergency Department Treatment and Disposition

Suspicion for frontal sinus fracture is best evaluated with CT. Fractures involving only the anterior table of the frontal sinus can be treated conservatively with referral to ENT or plastic surgery in 1 to 2 days. Fractures involving the posterior table require urgent neurosurgical consultation. Frontal sinus fractures are usually covered with broad-spectrum antibiotics against both skin and sinus flora. Emergency department management also includes control of epistaxis, application of ice packs, and analgesia.

Pearls

1. Explore every frontal laceration digitally before repair. Digital palpation is sensitive to identifying frontal fractures, although false positives from lacerations extending through the periosteum can occur.
2. Communication of irrigating solutions with the nose or mouth indicates a breach in the frontal sinus.
3. A head CT should be obtained if a frontal sinus fracture is suspected to evaluate for posterior wall injury, brain injury, and open fracture.

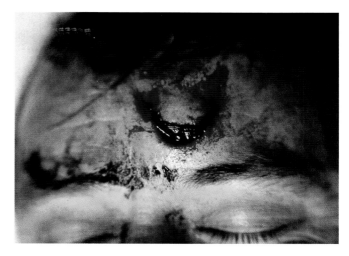

FIGURE 1.36 ■ Frontal Laceration. Any laceration over the frontal sinuses should be explored to exclude a fracture. This laceration was found to have an associated frontal fracture. (Photo contributor: David W. Munter, MD.)

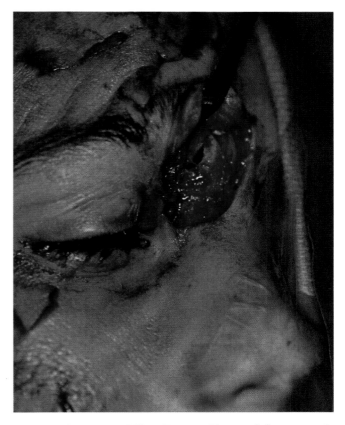

FIGURE 1.37 ■ Frontal Sinus Fracture. Fracture defect seen at the base of a laceration over the frontal sinus. (Photo contributor: Jeffrey Kuhn, MD.)

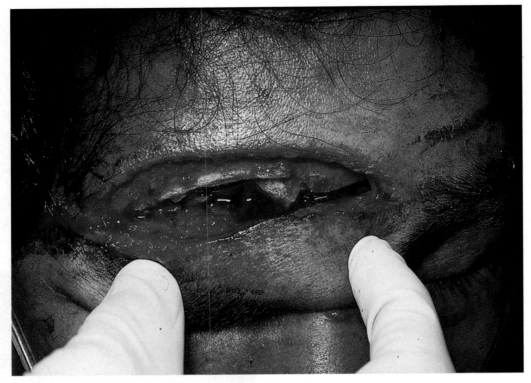

FIGURE 1.38 ■ Frontal Sinus Fracture. Fracture of the outer table of the frontal sinus is seen under this forehead laceration. (Photo contributor: Lawrence B. Stack, MD.)

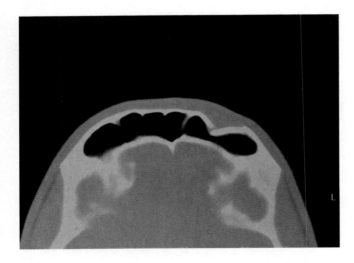

FIGURE 1.39 ■ Frontal Sinus Fracture. CT of the patient in Fig. 1.36 demonstrating a fracture of the anterior table of the frontal sinus. (Photo contributor: David W. Munter, MD.)

Clinical Summary

Traumatic exophthalmos develops as a retrobulbar hematoma pushes the globe outward. Patients present with periorbital edema, ecchymosis, a marked decrease in visual acuity, and an afferent pupillary defect in the involved eye. The exophthalmos, which may be obscured by periorbital edema, can be better appreciated from a superior view. Visual acuity may be affected by the direct trauma to the eye (retinal detachment, hyphema, globe rupture), compression of the retinal artery, or neuropraxia of the optic nerve. "Orbital compartment syndrome" occurs when intraorbital pressure exceeds central retinal artery pressure and ocular ischemia ensues. Causes are many with retrobulbar hematoma being the most common.

Emergency Department Treatment and Disposition

CT is the best modality to determine the presence and extent of a retrobulbar hematoma and associated facial or orbital fractures. Consultation of ENT and ophthalmology is indicated on an urgent basis. An emergent lateral canthotomy decompresses the orbit and can be performed in the emergency department and may be sight-saving.

Pearls

1. The retrobulbar hematoma and resultant exophthalmos may not develop for hours after the injury. Discharged patients with periorbital trauma should be instructed to be alert to change in vision.

2. Careful examination for globe injury should be conducted in all patients with periorbital trauma.

3. A subtle exophthalmos may be detected by looking down over the head of the patient and viewing the eye from the coronal plane.

4. Lateral canthotomy should be considered for emergent treatment of traumatic exophthalmos with associated afferent pupillary defect and decreased vision.

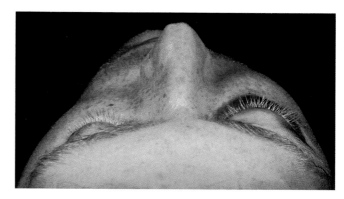

FIGURE 1.41 ■ Traumatic Exophthalmos. Superior view, demonstrating the right-sided exophthalmos. (Photo contributor: Frank Birinyi, MD.)

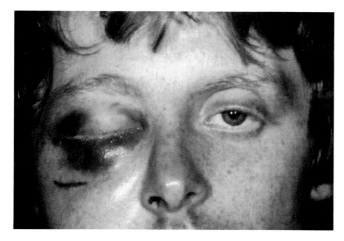

FIGURE 1.40 ■ Traumatic Exophthalmos. Blunt trauma resulting in periorbital edema and ecchymosis, which obscures the exophthalmos in this patient. The exophthalmos is not obvious in the AP view and can therefore be initially unappreciated. Figure 1.41 shows the same patient viewed in the coronal plane from over the forehead. (Photo contributor: Frank Birinyi, MD.)

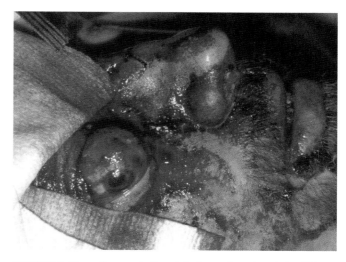

FIGURE 1.42 ■ Traumatic Exophthalmos. Anterior globe dislocation due to high energy head injury. (Photo contributor: Lawrence B. Stack, MD.)

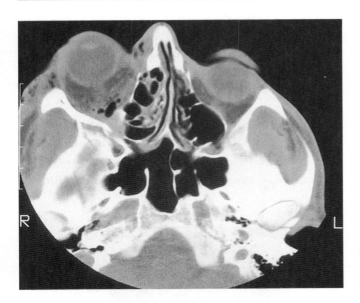

FIGURE 1.43 ■ Retrobulbar Hematoma. CT of the patient in Figs. 1.40 and 1.41 with right retrobulbar hematoma and traumatic exophthalmos. (Photo contributor: Frank Birinyi, MD.)

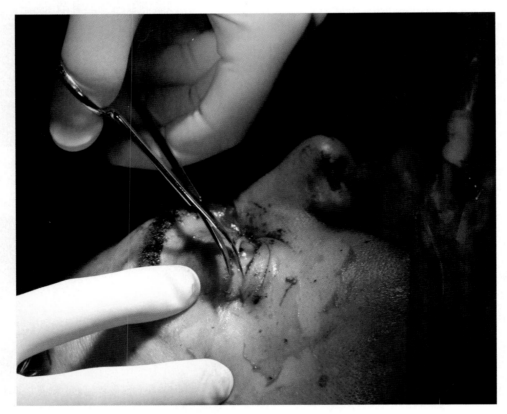

FIGURE 1.44 ■ Lateral Canthotomy. Lateral canthotomy with iris scissors is being performed to decrease intraorbital pressure. This step is preceded by crushing the tissue with a hemostat along the intended incision line. (Photo contributor: Kevin J. Knoop, MD, MS.)

Clinical Summary

Injury patterns of penetrating facial trauma can be somewhat predicted based on projectile type, by entry location, and path. Midface injuries extend from the oral commissure inferiorly, to the supraorbital rim superiorly, and to the external auditory meatus posteriorly. Mandibular injuries extend from the oral commissure superiorly and to the lower border of the mandible inferiorly. Shotgun wounds typically involve both facial zones and will involve one or both eyes in 50% of patients. Fifty percent of patients with gunshot wounds to the mandible will require an emergency airway. Stab wounds are less likely to require emergency airway than GSWs. Additional structures that require consideration during the emergency department evaluation include brain, blood vessels, and esophagus.

Emergency Department Treatment and Disposition

After the primary survey, elective intubation should be strongly considered in patients with any gunshot injury to the mandible, blood or swelling in the oropharynx, or any close range (<7 m) shotgun injury. If evidence suggests a projectile remains in the face or cranium, plain films in two planes may help guide subsequent evaluation such as CT-angiogram or fine cuts of the orbits. CT will provide more detailed information in the injured structures to guide therapy. Removal of any projectile should only be preformed after significant structure injury has been excluded and preparation for the consequences of removal is complete.

Pearls

1. Due to the likelihood of multisystem injury (vascular, ocular, cranial, face) penetrating facial trauma the patient should be transferred to a facility with comprehensive subspecialty trauma care.
2. Intubation should be strongly considered in all patients with GSWs to the mandible or in GSWs to the midface if there is any blood or swelling in the oral cavity.
3. Removal of any projectile is best done in the operating room.

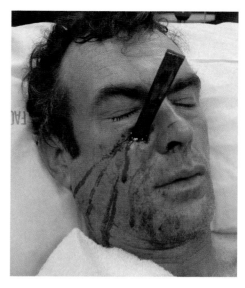

FIGURE 1.46 ■ Midface Injury. A jackhammer bit is lodged into the right maxillary sinus. (Photo contributor: R. Jason Thurman, MD.)

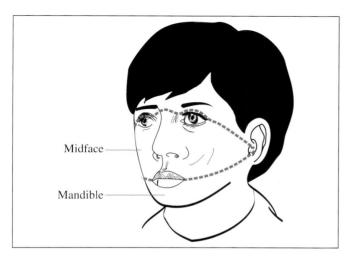

FIGURE 1.45 ■ Penetrating Facial Zones of Injury. (Described by Chen AY, Steward MG, Raup G. Penetrating injuries of the face. *Otolaryngol Head Neck Surg.* 1996;115:464-470.)

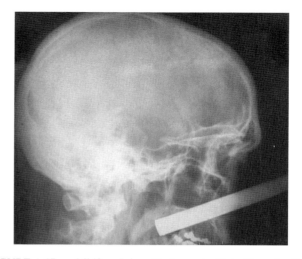

FIGURE 1.47 ■ Midface Injury Radiograph. Plain film of patient in Fig. 1.46. CT confirmed no other injury. Projectile was removed in the OR. (Photo contributor: R. Jason Thurman, MD.)

Clinical Summary

Severe head injury may result in extra axial hematoma, cerebral contusion, or diffuse cerebral edema which, in turn, may cause one of five brain herniation syndromes: uncal, central transtentorial, cerebellotonsillar, subfalcine, and external. Uncal herniation occurs when the uncus of the temporal lobe is displaced inferiorly through the medial edge of the tentorium. Compression of cranial nerve III can cause an ipsilateral dilated pupil. Typically patients with uncal herniation are unconscious and require intubation. A contusion to the eye may result in a dilated, nonresponsive pupil and arouse suspicion for severe head injury and uncal herniation.

Emergency Department Treatment and Disposition

Unconscious head trauma patients with a single dilated pupil should be intubated and transferred immediately to a facility capable of caring for traumatic brain injury. A noncontrast CT scan may reveal a subdural or epidural hematoma, diffuse edema, or temporal lobe contusion. These conditions may cause midline shift of cerebral structures and compression of the quadrigeminal cistern. Unilateral effacement of the quadrigeminal cistern confirms uncal herniation. Initial management focuses on maintaining cerebral perfusion pressure and normal tissue oxygenation as hypotension and hypoxia significantly contribute to secondary brain injury. Mannitol, burr holes, and hyperventilation should be carefully considered in emergency department patients with uncal herniation. Definitive care requires neurosurgical consultation.

Pearls

1. Uncal herniation is the most common of the five herniation syndromes.
2. If a patient has a unilateral dilated pupil after head and face trauma but is awake and talking, be suspicious for an eye contusion.
3. Steroids have no role in the emergency department management of traumatic brain injury.
4. A temporal lobe contusion in an initially neurologically intact patient may continue to expand and cause uncal herniation.

5. Excessive hyperventilation ($Paco_2 < 25$ mm Hg) in patients with severe traumatic brain injury is associated with cerebral ischemia.
6. Effacement of the quadrigeminal cistern is the hallmark CT finding of uncal herniation.

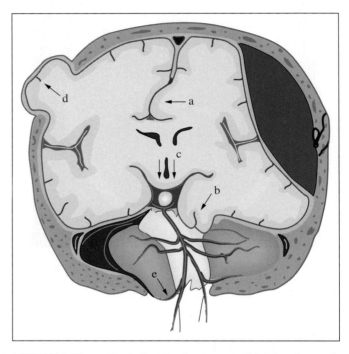

FIGURE 1.48 ■ Herniation Syndromes. **a.** subfalcine; **b.** uncal; **c.** central transtentorial; **d.** external; **e.** cerebellotonsillar.

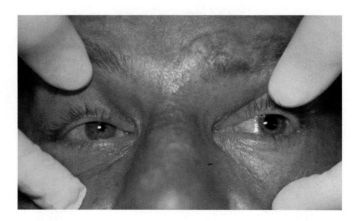

FIGURE 1.49 ■ Ipsilateral Dilated Pupil due to Uncal Herniation. CT reveals an epidural hematoma and unilateral effacement of the quadrigeminal cistern. (Photo contributor: Lawrence B. Stack, MD.)

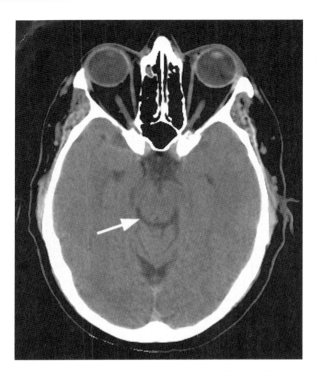

FIGURE 1.50 ■ Normal Quadrigeminal Cistern. The normal appearance of this CSF space is shaped like a baby's bottom (see arrow). It is located within two cuts superiorly of the dorsum sella. (Photo contributor: Lawrence B. Stack, MD.)

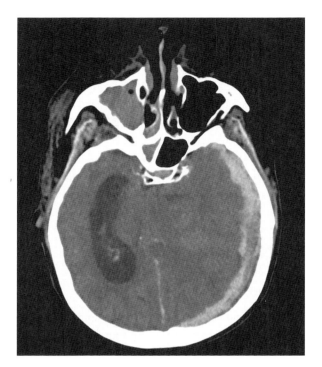

FIGURE 1.52 ■ Subdural Hematoma. A crescent-shaped subdural hematoma is seen on the left. The quadrigeminal cistern should be seen on this slice and is completely effaced, suggesting herniation. (Photo contributor: Lawrence B. Stack, MD.)

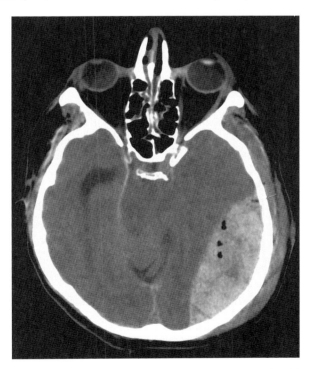

FIGURE 1.51 ■ Epidural Hematoma. A lens-shaped epidural hematoma is seen on the left. The quadrigeminal cistern should be seen on this slice and is completely effaced, suggesting herniation. (Photo contributor: Lawrence B. Stack, MD.)

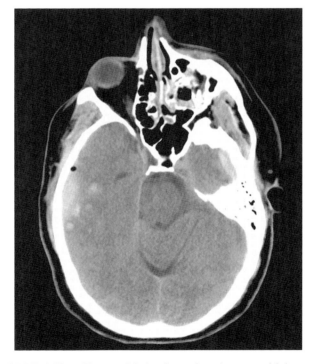

FIGURE 1.53 ■ Temporal Lobe Contusion. A temporal lobe contusion is seen on the right. The quadrigeminal cistern is partially effaced suggesting early herniation. (Photo contributor: Lawrence B. Stack, MD.)

Chapter 2

OPHTHALMOLOGIC CONDITIONS

Marc E. Levsky
Paul DeFlorio

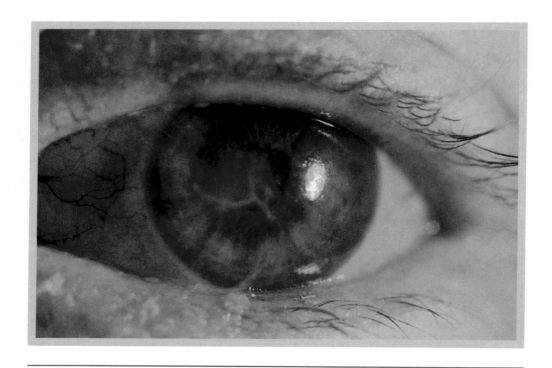

The authors acknowledge the contribution of Frank Birinyi, MD and Thomas F. Mauger, MD for portions of this chapter written for the previous editions of this book.

Clinical Summary

Neonatal conjunctivitis comprises a number of entities, including chemical irritation caused by antimicrobial prophylaxis (most common cause), infections acquired through direct contact between the neonate and the mother's cervix and vagina during delivery, and infections transmitted by cross-inoculation in the neonatal period. Common causative organisms include *Chlamydia trachomatis* (most common), *Neisseria gonorrhoeae* (most threatening), *Haemophilus* species, *Streptococcus* species, *Staphylococcus aureus,* and viruses such as *Herpes simplex* (HSV). Clinical findings in include drainage, conjunctival hyperemia, chemosis, and lid edema. Timing of presentation following birth and maternal findings often are useful in determining the most likely etiology.

Emergency Department Treatment and Disposition

As with any focal infection in the neonate, a careful evaluation for systemic involvement is indicated. When neonatal conjunctivitis is observed, cultures and smears are mandatory, and should be followed immediately by treatment, in consultation with a pediatrician or infectious disease specialist. Scrapings of the palpebral conjunctiva for cultures and Gram stain are more revealing than examination of the discharge itself. Corneal examination with fluorescein staining should be done to detect the dendritic lesions of HSV.

Pearls

1. Etiologies of neonatal conjunctivitis may be difficult to ascertain on clinical grounds, and though chemical irritation is most common, aggressive work-up and treatment

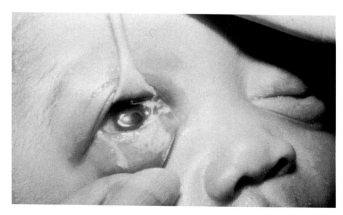

FIGURE 2.1 ■ Neonatal Conjunctivitis (Ophthalmia Neonatorum). Copious purulent drainage in a newborn with neonatal gonococcal conjunctivitis. (Reprinted with permission of the American Academy of Ophthalmology. Eye Trauma and Emergencies: A Slide-Script Program. San Francisco, 1985.)

TABLE 2.1 ■ SUMMARY OF ETIOLOGIES OF NEONATAL CONJUNCTIVITIS

Etiologic Agent	Time of Onset	Clinical Features	Treatment
Chemical	Day 1	Common with silver nitrate; erythromycin more commonly used now for this reason	Self-limited
N gonorrhoeae	Day 2-7	May cause hyperacute disease with profuse discharge	Ceftriaxone 25-50 mg/kg IV NTE 125 mg. Caution in hyperbilirubinemia. Topicals alone inadequate
C trachomatis	Day 3-14	Clinical severity varies. Common cause of blindness worldwide	Erythromycin 12.5 mg PO q6h × 14 days
HSV 1,2	Day 2-16	Should be suspected if child has any vesicular lesions on body	Vidarabine or trifluridine topically; consider adding systemic acyclovir
Other bacterial organisms	Day 2 and up	Empiric treatment based on Gram stain	Erythromycin ointment for gram-positive; gentamicin or tobramycin ointment for gram-negative

is mandatory in all cases due to the potentially devastating nature of gonococcal conjunctivitis.

2. The "rule of fives" is a mnemonic device for predicting the most likely bacterial etiology; however, there is considerable overlap in times to onset.

0 to 5 days:	*N gonorrhoeae*
5 days to 5 weeks:	*Chlamydia*
5 weeks to 5 years:	*Streptococcus* or *Haemophilus influenzae*

3. Although an uncommon cause of conjunctivitis, HSV may cause a concomitant life-threatening systemic infection in the neonate. A high index of suspicion should be maintained, especially in cases of known parental infection.

4. The cornea should be examined for involvement. Corneal ulcers, perforation, permanent scarring, and blindness can quickly result from gonococcal eye infection in the neonate. It is one of the few urgent "conjunctival" infections.

5. A detailed maternal history may help with the diagnosis of neonatal conjunctivitis secondary to *N gonorrhoeae*, *Chlamydia*, or herpes.

Clinical Summary

Bacterial conjunctivitis usually presents with painless conjunctival hyperemia and mucopurulent discharge of acute onset. Visual acuity is preserved, except for mild intermittent blurring from the film of discharge. Classically, patients describe the lids matted together, especially on awakening, though this finding is not specific for bacterial conjunctivitis. The most common causative organism is *S aureus; Streptococcus pneumoniae* and *Haemophilus influenzae* are found frequently in children. Hyperacute onset of copious purulent discharge in a sexually active adult should raise concern for gonococcal conjunctivitis, which unlike typical bacterial conjunctivitis, requires systemic therapy. *Neisseria* species can invade and rapidly perforate the cornea.

Emergency Department Treatment and Disposition

Gram stain and culture of conjunctival scrapings should be done if gonococcal or chlamydial conjunctivitis is suspected, as these types require systemic as well as topical therapy. Most other bacterial conjunctivitis responds well to fluoroquinolone drops or polymyxin—trimethoprim drops topically, and patients with these conditions can be discharged home with close follow-up.

Pearls

1. Slit-lamp microscopy and fluorescein stain should be done to rule out corneal ulcer or dendritic lesions. Increased level of suspicion of ulcer is warranted in all contact lens wearers.
2. Conjunctivitis should not be considered the primary diagnosis in a patient that has significant eye pain or decreased visual acuity, and another cause of the symptoms should be sought.
3. Worsening of symptoms after the use of topical antimicrobials, especially aminoglycosides or sulfonamides, suggests chemical conjunctivitis.
4. A patient with intense limbic injection (perilimbal "ciliary" flush) has an ongoing anterior chamber process, not conjunctivitis.

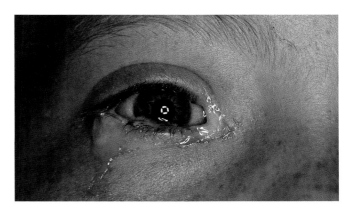

FIGURE 2.2 ■ Bacterial Conjunctivitis. Mucopurulent discharge, conjunctival injection, and lid swelling in a 10-year-old with *H influenzae* conjunctivitis. (Photo contributor: Frank Birinyi, MD.)

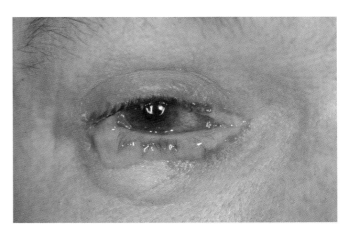

FIGURE 2.3 ■ Bacterial Conjunctivitis. Mucopurulent discharge, conjunctival in an adult with conjunctivitis. (Photo contributor: Lawrence B. Stack, MD.)

Clinical Summary

Viral conjunctivitis is a contagious infection most frequently caused by adenoviruses. Clinical features are usually mild and may include burning or irritation, injection, lid edema, chemosis, and a thin, watery discharge. Other than slight blurring caused by the discharge, visual acuity should not be impaired. One or both eyes may be involved, the latter from autoinoculation. Pharyngoconjunctival fever, a viral syndrome usually caused by adenovirus type 3, is highly infectious, and should be considered if there is fever, upper respiratory tract infection (cold, flu, or sore throat), and preauricular adenopathy.

Emergency Department Treatment and Disposition

Most cases are mild, self-limited, and do not require antibiotics. Cool compresses may help alleviate irritation. Meticulous hand washing and similar hygienic measures by patients and providers limit spread from person to person. Any atypical findings or disease that has not improved significantly in 7 days should prompt ophthalmologic referral.

Pearls

1. Significant eye pain or decreased visual acuity is not consistent with the diagnosis of viral conjunctivitis.
2. The hallmark of bacterial conjunctivitis is a continuous globular purulent discharge seen at the lid margins and in the corners of the eye. Viral conjunctivitis typically has a clear discharge with occasional scant mucoid discharge. Both may present with a history of the eye "matted shut" in the morning.
3. Patients who present with signs and symptoms consistent with viral conjunctivitis do not benefit from antibiotic therapy.

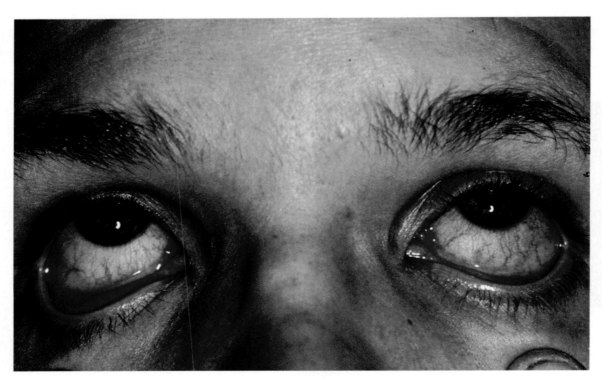

FIGURE 2.4 ■ Viral Conjunctivitis. Note the characteristic asymmetric conjunctival injection. Symptoms first developed in the left eye, with symptoms spreading to the other eye a few days later. A thin watery discharge is also seen. (Photo contributor: Kevin J. Knoop, MD, MS.)

Clinical Summary

Epidemic keratoconjunctivitis (EKC) is a highly contagious adenovirus infection, which is distinguished from typical viral conjunctivitis by involvement of the conjunctiva *and* cornea. EKC has an incubation period of about 8 days, and occurs most commonly in the fall and winter. Symptoms generally begin unilaterally; however, the other eye may become involved 4 to 5 days later. Clinical findings may resemble typical viral conjunctivitis and may also include a follicular (hyperplastic lymphoid tissue appearing as gray or white lobular elevations) and papillary (hyperplastic conjunctival epithelium being thrown into numerous folds and projections) conjunctival reaction. Pseudomembranes overlying the palpebral conjunctiva and tender preauricular nodes may be present. Papillae give the palpebral conjunctiva a velvety appearance. A painful keratitis, typically involving the central cornea, develops in about 80% of patients, usually around the eighth day. The keratitis initially appears as fine punctate epithelial lesions that stain faintly with fluorescein. After the second week, the lesions are replaced by subepithelial infiltrates located in the central cornea that no longer stain. Systemic symptoms are not present in EKC.

Emergency Department Treatment and Disposition

Although the symptoms caused by EKC are relatively severe for a viral conjunctivitis, they are self-limited and no specific treatment is indicated. Cool compresses and sunglasses may help with symptoms, and artificial tears or ointments may help to improve comfort. In severe cases, topical corticosteroids may provide improved symptomatic relief. However, these do not change the clinical outcome, and should be prescribed by or in close consultation with an ophthalmologist. Strict hand washing and hygienic measures are mandatory to limit spread.

Pearls

1. While nonspecific adenoviral conjunctivitis will generally resolve in 10 to 14 days, a virulent adenovirus causing EKC will peak in 5 to 7 days and may last 3 to 4 weeks.
2. EKC may be nosocomially transmitted by the physician's fingers and instruments. Adenovirus can be recovered for extended periods of time from these surfaces. Vigilant hygienic measures are mandatory.
3. Pharyngoconjunctival fever should be considered if there is an associated fever and upper respiratory tract infection.

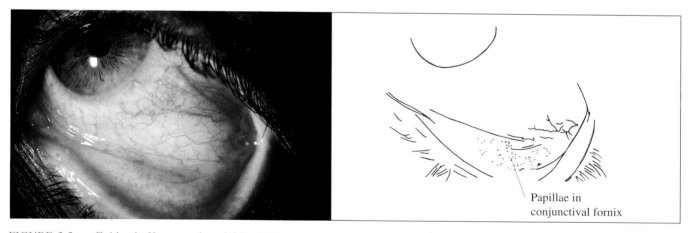

Papillae in conjunctival fornix

FIGURE 2.5 ■ Epidemic Keratoconjunctivitis (EKC). Diffuse injection of the bulbar conjunctiva is seen in addition to a papillary reaction of the palpebral conjunctiva—a classic finding in EKC. (Photo contributor: Department of Ophthalmology, Naval Medical Center, Portsmouth, VA.)

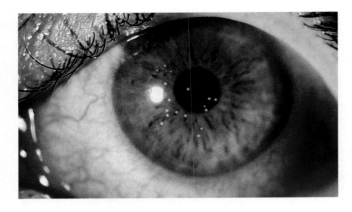

FIGURE 2.6 ■ Epithelial Keratitis. This usually develops after 5 to 7 days and is seen as a fine punctate abrasion pattern over the cornea. (Photo contributor: Department of Ophthalmology, Naval Medical Center, Portsmouth, VA.)

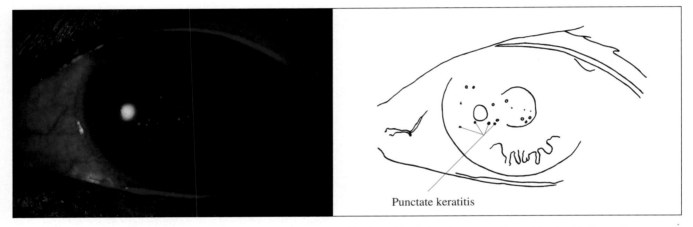

Punctate keratitis

FIGURE 2.7 ■ Fluorescein Stain. This demonstrates epithelial keratitis from Fig. 2.6. (Photo contributor: Katrina C. Santos.)

ALLERGIC CONJUNCTIVITIS

Clinical Summary

Allergic conjunctivitis comprises several classes of type-I hypersensitivity reactions. Many patients have a personal or family history of atopic disease such as asthma, allergic rhinitis, or eczema. Potential allergens are numerous, generally are airborne, and include any allergen that could trigger allergic rhinitis. The cardinal historical finding is itching; both eyes are usually involved and visual acuity is preserved. Other clinical findings include conjunctival hyperemia, chemosis, conjunctival papillae (cone-shaped areas that erupt on the surface of the conjunctiva in response to inflammation), and discharge, which is most frequently clear, but may be thicker mucus in some cases. Vernal conjunctivitis is a particularly severe variant of allergic conjunctivitis, which most frequently affects dark-skinned males during the summer months or in warm climates. Vernal conjunctivitis causes intense itching, and a thicker discharge. Giant conjunctival papillae that present a "cobblestone" appearance are the characteristic physical findings.

Emergency Department Treatment and Disposition

Identification and elimination of exposure to the allergen is important. Topical mast cell stabilizers, such as olopatadine or cromolyn, are useful for symptomatic relief, as are topical and systemic antihistamines, and nonsteroidal anti-inflammatory drugs. Cool compresses may help provide relief. In severe cases, topical steroids may be useful, but these should be used only in close consultation with an ophthalmologist.

Pearls

1. Itching is the hallmark of allergic conjunctivitis.
2. Conjunctival papillae are a common feature and are very prominent with vernal conjunctivitis. Small papillae give a velvety appearance, while giant papillae give a cobblestone appearance.
3. Other causes of red eye must be considered, and this diagnosis should be used cautiously, especially if involvement is unilateral, or concerning findings such as pain or decreased visual acuity are present.

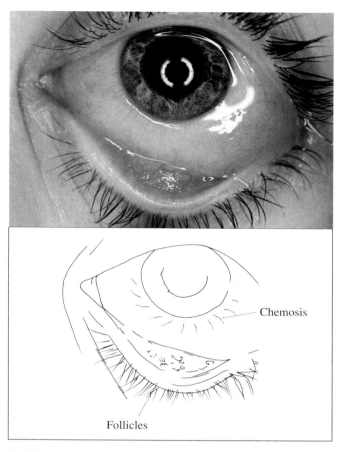

FIGURE 2.8 ■ Allergic Conjunctivitis. Conjunctival injection, chemosis, and a follicular response in the inferior palpebral conjunctiva in this patient with allergic conjunctivitis secondary to cat fur. (Photo contributor: Timothy D. McGuirk, DO.)

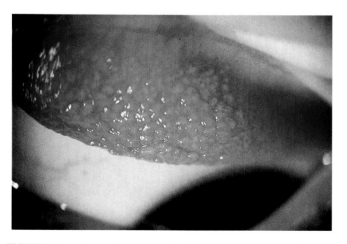

FIGURE 2.9 ■ Vernal Conjunctivitis. The tarsal conjunctiva demonstrates giant papillae and a cobblestone appearance pathognomonic for vernal conjunctivitis. (Photo contributor: William Beck.)

Clinical Summary

Dacryocystitis is inflammation of the medial lacrimal apparatus, which usually follows occlusion of the nasolacrimal duct. Age distribution is bimodal, with peaks in infancy and after 40 years. Clinical findings include, pain, erythema, and swelling over the medical lacrimal apparatus, tearing, and possibly mucopurulent discharge from the punctum. Dacryocystitis may develop in 4% to 7% of newborn infants who do not yet have a patent nasolacrimal passage, and may progress to periorbital cellulitis. Commonly implicated organisms include *S aureus, Streptococcus pneumoniae, Haemophilus influenza,* and *Pseudomonas aeruginosa.*

Emergency Department Treatment and Disposition

Acute dacryocystitis in otherwise well-appearing patients usually responds to an oral antibiotic such as amoxicillin-clavulanate, gentle massage, and warm compresses. In patients with systemic symptoms or significant periorbital cellulitis, intravenous antibiotics—usually third-generation cephalosporins—are indicated. A low threshold for admission must be maintained in the extremes of age and for patients with comorbidities. Culture of the discharge should be done to improve guide therapy, and especially to rule out MRSA as the cause. Ophthalmology referral is recommended for patients with severe, refractory, or recurrent disease.

Pearls

1. The lacrimal sac and punctum are located on the nasal aspect of the lower lid. This is the site where swelling will be found. This condition has been misdiagnosed as hordeolum.
2. Chronic or recurrent disease should raise suspicion of malignancy, causing nasolacrimal duct obstruction.
3. Many possible responsible organisms exist, so culture may be necessary to guide antibiotic therapy.

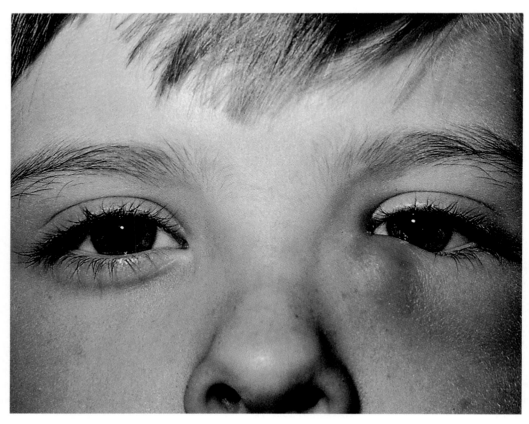

FIGURE 2.10 ■ Dacryocystitis. Swelling and erythema over the medial lid and lacrimal sac developed in this 10-year-old patient with streptococcal pharyngitis. (Photo contributor: Kevin J. Knoop, MD, MS.)

Clinical Summary

Dacryoadenitis is an uncommon inflammatory disorder of the lacrimal gland, located under the lateral portion of the upper lid. The most common causes are mumps and herpes virus. Bacterial causes include *Staphylococcus, Streptococcus,* gonorrhea, *Chlamydia,* and syphilis. Dacryoadenitis is associated with systemic inflammatory conditions such as sarcoidosis, and Sjögren syndrome. Clinical findings include painful swelling of the lateral third of the upper lid, conjunctival hyperemia, chemosis, and an S-shaped curve to the lid margin from ptosis of the upper lid. Diplopia may be present from involvement of the lateral rectus muscle.

Emergency Department Treatment and Disposition

If acute bacterial infection is suspected, oral antibiotics such as amoxicillin-clavulanate or cephalexin may be used pending culture results in mild cases, and intravenous antibiotics should be used in more severe cases. Viral and inflammatory dacryoadenitis is managed with cool compresses and analgesics. Nonemergent ophthalmology follow-up is generally appropriate. Patients with recurrent or refractory disease should undergo a thorough workup for local malignancies and systemic inflammatory disorders. Patients should be instructed to return to the emergency department for symptoms suggestive of orbital cellulitis.

Pearls

1. The swelling is usually unilateral and precisely located.
2. In children, mumps is the most likely etiology. Concurrent parotitis is suggestive.
3. Half of lacrimal gland masses are malignant; recommend close follow-up where suspected.

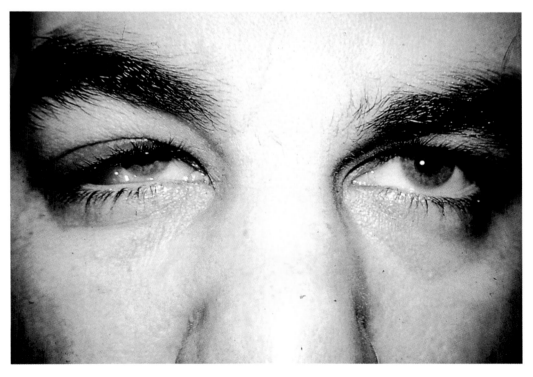

FIGURE 2.11 ■ Dacryoadenitis. Unilateral localized swelling and chemosis are present laterally secondary to inflammation of the lacrimal gland. (Used with permission from the American Academy of Ophthalmology. *External Disease and Cornea: A Multimedia Collection.* San Francisco, 1994.)

Clinical Summary

A pinguecula is a common degenerative lesion of the bulbar conjunctiva, and often appears as a partially translucent, colorless to light brown ridge adjacent to the limbus, usually on the nasal aspect. It may gradually enlarge with time, periodically become inflamed, or become a pterygium. Most pingueculae are asymptomatic. A pterygium is a benign proliferation of fibrovascular tissue found in a triangular shape, extending across the limbus, with the apex of the triangle pointing toward the center of the cornea. Pterygia, though often asymptomatic, may also become inflamed, causing a foreign body sensation. A pterygium may cause decreased visual acuity if it encroaches on the visual axis, or exerts a mechanical deforming force on the cornea. Both disorders are more common in males, and are associated with advanced age, and exposure to ultraviolet light, wind, and dust.

Emergency Department Treatment and Disposition

Though often concerning in appearance to the patient, most lesions are asymptomatic, and specific treatment in the emergency department is rarely necessary. Symptoms caused by inflamed lesions may improve with the use of sunglasses plus artificial tears or topical vasoconstrictors. Nonemergent referral to an ophthalmologist is appropriate. Persistently symptomatic or otherwise troublesome lesions may be excised by an ophthalmologist.

Pearls

1. Pterygia and pingueculae are usually found on the nasal conjunctiva, adjacent to the limbus, in the horizontal meridian.
2. Pterygia are a particular problem in sunny, hot, and dusty regions. Eye protection (goggles, sunglasses) and other conservative measures usually reduce symptoms when present.

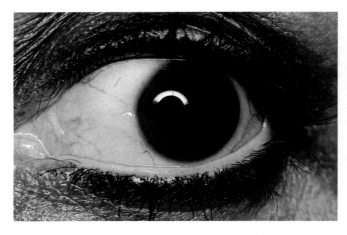

FIGURE 2.12 ■ Pinguecula. A small area of yellowish "heaped up" conjunctival tissue is seen adjacent to the limbus on the nasal aspect. (Photo contributor: Kevin J. Knoop, MD, MS.)

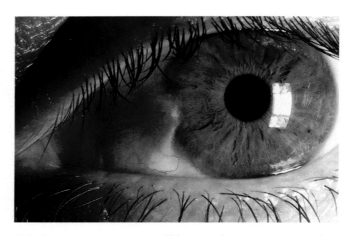

FIGURE 2.13 ■ Pterygium. This pterygium appears as a raised vascular triangular area of bulbar conjunctiva that encroaches on the cornea. (Photo contributor: Department of Ophthalmology, Naval Medical Center, Portsmouth, VA.)

Clinical Summary

A hordeolum is an acute inflammation and/or abscess involving the glandular structures of the eyelid and presents as an acute, tender swelling of the eyelid or eyelid margin. An internal hordeolum involves the meibomian glands, while an external hordeolum (stye) involves the glands of Zeis or Moll at the base of the eye lashes. When bacterial etiology is present, *S aureus* is the most frequently implicated pathogen. A chalazion is a firm, nontender lump that arises from obstruction of a meibomian gland. Tenderness, when present, occurs during lid swelling and cyst formation. Both hordeola and chalazia are associated with blepharitis, inflammation of the lid margins associated with plugging of the glandular ducts, and crusting around the lashes. Conditions such as seborrheic dermatitis of the eyelids, rosacea, or rarely eyelash infestation with lice can cause blepharitis and resultant blockage of the meibomian glands.

Emergency Department Treatment and Disposition

Chalazia are treated with excision or steroid injection by an ophthalmologist. External hordeola often resolve spontaneously with little or no specific management. Warm compresses may help to localize the inflammation and speed drainage. Internal hordeola that do not respond to conservative measures are treated with incision and or oral antibiotics. Eyelid hygiene by massaging with warm water and baby shampoo daily is recommended to help eliminate blepharitis and prevent recurrence. Topical ophthalmic antibiotic ointments such as erythromycin or bacitracin, while ineffective for abscesses and chronic inflammation, may serve as an adjunct to eyelid hygiene. If the mass persists beyond 3 weeks, is recurrent, or causes decreased visual acuity, referral to an ophthalmologist is appropriate.

Pearls

1. Blockage of the meibomian glands can form either chalazia or internal hordeola. If a chronic granulomatous reaction with cyst formation develops then a chalazion is formed. If an acute inflammation or abscess develops then an internal hordeolum is formed.
2. Management of hordeola and chalazia is usually conservative. Lid hygiene, warm compresses, and topical antibiotic ointments are usually adequate.

3. Optimal management of blepharitis will reduce recurrence of chalazia and hordeola.
4. Systemic antibiotics are generally unnecessary, unless significant cellulitis or an acute inflammation/infection involving the meibomian gland (meibomianitis) is present.
5. Excisional biopsy is indicated for recurrent chalazia to exclude malignancy.

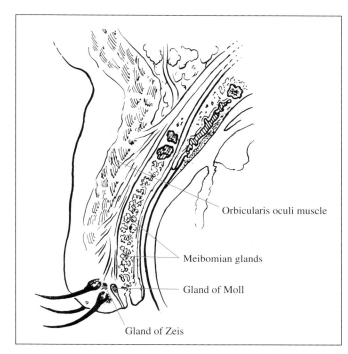

FIGURE 2.14A ■ Eyelid Anatomy. Anatomic structures related to eyelid pathology.

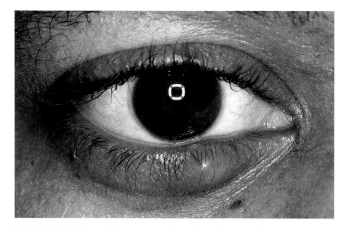

FIGURE 2.14B ■ Hordeolum. Focal swelling and erythema at the lid margin are seen in this hordeolum. (Photo contributor: Frank Birinyi, MD.)

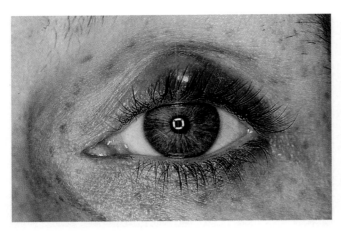

FIGURE 2.15 ■ Chalazion. This chalazion shows nodular focal swelling and erythema from meibomian cyst formation. Pain is present during swelling and cyst formation. (Photo contributor: Frank Birinyi, MD.)

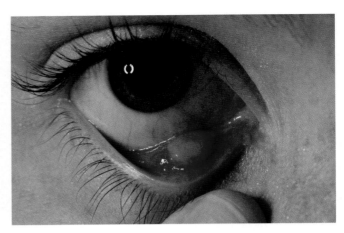

FIGURE 2.18 ■ Chalazion. This nontender lower lid chalazion was seen only with lid eversion. (Photo contributor: James Dahle, MD.)

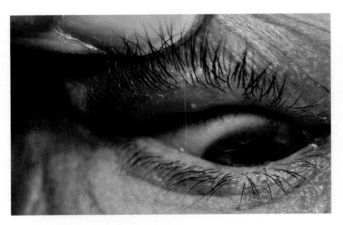

FIGURE 2.16 ■ Chalazion. This chalazion is in an early stage. Pointing of the chalazion to the inner tarsal conjunctiva is made evident with slight lid eversion. (Photo contributor: Kevin J. Knoop, MD, MS.)

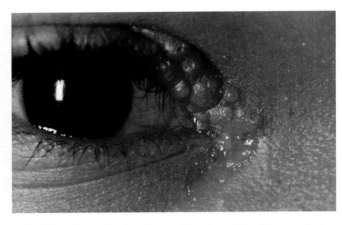

FIGURE 2.19 ■ Ocular Herpes Simplex. This 10-year-old has recurrent ocular herpes simplex since age 6. Vesicles should not be mistaken for hordeola. (Photo contributor: Lawrence B. Stack, MD.)

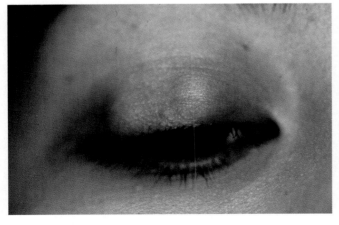

FIGURE 2.17 ■ Chalazion. A nontender bipartite chalazion is shown. (Photo contributor: Kevin J. Knoop, MD, MS.)

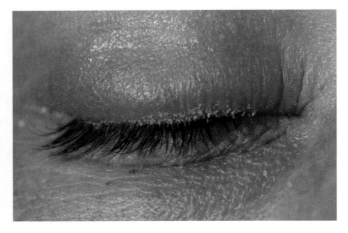

FIGURE 2.20 ■ Blepharitis. Inflamed, erythematous eyelid margins consistent with blepharitis. (Photo contributor: Kevin J. Knoop, MD, MS.)

Clinical Summary

Scleritis is an uncommon, but serious inflammatory condition involving the sclera. It is most often associated with systemic inflammatory conditions such as rheumatoid arthritis, and most commonly affects women. The onset is gradual and includes severe, deep eye pain, which may radiate over the distribution of the trigeminal nerve, as well as tearing and photophobia. There may be sectorial or diffuse involvement, with intense redness of the affected area. Bilateral involvement occurs in over half of cases. Sectorial scleritis may mimic the less-threatening condition episcleritis; however, in scleritis, the dilated blood vessels do not move with movement of the overlying conjunctiva with a cotton-tipped applicator, and do not blanch with topical 2.5% phenylephrine drops. The associated pain often responds poorly to topical anesthetic drops, and the globe is notably tender on palpation. Associated iritis and keratitis are common, and secondary glaucoma may occur; these may cause decreased visual acuity.

Emergency Department Treatment and Disposition

Urgent ophthalmology consultation and systemic therapy are required. Oral nonsteroidal anti-inflammatory drugs are useful; however, steroids and other immunosuppressive agents may be required, and management is best left to an ophthalmologist. Diagnosis and treatment of underlying systemic conditions is mandatory.

Pearls

1. Scleritis, unlike episcleritis, and like other causes of deep eye pain, is a severe and sight-threatening condition, and requires prompt management by an ophthalmologist.
2. Scleritis should be assumed to be a sign of a systemic disease.

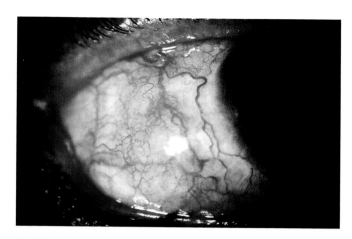

FIGURE 2.21 ■ Scleritis. A prominent generalized vascular injection is present. These vessels do not move when the overlying conjunctiva is moved with a cotton-tipped applicator. (Photo contributor: Thomas F. Mauger, MD.)

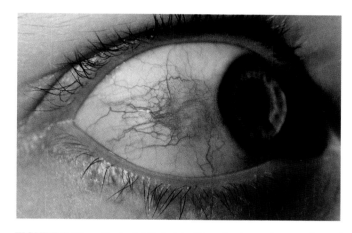

FIGURE 2.22 ■ Sectorial Scleritis. Deep-boring pain experienced by this patient distinguishes this segmental area of erythema from episcleritis. (Photo contributor: Kevin J. Knoop, MD, MS.)

Clinical Summary

Episcleritis is a common, benign inflammatory condition of the episclera. It most often affects young adults. Most cases are idiopathic, though up to a third may be associated with systemic conditions, and some cases may also be caused by exogenous irritants or inflammatory stimuli. Associated systemic disorders include gout, systemic lupus erythematosus, rheumatoid arthritis, inflammatory bowel disease, and herpes zoster. The symptoms, which include foreign body sensation, mild pain, photophobia, and lacrimation, are generally self-limited. Visual acuity is normal.

Emergency Department Treatment and Disposition

Generally the condition is mild and self-limited, but ophthalmology referral is advisable for confirmation and treatment. The main role of the emergency physician is to rule out more threatening causes of the red eye. Topical vasoconstrictors and oral nonsteroidal anti-inflammatory drugs may be helpful for symptoms. Resolution should be expected in 1 to 2 weeks. Any underlying systemic disorders should be diagnosed and treated.

Pearls

1. The differentiation of episcleritis from more threatening disorders such as scleritis is paramount.
2. The bulbar hyperemia of episcleritis is unilateral in two-thirds of cases, usually sectorial, on the eye, and blanches with topical 2.5% phenylephrine drops.
3. In episcleritis, dilated vessels in the superficial episcleral plexus will blanch with topical 2.5% phenylephrine.

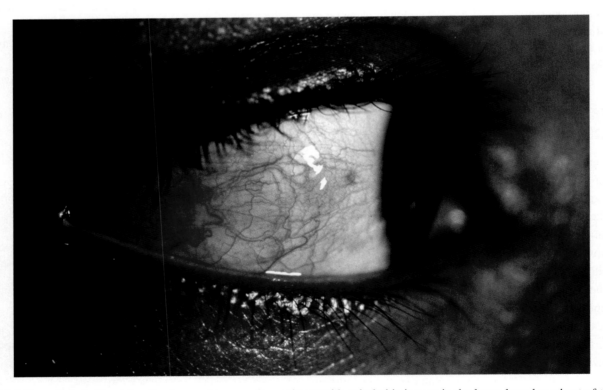

FIGURE 2.23 ■ Episcleritis. A localized area of hyperemia consistent with episcleritis is seen in the lower lateral quadrant of the eye. (Photo contributor: Robert Trieff, MD.)

Clinical Summary

Like other forms of glaucoma, acute angle closure glaucoma (ACG) is a disease process involving increased intraocular pressure (IOP) and damage to the retina and optic nerve. This condition; however, is unique in its acute presentation and ability to rapidly progress to vision loss. In ACG, the peripheral iris blocks outflow of aqueous humor from the anterior chamber into the canal of Schlemm. This is associated with papillary dilation. As a result, IOP rises rapidly from its normal value between 10 and 21 mm Hg to over 50 mm Hg. As IOP rises, it causes the cornea to become edematous. Patients with ACG complain of acute eye pain, redness, and decreased visual acuity, typically occurring after remaining in a darkened room, such as a theater. Nausea, vomiting, and headache are common complaints and may be the chief reason for the emergency department visit. Persons at increased risk of ACG include the elderly, due to increased volume of the lens and subsequent shallower anterior chamber and persons of Asian descent and hyperopes, due to an anatomically shallower anterior chamber. Examination findings include decreased visual acuity; a cloudy, steamy, or stippled-appearing cornea; conjunctival hyperemia with ciliary flush; a fixed, mid-dilated pupil; a shallow anterior chamber; and elevated IOP.

Emergency Department Treatment and Disposition

Treatment of ACG is aimed at quickly reducing IOP and opening the outflow track for the aqueous humor. First-line topical agents decrease aqueous humor production and include β-blockers (timolol, betaxolol, levobunolol), α-antagonists (brimonidine, apraclonidine), and prostaglandin analogues (latanoprost). Pilocarpine (1% or 2%), a topical miotic, is used only when IOP is below 40 to 50 mm Hg, as it will often be ineffective when the IOP is above this level. Pilocarpine is also ineffective when the attack is many hours old, because of ischemia of the iris. One drop every 5 minutes for 3 to 6 doses, then one drop hourly until the pressure has normalized, acts to open the outflow track. Additional adjunct agents include topical (dorzolamide) and systemic carbonic anhydrase inhibitors (acetazolamide) and osmotic diuretics (mannitol, glycerol, isosorbide). Corneal indentation may be used in situations where the IOP is 50 mm Hg or greater and first-line topical agents and pilocarpine are ineffective.

Indentation of the cornea displaces the aqueous to the peripheral anterior chamber, temporarily opening the angle. Corneal indentation is performed with topical anesthetics and any smooth instrument such as the Goldmann applanation prism. The prism is held with the fingers and firm pressure is applied for 30 seconds. This may successfully decrease the IOP and abort the attack; however, if the IOP has been long standing, however, it is more likely to be unsuccessful. Patients should also receive opiate analgesia as needed for pain. The definitive treatment of ACG is by laser iridotomy or incisional peripheral iridectomy by an ophthalmologist. Emergent ophthalmologic consultation is advised, as ACG is a true ophthalmologic emergency.

Pearls

1. Patients with acute, atraumatic eye pain or decreased visual acuity should have their IOP checked, to rule out ACG. Tactile tonometry, using the examiner's fingers to ballot the globe, can easily detect markedly elevated IOP.
2. IOP should be checked in at risk patients with headache and vomiting, as ACG is a possible cause.
3. The unaffected eye also will have a shallow anterior chamber.
4. ACG may be precipitated iatrogenically by mydriatic/cycloplegic agents in susceptible individuals.
5. Pilocarpine will often be ineffective with severe or prolonged elevated IOP.

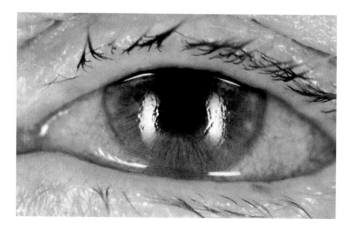

FIGURE 2.24 ■ Acute Angle Closure Glaucoma. The cornea is edematous, manifest by the indistinctness of the iris markings and the irregular corneal light reflex. Conjunctival hyperemia is also present. (Photo contributor: Kevin J. Knoop, MD, MS.)

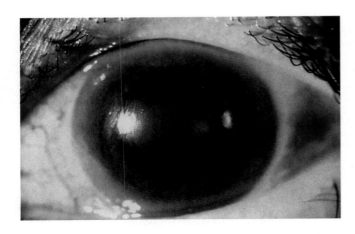

FIGURE 2.25 ▪ Acute Angle Closure Glaucoma. Note the cloudy or "steamy" appearance of the cornea and the midposition pupil. Conjunctival hyperemia is not as evident. (Photo contributor: Gary Tanner, MD.)

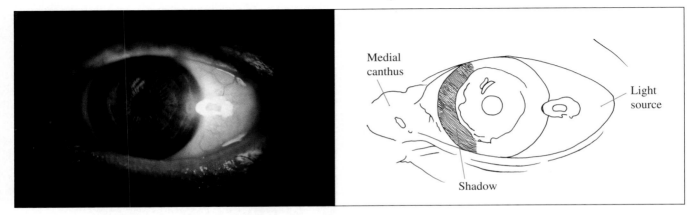

FIGURE 2.26 ▪ Penlight Test. A penlight, held laterally and directed nasally, projects a shadow on the nasal side of an iris with a shallow anterior chamber. This patient presented with acute angle closure glaucoma. (Photo contributor: Alan B. Storrow, MD.)

Clinical Summary

Anterior uveitis, or iritis, is an inflammation of the anterior portions of the uvea (iris, ciliary body, and choroid). It is often idiopathic, but approximately half of cases are associated with systemic diseases. These include inflammatory disorders (juvenile rheumatoid arthritis, rheumatoid arthritis, sarcoidosis, Behçet disease, Sjögren syndrome), conditions associated with HLA-B27 (ankylosing spondylitis, inflammatory bowel disease, Reiter syndrome), and infectious diseases (tuberculosis, toxoplasmosis, herpes simplex, herpes zoster, cytomegalovirus, syphilis, AIDS, Lyme disease).

Patients report pain, tearing, photophobia, and may have decreased visual acuity. While the eyelids appear normal, inspection may reveal hyperemia of the conjunctiva and the perilimbal vessels ("ciliary flush"). The pupil is often miotic and may be distorted due to the formation of synechiae. Slit-lamp examination may reveal iris nodules, hypopyon, cells, or flare. In addition, inflammatory cells may clump and adhere to the corneal endothelium. These keratic precipitates appear either as fine gray-white deposits, or larger, flat, greasy-looking areas ("mutton fat"). IOP may be decreased due to compromised aqueous production, or increased due to inflammatory debris clogging the outflow tract.

Emergency Department Treatment and Disposition

A thorough history and physical examination may suggest a systemic cause and should drive further workup. Prompt ophthalmologic referral is the key so that topical cycloplegics and steroids (after infection is ruled out) can be administered and titrated to symptoms.

Pearls

1. Key diagnostic features of anterior uveitis are a miotic pupil, ciliary flush, and the finding of cells and flare in the anterior chamber.
2. Consider consensual response to light causing photophobia as pathognomonic for iritis.
3. The presence of anterior uveitis requires a search for associated systemic illness.
4. Topical analgesics do not significantly ameliorate the pain of anterior uveitis.

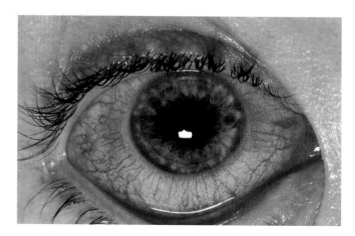

FIGURE 2.27 ■ Anterior Uveitis. Marked conjunctival injection and perilimbal hyperemia ("ciliary flush") are seen in this patient with recurrent iritis. (Photo contributor: Frank Birinyi, MD.)

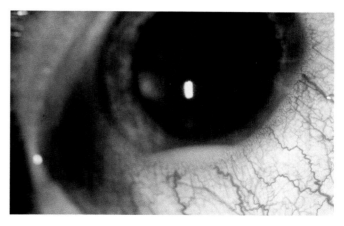

FIGURE 2.28 ■ Hypopyon. A thin layering of white blood cells is present in the inferior anterior chamber. (Used with permission from Spalton DJ, Hitchings RA, Hunter PA (eds). *Atlas of Clinical Ophthalmology*. 2nd ed. London, UK: Mosby-Wolfe Limited; 1994.)

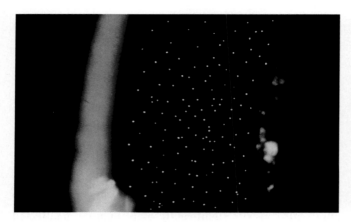

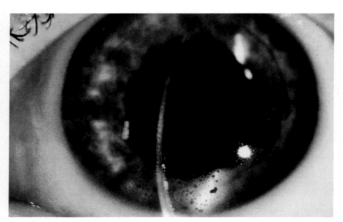

FIGURE 2.29 ■ Anterior Chamber Cells. Cells in the anterior chamber are a sign of inflammation or bleeding and appear similar to particles of dust in a sunbeam. They are best seen with a narrow slit-lamp beam directed obliquely across the anterior chamber. (Used with permission from Spalton DJ, Hitchings RA, Hunter PA (eds). *Atlas of Clinical Ophthalmology*. 2nd ed. London, UK: Mosby-Wolfe Limited; 1994.)

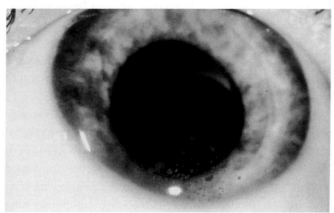

FIGURE 2.31 ■ Keratic Precipitates. Deposits of cells on the *endothelial* layer of the cornea are seen in these photographs. (Used with permission from Spalton DJ, Hitchings RA, Hunter PA (eds). *Atlas of Clinical Ophthalmology*. 2nd ed. London, UK: Mosby-Wolfe Limited; 1994.)

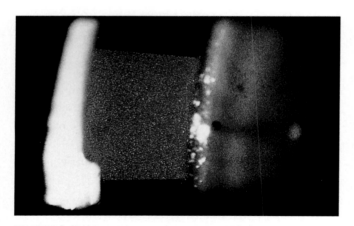

FIGURE 2.30 ■ Anterior Chamber Flare. Flare in the anterior chamber represents an elevated concentration of plasma proteins from inflamed, leaking intraocular blood vessels. Flare seen in a slit-lamp beam appears similar to a car headlight cutting through the fog. (Used with permission from Spalton DJ, Hitchings RA, Hunter PA (eds). *Atlas of Clinical Ophthalmology*. London, UK: Mosby-Wolfe Limited; 1984.)

Clinical Summary

Anisocoria is a disparity of pupil size. Five to twenty percent of people have physiologic anisocoria, usually of less than 2 mm. This asymmetry is preserved in both light and dark conditions, and no other ocular abnormalities are present.

If pathologic anisocoria is suspected, examine pupil size in both light and dark to determine which eye is affected; anisocoria increases in the direction of action of the paretic iris muscle. A weakened iris sphincter muscle is accentuated by bright light. Because constriction is impaired, the abnormal pupil will appear much bigger. Conversely, if the iris dilator muscle is paretic, the anisocoria will be accentuated in darkness, with an unusually small pupil.

In the setting of trauma, severe headache, or following intracranial surgery, a dilated, nonreactive pupil with third-nerve palsy represents an expanding supratentorial mass with tentorial herniation.

An Adie pupil is dilated because postganglionic nerve supply to the iris sphincter is compromised, often in a segmental manner that can be visualized on slit-lamp microscopy. Patients may note difficulty in focusing, as well as the dilated pupil; most often these are idiopathic and benign, but consider orbital trauma, infection, diabetes, autonomic neuropathies, and Guillain-Barré syndrome. Although an Adie pupil is initially dilated, it may become miotic over time.

A pupil enlarged by atropine (or contaminated by a scopolamine patch) will not react to light, while sympathomimetics eye drops such as phenylephrine result in a dilated pupil that still has some response to light.

Ocular trauma can tear the iris sphincter, and examination may show a frankly torn iris, an irregularly shaped pupil, hyphema, or lens dislocation.

An abnormally small pupil may be secondary to Horner syndrome, chronic Adie pupil, iritis, and eye drops. Ocular trauma can cause spasm of the papillary sphincter, followed by mydriasis.

Emergency Department Treatment and Disposition

The evaluation of anisocoria in the emergency department is dependent on the clinical presentation. A patient with acute onset of a third-nerve palsy and associated headache or trauma should be aggressively evaluated and treated as a neurosurgical emergency. Pilocarpine may be helpful to differentiate pharmacologic pupil dilation from other causes of an abnormally dilated pupil, such as Adie pupil and third-nerve palsy. With low concentrations of pilocarpine (0.125%), an Adie pupil will constrict significantly more than the unaffected pupil because of denervation supersensitivity. With higher concentrations (1%), a pupil will constrict even if there is third-nerve palsy. If a thorough history and physical examination fails to reveal a concerning underlying pathology, outpatient referral is appropriate.

Pearls

1. An old photograph, ID badge, or driver's license can reveal a prior anisocoria.
2. Some brands of eye makeup contain belladonna alkaloids, which can cause mydriasis.
3. A pupil that fails to constrict with 1% pilocarpine localizes the etiology to the iris sphincter muscle itself. In this situation, the most likely diagnosis is the use of topical anticholinergic mydriatics.
4. In physiologic or normal anisocoria, the disparity in pupil size is the same in light as in dark.

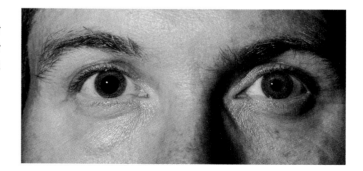

FIGURE 2.32 ■ Posttraumatic Anisocoria. Marked chronic anisocoria secondary to prior trauma. (Photo contributor: Kevin J. Knoop, MD, MS.)

Clinical Summary

Varicella zoster virus lying dormant within the trigeminal ganglion can reactivate and spread through the ophthalmic division of the trigeminal nerve. While almost any ophthalmic abnormality can occur as a result, grouped vesicles in a dermatomal distribution are a classic finding. Skin lesions on the tip of the nose (Hutchinson sign) can indicate risk of ocular involvement, as this area is innervated by the nasociliary branch of the ophthalmic division of cranial nerve V.

The most common corneal lesion is punctate epithelial keratitis, in which the cornea has a ground-glass appearance because of stromal edema. Pseudodendrites, formed by the deposition of mucus, are usually peripherally located and stain poorly with fluorescein. Pseudodendrites lack rounded terminal bulbs, are broader, and more plaque-like than the true dendrites of herpes simplex infection. While herpes simplex dendritic lesions are full-thickness, pseudodendrites can be wiped from the cornea to uncover a layer of intact epithelium.

A number or late-term sequelae may follow acute disease. Single or multiple anterior stromal infiltrates can appear 2 or 3 weeks after acute disease and are likely due to an immune response to viral antigen diffusing into the anterior stroma. Corneal anesthesia or hypoesthesia is a frequent complication of herpes zoster keratitis. While some 60% of patients will recover essentially normal sensitivity within 2 to 3 months, about a quarter suffer permanent anesthesia. Anterior uveitis may develop early, or follow years after the acute disease.

Emergency Department Treatment and Disposition

In patients with epithelial defects, topical broad-spectrum antibiotics should be administered to prevent secondary infection. Oral antiviral agents have particular benefit if started within the first 3 days of disease. Artificial tears and ointment may be soothing, but both nonsteroidal anti-inflammatory drugs and narcotic analgesics may be needed. An ophthalmology consult is appropriate.

Pearls

1. The severity of the cutaneous disease does not necessarily correlate with the severity of the ocular disease.
2. The prognosis is good, and recurrences—unlike those for herpes simplex keratitis–are rare.

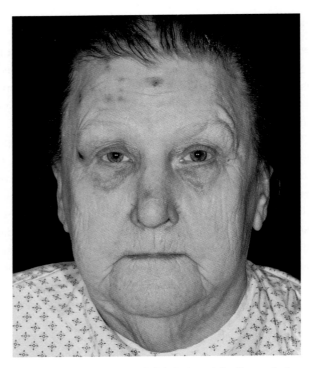

FIGURE 2.33 ■ Herpes Zoster Ophthalmicus. A healing vesicular rash in the distribution of the ophthalmic division (V1) of the trigeminal nerve is present in this 72-year-old diabetic patient. The presence of the lesion near the tip of the nose (Hutchinson sign) increases the risk of ocular involvement. (Photo contributor: Frank Birinyi, MD.)

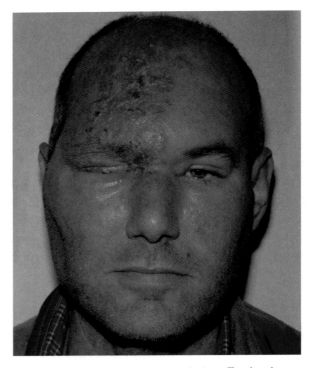

FIGURE 2.34 ■ Herpes Zoster Ophthalmicus. Eye involvement is present in this patient with moderate HZV in the V1 distribution. (Photo contributor: Lawrence B. Stack, MD.)

Clinical Summary

Herpes simplex virus (HSV) infection of the eye can result in varying presentations, from conjunctivitis to blindness. Neonatal infection, from passage through the birth canal, should be treated aggressively, and potentially life-threatening systemic disease should be ruled out.

Three to nine days after inoculation, primary ocular herpes may present as a vesicular blepharitis, conjunctivitis, or keratoconjunctivitis with significant periorbital skin involvement. Patients report pain, irritation, foreign-body sensation, redness, photophobia, tearing, and, occasionally, decreased visual acuity. Examination findings include follicles and preauricular adenopathy. Initially the keratitis is diffuse and punctate, but after 24 hours, fluorescein stain reveals serpiginous ulcers without clear-cut branching, or multiple diffuse microdendritic epithelial defects. True dendritic ulcers are rare in primary disease.

Recurrent disease is a much more common presentation. Triggered by immunosuppression, fever, ultraviolet light exposure, trauma, systemic illness, stress, or menstruation, recurrences often involve the cornea, and may also involve keratoconjunctivitis, blepharitis, or iritis. Blepharitis in recurrent disease consists of more focal vesicular clusters, with less skin involvement than primary infection. Corneal involvement may start as punctate lesions before progressing into characteristic dendritic keratitis. The branches of dendritic ulcers end in bead-like extensions called terminal bulbs, best seen with rose Bengal stain, which stains both the epithelial defect and the infected cells surrounding it. Fluorescein reveals the corneal defect with punctate uptake in surrounding damaged epithelium; particularly if steroids have been incorrectly prescribed, fluorescein may reveal geographic ulcerations.

Eighty percent of herpes simplex keratitis cases feature decreased or absent corneal sensation in the area of the dendrite or geographic ulceration. Protracted or repeated episodes of HSV keratitis can scar the cornea and permanently compromise vision. In the worst cases, structural compromise of the cornea leads to melting and perforation.

Emergency Department Treatment and Disposition

Because neonatal ocular herpes infections are so frequently associated with potentially lethal neurologic or systemic involvement, an emergent pediatric or infectious disease consultation is essential. Intravenous acyclovir should be started in the emergency department. Ocular involvement is treated with topical antivirals.

Adult patients with primary ocular herpes need both symptom control and antimicrobials. Blepharitis or periocular dermatitis is relieved by twice daily warm wet soaks. Meticulous hygiene will help prevent infecting the other eye, as will prophylactic topical antivirals, which should continue until skin lesions scab and dry. Corneal involvement requires 2 to 3 weeks of topical antivirals with concomitant topical antibiotics to prevent secondary bacterial infection.

While recurrent disease results in less severe periorbital lesions, the globe is at much higher risk, and an ophthalmologist should be involved early. Treat involved skin with topical antivirals five to six times a day until the lesions have scabbed. While unproven, oral acyclovir five times a day for 5 days may help if started at the first sign of recurrence. Corneal involvement is treated with frequent topical antivirals, such as 1% trifluorothymidine nine times a day for 2 or 3 weeks. Administer topical prophylactic antibiotics until the corneal defect is healed.

Pearls

1. The diagnosis of acute neonatal ocular HSV should be entertained in any infant with nonpurulent conjunctivitis or keratitis.
2. HSV is a common cause of corneal ulceration and the most common infectious cause of corneal blindness in the western hemisphere.
3. In primary infection and early recurrent HSV, fluorescein may show only punctate keratitis. True dendrites are marked by terminal bulbs, and are not seen in herpes zoster.
4. Because of increasing corneal hypoesthesia, recurrent attacks may be less painful than prior episodes.

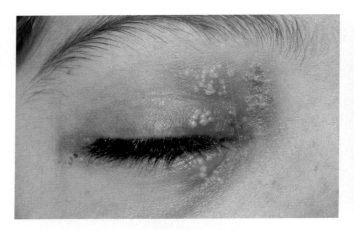

FIGURE 2.35 ■ Ocular Herpes Simplex. This 18-year-old has a history of ocular herpes simplex since childhood. Grouped vesicles on an erythematous base with periorbital erthythema are seen. Honey-colored crusts suggest secondary impetigo. (Photo contributor: Lawrence B. Stack, MD.)

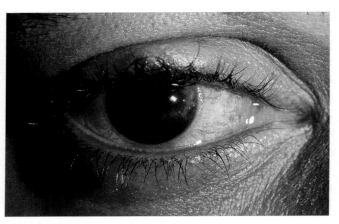

FIGURE 2.37 ■ Herpes Simplex Keratitis. A large dendritic lesion after fluorescein staining. The patient had been diagnosed with "pink eye" in a prior visit. (Photo contributor: Kevin J. Knoop, MD, MS.)

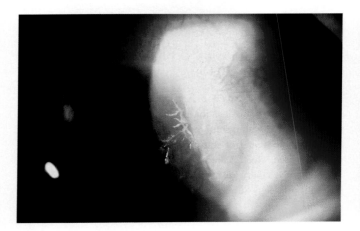

FIGURE 2.36 ■ Herpes Simplex Keratitis. A slit-lamp view of unstained dendritic lesions. (Photo contributor: Lawrence B. Stack, MD.)

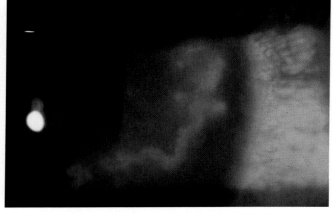

FIGURE 2.38 ■ Herpes Simplex Keratitis. A magnified view via slit-lamp biomicroscopy shows the classic terminal bulbs pathognomonic for ocular HSV infection. (Photo contributor: Department of Ophthalmology, Naval Medical Center, Portsmouth, VA.)

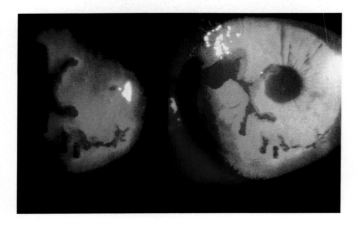

FIGURE 2.39 ■ Herpes Simplex Keratitis. Fluorescein (*left*) and rose Bengal (*right*) stains demonstrate characteristic dendritic patterns. Whereas fluorescein staining is used to detect epithelial defects, rose Bengal staining additionally demonstrates degenerating or dead epithelial cells and is particularly good for demonstrating the club-shaped terminal bulbs at the end of each branch. (Used with permission from the American Academy of Ophthalmology. *External Disease and Cornea: A Multimedia Collection.* San Francisco; 1994.)

Clinical Summary

A number of infections and inflammatory conditions can ulcerate the cornea. Common bacterial causes include *Staphylococcus, Streptococcus,* and *Pseudomonas.* Herpes simplex virus can also ulcerate the cornea, as can Acanthamoeba, a ubiquitous protozoan. Because contacts lens and contaminated solutions can permit microbial invasion, lens wear should raise clinical suspicion for a serious bacterial or protozoan infection. Fungal infections are rare but possible when either vegetable matter (such as a tree branch) contacts the eye, in chronic corneal conditions, or steroids are used.

Patient with corneal ulcers report pain, photophobia, decreased vision, discharge, and a foreign-body sensation. The ulcer appears as a corneal stromal infiltrate associated with conjunctival hyperemia, ciliary flush, a miotic pupil, and chemosis, along with lid edema and erythema. Slit-lamp microscopy reveals fluorescein uptake over the epithelial defect. The anterior chamber may have cells and flare, keratic precipitates, or frank hypopyon.

Emergency Department Treatment and Disposition

Corneal ulcers represent a sight-threatening bacterial infection until proven otherwise. Immediate ophthalmology consultation is essential. Stains and cultures should be taken as soon as possible to allow the expeditious administration of topical antibiotics. Intensive topical treatment is the most effective way to treat corneal infections. While single-agent fluoroquinolone therapy may suffice for mild cases of infectious keratitis, dual therapy with fortified cephalosporins or vancomycin combined with an aminoglycoside may be required, with administration intervals starting as frequent as every half hour. Systemic antibiotics are needed only when invasion of the sclera is expected (*Pseudomonas*), or if there is a high risk of concurrent systemic disease (*Neisseria, Haemophilus*). Cycloplegics may alleviate symptoms if iritis is present; steroids and eye-patching are contraindicated. All lens wearers must discontinue lens wear, discard opened lens and solutions, and sterilize contact lens equipment.

Pearls

1. *Pseudomonas* is capable of destroying the cornea within 6 to 12 hours. Suspect *Pseudomonas* if there is aggressive progression, with thick yellow-green or blue-green mucopurulent exudate, and ground-glass edema surrounding the ulcer.

2. Contact lens wears, and particularly those wearing them underwater, are at risk for *Acanthamoeba* infection. Typically, these patients have pain out-of-proportion to findings on examination.

3. Infectious ulcers tend to develop centrally, away from the vascular supply and immune system of the limbus.

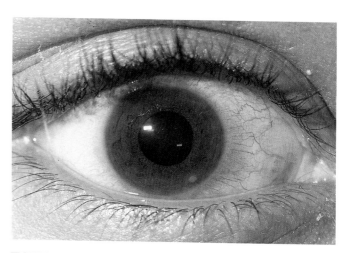

FIGURE 2.40 ■ Corneal Ulcer. An elliptical ulcer at 5 o'clock near the periphery is seen. This location is atypical for a bacterial ulcer. The patient presented with painful red eyes and normal uncorrected vision, but was a new wearer of soft contact lenses. Bilateral corneal ulcers were diagnosed, which cleared after treatment with topical ciprofloxacin. The impressive ciliary flush is pathognomonic for corneal (versus conjunctival) pathology. (Photo contributor: Kevin J. Knoop, MD, MS.)

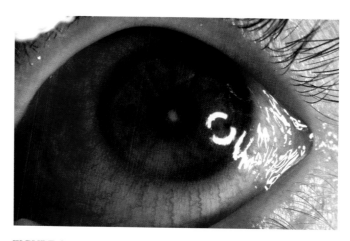

FIGURE 2.41 ■ Corneal Ulcer. A white circular corneal infiltrate is seen at 12 o'clock directly in the central visual access. This area of the cornea is typical for ulcers due to soft contact lens use. (Photo contributor: Kevin J. Knoop, MD, MS.)

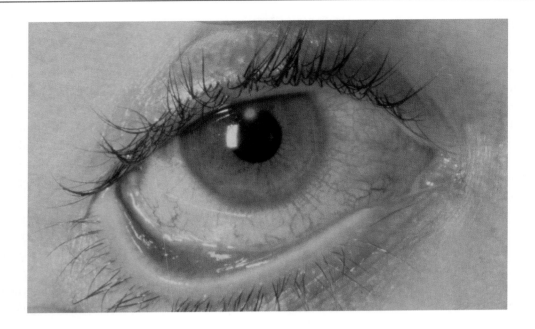

FIGURE 2.42 ■ Corneal Ulcer. A small circular corneal infiltrate is seen adjacent to the white flash photography reflection. Diffuse conjunctival hyperemia with ciliary flush is present. (Photo contributor: Lawrence B. Stack, MD.)

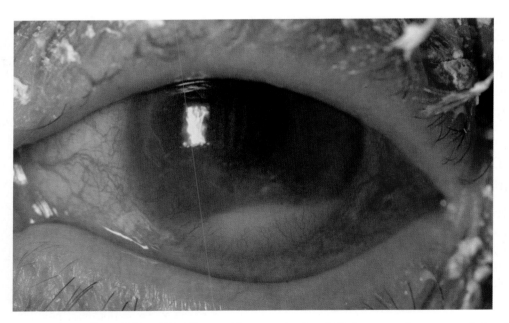

FIGURE 2.43 ■ Hypopyon due to Corneal Ulcer. This 78-year-old woman developed this hypopyon from a corneal ulcer (seen just inferior to the visual axis) that developed from a corneal abrasion. Corneal neovascularization and intense limbic injection is seen. (Photo contributor: Lawrence B. Stack, MD.)

Clinical Summary

In the normal eye, a light stimulus is transmitted to both pupils by bilateral output, resulting in direct and consensual pupil contraction. When pathology exists that prevents the detection of this stimulus, pupil contraction is decreased. However, when the contralateral healthy eye is stimulated with light, the abnormal pupil's consensual response is normal, since the afferent light stimulus is normal. In this situation, the diseased eye is said to demonstrate an afferent pupillary defect (APD), also called a Marcus Gunn pupil.

The best examination technique for an APD is the swinging flashlight test. In a darkened room, with the patient looking at an object across the room (to avoid the normal papillary constriction associated with accommodation), a flashlight is directed onto one pupil and then the other. In a normal examination, the first eye will trigger prompt bilateral constriction, followed by slight "release" dilation. During the brief interval between stimulation of the first and second eyes, both pupils dilate enough that by the time the contralateral eye is illuminated, reflex constriction occurs. With a diseased second eye, however, light perception is muted compared to the normal eye, and the midbrain therefore sets pupil size to be larger.

Although sensitive, the swinging flashlight test is not specific since the pathology may be anywhere in the visual pathway from the retina to the midbrain. An APD is best seen in conditions involving the optic nerve, such as ischemic optic neuropathy, optic neuritis, and glaucoma.

Emergency Department Treatment and Disposition

Because an APD is nonspecific, a thorough ocular and neurologic examination may fail to reveal a cause. In the absence of gross ocular or neurologic disease, a clinically stable patient may be discharged from the emergency department with ophthalmology follow-up.

Pearls

1. Dim room illumination may be helpful in performing the swinging flashlight test. The patient should focus on an object 15 ft away to avoid the pupillary constriction normally seen with accommodation.

2. The normal pupillary response to bright light is an initial constriction followed by a small amount of dilation. In performing the swinging flashlight test, it is important to assess the initial reaction. In the Marcus Gunn pupil, this initial reaction is dilation.

3. A "subjective" APD can be seen in mild cases of optic neuritis. Patients report decreased light perception and may have slightly decreased visual acuity when no objective APD is present.

4. If an eye is damaged, paralyzed, or anisocoria is present, an APD can still be assessed by observing pupillary response in the normal eye as light is shined alternately in each eye. Because the pathologic eye perceives less light, the normal pupil will have a decreased consensual response, and dilate.

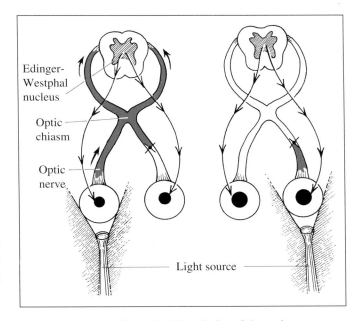

FIGURE 2.44 ■ Afferent Pupillary Defect. Schematic representation of an afferent pupillary defect (APD) due to neurologic lesion in the anterior visual pathway.

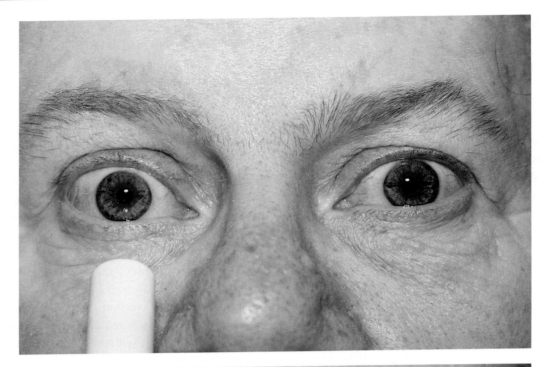

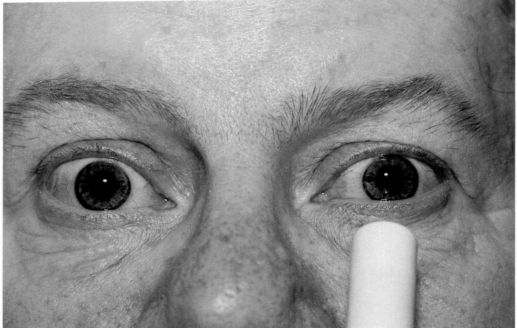

FIGURE 2.45 ■ Marcus Gunn Pupil. These photographs demonstrate an afferent pupillary defect of the left pupil. When the light shines in the affected left eye, the pupils are less constricted than when the light shines in the right eye. Thus, when the light is swung from the right pupil to the left, the pupils appear to dilate. The anisocoria here is subtle. (Photo contributor: Frank Birinyi, MD.)

Clinical Summary

Horner syndrome is the loss of ocular sympathetic innervation. This pathway begins in the hypothalamus, and runs down through the brainstem and spinal cord to the apex of the chest and back up along the carotid sheath through the cavernous sinus to the orbit. Compromise of sympathetic innervation leads to the clinical triad of miosis, ptosis, and facial anhidrosis.

Pupillary dilation lag is specific to Horner syndrome, resulting from weakened dilation with a normal sphincter. This anisocoria is maximal after about 5 seconds, with resolution after 10 to 20 seconds, as the intact sphincter muscles slowly relaxes.

Emergency Department Treatment and Disposition

Horner syndrome is often caused by vascular disease, trauma, or tumor; associated signs and symptoms that help to localize the lesion. Cranial nerve abnormalities suggest brainstem or intracavernous pathology. Immobilize and image trauma patients with Horner syndrome. Because Horner syndrome is a primary presentation for malignancy, consider a chest x-ray in patients with risk factors. Neck pain in association with Horner syndrome raises the possibility of carotid artery dissection.

Pearls

1. Upper eyelid ptosis and high-riding lower eyelid position ("reverse ptosis") causes a narrowed palpebral fissure in Horner syndrome. Loss of sympathetic innervation to Müller muscle of the upper eyelid, and the inferior tarsal muscle of the lower eyelid, causes this effect.
2. The ptosis of Horner syndrome is moderate and never complete.
3. Carotid artery dissection should be entertained in the patient with neck pain and an ipsilateral Horner syndrome.
4. Cluster headaches, with autonomic sympathetic system dysfunction, are capable of producing an ipsilateral Horner syndrome.

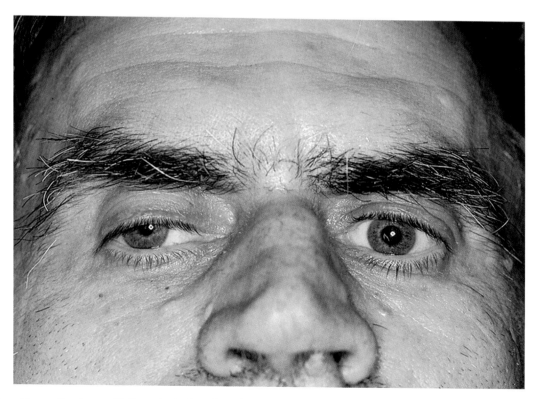

FIGURE 2.46 ■ Horner Syndrome. Unilateral miosis and ptosis are seen in this patient with Horner syndrome and sarcoma metastatic to the spine. (Photo contributor: Frank Birinyi, MD.)

Clinical Features

The abducens nerve innervates the lateral rectus muscle and is the most common single-muscle palsy, causing loss of abduction and horizontal diplopia. Other associated findings depend on the location of the lesion. This can involve brainstem structures, resulting in hemiparesis; be a part of Wernicke encephalopathy; or result from trauma. The sixth nerve's length makes it vulnerable to stretching from compression or movement of the brainstem secondary to elevated intracranial pressure, trauma, neurosurgical manipulation, and cervical traction. While aneurysmal compression is uncommon, any meningeal process (infectious, inflammatory, or neoplastic) can compromise sixth nerve function.

Cavernous sinus pathology is suggested by involvement of other structures that course through the sinus: the internal carotid artery, the venous drainage of the eye and orbit, the trochlear and oculomotor nerves, the first division of the trigeminal nerve, and the ocular sympathetic nerves. Microvascular changes secondary to diabetes, hypertension, giant cell arteritis, or arteriosclerosis can also compromise function. In children, transient sixth-nerve palsy may follow a virus infection.

Emergency Department Treatment and Disposition

Associated signs and symptoms guide emergency department workup. If involvement of the brainstem or cavernous sinus is suspected, it should be imaged with CT or MRI. Pathology localizing to the subarachnoid space should trigger CT scanning and subsequent spinal tap. Children with antecedent viral illness and normal CT scan may be discharged provided that close follow-up is arranged. In the elderly, an isolated sixth-nerve palsy is likely ischemic, transient, and not indicative of underlying neurologic disease. After screening for glucose and erythrocyte sedimentation rate (for diabetes and giant cell arteritis), these patients may get an out-patient workup.

Treatment is supportive. If diplopia is particularly bothersome, the affected eye may be patched.

Pearls

1. Isolated sixth-nerve palsy is unlikely to be due to an aneurysm.

2. Sixth-nerve palsy with an ipsilateral Horner syndrome is usually localized to the cavernous sinus, since sympathetic fibers, as they traverse from the internal carotid artery to the oculomotor nerve, may briefly accompany the abducens nerve.

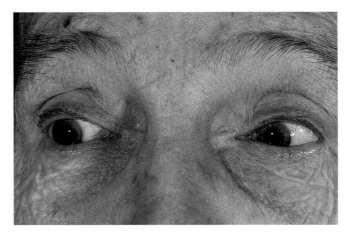

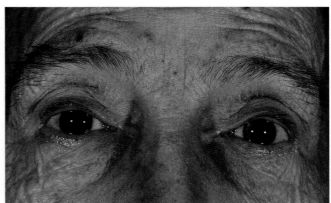

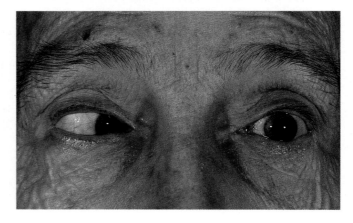

FIGURE 2.47 ■ Sixth-Nerve Palsy. Loss of abduction of the left eye is seen in lateral gaze, demonstrating an isolated sixth-nerve palsy. (Photo contributor: Frank Birinyi, MD.)

Clinical Summary

The third cranial nerve controls all extraocular muscles (except the lateral rectus and superior oblique), and the levator palpebrae muscle. It also supplies parasympathetic input to the pupillary constrictor and ciliary muscles. Thus symptoms of third-nerve palsy include double vision, droopy lid, an enlarged pupil, and blurred vision at near range. On examination, the pupil is dilated and nonreactive, with limited extraocular movements and ptosis. The affected pupil deviates laterally (exotropia) because the lateral rectus muscle is now unopposed.

Third-nerve palsy can result from a lesion anywhere along its anatomic path, which begins in the brainstem nucleus, continues within the subarachnoid space, traverses the cavernous sinus, and terminates within the orbit. Contralateral hemiplegia suggests brainstem involvement. In cases of isolated oculomotor palsy, the subarachnoid space is the most likely site of pathology. The differential includes a posterior communicating artery aneurysm, uncal herniation, compressive neoplasms, inflammatory lesions, or trauma.

Causes for third-nerve palsy within the cavernous sinus include neoplasms, carotid artery aneurysm, cavernous sinus thrombosis, and carotid-cavernous fistula. Orbital lesions causing third-nerve palsies may be due to inflammation, trauma, neoplasms, and mucoceles. In addition, isolated third-nerve palsy is common with diabetic or hypertensive disease, likely due to microvascular ischemia. In this situation, the palsy rarely affects the pupil, and may be extremely painful.

Emergency Department Treatment and Disposition

Careful documentation of associated signs and symptoms will help in locating the specific area of third-nerve compromise. In patients with brainstem involvement, CT or MRI is indicated. Consider CT and lumbar puncture when fever, headache, altered consciousness, or next stiffness is present.

If cavernous sinus involvement is suspected, MRI with gadolinium is the study of choice. For orbital pathology, CT scanning is recommended. A sudden onset of a third-nerve palsy accompanied by thunderclap headache, stiff neck, and a depressed level of consciousness is a neurosurgical emergency, even with papillary sparing. Emergent neuroimaging is needed to rule out an aneurysm with uncal herniation. Similarly, patients with head trauma with an oculomotor palsy should be worked up expeditiously, while efforts to reduce intracranial pressure are initiated.

Vasculopathic patients over 50 who present with isolated pupil-sparing third-nerve palsies, felt to be secondary to an ischemic neuropathy, should have a blood pressure and glucose check. They can be discharged from the emergency department with close follow-up for pupillary involvement, and strict return precautions.

Pearls

1. A third-nerve palsy can result from pathology anywhere along its anatomic pathway, beginning with the brainstem, continuing within the subarachnoid space, traversing the cavernous sinus, and terminating within the orbit itself.

2. Patients with the abrupt onset of "thunderclap" headache and third-nerve palsy require immediate neurosurgical evaluation for an aneurysm. (Posterior communicating artery is a common cause.)

3. In patients over 50 years of age with pupil-sparing third-nerve palsies, the etiology is usually hypertensive or diabetic vascular disease.

4. In the patient who presents with diplopia and possible third-nerve palsy, the emergency department physician should confirm the binocularity of the diplopia. Monocular diplopia is optical in origin.

5. Eighty percent of carotid-cavernous fistulas result from trauma, and may present weeks after minor mechanisms. Findings include an ocular bruit, pain, pulsatile exophthalmos, and chemosis.

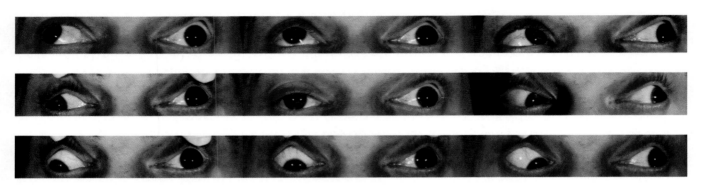

FIGURE 2.48 ▪ Third-Nerve Palsy. This composite shows the classic defects of a third cranial nerve palsy in all fields of gaze. The pupil is dilated. Conjugate eye movement is present in only one position, when the affected eye gazes laterally to the affected side (intact lateral rectus). When gaze is directly ahead, exotropia is seen secondary to the unopposed lateral rectus muscle of the affected side. (Photo contributor: Frank Birinyi, MD.)

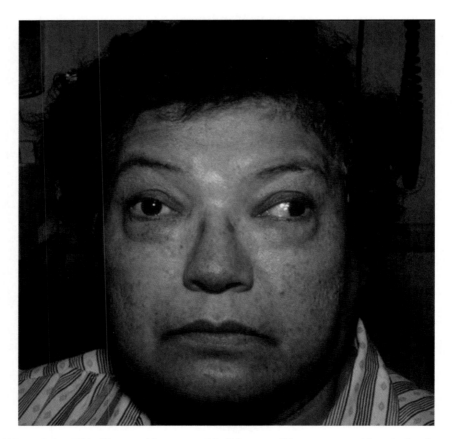

FIGURE 2.49 ▪ Third-Nerve Palsy. This 60-year-old woman with diabetes mellitus presents with an isolated cranial nerve III palsy due to diabetic mononeuropathy. She is currently attempting to look leftward. Her symptoms began as an isolated pain above her right orbit 10 days prior at which time her double vision with leftward gaze began. (Photo contributor: Lawrence B. Stack, MD.)

Chapter 3

FUNDUSCOPIC FINDINGS

David Effron
Beverly C. Forcier
Richard E. Wyszynski

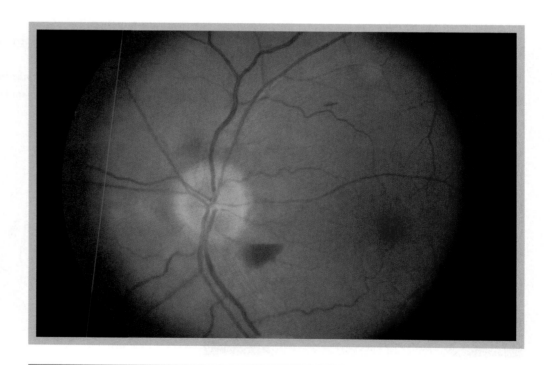

Clinical Summary

Disk

The disk is pale pink, approximately 1.5 mm in diameter, with sharp, flat margins. The physiologic cup is located within the disk and usually measures less than six-tenths the disk diameter. The cups should be approximately equal in both eyes.

Vessels

The central retinal artery and central retinal vein travel within the optic nerve, branching near the surface into the inferior and superior branches of arterioles and venules, respectively. Normally the walls of the vessels are not visible; the column of blood within the walls is visualized. The venules are seen as branching, dark red lines. The arterioles are seen as bright red branching lines, approximately two-thirds or three-fourths the diameter of the venules.

Macula

This is an area of the retina located temporal to the disk; it is void of visible vessels. The fovea is an area of depression approximately 1.5 mm in diameter (similar to the optic disk) in the center of the macula. The foveola is a tiny pit located in the center of the fovea. These areas correspond to central vision.

Background

The background fundus is red; there is some variation in the color, depending on the amount of individual pigmentation and the visibility of the choroidal vessels beneath the retina.

Pearls

1. Fundal examination should be an integral part of any eye examination.
2. The cup/disk ratio is slightly larger in the African American population.
3. The normal fundus should be void of any hemorrhages, exudates, or tortuous vasculature.

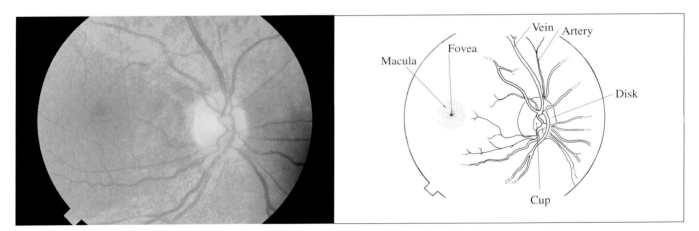

FIGURE 3.1 ■ Normal Fundus. The disk has sharp margins and is normal in color, with a small central cup. Arterioles and venules have normal color, sheen, and course. Background is in normal color. The macula is enclosed by arching temporal vessels. The fovea is located by a central pit. (Photo contributor: Beverly C. Forcier, MD.)

Clinical Summary

Age-related macular degeneration increases in incidence with each decade over 50 and is evidenced by accumulation of either hard drusen (small, discrete, round, punctate nodules), or soft drusen (larger, pale yellow or gray, without discrete margins that may be confluent). Most patients with drusen have good vision, although there may be decreased visual acuity and distortion of vision. There may be associated pigmentary changes and atrophy of the retina. Vision may slowly deteriorate if atrophy occurs.

Patients with early or late degenerative changes of the macula are at risk of developing choroidal neovascularization (CNV), which is associated with distortion of vision, blind spots, and decreased visual acuity. Macular appearance may show dirty gray lesions, hemorrhage, retinal elevation, and exudation.

Emergency Department Treatment and Disposition

Patients with drusen need ophthalmologic evaluation every 6 to 12 months or sooner if visual distortion or decreasing visual acuity develops. If a patient complains of deterioration of visual acuity or image distortion; prompt ophthalmic evaluation is warranted.

Pearls

1. Age-related macular degeneration is the leading cause of blindness in the United States in patients above 65 years of age.
2. Patient may have normal peripheral vision.
3. Untreated CNV can lead to visual loss within a few days.
4. Patients frequently complain of distortion with CNV.

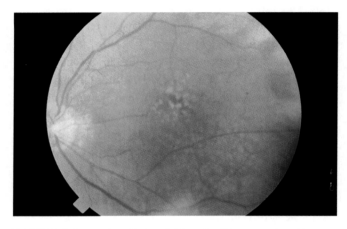

FIGURE 3.3 ■ Age-Related Macular Degeneration, Drusen. Drusen are clustered in the center of the macula. (Photo contributor: Richard E. Wyszynski, MD.)

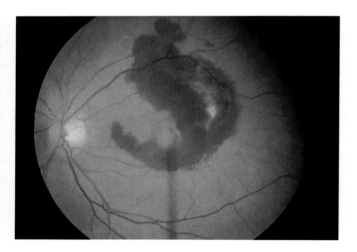

FIGURE 3.2 ■ Age-Related Macular Degeneration, Drusen. Typical macular drusen and retinal pigment epithelial (RPE) atrophy (scalloped pigment loss) in age-related macular degeneration. (Photo contributor: Richard E. Wyszynski, MD.)

FIGURE 3.4 ■ Age-Related Macular Degeneration. Hemorrhage seen beneath the retina in association with subretinal neovascularization. Note the retinal vessels are superficial to the hemorrhage, which lies just beneath the retina. (Photo contributor: Richard E. Wyszynski, MD.)

Clinical Summary

Hard exudates are refractile, yellowish deposits with sharp margins composed of fat-laden macrophages and serum lipids. Occasionally the lipid deposits form a partial or complete ring (called a circinate ring) around the leaking area of pathology. If the lipid leakage is located near the fovea, a spoke or star-type distribution of the hard exudates may be seen.

Cotton wool spots, or soft "exudates," are actually microinfarctions of the retinal nerve-fiber layer, and appear white with soft or fuzzy edges.

Inflammatory exudates are secondary to retinal or chorioretinal inflammation.

Hard exudation and cotton wool spots are associated with vascular diseases such as diabetes mellitus, hypertension, and collagen vascular diseases but can be seen with papilledema and other intrinsic ocular conditions. Inflammatory exudates are seen in patients with such diseases as sarcoidosis and toxoplasmosis.

Emergency Department Treatment and Disposition

Routine referral for ophthalmologic and medical workup is appropriate.

Pearl

1. Hard exudates that are intraretinal may easily be confused with drusen occurring near Bruchs membrane, which separates the retina from the choroid.

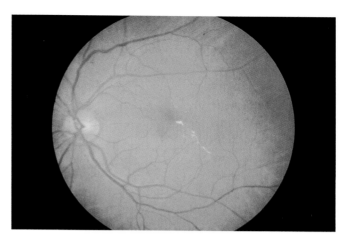

FIGURE 3.5 ■ Hard Exudates. Linear collection of yellow lipid deposits with sharp margins in macula. (Photo contributor: Beverly C. Forcier, MD.)

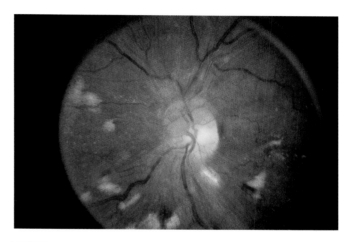

FIGURE 3.6 ■ Cotton Wool Spots. White lesions with fuzzy margins, seen here approximately one-fifth to one-fourth disk diameter in size. Orientation of cotton wool spots generally follows the curvilinear arrangement of the nerve fiber layer. Intraretinal hemorrhages and intraretinal vascular abnormalities are also present. (Photo contributor: Richard E. Wyszynski, MD.)

Clinical Summary

Roth spots are retinal hemorrhages with a white or yellow center. They may be seen in patients with a host of diseases such as anemia, leukemia, multiple myeloma, diabetes mellitus, collagen vascular disease, other vascular diseases, intracranial hemorrhage in infants, septic retinitis, and carcinoma. Flame-shaped or splinter hemorrhages or dot-blot hemorrhages may resemble Roth spots.

Emergency Department Treatment and Disposition

Routine referral for general medical evaluation is appropriate.

Pearls

1. Roth spots are not pathognomonic for any particular disease process and can represent a variety of clinical conditions.
2. These lesions represent red blood cells surrounding inflammatory cells.

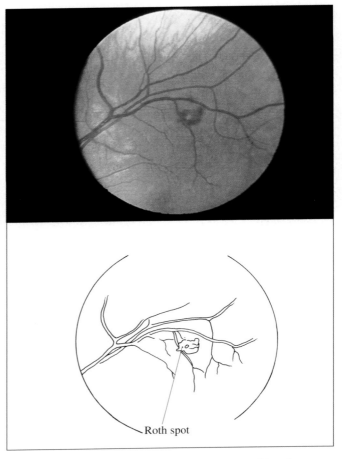

FIGURE 3.7 ■ Roth Spot. Retinal hemorrhage with pale center. (Photo contributor: William E. Cappaert, MD.)

Clinical Summary

Plaques, if present, are often found at arteriolar bifurcations. Patients may have signs and symptoms of vascular disease such as carotid bruits or stenosis, aortic stenosis, aneurysms, or atrial fibrillation. Amaurosis fugax, a transient loss of vision often described as a curtain of darkness obscuring vision with sight restoration within a few minutes, may be present in the history.

Cholesterol emboli (Hollenhorst plaques), associated with generalized atherosclerosis, often from carotid atheroma which are bright, highly refractile plaques. Platelet emboli (carotid artery or cardiac thrombus) are white and very difficult to visualize. Calcific emboli (cardiac valvular disease) are irregular and white or dull gray and much less refractile.

Emergency Department Treatment and Disposition

Referral for routine general medical evaluation is appropriate unless the patient presents with signs or symptoms consistent with showering of emboli, transient ischemic attack, or cerebrovascular accident, in which case admission should be considered.

Pearls

1. Retinal emboli may produce a loss of vision, either transient or permanent in nature.
2. Arteriolar occlusion may occur either in a central or peripheral branch location.
3. Occurrence of retinal emboli should prompt the clinician to search for an embolic source as the event may be a precursor to impending ischemic stroke.

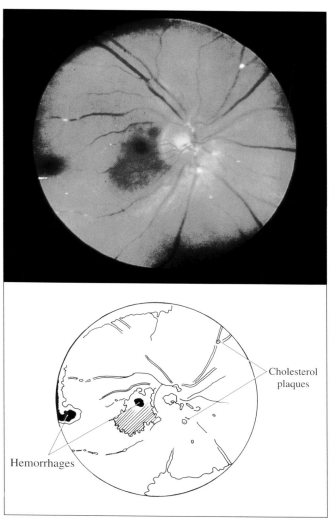

FIGURE 3.8 ■ Emboli. Refractile cholesterol plaques usually lodge at vessel bifurcations. (Photo contributor: William E. Cappaert, MD.)

Clinical Summary

In central retinal artery occlusion (CRAO), the typical patient experiences a sudden painless monocular loss of vision, either segmental or complete. Visual acuity may range from finger counting or light perception to complete blindness. Fundal findings may include the following: fundal paleness caused by retinal edema; the fovea does not have the edema and thus appears as a cherry-red spot; narrow and irregular retinal arterioles; and a "boxcar" appearance of the retinal venules.

Emergency Department Treatment and Disposition

Attempts to restore retinal blood flow may be beneficial if performed in a very narrow time window after the acute event. This may be accomplished by (1) decreasing intraocular pressure with topical β-blocker eye drops or intravenous acetazolamide; (2) ocular massage, applied with cyclic pressure on the globe for 10 seconds, followed by release and then repeated. Urgent consultation with an ophthalmologist is indicated to determine if more aggressive acute therapy (paracentesis) is warranted. However, such aggressive treatment rarely alters the poor prognosis. Medical evaluation and treatment of associated findings may be warranted. Tissue plasminogen activator may be considered for lysis of an occluding thrombus.

Pearls

1. Visual decrement may be caused by a "low flow" state (vs total occlusion). As this cannot be identified on presentation and can present hours later, immediate treatment and consultation is indicated regardless of the time of onset.
2. Sudden, painless monocular vision loss is typical.
3. CRAO may be associated with temporal arteritis. This diagnosis should be strongly considered in all patients presenting with signs and symptoms of CRAO who are older than 55 years.

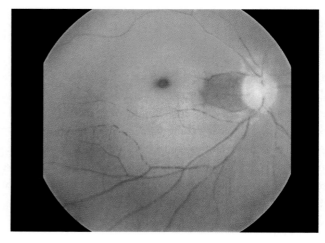

FIGURE 3.10A ■ CRAO with Cilioretinal Artery Sparing. "Hyperemia" of the fundus on the temporal side of the disc and sparing of the macular region is owing to the presence of a patent cilioretinal artery. (Photo contributor: Thomas R. Hedges III, MD.)

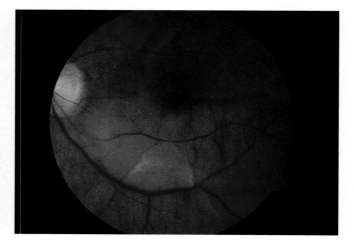

FIGURE 3.9 ■ Central Retinal Artery Occlusion. The retinal pallor caused by retinal edema is well demonstrated, contrasting with the "cherry red spot" of the nonedematous fovea. Note the vascular narrowing and the "boxcar" appearance of the venules. (Photo contributor: Aaron Sobol, MD.)

FIGURE 3.10B ■ Branch Central Retinal Artery Occlusion. Retinal whitening (owing to ischemia) and absence of blood flow in the infero termporal branch retinal arteriole. (Photo contributor: Arun D. Singh, MD.)

Clinical Summary

Patients are usually older individuals and complain of sudden, painless visual loss in one eye. The vision loss is usually not as severe as CRAO and may vary from normal to hand motion. Funduscopy in a classic, ischemic central retinal vein occlusion (CRVO) shows a "blood and thunder" fundus: hemorrhages (including flame, dot or blot, preretinal, and vitreous) and dilation and tortuosity of the venous system. The arterial system often shows narrowing. The disk margin may be blurred. Cotton wool spots and edema may be seen.

Emergency Department Treatment and Disposition

Treatment is rarely effective in preventing or reversing the damage done by the occlusion and is directed toward systemic evaluation to identify and treat contributing factors, hopefully decreasing the chance of contralateral CRVO. Ophthalmologic evaluation is necessary to confirm the diagnosis, estimate the amount of ischemia, and follow the patient so as to minimize sequelae of possible complications such as neovascularization and neovascular glaucoma.

Pearls

1. Sudden, painless visual loss in one eye should be evaluated promptly to determine its etiology.
2. Look for the classic "blood and thunder" funduscopic findings.
3. Consider the differential diagnosis of acute *painful* (glaucoma, retrobulbar neuritis) versus *painless* vision loss (CRAO, anterior ischemic optic neuropathy, retinal detachment, subretinal neovascularization, and vitreous hemorrhage).

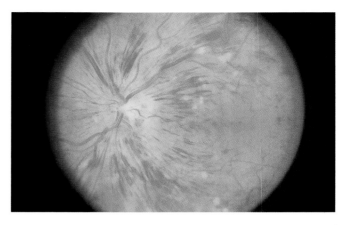

FIGURE 3.11 ■ Central Retinal Vein Occlusion. The amount of hemorrhage is the most striking feature in this photograph. Also note the blurred disk margin, the dilation and tortuosity of the venules, and the cotton wool spots. Retinal edema is suggested by blurring of the retinal details. (Photo contributor: Department of Ophthalmology, Naval Medical Center, Portsmouth, VA.)

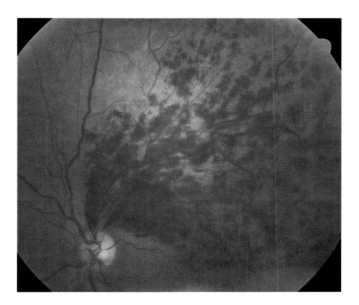

FIGURE 3.12 ■ Central Retinal Vein Branch Occlusion. The hemorrhage seen is limited to a sector of the fundus, indicating that a branch occlusion has occurred. There is less edema, and a large portion of the fundus is unaffected. (Photo contributor: Richard E. Wyszynski, MD.)

Clinical Summary

Fundus changes that may be seen with hypertension include generalized and focal narrowing of arterioles, generalized arteriolar sclerosis (resembling copper or silver wiring), arteriovenous crossing changes, hemorrhages (usually flame-shaped), retinal edema and exudation, cotton wool spots, microaneurysms, and disk edema.

Diabetic retinopathy, many hematologic and vascular diseases, traumas, localized ocular pathology, and papilledema should all be considered.

Emergency Department Treatment and Disposition

The patient's hypertension should be appropriately treated, and a search for other end-organ damage should be considered. The patient should be referred for appropriate long-term blood pressure management.

Pearls

1. Hypertensive arteriolar findings may be reversible if organic changes have not occurred in the vessel walls.
2. Always consider hypertensive retinopathy in the differential diagnosis of papilledema.

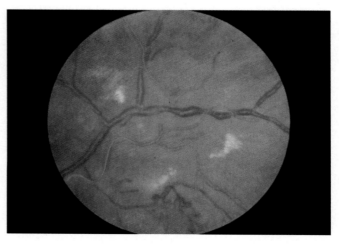

FIGURE 3.13 ■ Hypertension. Chronic, severe systemic hypertensive changes are demonstrated by hard exudates, increased vessel light reflexes, and sausage-shaped veins. (Photo contributor: Richard E. Wyszynski, MD.)

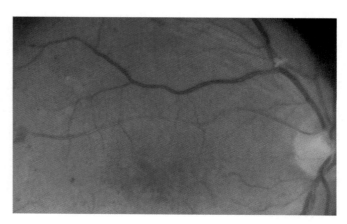

FIGURE 3.14 ■ Copper and Silver Wiring. Arteriolar changes seen in hypertensive retinopathy resemble copper (light reflex occupies most of the width) and silver (light reflex occupies the entire width of the arteriole) wiring. (Photo contributor: Aaron Sobol, MD.)

Clinical Summary

The early ocular manifestations of diabetes mellitus are referred to as background diabetic retinopathy (BDR). Fundus findings include flame or splinter hemorrhages (located in the superficial nerve fiber layer) or dot and blot hemorrhages (located deeper in the retina), hard exudates, retinal edema, and microaneurysms. If these signs are located in the macula, the patient's visual acuity may be decreased or at risk of becoming compromised, requiring laser treatment. Preproliferative diabetic retinopathy can show BDR changes plus cotton wool spots, intraretinal microvascular abnormalities, and venous beading. Proliferative diabetic retinopathy is demonstrated by neovascularization at the disk (NVD) or elsewhere (NVE). These require laser therapy owing to risk of severe visual loss from sequelae: vitreous hemorrhage, tractional retinal detachment, and severe glaucoma.

Many vascular and hematologic diseases—such as collagen vascular disease, sickle cell trait, hypertension, hypotension, anemia, leukemia, inflammatory and infectious states—and ocular conditions can be associated with some or of all the above signs.

Emergency Department Treatment and Disposition

Routine ophthalmologic referral for laser or surgical treatment is indicated.

Pearls

1. Periodic ophthalmologic evaluations are recommended for all diabetic patients.
2. Microaneurysms typically appear 10 years after the initial onset of diabetes, although they may appear earlier in patients with juvenile diabetes.
3. Control of blood sugar alone does not prevent the development of retinopathy.
4. Blurred vision can also occur from acute increases in serum glucose, causing lens swelling and a refractive shift even in the absence of retinopathy.

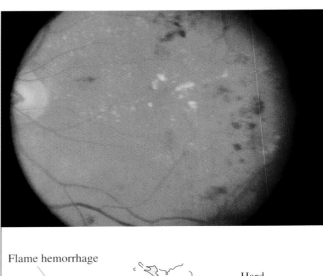

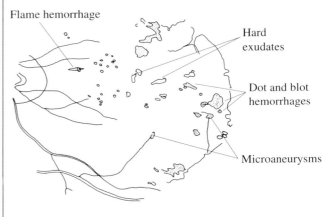

FIGURE 3.15 ■ Background Diabetic Retinopathy. Hard exudates, dot hemorrhages, blot hemorrhages, flame hemorrhages, and microaneurysms are present. Because these changes are located within the macula, this is classified as diabetic maculopathy. (Photo contributor: Richard E. Wyszynski, MD.)

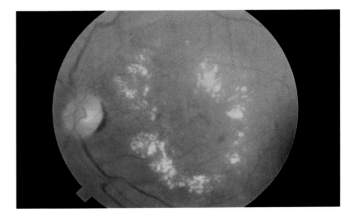

FIGURE 3.16 ■ Background Diabetic Retinopathy. An example of diabetic maculopathy with a typical circinate lipid ring. (Photo contributor: Richard E. Wyszynski, MD.)

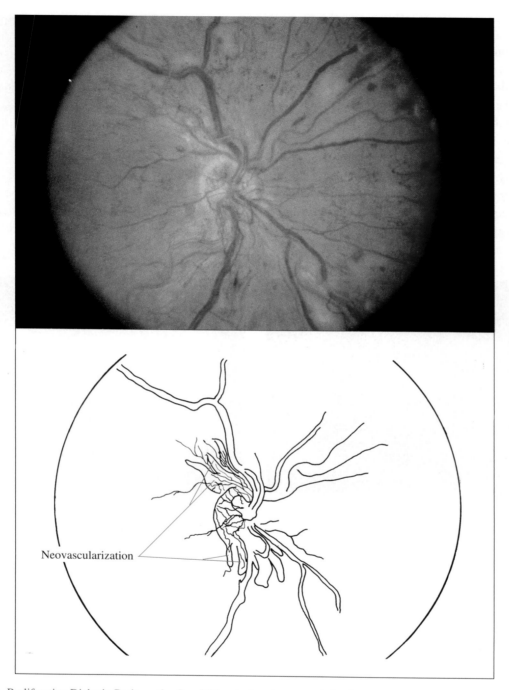

FIGURE 3.17 ■ Proliferative Diabetic Retinopathy. In addition to the signs seen in background and preproliferative diabetic retinopathy, neovascularization is seen here coming off the disk. (Photo contributor: Richard E. Wyszynski, MD.)

Clinical Summary

Patients may complain of floaters followed by the sudden loss or deterioration of vision in the affected eye, although bilateral hemorrhage can occur. The red reflex is diminished or absent, and the retina is obscured because of the bleeding. Large sheets or three-dimensional collections of red to red-black blood may be detected.

Multiple underlying etiologies include proliferative diabetic retinopathy, retinal or vitreous detachments, hematologic diseases, trauma (ocular or shaken impact syndrome), subarachnoid hemorrhage, collagen vascular disease, infections, macular degeneration, and tumors.

Emergency Department Treatment and Disposition

Refer to an ophthalmologist and an appropriate physician for associated conditions. Ophthalmic observation, photocoagulation, and surgery are all therapeutic options. Bed rest may help to increase visualization of the fundus.

Pearl

1. The patient's vision may improve somewhat after a period of sitting or standing as the blood layers out.

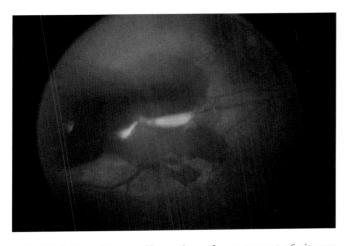

FIGURE 3.18 ■ Vitreous Hemorrhage. Large amount of vitreous hemorrhage associated with metallic intraocular foreign body. The large quantity of blood obscures visualization of retinal details. (Photo contributor: Richard E. Wyszynski, MD.)

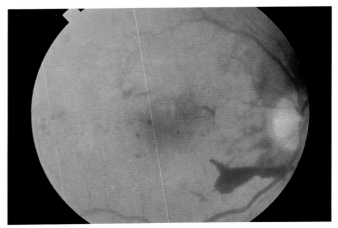

FIGURE 3.19 ■ Vitreous Hemorrhage. A smaller amount of vitreous hemorrhage is more easily photographed. Gravitational effect on the vitreous blood creates the appearance of a flat meniscus (keel-shaped blood) in this patient with vitreous hemorrhage associated with proliferative diabetic retinopathy. (Photo contributor: Richard E. Wyszynski, MD.)

Clinical Summary

Patients often complain of monocular, decreased visual function and may describe a shadow or curtain descending over the eye. Other complaints include cloudy or smoky vision, floaters, or momentary flashes of light. Monocular visual filed defects may be noted, and central visual acuity is diminished with macular involvement. Fundal examination may reveal a billowing or tentlike elevation of retina compared with adjacent areas. The elevated retina often appears gray. Retinal holes and tears may be seen, but often the holes, tears, and retinal detachment cannot be seen without indirect ophthalmoscopy.

Retinal detachments caused by retinal tears or holes can be associated with trauma, previous ocular surgery, near-sightedness, family history of retinal detachment, and Marfan disease. Retinal detachments caused by traction on the retina by an intraocular process can be because of systemic influences in the eye, such as diabetes mellitus or sickle cell trait. Occasionally retinal detachments are caused by tumors or exudative processes that elevate the retina. Symptoms of "light flashes" may occur with vitreous changes in the absence of retinal pathology. Patients may note flashes of light occurring only in a darkened environment because of the mechanical stimulation of the retina from the extraocular muscles, usually in a nearsighted individual.

Emergency Department Treatment and Disposition

Urgent ophthalmologic evaluation and treatment are warranted.

Pearls

1. Often patients have had sensation of flashes of light that occur in a certain area of a visual field in one eye, corresponding to the pathologic pulling on the corresponding retina.
2. Visual loss may be gradual or sudden.

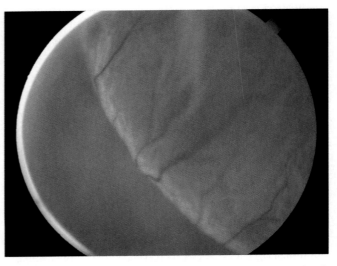

FIGURE 3.20 ■ Retinal Detachment. A fold of detached retina is seen drooping well in front of the posterior pole giving the appearance of a "three-dimensional" fundus. (Photo contributor: Department of Ophthalmology, Naval Medical Center, Portsmouth, VA.)

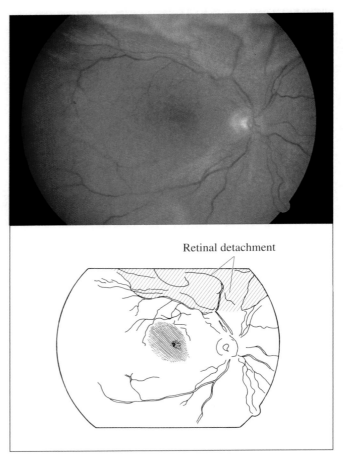

FIGURE 3.21 ■ Retinal Detachment. Undulating, out-of-focus, elevated retina is seen with few vessels in focus. (Photo contributor: Richard E. Wyszynski, MD.)

Clinical Summary

Patients may complain of the gradual and usually painless onset of the following visual sensations: floaters, scintillating scotomas (quivering blind spots), decreased peripheral visual field, and metamorphopsia (wavy distortion of vision). Cytomegalovirus (CMV) infiltrates appear as focal, small (but may be larger, confluent) white lesions in the retina that look like cotton wool spots. CMV is a necrotizing virus that is spread hematogenously, so that damage is concentrated in the retina adjacent to the major vessels and the optic disk. Often hemorrhage is involved with significant retinal necrosis (dirty white with a granular appearance), giving the "pizza pie" or "cheese and ketchup" appearance. Optic nerve involvement and retinal detachments can be present.

The differential includes other infections such as toxoplasmosis, other herpesviruses, syphilis, and occasionally other opportunistic infections.

Emergency Department Treatment and Disposition

Reversal, if possible, of immunosuppression; antiviral agents have been used effectively to threat this condition.

Pearls

1. HIV retinopathy consists of scattered retinal hemorrhages and scattered, multiple cotton wool spots that resolve over time, whereas CMV lesions will typically progress.
2. Although exposure to the CMV virus is widespread, the virus rarely produces a clinically recognized disease in nonimmunosuppressed individuals.

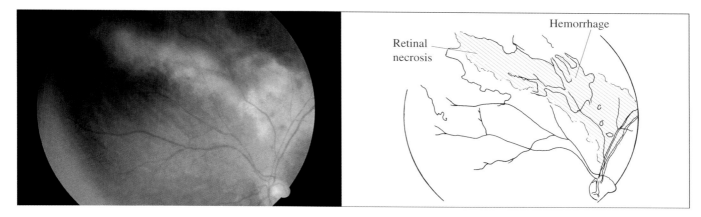

FIGURE 3.22 ■ CMV Retinitis. "Pizza pie" or "cheese and ketchup" appearance is demonstrated by hemorrhages and the dirty, white, granular-appearing retinal necrosis adjacent to major vessels. (Photo contributor: Richard E. Wyszynski, MD.)

Clinical Summary

Papilledema involves swelling of the optic nerve head, usually in association with elevated intracranial pressure. The optic disks are hyperemic with blurred disk margins; the venules are dilated and tortuous. The optic cup may be obscured by the swollen disk. There may be flame hemorrhages and infarctions (white, indistinct cotton wool spots) in the nerve fiber layer and edema in the surrounding retina.

Ocular inflammation (eg, papillitis), tumors or trauma, central retinal artery or vein occlusion, optic nerve drusen, and marked hyperopia may present with similar findings.

Emergency Department Treatment and Disposition

Expeditious ophthalmologic and medical evaluation is warranted.

Pearls

1. The top of a swollen disk and the surrounding unaffected retina will not both be in focus on the same setting on direct ophthalmoscopy.
2. Papilledema is a bilateral process, though it may be slightly asymmetric. A unilateral swollen disk suggests a localized ocular or orbital process.
3. Vision is usually normal acutely, though the patient may complain of transient visual changes. The blind spot is usually enlarged.
4. Diplopia from sixth cranial nerve palsy can be associated with increased intracranial pressure and papilledema.

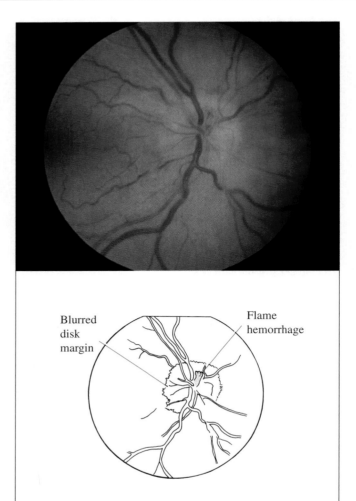

FIGURE 3.23 ■ Papilledema. Disk is hyperemic and swollen with loss of sharp margins. The venules are dilated and tortuous. The cup is obscured. A small flame hemorrhage is seen at 12 to 1 o'clock on the disk margin. (Photo contributor: Department of Ophthalmology, Naval Medical Center, Portsmouth, VA.)

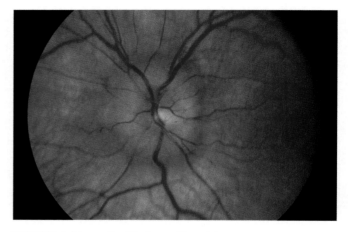

FIGURE 3.24 ■ Papilledema. Note blurred disk margins and congested disk. (Photo contributor: Arun D. Singh, MD.)

71

Clinical Summary

Most cases of optic neuritis are retrobulbar and involve no changes in the fundus, or optic disk, during the acute episode. With time, variable optic disk pallor may develop. Typical retrobulbar optic neuritis presents with sudden or rapidly progressing monocular vision loss in patients younger than 50 years. There is a central visual field defect that may extend to the blind spot. There may be pain on movement of the globe. The pupillary light response is diminished in the affected eye. Over time the vision improves partially or completely; minimal or severe optic atrophy may develop. Papillitis, inflammation of the intraocular portion of the optic nerve, will accompany disk swelling, with a few flame hemorrhages and possible cells in the vitreous.

Optic neuritis must be differentiated from papilledema (bilateral disk swelling, typically with no acute visual loss with the exception of transient visual changes), ischemic neuropathy (pale, swollen disk in an older individual with sudden monocular vision loss), tumors, metabolic or endocrine disorders. Most cases of optic neuritis are of unknown etiology. Some known causes of optic neuritis include demyelinating disease, infections (including viral, syphilis, tuberculosis, sarcoidosis), or inflammations from contiguous structures (sinuses, meninges, orbit).

Emergency Department Treatment and Disposition

Treatment is controversial; often none is recommended. Oral steroids may worsen prognosis in certain cases. Intravenous steroids may be considered after consultation with an ophthalmologist.

Pearls

1. Monocular vision loss with pain on palpation of the globe or with eye movement are clinical clues to the diagnosis.
2. Sudden or rapidly progressing central vision loss is characteristic.
3. Most cases of acute optic neuritis are retrobulbar. Thus ophthalmoscopy shows a normal fundus.
4. Suspect temporal arteritis in older patients.

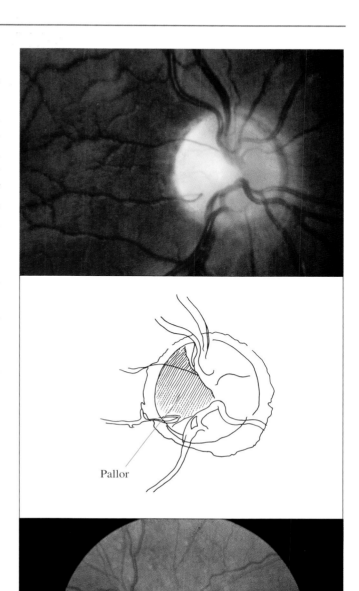

FIGURE 3.25 ■ Optic Nerve Pallor. Optic nerve pallor, either segmental (*top*) or generalized (*bottom*), is a nonspecific change that may be associated with a previous episode of optic neuritis or other insults to the optic nerve. (Photo contributor: Richard E. Wyszynski, MD.)

Clinical Summary

Anterior ischemic optic neuropathy (AION) presents with a sudden loss of visual field (often altitudinal), usually involving fixation, in an older individual. The loss is usually stable after onset, with no improvement, and only occasionally, progressive over several days to weeks. Pale disk swelling is present involving a sector or the full disk, with accompanying flame hemorrhages. The cup to disc ratio is typically small (0.1-0.2) bilaterally.

The common, nonarteritic causes of AION (probably arteriosclerosis) need to be differentiated from arteritic ones, such as giant cell arteritis. If untreated, the latter will involve the other eye in 75% of cases, often in a few days to weeks. These elderly individuals often have weight loss, masseter claudication, weakness, myalgias, elevated sedimentation rate, and painful scalp, temples, or forehead.

Emergency Department Treatment and Disposition

Routine ophthalmologic and medical evaluation is appropriate.

Pearls

1. Consider AION in an elderly patient with sudden, usually painless, visual field loss.
2. Rule out giant cell arteritis. These patients tend to be older (age > 55) and may have associated CRAO or cranial nerve palsies (III, IV, or VI) with diplopia.

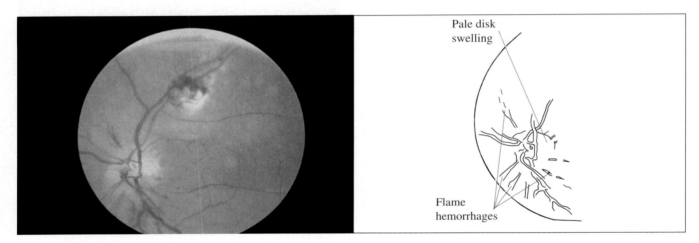

FIGURE 3.26 ■ Anterior Ischemic Optic Neuropathy. Pale disk swelling and flame hemorrhages are present. This patient also has an unrelated retinal scar owing to toxoplasmosis. (Photo contributor: William E. Cappaert, MD.)

Clinical Summary

Acute narrow or closed-angle glaucoma (ACG) results from a physical impedance of aqueous humor outflow. Symptoms range from colored halos around lights and blurred vision to severe pain (described as a headache or brow ache) with nausea and vomiting. Intraocular pressure (IOP) is markedly elevated. Perilimbal vessels are injected, the pupil is middilated and poorly reactive to light, and the cornea may be hazy and edematous.

Two-thirds of glaucoma patients have open-angle glaucoma. Often they are asymptomatic. They may have a family history of glaucoma. Funduscopy may show asymmetric cupping of the optic nerves. The optic nerve may show notching, local thinning of tissue, or disk hemorrhage. Optic cups enlarge, especially vertically, with progressive damage. Tissue loss is associated with visual field abnormalities. The IOP is often but not always greater than 21 mm Hg.

Emergency Department Treatment and Disposition

Acute ACG requires emergent ophthalmologic consultation and administration of medications to decrease intraocular pressure such as β-blocker drops (timolol), carbonic anhydrase inhibitors (acetazolamide), cholinergic-stimulating drops (pilocarpine), hyperosmotic agents (osmoglyn), and α-adrenergic agonists (apraclonidine). *Open-angle glaucoma is treated with* long-term ophthalmic evaluation and treatment with medications and laser or surgery.

Pearls

1. Nausea, vomiting, and headache may obscure the diagnosis. Use digital globe palpation routinely in patients with these complaints.
2. Open-angle glaucoma usually causes no symptoms other than gradual loss of vision.
3. Congenital glaucoma is rare. However, because of prognosis if diagnosis is delayed, consider congenital glaucoma in infants and children with tearing, photophobia, enlarged eyes, or cloudy corneas.
4. Asymmetric cupping, enlarged cups, and elevated IOP are hallmarks of open-angle glaucoma.

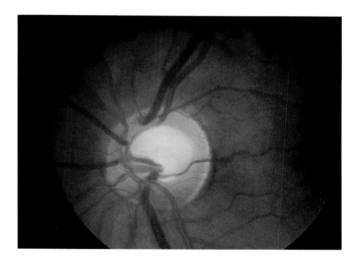

FIGURE 3.27 ■ Glaucomatous Cupping. The cup is not central; it is elongated toward the rim superotemporally. (Photo contributor: Department of Ophthalmology, Naval Medical Center, Portsmouth, VA.)

Clinical Summary

Subhyaloid hemorrhage appears as extravasated blood beneath the retinal layer. These are often described as "boat-shaped" hemorrhages to distinguish them from the "flame-shaped" hemorrhages on the superficial nerve fiber layer of the retina. They may occur as a result of blunt trauma but are perhaps best known as a marker for subarachnoid hemorrhage (SAH). In SAH, the hemorrhages appear as a "puff" of blood emanating from the central disk.

SAH, shaken impact syndrome, hypertensive retinopathy, and retinal hemorrhage should all be considered and aggressively evaluated.

Emergency Department Treatment and Disposition

No specific treatment is required for subhyaloid hemorrhage. Treatment is dependent on the underlying etiology. Appropriate specialty referral should be made in all cases.

Pearls

1. A funduscopic examination looking for subhyaloid hemorrhage should be included in all patients with severe headache, unresponsive pediatric patients, or those with altered mental status.

2. The appearance of a retinal hemorrhage indicates its anatomic location. A subhyaloid hemorrhage lies over the retinal vessels—thus they cannot be seen on funduscopic examination. In a subretinal hemorrhage (see Fig. 3.4), the vessels lie superficial to the hemorrhage, and thus are easily seen.

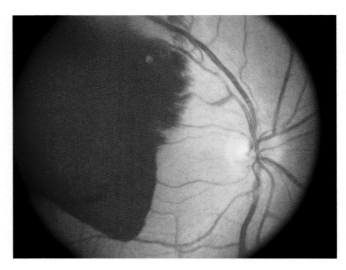

FIGURE 3.28 ■ Subhyaloid Hemorrhage. Subhyaloid hemorrhage seen on funduscopic examination in a patient with subarachnoid hemorrhage. (From Edlow and Caplan. Primary care: avoiding pitfalls in the diagnosis of subarachnoid hemorrhage. *N Engl J Med.* 2000;342:29-36, with permission.)

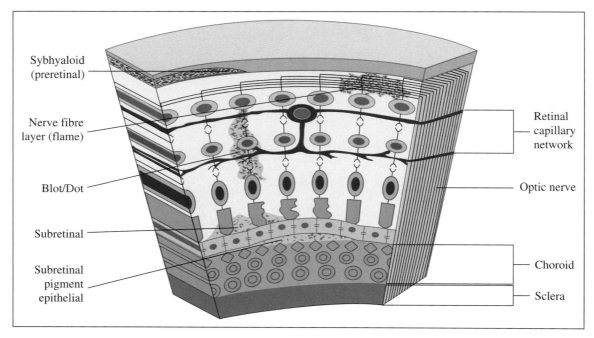

FIGURE 3.29 ■ Retinal Hemorrhages—Anatomic Location.

Chapter 4

OPHTHALMIC TRAUMA

Dallas E. Peak
Christopher S. Weaver
Kevin J. Knoop

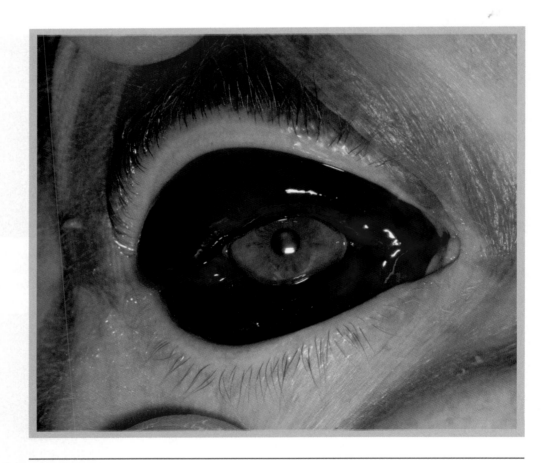

The authors acknowledge the special contributions of Carey D. Chisholm for contributions to prior editions.

Clinical Summary

Corneal abrasions present with acute onset of eye discomfort, tearing, and often a foreign-body sensation. A "ciliary flush" (conjunctival injection hugging the limbus) may be seen. Visual acuity may be affected by large abrasions or those in the central visual axis. Photophobia and headache from ciliary muscle spasm may be present. Associated findings or complications include traumatic iritis, hypopyon, or a corneal ulcer. Fluorescein examination, preferably with a slit lamp, reveals the defect.

Emergency Department Treatment and Disposition

Instillation of topical anesthetic drops (ie, 0.5% solution of either proparacaine or tetracaine) facilitates examination while relieving pain and blepharospasm. A short-acting cycloplegic (eg, cyclopentolate 1%, homatropine 5%) may further reduce pain from ciliary spasm and should be considered in patients who complain of headache or photophobia. Oral opioid analgesics may be needed for pain control. NSAID eye drops (eg, diclofenac or ketorolac) are equally effective and avoid risks of sedation. Neither treatment with topical antibiotics nor patching has been scientifically validated. Routine use of these practices has been called into question. Tetanus prophylaxis is indicated. Follow-up is required for any patient who is still symptomatic after 12 to 24 hours.

Pearls

1. Mucus may simulate fluorescein uptake, but its position changes with blinking.
2. Multiple linear corneal abrasions, the "ice-rink sign," may result from an embedded foreign body adhered to the upper lid. The lid should always be everted to rule this out.
3. A high index of suspicion for penetrating injury should be maintained whenever mechanism includes grinding or striking metal, or high-velocity injuries from mowers or string trimmers. Fluorescein streaming away from an "abrasion" (Seidel test) may be an indication of a corneal perforation.
4. Routine prophylactic treatment with topical antibiotics remains controversial. When used, inexpensive broad-spectrum antibiotic drops (sulfacetamide sodium or trimethoprim/polymyxin B) allow clearer vision than

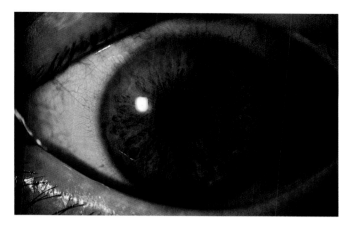

FIGURE 4.1 ■ Corneal Abrasion. Seen under magnification from the slit lamp, corneal abrasion can sometimes be appreciated without fluorescein staining. This abrasion is seen without using the cobalt blue light. (Photo contributor: Harold Rivera.)

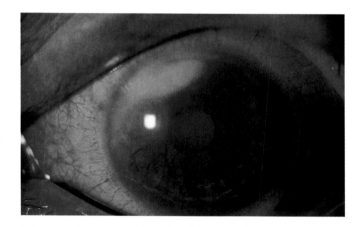

FIGURE 4.2 ■ Corneal Abrasion. The same abrasion as Fig. 4.1 is seen under magnification from the slit lamp with fluorescein stain using the cobalt blue light. (Photo contributor: Harold Rivera.)

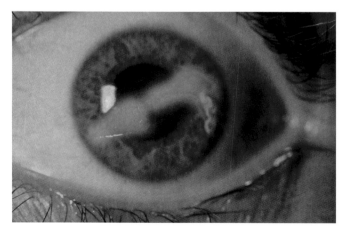

FIGURE 4.3 ■ Corneal Abrasion. Abrasions obscuring the visual axis benefit from close follow up with an ophthalmologist to ensure adequate healing. (Photo contributor: Lawrence B. Stack, MD.)

lubricating ointments, which cause visual blurring. Topical neomycin antibiotics should be avoided owing to high risk of irritant allergy symptoms in the general population.

5. An "abrasion" in a contact lens wearer should alert one to suspect a corneal ulcer.

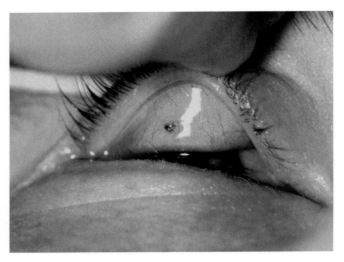

FIGURE 4.4 ■ Foreign Body under the Upper Lid. Lid eversion is an essential part of the eye examination to detect foreign bodies. (Photo contributor: Lawrence B. Stack, MD.)

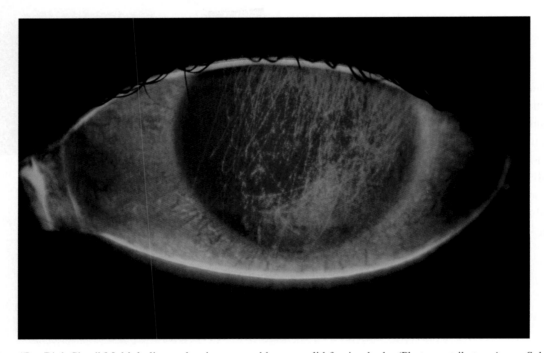

FIGURE 4.5 ■ "Ice-Rink Sign." Multiple linear abrasions caused by upper lid foreign body. (Photo contributor: Aaron Sobol, MD.)

Clinical Summary

A subconjunctival hemorrhage or hematoma occurs with often trivial events such as a cough, sneeze, Valsalva maneuver, or minor blunt trauma. The patient may present with some degree of duress secondary to the appearance of the bloody eye. The blood is usually bright red and appears flat. It is limited to the bulbar conjunctiva and stops abruptly at the limbus. This appearance is important to differentiate the lesion from bloody chemosis, which can occur with scleral rupture or nontraumatic conditions. Aside from appearance, this condition does not cause the patient any pain or diminution in visual acuity.

Emergency Department Treatment and Disposition

No treatment is required. The patient should be told to expect the blood to be resorbed in 2 to 3 weeks.

Pearls

1. Subconjunctival hematoma may be differentiated from bloody chemosis by the flat appearance of the conjunctival membranes.
2. A subconjunctival hematoma involving the extreme lateral globe after blunt trauma is very suspicious for zygomatic arch fracture.
3. Patients with nontraumatic bloody chemosis should be evaluated for an underlying metabolic (coagulopathy) or structural (cavernous sinus thrombosis) disorder.

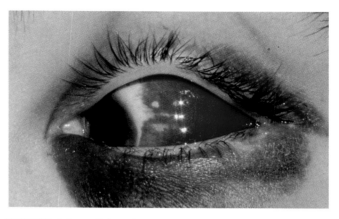

FIGURE 4.6 ■ Subconjunctival Hemorrhage. Subconjunctival hemorrhage in a patient with blunt trauma. The flat appearance of the hemorrhage indicates its benign nature. (Photo contributor: Dallas E. Peak, MD.)

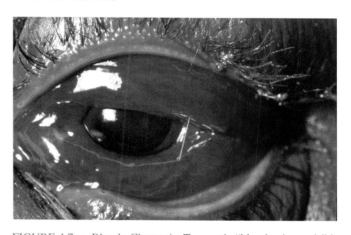

FIGURE 4.7 ■ Bloody Chemosis. Traumatic "bloody chemosis" is suspicious for globe penetration. Open globe was ruled out in this patient. Bedside ultrasonography is a useful adjunct. Dilated pupil is a result of pharmacologic agent. (Photo contributor: Lawrence B. Stack, MD.)

Clinical Summary

Patients typically report getting something in the eye or complain of foreign body (FB) sensation. Vision may be affected if the FB overlies the cornea. Tearing, conjunctival injection, headache, and photophobia may also be present. The most important consideration is the possibility of a penetrating globe injury. A meticulous history about the mechanism of injury must be elicited.

Emergency Department Treatment and Disposition

Topical anesthetic drops (eg, 0.5% proparacaine or tetracaine) facilitate examination and removal. If superficial, removal with saline flush may be attempted before using a sterile eye spud or small (25-gauge) needle. Consider topical antibiotic drops or ointment for the residual corneal abrasion. Tetanus prophylaxis is indicated. A "short-acting" cycloplegic (eg, cyclopentolate 1% or homatropine 5%) may benefit patients with headache or photophobia. FB or "rust ring" removal should be conducted using slit-lamp microscopy, *only* by a physician skilled in rust ring removal due to the risk of corneal perforation or scarring.

Pearls

1. Always evert the upper lid and search carefully for a foreign body. An FB adherent to the upper lid abrades the cornea, producing the "ice-rink" sign, caused from multiple linear abrasions.
2. Vigorous attempts to remove the entire rust ring are not warranted. This may await emergency department or ophthalmology follow-up in 24 hours.
3. Use of cotton-tipped applicators to attempt FB removal should be discouraged (large surface area and potential to cause a larger corneal defect).

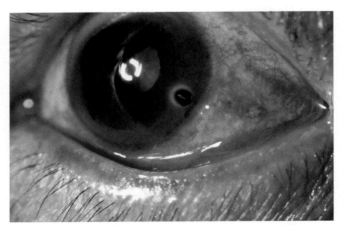

FIGURE 4.8 ■ Foreign Body on the Cornea. A small foreign body is lodged at 4 o'clock on the cornea. (Photo contributor: Kevin J. Knoop, MD, MS.)

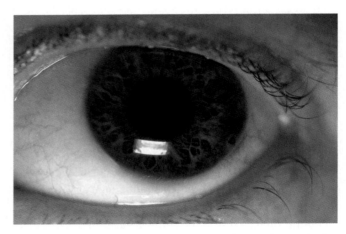

FIGURE 4.9 ■ "Rust Ring." A rust ring has formed from a foreign body (likely metallic) in this patient. A burr drill can be used for attempted removal, which, if unsuccessful, can be reattempted in 24 hours. (Photo contributor: R. Jason Thurman MD.)

Clinical Summary

Injury to the anterior chamber that disrupts the vasculature supporting the iris or ciliary body results in a hyphema. The blood tends to layer with time, and left undisturbed, gravity will form a visible meniscus. Symptoms can include pain, photophobia, and possibly blurred vision secondary to obstructing blood cells. Nausea and vomiting may signal a rise in intraocular pressure (glaucoma) caused by blood cells clogging the trabecular meshwork.

Emergency Department Treatment and Disposition

Prevention of further hemorrhage is the foremost treatment goal. Most rebleeding occurs within the first 72 hours and is usually more extensive than the initial event. The patient should be kept at rest in the supine position with the head elevated slightly. A hard eye shield should be used to prevent further trauma from manipulation. Oral or parenteral pain medication and sedatives are appropriate, but avoid agents with antiplatelet activity such as nonsteroidal anti-inflammatory drugs (NSAIDs). Antiemetics should be used if the patient has nausea. Further treatment is at the discretion of specialty consultants but may include topical and oral steroids, anti-fibrinolytics such as aminocaproic acid, or surgery. Intra-ocular pressure (IOP) should be measured in all patients unless there is a suspicion of penetrating injury to the globe. If elevated, IOP should be treated with appropriate agents, including topical β-blockers, pilocarpine, and, if needed, osmotic agents (mannitol, sorbitol) and acetazolamide. The need for admission for hyphema is variable. Ophthalmologic consultation is warranted to determine local practices.

Pearls

1. The patient should be told specifically not to read or watch television, as these activities result in greater than usual ocular activity.
2. Rebleeding may occur in 10% to 20% of patients, most commonly in the first 2 to 5 days when the blood clots start to retract.
3. An "eight-ball" or total hyphema occurs when blood fills the entire anterior chamber. These more often lead to elevated IOP and corneal bloodstaining and typically require surgical evacuation.
4. Patients with sickle cell and other hemoglobinopathies are at risk for sickling of blood inside the anterior chamber. This can cause a rise in IOP caused by obstruction of the trabecular meshwork even if only small amount of blood is present.
5. An abnormally low IOP should prompt consideration for presence of penetrating globe injury.
6. Trauma patients should be evaluated for slight differences in iris color while supine, indicating a hyphema is present.

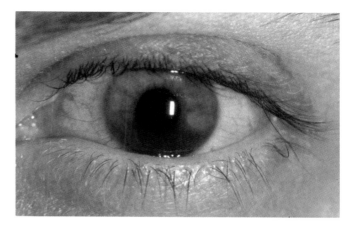

FIGURE 4.10 ■ Hyphema. This hyphema is just beginning to layer out reflecting its acute nature. (Photo contributor: Lawrence B. Stack, MD.)

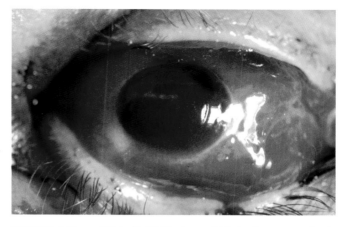

FIGURE 4.11 ■ "Eight-Ball" Hyphema. This hyphema completely fills the anterior chamber. (Photo contributor: Lawrence B. Stack, MD.)

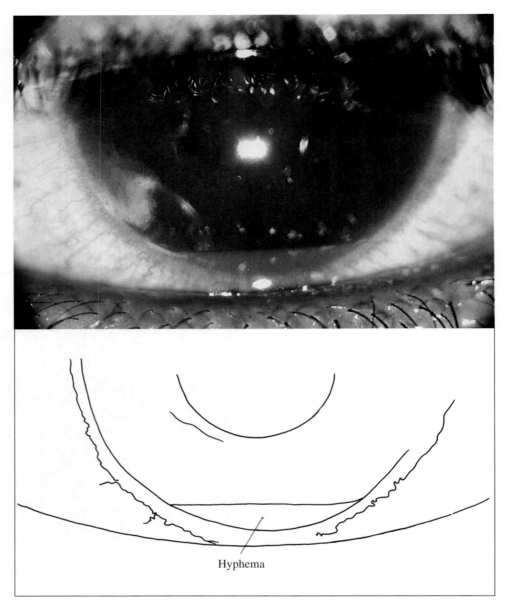

FIGURE 4.12 ■ Hyphema. A small hyphema (about 5%) in a patient with sickle cell disease. (Photo contributor: Dallas E. Peak, MD.)

Clinical Summary

The most important consideration with any eye injury is the possibility of a penetrating globe injury with residual intraocular foreign body (IO FB). Patients may report FB sensation, but subtle presentations occur. A meticulous history about the mechanism of injury (grinding or metal on metal) must be elicited.

Emergency Department Treatment and Disposition

For suspected subtle injury a careful examination is required. Bedside, ultrasound can be a useful adjunct and allow rapid identification of an IO FB. Care must be taken to avoid any pressure on the globe. A slit lamp examination with Seidel test (copious amounts of fluorescein instilled and observed for streaming away from the site of perforation) may reveal a microperforation.

Pearls

1. Always maintain a high index of suspicion for penetrating globe injury. Be particularly wary in mechanisms involving use of "metal on metal" such as grinding or hammering. A positive Seidel test demonstrates corneal microperforation.

2. If ocular penetration is suspected, a diligent search for a retained foreign body is indicated, beginning with bedside ultrasound using a high-frequency transducer. Computed tomography (CT) is the diagnostic study of choice (avoid MRI) with indeterminate results or when confirmation is desired.

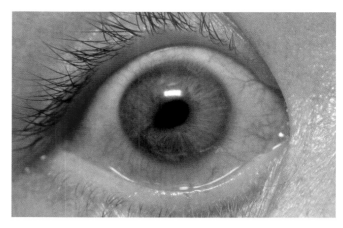

FIGURE 4.13 ■ Anterior Chamber Foreign Body. A shard from a nail is seen embedded in the anterior chamber. A "teardrop" pupil is present, indicating perforation. (Photo contributor: Lawrence B. Stack, MD.)

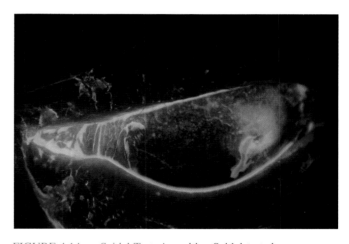

FIGURE 4.14 ■ Seidel Test. A positive Seidel test shows aqueous leaking through a corneal perforation while being observed with the slit lamp. (Photo contributor: Aaron Sobol, MD.)

Clinical Summary

Traumatic iridodialysis is the result of an injury, typically blunt trauma, that pulls the iris away from the ciliary body. The resulting deformity appears as a lens-shaped defect at the outer margin of the iris. Patients may present complaining of a "second pupil." As the iris pulls away from the ciliary body, a small amount of bleeding may result. Look closely for associated traumatic hyphema.

Penetrating injury to the globe, scleral rupture, intraocular foreign body, and lens dislocation causing billowing of the iris should all be considered.

Emergency Department Treatment and Disposition

A remote traumatic iridodialysis requires no specific treatment in the emergency department. Recent history of ocular trauma should prompt a diligent slit-lamp examination for associated hyphema or lens dislocation. If hyphema is present, it should be treated as discussed (see "Hyphema"). Pure cases of iridodialysis may be referred for specialty consultation to exclude other injuries; if the defect is large enough to result in monocular diplopia, surgical repair may be necessary.

Pearls

1. The examination should carefully exclude posterior chamber pathology and hyphema. Consider bedside ultrasonography to rule out posterior pole injuries (retinal detachment, vitreous hemorrhage, lens dislocation, or foreign body).
2. A careful review of the history to exclude penetrating trauma should be made. If the history is unclear, CT scan may be used to exclude the presence of intraocular foreign body.
3. A careful examination includes searching for associated lens dislocation.

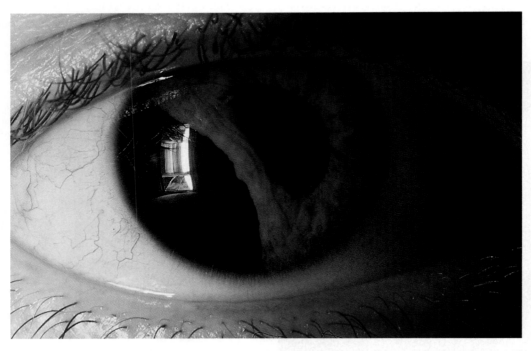

FIGURE 4.15 ■ Traumatic Iridodialysis. The iris has pulled away from the ciliary body as a result of blunt trauma. (Photo contributor: Department of Ophthalmology, Naval Medical Center, Portsmouth, VA.)

LENS DISLOCATION

Clinical Summary

Lens dislocation may result from blunt trauma to the globe. As the anterior surface of the eye is struck, there is compression in the AP dimension with resultant stretching of the globe along its equator in the medial-lateral plane. As this occurs, the zonule fibers, which suspend the lens in place, are stretched and along with lens capsule may become disrupted. The patient may experience symptoms of monocular diplopia or gross blurring of images, depending on the severity of the injury. Occasionally there can be dramatic visual fluctuations caused by the lens changing position with resultant phakic and aphakic vision. There is generally a lack of pain except if secondary angle closure glaucoma occurs from the lens causing pupillary block. On slit-lamp examination, the displaced crystalline lens appears as a crescent shape along its edge against a backdrop of the red reflex from the fundus. The edge of the subluxed lens may be visible only when the pupil is dilated. Caution should be used in dilating the pupil as this may cause the lens to sublux into the anterior chamber, which occurs if all the zonule fibers are torn. Chronically, the lens may lodge in either the anterior chamber or the vitreous. Marfan syndrome, tertiary syphilis, and homocystinuria may be present and should be considered in patients presenting with lens dislocation.

Emergency Department Treatment and Disposition

A subluxed lens does not always require surgery; partial subluxations may require only a change in refraction. Surgery is required if anterior dislocation of the lens results in papillary block and angle closure glaucoma results.

Pearls

1. Patients may experience lens dislocation with seemingly trivial trauma if they have an underlying coloboma of the lens, Marfan syndrome, homocystinuria, or syphilis.
2. Iridodonesis is a trembling movement of the iris noted after rapid eye movements and is a sign of occult posterior lens dislocation.
3. Phacodonesis is a tremulousness of the lens itself caused by disruption of the zonule fibers.
4. Lens dislocation or subluxation is commonly associated with traumatic cataract formation.
5. Other associated injuries include hyphema, vitreous hemorrhage, and globe rupture.

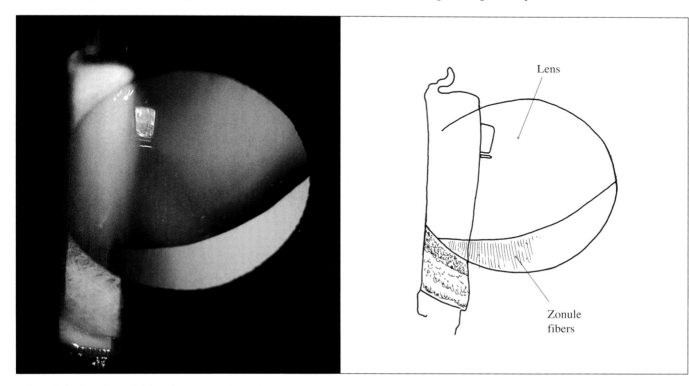

FIGURE 4.16 ■ Lens Dislocation. Lens dislocation revealed during slit-lamp examination. Note the zonule fibers, which normally hold the lens in place. (Photo contributor: Department of Ophthalmology, Naval Medical Center, Portsmouth, VA.)

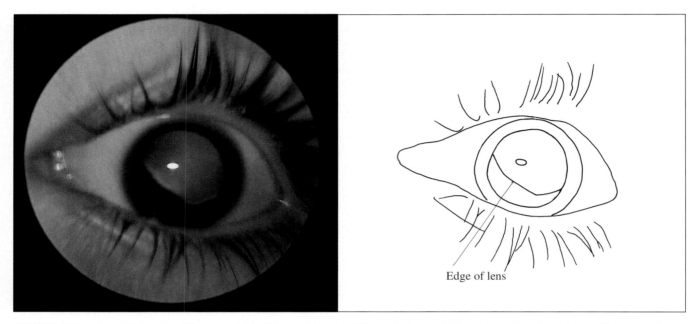

Edge of lens

FIGURE 4.17 ■ Lens Dislocation. The edge of this dislocated lens is visible with the pupil dilated as an altered red reflex. (Photo contributor: Department of Ophthalmology, Naval Medical Center, Portsmouth, VA.)

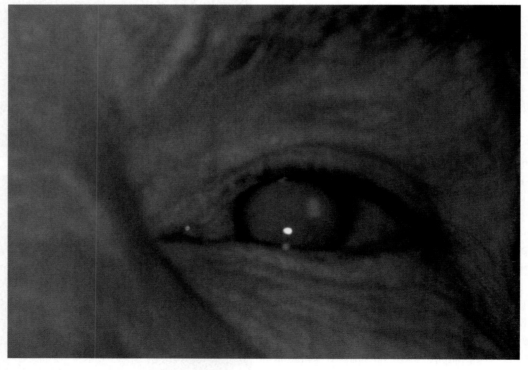

FIGURE 4.18 ■ Lens Dislocation. Complete lens dislocation prolapsed into the anterior chamber. (Photo contributor: R. Jason Thurman, MD.)

Clinical Summary

Penetrating globe injuries can be subtle and easily overlooked. All are serious injuries. Signs to look for are loss of anterior chamber depth caused by leakage of aqueous humor, a teardrop-shaped ("peaked") pupil, or prolapse of choroid through the wound.

Emergency Department Treatment and Disposition

All open globe injuries require urgent specialty consultation. A rigid eye shield should be immediately placed over the affected eye. If a specifically designed rigid shield (eg, Fox metal eye shield) is unavailable, the bottom of a Styrofoam cup may be used. Do not use a pressure patch. Tonometry to measure pressures is strictly contraindicated. The utmost care should be exercised in any attempts to examine the injured eye. It is imperative to avoid inadvertent pressure on the globe with resulting irreversible expulsion of choroid through the wound. Intravenous antibiotics appropriate to cover gram-positive organisms are indicated. Consider adding gram-negative coverage for injuries that involve organic foreign bodies. Sedation and aggressive pain management are crucial and should be used liberally to prevent or decrease expulsion of intraocular contents caused by crying, activity, or vomiting. Antiemetics should be given as prophylaxis. Tetanus status should be updated as necessary. Penetrating globe injuries may be accompanied by other significant blunt trauma. Always consider the possibility that foreign bodies may have penetrated through the globe into the posterior orbit and possibly extend into the cranial vault.

Pearls

1. Protruding foreign bodies should be stabilized without manipulation until definitively treated in the operating room.
2. Control of pain, activity, and nausea may be sight saving and requires proactive use of appropriate medications.
3. Use of lid retractors is preferred to open the eyelids of trauma victims with blepharospasm or massive swelling when such examination is indicated. Attempts to use fingers can inadvertently increase the pressure on the globe.
4. Emergency department ultrasound with a high-frequency probe using no pressure technique can be a useful adjunct to detect posterior pole injury at the bedside.

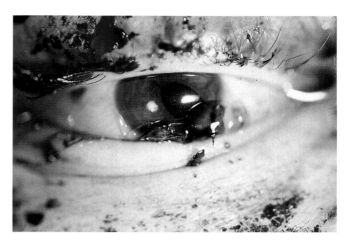

FIGURE 4.19 ■ Open Globe. This injury is not subtle; extruded ocular contents (vitreous) can be seen; a teardrop pupil is also present. (Photo contributor: Alan B. Storrow, MD.)

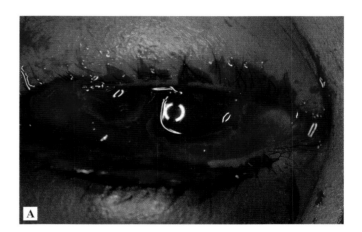

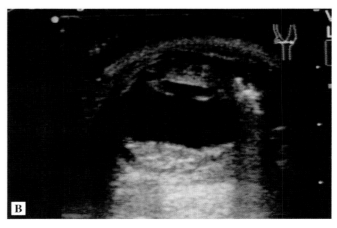

FIGURE 4.20A and B ■ Penetrating Globe. (A) This penetrating injury shows an "eight-ball" hyphema. (B) Bedside ultrasound shows both intraocular and anterior chamber hemorrhage. (Photo contributor: Kevin J. Knoop, MD, MS.)

5. Penetrating globe injuries are a relative contraindication to the sole use of depolarizing neuromuscular blockade (eg, succinylcholine). Consider a "de-fasciculating" dose of a nondepolarizing agent as a pretreatment to avoid increasing intraocular pressure.

6. CT scanning is the most readily available and sensitive modality to evaluate penetrating injuries. Some nonmetallic objects such as wood, glass, or plastic may be difficult to visualize with CT. MRI is preferable in these cases and is excellent at demonstrating associated soft-tissue injuries to the globe and orbit. MRI is contraindicated when a metallic foreign body is suspected.

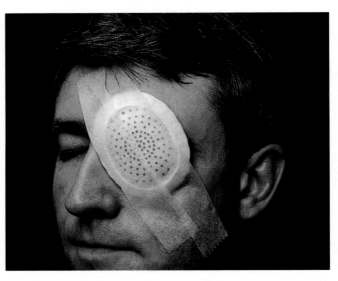

FIGURE 4.22 ■ Protective Metal (Fox) Shield. A protective shield is used in the setting of a suspected or confirmed perforating injury. (Photo contributor: Kevin J. Knoop, MD, MS.)

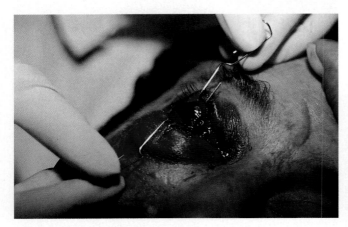

FIGURE 4.21 ■ Eyelid Retractors. Retractors fashioned from paper clips can safely be used when standard retractors are not available. (Photo contributor: Kevin J. Knoop, MD, MS.)

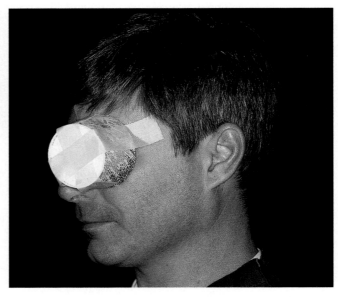

FIGURE 4.23 ■ Protective Shield. A protective shield is readily fashioned from a paper cup if a metal shield is not available. (Photo contributor: Kevin J. Knoop, MD, MS.)

Clinical Summary

A forceful blow to the eye may result in a ruptured globe. The diagnosis is obvious when orbital contents are seen spilling from the globe itself. Occult presentations occur when there is only a tiny rent in the sclera. Ruptures at the limbus, the margin between the cornea and sclera, may cause a small amount of iris to herniate resulting in an irregularly shaped "teardrop pupil." A "peaked" or teardrop pupil may also result from a penetrating foreign body. Mechanism of injury is the key to distinguishing these two causes. Another associated finding is bloody chemosis involving the bulbar conjunctiva. This may be distinguished from a simple subconjunctival hemorrhage by bulging of the conjunctiva over the wound. A rupture should also be suspected when severe conjunctival hemorrhage exists (covering 360° of the bulbar conjunctiva) following trauma.

Subconjunctival hemorrhage, nontraumatic bloody chemosis, corneal-scleral laceration, intraocular foreign body, iridodialysis, and traumatic lens dislocation may have a similar presentation. A coloboma of the iris may appear similar to a teardrop pupil.

Emergency Department Treatment and Disposition

Urgent specialty consultation and operative management are mandatory. The eye should be protected by a rigid eye shield, and all further examination and manipulation of the eye should be discouraged to prevent prolapse or worsening prolapse of choriouveal structures. Tetanus status should be addressed. Intravenous antibiotics to cover suspected organisms are appropriate. Adequate sedation and use of parenteral analgesics is encouraged. Antiemetics should be given proactively, since vomiting may result in further prolapse of intraocular contents. CT scanning should be considered if the presence of a foreign body is suspected.

Pearls

1. The eyeball may appear deflated or the anterior chamber excessively deep. Intraocular pressure will likely be decreased, but measurement is contraindicated, since this may worsen herniation of intraocular contents.
2. Rupture usually occurs where the sclera is the thinnest, at the point of attachment of extraocular muscles and at the limbus.

3. A teardrop pupil may easily be overlooked in the triage process or in the setting of multiple traumatic injuries.
4. Seidel test (see Fig. 4.14) (instillation of fluorescein and observing for fluorescein streaming away from the injury) may be used to diagnose subtle perforation.
5. Penetrating globe injuries are a relative contraindication to the sole use of depolarizing neuromuscular blockade (eg, succinylcholine). Consider a "de-fasciculating" dose of a nondepolarizing agent as a pretreatment to avoid increasing intraocular pressure.

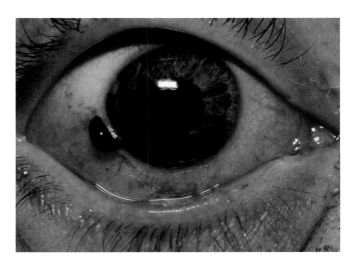

FIGURE 4.24 ■ Prolapsed Iris. A teardrop pupil is present, with a small amount of iris herniating from a rupture at 8 o'clock on the limbus. (Photo contributor: Lawrence B. Stack, MD.)

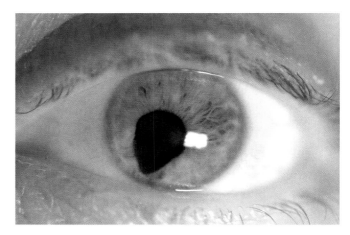

FIGURE 4.25 ■ Iris Coloboma. Iris coloboma is a congenital finding resulting from incomplete closure of the fetal ocular cleft. It appears as a teardrop pupil and may be mistaken for a sign of scleral rupture. (Photo contributor: R. Jason Thurman, MD.)

Clinical Summary

Any trauma to the eye that disrupts the normal architecture of the lens may result in the development of a traumatic cataract—a lens opacity. The mechanism behind cataract formation involves fluid infiltration into the normally avascular and acellular lens stroma. The lens may be observed to swell with fluid and become cloudy and opacified. The time course is usually weeks to months following the original insult. Cataracts that are large enough may be observed by the naked eye. Those that are within the central visual field may cause blurring of vision or distortion of light around objects (eg, halos).

Emergency Department Treatment and Disposition

No specific treatment is rendered in the emergency department for cases of delayed traumatic cataract. Routine ophthalmologic referral is indicated for most cases.

Pearls

1. Traumatic cataracts are frequent sequelae of lightning injury. All victims of lightning strike should be warned of this possibility.
2. Cataracts may also occur as a result of electric current injury to the vicinity of the cranial vault.
3. Leukocoria results from a dense cataract, which causes loss of the red reflex.
4. If a cataract develops sufficient size and "swells" the lens, the trabecular meshwork may become blocked, producing glaucoma.

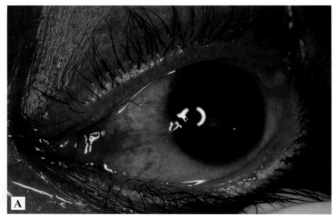

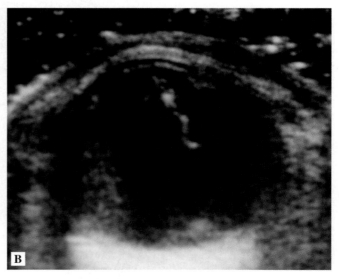

FIGURE 4.27A and B ■ Traumatic Cataract. (**A**) This acute traumatic cataract is seen as a milky cornea at the time of injury. (**B**) Bedside ultrasound shows a collapsed anterior chamber and intraocular foreign body. (Photo contributor: Kevin J. Knoop, MD, MS.)

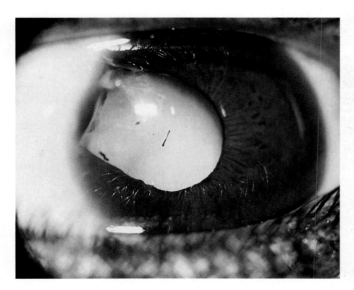

FIGURE 4.26 ■ Traumatic Cataract. This mature traumatic cataract is seen as a large lens opacity overlying the visual axis. A traumatic iridodialysis is also present. (Photo contributor: Dallas E. Peak, MD.)

Clinical Summary

Eyelid lacerations should always prompt a thorough search for associated injury to the globe, penetration of the orbit, or involvement of other adnexal structures (eg, lacrimal glands, canaliculi, puncta). Depending on the mechanism of injury, a careful exclusion of foreign body may be indicated.

Emergency Department Treatment and Disposition

Eyelid lacerations involving superficial skin can be repaired with 6-0 nonabsorbable interrupted sutures, which should remain in place for 3 to 5 days. Lacerations through an anatomic structure called the gray line, situated on the palpebral edge, require diligent reapproximation and should be referred. Other injuries that require specialty consultation for repair include:

— Lacerations through the lid margins: these require exact realignment to avoid entropion or ectropion.

— Deep lacerations through the upper lid that divide the levator palpebrae muscles or their tendinous attachments: these must be repaired with fine absorbable suture to avoid ptosis.

— Lacrimal duct injuries: these are repaired by stenting of the duct to avoid permanent epiphora.

— Medial canthal ligaments: these must be repaired to avoid drooping of the lids and telecanthus.

— The most important objectives are to rule out injury to the globe and to search diligently for foreign bodies.

Pearls

1. Lacerations of the medial one-third of the lid or epiphoria (tearing) raises suspicion for injury to the lacrimal system or the medial canthal ligament.

2. A small amount of adipose tissue seen within a laceration is a sign that perforation of the orbital septum has occurred (there is no subcutaneous fat in the eyelids).

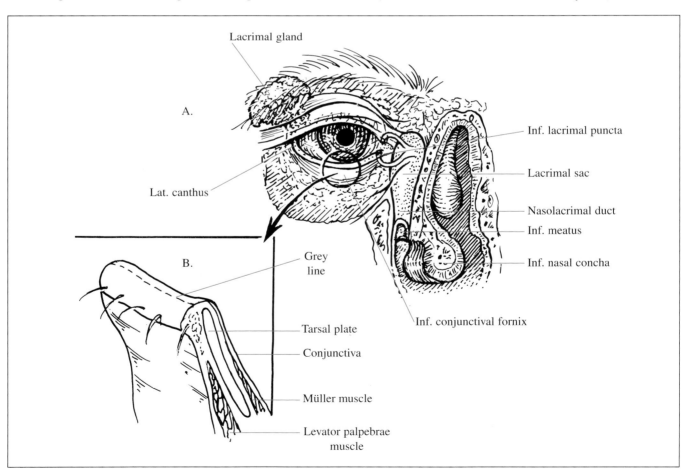

FIGURE 4.28 ■ Eyelid and Adnexa Anatomy. Ocular trauma should prompt examination of surrounding anatomic structures for associated injuries.

3. Laceration of the levator palpebrae musculature or tendinous attachments may result in traumatic ptosis.

4. Laceration of the canthal ligamentous support is suggested when there is rounding of the lid margins or telecanthus (widening of the distance between the medial canthi).

5. Anesthesia of the forehead may result from supraorbital nerve injury and should be sought prior to instilling local anesthetics.

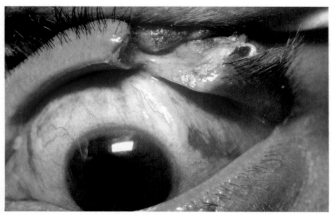

FIGURE 4.30 ■ Eyelid Laceration. Laceration involving the lid margin requires anatomic closure, ideally by a specialist. Careful approximation of the lid margins is required for adequate function. (Photo contributor: Kevin J. Knoop, MD, MS.)

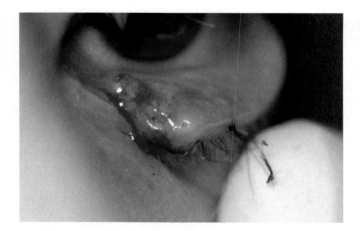

FIGURE 4.29 ■ Eyelid Laceration. This laceration from a dog bite clearly violates the canalicular structures. (Photo contributor: Lawrence B. Stack, MD.)

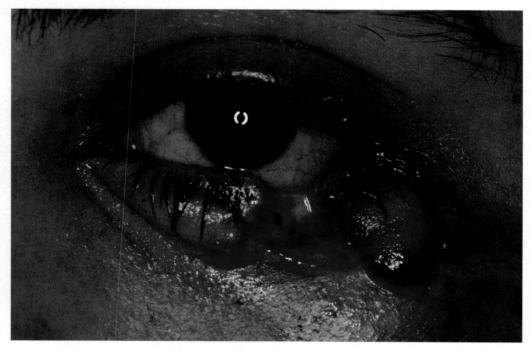

FIGURE 4.31 ■ Eyelid Laceration. Assault resulting in laceration to upper lid involving the tarsal plate. The assailant was wearing a ring. (Photo contributor: Lawrence B. Stack, MD.)

Clinical Summary

Symptomatic ocular exposures involve either immediate or delayed onset of eye discomfort accompanied either by itching, tearing, redness, photophobia, blurred vision, and/or by foreign-body sensation. Conjunctival injection or chemosis may be seen. Abrupt onset of severe symptoms may indicate exposure to caustic alkaline or acidic substances and represent a true ocular emergency. Exposure to defensive sprays or riot-control agents (eg, Mace or tear gas) causes immediate onset of severe burning, intense tearing, blepharospasm, and nasal and oropharynx irritation.

Emergency Department Treatment and Disposition

Copious irrigation should begin immediately at the scene. Acute caustic exposures are triaged to immediate treatment. The conjunctival sac pH should be determined with a broad-range pH paper without delaying treatment. Topical anesthetic drops permit examination and facilitate irrigation. Upper lid conjunctiva is everted to examine for concretions. If pH reads acid or alkali, irrigation with warmed normal saline (NS) or lactated ringers (LR; preferred) solution should be instilled (2-L minimum). Following a short delay for re-equilibration, the pH and symptoms are reassessed. If a normal tear film pH of 7.4 has not been achieved, irrigation is continued. Alkali exposures cause more severe injury (liquefaction necrosis), which penetrates deeper into tissues. Acids are less damaging (coagulation necrosis), which creates a barrier to further penetration. The exception is hydrofluoric acid, which acts as an alkali exposure.

Irrigation should be performed after all exposures. Many chemicals merely cause irritative symptoms; however, some may also denude the corneal epithelium and inflame the anterior chamber. All should undergo slit-lamp examination to document corneal epithelial defects or anterior chamber inflammation. Cycloplegics may benefit to reduce ciliary spasm and pain. Tetanus status should be addressed.

Pearls

1. Immediate onset of severe symptoms calls for immediate treatment and should prompt consideration of alkali or acid exposure.
2. Prolonged (up to 24 hours) irrigation may be needed for alkaline exposures.
3. Concretions from the exposure agent may form deep in the conjunctival fornices and must be removed to prevent ongoing injury.
4. A Morgan lens or other eye irrigation system is ideal for effective treatment as blepharospasm severely limits effectiveness of IV tubing alone.

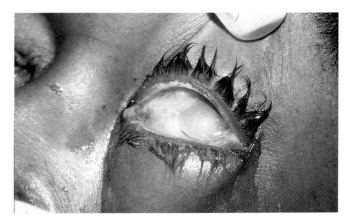

FIGURE 4.32 ■ Alkali Burn. Diffuse opacification of the cornea occurred from a "lye" burn to the face. (Photo contributor: Stephen W. Corbett, MD.)

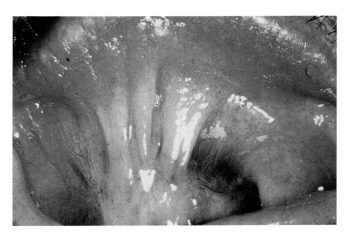

FIGURE 4.33 ■ Caustic Burn Adhesions (Symblepharon). Scarring of both palpebral and bulbar conjunctivae results in severe adhesions between the lids and the globe. (Photo contributor: Arden H. Wander, MD.)

Chapter 5

EAR, NOSE, AND THROAT CONDITIONS

Edward C. Jauch
Sean P. Barbabella
Francisco J. Fernandez
Kevin J. Knoop

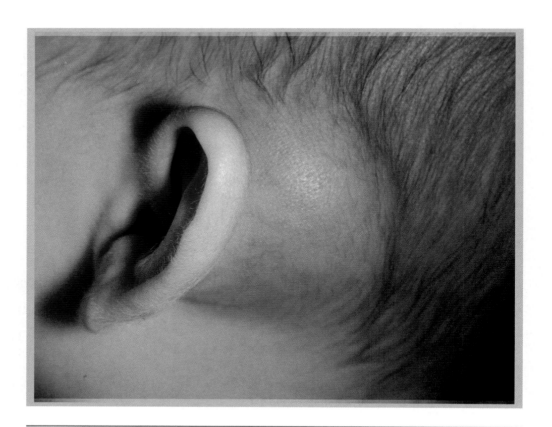

Clinical Summary

Children between the ages of 6 months and 2 years are at highest risk of developing acute otitis media (AOM). Children at increased risk of recurrent AOM contract their first episode prior to 12 months, have a sibling with a history of recurrent AOM, are in day care, or have parents who smoke.

AOM is an acute inflammation and effusion of the middle ear. Otoscopy should focus on color, position, translucency, and mobility of the tympanic membrane (TM). Compared with the TM of a normal ear, AOM causes the TM to appear dull, erythematous or injected, bulging, and less mobile. The light reflex, normal TM landmarks, and malleus become obscured. Pneumatic otoscopy and tympanometry enhance accuracy in diagnosing AOM.

The pathogenesis of AOM is eustachian tube dysfunction, allowing retention of secretions (serous otitis) and seeding of bacteria.

Viral, bacterial, and fungal pathogens cause AOM. The most common bacterial isolates are *Streptococcus pneumoniae*, *Haemophilus influenzae*, *Moraxella catarrhalis*, and *Streptococcus pyogenes*. There is an increased prevalence of antimicrobial resistance for *S pneumoniae* and β-lactamase producing strains of *H influenzae*.

Patient presentations and complaints vary with age. Infants with AOM have vague, nonspecific symptoms (irritability, lethargy, and decreased oral intake). Young children can be irritable, often febrile, and frequently pull at their ears, but they may also be completely asymptomatic. Older children and adults note ear pain, decreased auditory acuity, and occasionally otorrhea.

Emergency Department Treatment and Disposition

Although AOM generally resolves spontaneously, most patients are treated with antibiotics and analgesics. Steroids, decongestants, and antihistamines do not alter the course in AOM but may improve upper respiratory tract symptoms.

Patients should follow up in 10 to 14 days or return if symptoms persist or worsen after 48 hours. Refer patients who have significant hearing loss, have failed two complete courses of outpatient antibiotics during a single event, have chronic otitis media (OM) with or without acute exacerbations, or have failed prophylactic antibiotics to an otolaryngologist for further evaluation, an audiogram, and possible tympanostomy tubes.

Pearls

1. In children, recurrent OM may be due to food allergies.
2. Only 4% of children less than 2 years with OM develop temperatures greater than 104°F. Those with fever higher than 104°F or with signs of systemic toxicity should be closely evaluated for other causes before attributing the fever to OM.
3. Some children over 2 years may qualify for observation for 48 hours prior to initiation of antibiotics.
4. Management of AOM may require narcotic analgesia.
5. Topical Auralgan may decrease pain.

TABLE 5.1	AOM TREATMENT BASED ON AGE, SEVERITY OF ILLNESS, AND CERTAINTY OF DIAGNOSIS	
Age	**Certain Diagnosis**	**Uncertain Diagnosis**
<6 mo	Antibacterial therapy	Antibacterial therapy
6 mo-2 yr	Antibacterial therapy	Antibacterial therapy; observation option if nonsevere
>2 yr	Antibacterial therapy if severe illness: observation option if nonsevere illness	Observation option

Nonsevere illness is mild otalgia and fever <39°C in past 24 hours. Severe illness is moderate to severe otalgia or fever ≥39°C. A certain diagnosis meets all three criteria: (1) rapid onset, (2) signs of middle ear effusion, (3) signs and symptoms of middle ear inflammation.

From American Academy of Pediatrics Subcommittee on Management of Acute Otitis Media. Diagnosis and management of acute otitis media. *Pediatrics.* 2004;113:1451.

TABLE 5.2 ■ TREATMENT RECOMMENDATIONS FOR SEVERE AOM

Temperature ≥39°C or Severe Otalgia or Both	At Diagnosis —Patients Being Treated Initially With Antibacterial Agents		Observation Option —48-72 hours After Initial Management —Clinically Defined Treatment Failure		Antibacterial Agents —48-72 hours After Initial Management —Clinically Defined Treatment Failure	
	Recommended	PCN Allergy	Recommended	PCN Allergy	Recommended	PCN Allergy
No	AMOX 80-90 mg/kg/day	Non-type 1: Cefdinir, cefuroxime, cefpodoxime	AMOX 80-90 mg/kg/day	Non-type 1: Cefdinir, cefuroxime, cefpodoxime	AMOX-CL: 90 mg/kg/day of AMOX with 6.4 mg/kg/day of CLAV	Non-type 1: Ceftriaxone 3 days
		Type 1: Azithromycin, clarithromycin		Type 1: Azithromycin, clarithromycin		Type 1: Clindamycin
Yes	AMOX-CL: 90 mg/kg/day of AMOX with 6.4 mg/kg/day of CLAV	Ceftriaxone 1 or 3 days	AMOX-CL: 90 mg/kg/day of AMOX with 6.4 mg/kg/day of CLAV	Ceftriaxone 1 or 3 days	Ceftriaxone 3 days	Tympano-centesis, clindamycin

Type 1 sensitivity—urticaria or anaphylaxis.

AMOX = Amoxicillin (80-90 mg/kg/day);

AMOX-CLAV = Amoxicillin-clavulanate (90 mg/kg/day AMOX + 6.4 mg/kg/day CLAV).

From American Academy of Pediatrics Subcommittee on Management of Acute Otitis Media. Diagnosis and management of acute otitis media. *Pediatrics*. 113: 2004;1451.

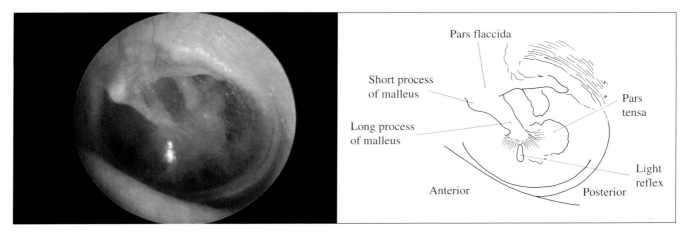

FIGURE 5.1 ■ Normal Tympanic Membrane. Normal tympanic membrane anatomy and landmarks. (Photo contributor: Richard A. Chole, MD, PhD.)

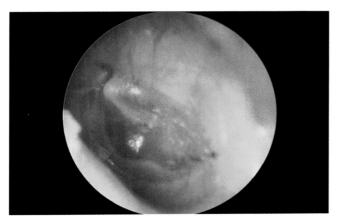

FIGURE 5.2 ■ Early Acute Otitis Media. A mildly erythematous tympanic membrane is seen with a small purulent effusion in the middle ear. (Photo contributor: C. Bruce MacDonald, MD.)

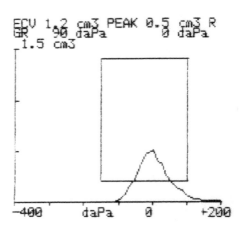

FIGURE 5.4 ■ Tympanogram of Normal Ear. The compliance tracing of a normal ear. (Photo contributor: Lawrence B. Stack, MD.)

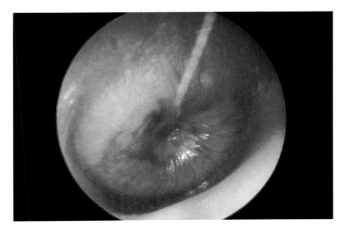

FIGURE 5.3 ■ Acute Otitis Media. The middle ear is filled with purulent material behind an erythematous, bulging tympanic membrane. (Photo contributor: Richard A. Chole, MD, PhD.)

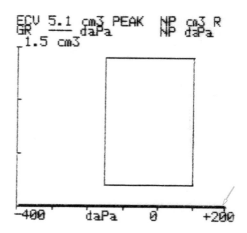

FIGURE 5.5 ■ Tympanogram of Otitis Media. The compliance tracing of an ear with otitis media. The line is flat (arrow). (Photo contributor: Lawrence B. Stack, MD.)

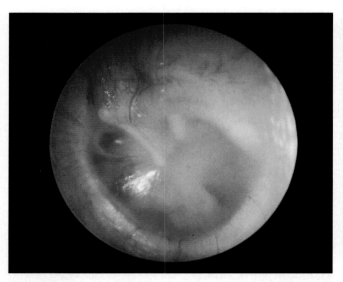

FIGURE 5.6 ■ Serous Otitis Media with Effusion (OME). Serous OME is commonly seen after AOM, but it is also common without this history. Any process that leads to obstruction of a Eustachian tube may cause OME. A clear amber-colored effusion with a single air-fluid level is seen in the middle ear behind a normal tympanic membrane. (Photo contributor: C. Bruce MacDonald, MD.)

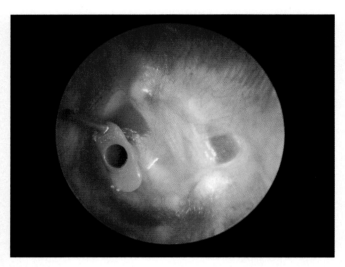

FIGURE 5.8 ■ Tympanostomy Tube. Typical appearance of a tympanostomy tube in the tympanic membrane. These tubes will migrate to the periphery and eventually drop out. Occasionally, they will be found in the external ear canal. (Photo contributor: C. Bruce MacDonald, MD.)

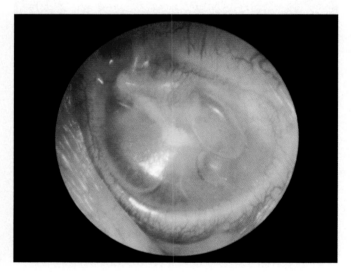

FIGURE 5.7 ■ Serous OME. A clear, amber-colored effusion with multiple air-fluid levels is seen in the middle ear behind a normal tympanic membrane. (Photo contributor: C. Bruce MacDonald, MD.)

Clinical Summary

Bullous myringitis is a direct inflammation and infection of the tympanic membrane (TM) secondary to a viral or bacterial agent. Vesicles or bullae filled with blood or serosanguinous fluid on an erythematous TM are the hallmark of bullous myringitis. Frequently a concomitant otitis media with effusion is noted. Common bacterial agents are *Mycoplasma pneumoniae, Streptococcus pneumoniae,* and *Haemophilus influenzae.*

The onset of bullous myringitis is preceded by an upper respiratory tract infection and is heralded by sudden onset of severe ear pain, scant serosanguinous drainage from the ear canal, and frequently some degree of hearing loss. Otoscopy reveals bullae on either the inner or outer surface of the TM, often filled with bloody fluid. Patients presenting with fever, hearing loss, and purulent drainage are more likely to have other concomitant infections, such as otitis media and otitis externa.

Emergency Department Treatment and Disposition

Differentiation between viral and bacterial etiologies for TM bullae is seldom necessary. Although most episodes resolve spontaneously, many physicians prescribe antibiotics such as trimethoprim-sulfamethoxazole or a macrolide. Warm compresses, topical or strong systemic analgesics, and oral decongestants may provide symptomatic relief. Referral is not necessary in most cases unless rupture of the bullae is required for pain relief.

Pearls

1. Instruct parents that TM rupture may occur with sudden resolution of the pain, purulent drainage, and/or bleeding from the ear canal.
2. Carefully differentiate TM bullae from "bullae" of the ear canal that may mimic cholesteatomas or herpetic vesicles.
3. Facial nerve paralysis associated with clear, fluid-filled TM vesicles is characteristic of herpes zoster oticus.

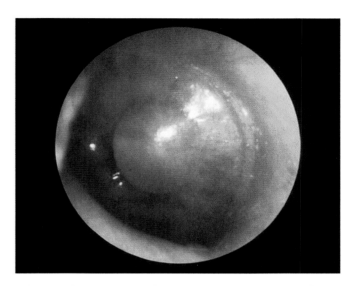

FIGURE 5.9 ■ Bullous Myringitis. A large fluid-filled bulla is seen distorting the surface of the tympanic membrane. (Photo contributor: Richard A. Chole, MD, PhD.)

Clinical Summary

Cholesteatomas are collections of desquamating stratified squamous epithelium found in the middle ear or mastoid air cells. Congenital cholesteatomas are most frequently found in children and young adults. Acquired cholesteatomas originate from perforations of the tympanic membrane, usually marginally or in the pars flaccida, allowing migration of stratified squamous epithelium from the external auditory canal (EAC) into the middle ear.

Cholesteatomas can be locally destructive of the middle ear ossicles and tympanic membrane through the production of collagenases. They may also erode into the temporal bone, inner ear structures, mastoid sinus, or posterior fossa dura. Delays in treatment can lead to permanent conductive hearing loss or infectious complications.

Patients present with progressive hearing loss, foul-smelling ear drainage, and, in advanced stages, pain, headache, dizziness, facial paralysis, fever, or vertigo. Many cholesteatomas have an insidious progression without associated pain or symptoms. Cholesteatomas are seen on otoscopy as either retraction pocket containing white debris or a yellow crust on the tympanic membrane with or without a perforation. A middle ear cholesteatoma appears as a pearly white or yellow middle ear mass behind the tympanic membrane, producing a focal bulge, in contrast to the more diffuse displacement of the tympanic membrane seen in otitis media. Computed tomography (CT) scans may reveal bony destruction.

Osteomas (sometimes called exostoses) are benign bone overgrowths of the external auditory canal found deep in the meatus. Osteomas are often seen in patients with recurrent cold water exposures, such as swimmers and divers. Osteomas are seen on otoscopy as single or multiple round shiny swellings of the bony external auditory canal. A secondary cerumen impaction or an otitis externa may obscure the examination.

Emergency Department Treatment and Disposition

Early diagnosis of cholesteatomas is essential for proper referral. Small cholesteatomas found in retraction pockets

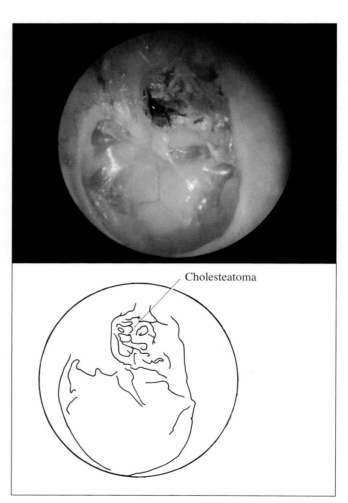

FIGURE 5.11 ■ Acquired Cholesteatoma. A cholesteatoma is seen in this ear. Primary acquired cholesteatomas are thought to arise from gradual invagination of the pars flaccida, usually secondary to trauma. Note the yellow epithelial debris from the cholesteatoma in the area of the pars flaccida. Often there is an effusion and debris, which can distort the anatomy on otoscopy. (Photo contributor: C. Bruce MacDonald, MD.)

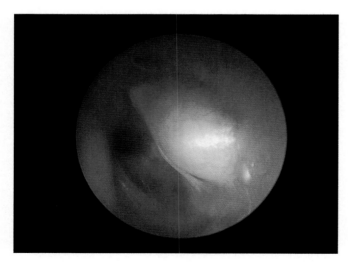

FIGURE 5.10 ■ Congenital Cholesteatoma. A congenital cholesteatoma is seen behind an intact tympanic membrane. (Photo contributor: C. Bruce McDonald, MD.)

can be excised and a tympanostomy tube placed to equilibrate middle ear pressures. More extensive cholesteatomas may require surgical excision, tympanoplasty, and radical mastoidectomy. Osteomas require no medical or surgical management unless they become symptomatic.

Pearls

1. Persistent pain associated with headache, facial motor weakness, nystagmus, or vertigo suggests inner ear or intracranial involvement.
2. Polyps found on the tympanic membrane can indicate the presence of a cholesteatoma and require further evaluation to exclude its presence.

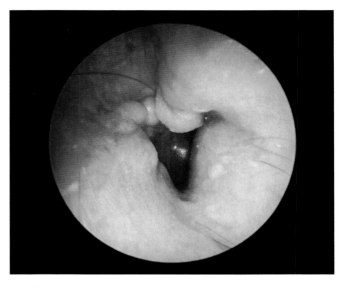

FIGURE 5.12 ▪ Osteomas. Multiple osteomas almost occlude the external auditory canal. The tympanic membrane can be seen in the center, past the osteomas. These lesions are often seen in patients who are cold water swimmers. (Photo contributor: C. Bruce MacDonald, MD.)

Clinical Summary

Acute tympanic membrane (TM) perforations are caused by direct penetrating trauma, barotrauma, otitis media, corrosives, thermal injuries, and iatrogenic causes (foreign-body removal, tympanostomy tubes). TM perforations are occasionally accompanied by injuries to the ossicular chain and temporal bone.

Patients complain of a sudden onset of ear pain, vertigo, tinnitus, and altered hearing after a specific event. Physical examination of the TM reveals a slit-shaped tear or a larger perforation with an irregular border. An acute perforation can have blood on the perforation margin and blood or clot in the canal. Subacute or chronic perforations have smooth margins and a round or ovoid shape.

Emergency Department Treatment and Disposition

Treatment of acute TM perforations is tailored to the mechanism of injury. All easily removable foreign bodies should be extracted. Corrosive exposures require face, eye, and ear decontamination. Antibiotics and irrigation do not improve the rate or completeness of healing unless the injury is associated with OM. Systemic antibiotics should be reserved for perforations associated with OM, penetrating injury, and possibly water-sport injuries (see "Otitis Media" above). Topical steroids impede perforation healing.

Patients are instructed to avoid allowing water to get into the ear while the perforation is healing and to return if symptoms of infection appear. Even though nearly 80% of all TM perforations heal spontaneously, all TM perforations should be referred to an otolaryngologist for follow-up for possible myringoplasty.

Pearls

1. Cortisporin eardrops of any formulation retard spontaneous healing and should be avoided.
2. Traumatic TM perforation associated with cranial nerve deficits or persistent vertigo requires immediate otolaryngology consultation for possible temporal bone fractures or injury to the round or oval window.
3. TM ruptures associated with blast injuries should increase the suspicion for associated injuries such as lung or intra-abdominal injury.

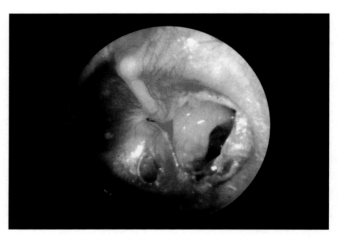

FIGURE 5.13 ■ Acute Tympanic Membrane Perforation. An acute tympanic membrane perforation is seen. Note the sharp edges of the ruptured tympanic membrane. (Photo contributor: Richard A. Chole, MD, PhD.)

Clinical Summary

Otitis externa (OE), or "swimmer's ear," is an inflammation and infection (bacterial or fungal) of the auricle and external auditory canal (EAC). Typical symptoms include otalgia, pruritus, otorrhea, and hearing loss. Physical examination reveals EAC hyperemia and edema, otorrhea, malodorous discharge, occlusion from debris and swelling, pain with manipulation of the tragus, and periauricular lymphadenopathy.

Several factors predispose the EAC to infection: increased humidity and heat, water immersion, foreign bodies, trauma, hearing aids, and cerumen impaction. Bacterial OE is primarily an infection due to *Pseudomonas* species or *Staphylococcus aureus*. Diabetics are particularly prone to infections by *Pseudomonas, Candida albicans,* and, less commonly, *Aspergillus niger*.

Emergency Department Treatment and Disposition

Saline irrigation and suctioning is recommended to thoroughly evaluate the EAC. Topical antibiotic *suspensions* containing polymyxin, neomycin, and hydrocortisone or ciprofloxacin with ear wicks are effective. Topical *solutions* are not pH-balanced and thus are irritating and may cause inflammation in the middle ear if a perforation is present. The new fluoroquinolones can be less irritating and are only given twice a day. Systemic antibiotics are not indicated unless extension into the periauricular tissues is noted. Patients should avoid swimming and prevent water from entering the ear while bathing. Dry heat aids in resolution, and analgesics provide symptomatic relief. Follow-up should be arranged in 10 days for routine cases.

Pearls

1. Resistant cases may have an allergic or edematous component. These typically present with a dry, scaly, itchy EAC and are recurrent and chronic in nature.
2. Drying the EAC after water exposure with a 50:50 mixture of isopropyl alcohol and water or with acetic acid (white vinegar) minimizes recurrence. If the TM is possibly perforated, isopropyl alcohol should be avoided.
3. Often the symptoms are out of proportion to the visible findings, necessitating narcotic analgesia.
4. If a TM perforation is suspected and antibiotic drops are indicated, a suspension is recommended.
5. Consider malignant otitis externa, typically caused by *Pseudomonas aeruginosa* in elderly, diabetics, and immunocompromised patients.

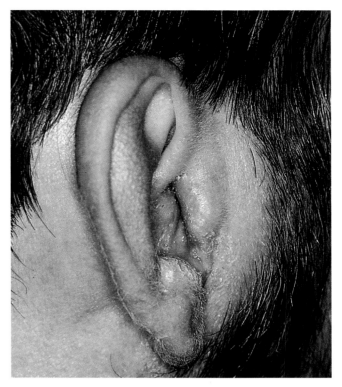

FIGURE 5.14 ■ Otitis Externa. A discharge is seen coming from the external auditory canal, which is swollen and almost completely occluded. An ear wick placed in the EAC facilitates delivery of topical antibiotic suspension and drainage of debris. (Photo contributor: Frank Birinyi, MD.)

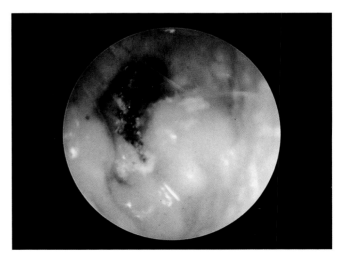

FIGURE 5.15 ■ Aspergillus Otitis Externa. Chronic otitis externa with copious debris, including black spores from *Aspergillus niger*, cottony fungal elements, and wet debris. This patient had been treated with topical and systemic antibiotics. (Photo contributor: C. Bruce MacDonald, MD.)

Clinical Summary

Mastoiditis is an infection or inflammation of the mastoid air cells that usually results from extension of purulent otitis media with progressive destruction and coalescence of air cells. Medial wall erosion can cause cavernous sinus thrombosis, facial nerve palsy, meningitis, brain abscess, and sepsis. With the use of antibiotics for acute otitis media, the incidence of mastoiditis has fallen sharply.

Patients present with fever, chills, postauricular ear pain, and frequently discharge from the external auditory canal. Patients may have tenderness, erythema, swelling, and fluctuance over the mastoid process; proptosis of the pinna; erythema of the posterior-superior external auditory canal wall; and purulent otorrhea through a tympanic membrane perforation.

Emergency Department Treatment and Disposition

Initial evaluation includes a thorough head, neck, and cranial nerve examination. Contrasted computed tomography of the head or mastoid may reveal bony extension and intracranial involvement.

Penicillinase-resistant penicillins, amoxicillin-clavulanic acid, third-generation cephalosporins, and the newer macrolides are effective in mild cases of mastoiditis. Severe cases require parenteral semisynthetic penicillins, cephalosporins, or vancomycin. Mastoiditis requires close follow-up and prompt consultation.

Pearls

1. Most patients require admission for parenteral antibiotics to cover *Haemophilus influenzae, Moraxella catarrhalis,* streptococcal species, and *Staphylococcus aureus.*
2. Surgical irrigation and debridement and possibly mastoidectomy are reserved for refractory cases.
3. Delays in treatment can result in significant morbidity and mortality.
4. Chronic mastoiditis describes chronic otorrhea of at least 2 months duration. It is often associated with craniofacial anomalies.

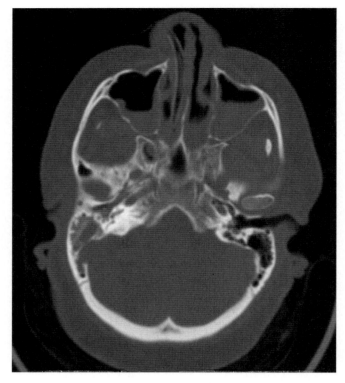

FIGURE 5.16 ■ Acute Mastoiditis. Postauricular swelling, redness, and proptosis in a young girl with acute mastoiditis and sinusitis. (Photo contributor: Lawrence B. Stack, MD.)

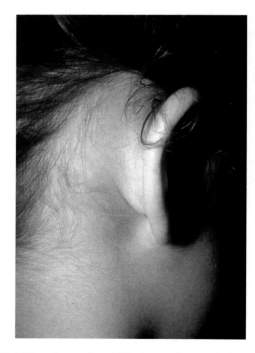

FIGURE 5.17 ■ Acute Mastoiditis. Bone window of a head CT scan which demonstrates fluid in the right mastoid air cells. Maxillary sinus disease is also present. (Photo contributor: Lawrence B. Stack, MD.)

Clinical Summary

Auricular perichondritis is a bacterial infection of the overlying skin and perichondrium of the ear. By definition, it spares the auricular cartilage. Causative organisms include *Pseudomonas aeruginosa*, *Staphylococcus aureus*, and *Streptococcus pyogenes*. Activities predisposing to auricular perichondritis include surgery, ear piercing, burns, frostbite, insect bites, and contact sports. Auricular perichondritis may be an extension of otitis externa. The clinical diagnosis includes a swollen, tender, erythematous, and warm auricle, which may involve the ear lobule. The tympanic membrane is unaffected. Fever may be present. Infectious perichondritis may be confused with relapsing polychondritis, an autoimmune condition which typically involves the cartilage of the ears, nose and trachea.

Emergency Department Treatment and Disposition

Outpatient management of the healthy patient includes an oral fluoroquinolone and follow-up in 48 hours. Hospitalization for IV antibiotics in the immunocompromised and diabetic patient is advised. Ciprofloxacin or ofloxacin otic drops should be used if the external canal is involved. Relapsing polychondritis is treated as an outpatient with prednisone if it involvement is confined to the ear.

Pearls

1. *P aeruginosa* is the most common bacteria causing auricular perichondritis.
2. Ear piercing is the most common activity resulting in auricular perichondritis.
3. Findings of fluctuance and auricular deformity suggest auricular chondritis, a complication of perichondritis.

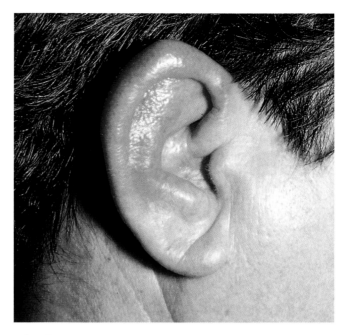

FIGURE 5.18 ■ Perichondritis. The pinna is swollen and erythematous. No concomitant otitis externa, mastoiditis, or furuncle is noted. (Photo contributor: Lawrence B. Stack, MD.)

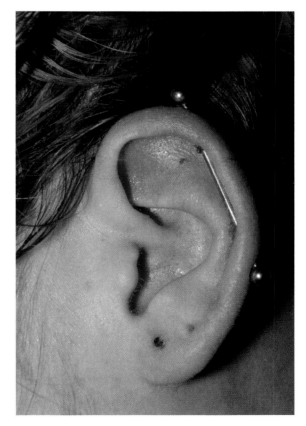

FIGURE 5.19 ■ Perichondritis. Erythema is seen surrounding the piercing sites of the ear this patient in DKA. (Photo contributor: Lawrence B. Stack, MD.)

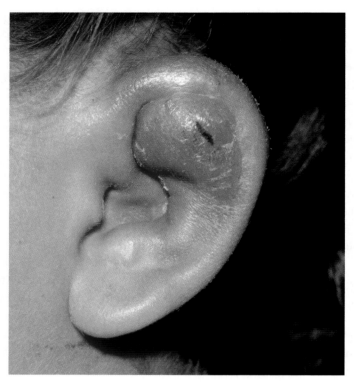

FIGURE 5.20 ■ Auricular Chondritis. Deformity of the auricular cartilage is seen in this patient with chondritis. Ear piercing caused the initial insult to this pinna. (Photo contributor: Lawrence B. Stack, MD.)

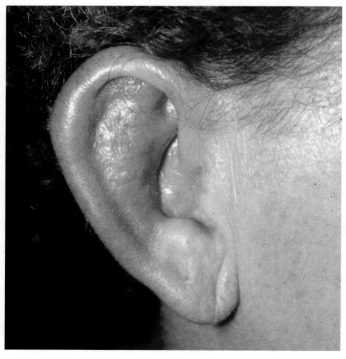

FIGURE 5.21 ■ Relapsing Polychondritis. Erythema of the right pinna that spares the lobe. A month prior the left pinna was involved and was treated as infectious perichondritis. (Photo contributor: Lawrence B. Stack, MD.)

Clinical Summary

Herpes zoster oticus (HZO), or Ramsay Hunt syndrome, is the second most common cause of facial paralysis, representing 3% to 12% of cases. The syndrome consists of facial and neck pain, auditory symptoms, and facial palsy associated with the reactivation of latent varicella zoster virus in the facial nerve and geniculate ganglion. Patients first note pruritus, followed by pain out of proportion to the physical examination over the face and ear. Patients may have vertigo, hearing loss from involvement of the eighth cranial nerve, tinnitus, rapid onset of facial paralysis, decrease in salivation, loss of taste sensation over the posterolateral tongue, and vesicles on the ear, external auditory canal, and face.

Emergency Department Treatment and Disposition

The diagnosis of HZO is based largely on history and physical examination. Tzanck preparations may be difficult because of the vesicles' location. Magnetic resonance imaging (MRI) with contrast may show enhancement of the geniculate ganglion and facial nerve, but it is not required to make the diagnosis.

Oral acyclovir, 800 mg five times a day for 7 to 10 days, famciclovir, 500 mg tid for 7 days, or valacyclovir 1 g po bid for 10 days and oral steroids (prednisone 60 mg/day) in combination with antivirals are mainstays of treatment. It is important to protect the involved eye from corneal abrasions and ulcerations by using lubricating drops. Referral to a specialist should be made for follow-up care.

Pearls

1. The prognosis for facial paralysis due to HZO is worse than that for Bell palsy. Approximately 10% and 66% of patients with full and partial facial paralysis, respectively, recover fully. The prognosis improves if the symptoms of HZO are preceded by the vesicular eruption.
2. The combination of acyclovir with prednisone produces better outcomes than with either agent alone.

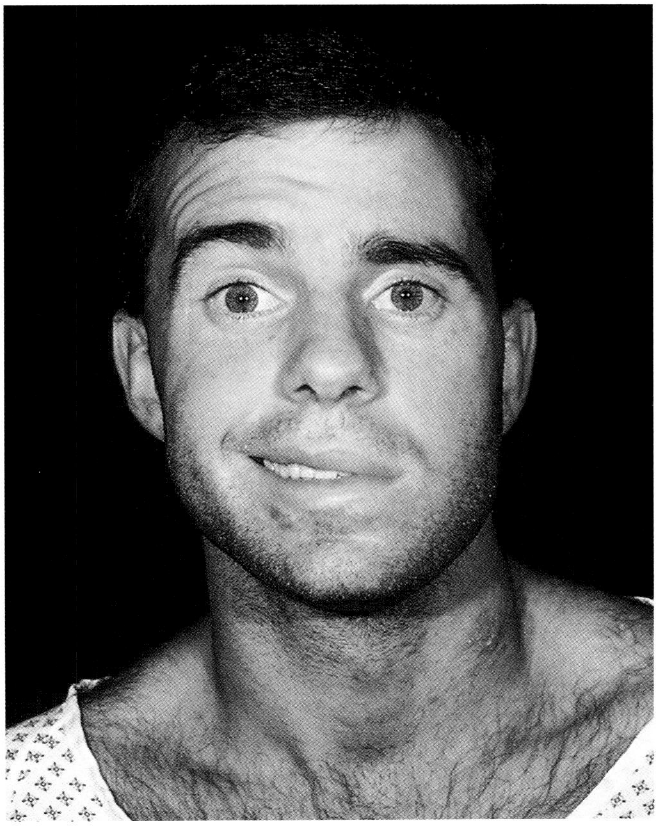

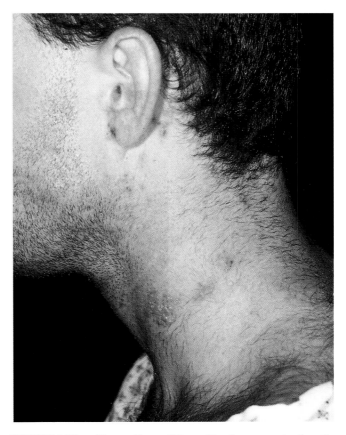

FIGURE 5.22 ■ Herpes Zoster Oticus. Facial palsy in a young adult. Note the vesicular eruptions on the neck. (Photo contributor: Frank Birinyi, MD.)

FIGURE 5.23 ■ Herpes Zoster Oticus. On closer examination, the vesicles extend up the neck to the external auditory canal. (Photo contributor: Frank Birinyi, MD.)

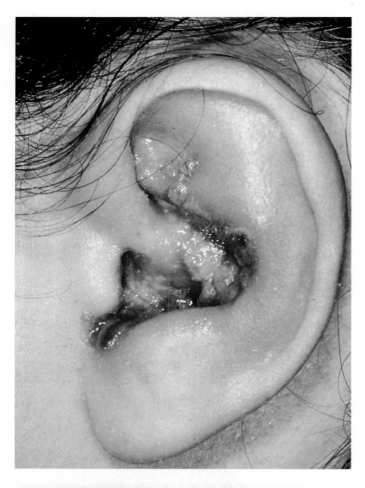

FIGURE 5.24 ■ Herpes Zoster Oticus. Erythema and drainage coming from the EAC is seen in this patient with herpes zoster oticus. Otitis externa can have a similar appearance but does not have vesicles, as seen in this patient. (Photo contributor: Robin T. Cotton, MD.)

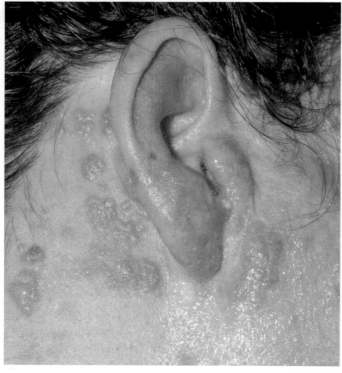

FIGURE 5.25 ■ Herpes Zoster Oticus. Vesicles of zoster are clearly seen in this patient. (Photo contributor: Lawrence B. Stack, MD.)

Clinical Summary

Cranial nerve (CN) VII innervates the facial muscles via the five branches of the motor root, the submandibular, sublingual, and lacrimal glands, and the taste organs on the anterior two-thirds of the tongue; and it provides sensation to the pinna of the ear. CN VII (facial) palsy may occur as an isolated finding or as part of a constellation of symptoms. Facial palsies are either central or peripheral. Central lesions occur before or proximal to the CN VII nucleus in the pons. Lesions distal to the nucleus are classified as peripheral lesions. The ipsilateral frontalis muscle is functional or "spared" in central lesions, since it receives innervation in the nucleus from both ipsilateral and contralateral motor cortices. Peripheral injuries involve the entire side of the face, including the forehead, thus the forehead is not "spared."

The most common etiology of seventh-nerve dysfunction is idiopathic and called Bell palsy. Sixty percent have a viral prodrome. There is no age, sex, or racial predilection. The incidence is higher in pregnant women, diabetics, and those with a family history of Bell palsy. It is bilateral in less than 1% of patients. Patients have an acute onset of facial weakness and may have numbness or pain on the ipsilateral face, ear, tongue, and neck as well as a decrease or loss of ipsilateral tearing and saliva flow. Hearing is preserved.

The prognosis is variable. Facial weakness has a better prognosis for full recovery than complete paralysis. Palsies due to herpes zoster have a protracted course, and many do not fully resolve. In comparison, 80% of patients with Bell palsy due to other causes completely recover within 3 months. The recurrence rate is 7% to 10%.

Emergency Department Treatment and Disposition

Initial evaluation is directed by the history. The examination should include a thorough examination of the ear (including sensorineural or conductive hearing loss), the eye (including lacrimation), and the cranial nerves—especially extraocular muscles (EOMs). Motor function of the seventh cranial nerve is evaluated by having the patient raise their eyebrows, smile, pucker, and frown. No single laboratory test is diagnostic. Screening CT or MRI of the head is of little value in the absence of additional findings on physical examination.

Current recommendations include steroids with antiherpetic antivirals. A typical regimen is prednisone, 60 mg a day and valcyclovir 1000 mg three times daily, for 7 days. If treated within the first 3 weeks, steroids may decrease the sequelae of

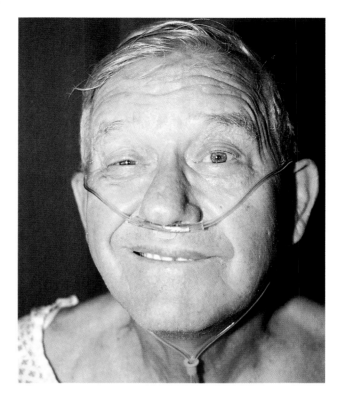

FIGURE 5.26 ■ Central Seventh-Nerve Palsy. Central facial nerve paralysis with forehead sparing. (Photo contributor: Frank Birinyi, MD.)

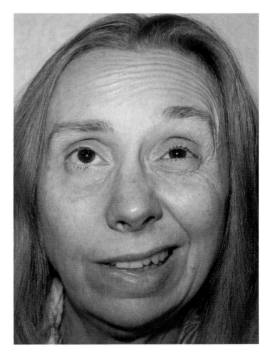

FIGURE 5.27 ■ Peripheral Seventh-Nerve Palsy. A peripheral nerve paralysis involving the entire ipsilateral face, including the forehead, is seen in this patient with Bell palsy. (Photo contributor: Lawrence B. Stack, MD.)

Bell palsy. Eye lubricants (Celluvisc, Lacrilube) and taping or patching of the eye at night help prevent keratitis and ulceration. Referral to a neurologist should be made for follow-up care.

Pearls

1. Facial nerve paralysis is a symptom, not a diagnosis. The etiology of the paralysis must be known before a diagnosis can be made.
2. If a provisional diagnosis of Bell palsy is made and no resolution of symptoms occurs, the diagnosis must be reconsidered. In patients misdiagnosed with Bell palsy, tumors are the most common missed etiology.
3. The finding of CN VI (lateral rectus) palsy along with CN VII palsy is diagnostic of a CN VI stroke, which involves the ipsilateral CN VII as it partially surrounds the CN VI nucleus. Hence, always evaluate for CN VI palsy when evaluating CN VII palsy.
4. Further emergency department evaluation is required for facial palsy presenting with sparing of the ipsilateral frontalis muscle as this represents a central lesion that may be caused by neoplasm or stroke.

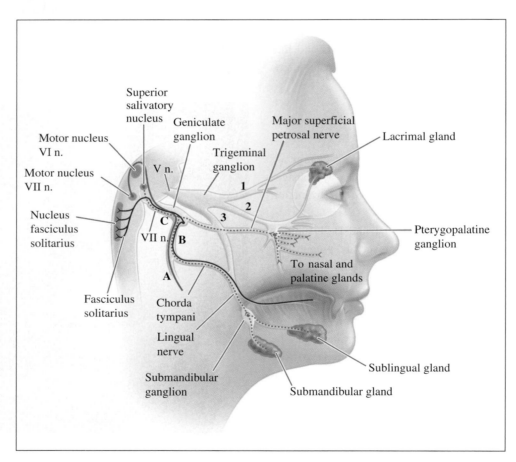

FIGURE 5.28 ■ Cranial Nerve VII Neuropathway. (Reproduced with permission from Fauci AS, Braunwald E, Kasper DL, et al. *Harrison's Principles of Internal Medicine*, 17th ed. New York: McGraw-Hill; 2008, p. 2584.)

Clinical Summary

Angioedema is clinically characterized by acute onset of well-demarcated cutaneous swelling of the face, lips, and tongue; edema of the mucous membranes of the mouth, throat, or abdominal viscera; or nonpitting edema of the hands and feet (often asymmetric). It is either hereditary, allergic, or idiopathic. Hereditary angioedema is an autosomal dominant trait associated with a deficiency of serum inhibitor of the activated first component of complement (C1). Allergic angioedema can result from medications or contrast agents, environmental antigens such as hymenoptera, or local trauma. Complications range from dysphagia and dysphonia to respiratory distress, airway obstruction, and death. Angiotensin converting enzyme (ACE) inhibitor–induced angioedema has a predilection for involvement of the lips, face, tongue, and glottis and like hereditary angioedema, is often refractory to medical therapy.

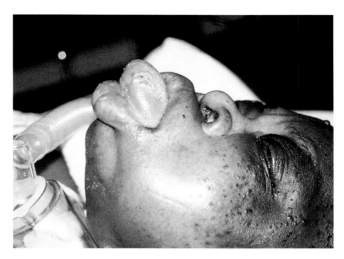

FIGURE 5.29 ■ Angioedema. Severe angioedema of the face and tongue requiring emergent cricothyrotomy. (Photo contributor: W. Brian Gibler, MD.)

Emergency Department Treatment and Disposition

Airway protection remains the primary focus of emergency treatment. Frequent reassessment and early airway management is mandatory as deterioration due to edema formation can be rapid.

Medical therapy includes steroids, H_1 and H_2 histamine blockers, and subcutaneous or intramuscular epinephrine. Chronic angioedema responds better to corticosteroids and H_2 blockers.

Disposition depends on the severity and resolution of symptoms. Patients with symptomatic improvement or showing no worsening after 4 hours of observation may be discharged home. Discontinue suspect medications. Airway involvement requires admission to a monitored environment with surgical airway equipment at the bedside.

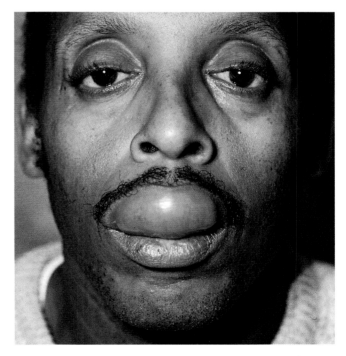

FIGURE 5.30 ■ ACE Inhibitor–Induced Angioedema. Angioedema of the upper lip in a man who had been taking an ACE inhibitor for 2 years. The patient had no previous episodes. (Photo contributor: Kevin J. Knoop, MD, MS.)

Pearls

1. Do not underestimate the degree of airway involvement; act early to preserve airway patency.
2. Angioedema can also cause gastrointestinal and neurologic involvement.
3. Early response to medical intervention does not preclude rebound of symptoms to a greater extent than at presentation.
4. Patients who have been using ACE inhibitors for months or years can still develop angioedema from these agents.

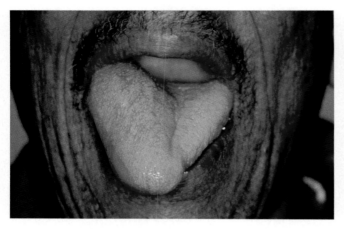

FIGURE 5.31 ▪ ACE Inhibitor–Induced Angioedema. Unilateral tongue swelling in a man who had been taking ACE inhibitors for 5 years. (Photo contributor: Lawrence B. Stack, MD.)

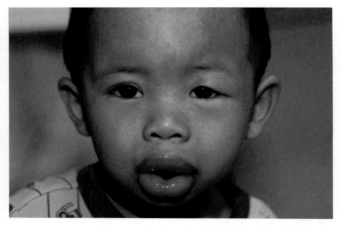

FIGURE 5.32 ▪ Angioedema. Severe lip swelling in a patient with hereditary angioedema. (Photo contributor: Clay B. Smith, MD.)

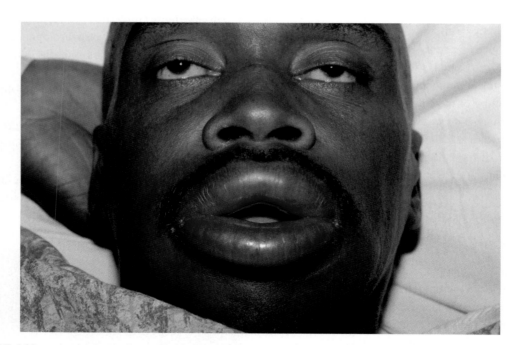

FIGURE 5.33 ▪ Angioedema. Severe lip swelling from an unknown cause. (Photo contributor: Clay B. Smith, MD.)

Clinical Summary

Pharyngitis is an inflammation and commonly an infection of the pharynx and its lymphoid tissues. Viral causes account for 90% of all cases. Group A β-hemolytic streptococci (GABHS) is responsible for up to 50% of bacterial infections. Other bacterial causes include other streptococci, *Mycoplasma pneumoniae, Neisseria gonorrhea,* and *Corynebacterium diphtheriae.* In immunocompromised patients and patients on antibiotics, *Candida* species can cause thrush. Sore throats that last longer than 2 weeks should increase suspicion for either a deep-space neck infection or a neoplastic cause.

Patients with bacterial and especially GABHS pharyngitis present with an acute onset of sore throat, fever and frequently with nausea, vomiting, headache, and abdominal cramping. They may have a mild to moderate fever, an erythematous posterior pharynx and palatine tonsils, tender cervical lymphadenopathy, and palatal petechiae. Classically, the tonsils have a white or yellow exudate with debris in the crypts; however, many patients may not have exudate on examination. Viral pharyngitis is typically more benign, with a gradual onset, lower temperature, and less impressive erythema and swelling of the pharynx. Except for infectious mononucleosis, which can take weeks to resolve, most cases of viral pharyngitis are self-limited, with spontaneous resolution in a matter of days. Lingual and adenoid tonsillitis may also be present.

Emergency Department Treatment and Disposition

Treatment is largely symptomatic except for antibiotics and rehydration. Analgesics, antipyretics, and throat sprays or gargles can provide symptomatic relief. Patients with known or suspected GABHS require antibiotics primarily to prevent rheumatic fever and suppurative complications. The Centor criteria are clinical decision rules developed to help guide physicians in testing and prescribing of antibiotics. Criteria include: (1) tonsillar exudates, (2) tender anterior cervical adenopathy, (3) fever by history, and (4) absence of cough. Patients with fewer than two criteria should not receive either antibiotic treatment or diagnostic testing. Most authorities now favor evaluation using a sensitive rapid streptococcal antigen test (RSAT) for identification of group A β-hemolytic streptococci, without throat culture for negative results, in adult patients with two or more Centor criteria. However, in children it is recommended that all negative RSAT be followed up with a throat culture. Current first-line antibiotic therapies remain a single dose of intramuscular benzathine penicillin or oral penicillin for 10 days. Patients allergic to penicillin should receive erythromycin for primary prophylaxis against rheumatic fever. Other suitable antibiotics include azithromycin, clarithromycin, and second-generation cephalosporins.

Pearls

1. Other manifestations of pharyngitis should be sought in patients with sore throat. Sandpaper rash, Pastia lines, and desquamation are suggestive of scarlet fever. Hepatomegaly and/or splenomegaly should raise suspicion for infectious mononucleosis.

2. Sore throat or chronic pharyngitis that lasts more than 2 weeks must be referred for further evaluation to rule out possible neoplastic or neurologic causes, especially in patients over 50 years old who have a smoking or chewing tobacco history.

3. Recurrent tonsillitis in children merits referral for possible adenoid-tonsillectomy.

4. Amoxicillin should be avoided if infectious mononucleosis is a possibility, as a diffuse maculopapular rash will occur in up to 80% of patients.

5. Pharyngitis itself may be a prodrome for other pathologic conditions, such as measles, scarlet fever, and influenza.

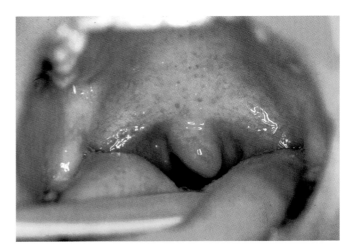

FIGURE 5.34 ■ Palatal Petechiae. Palatal petechiae and erythema of the tonsillar pillars in a patient with streptococcal pharyngitis. (Photo contributor: Kevin J. Knoop, MD, MS.)

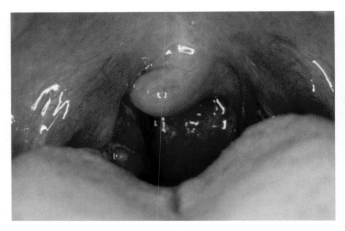

FIGURE 5.35 ■ Exudative Pharyngitis. Intense erythema with scant exudates is seen in this early (<24 hours) case of GABH pharyngitis. (Photo contributor: Kevin J. Knoop, MD, MS.)

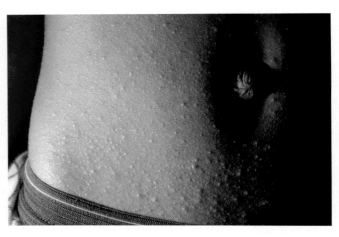

FIGURE 5.38 ■ Scarlet Fever. This sandpaper rash started 2 days after sore throat and fever began in this 6-year-old child. (Photo contributor: Lawrence B. Stack, MD.)

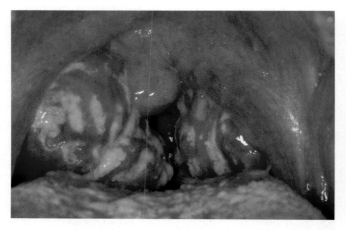

FIGURE 5.36 ■ Tonsilar Exudate. White and yellow cryptic exudates are seen in this patient with rapid strep test proven streptococcal pharyngitis. (Photo contributor: Lawrence B. Stack, MD.)

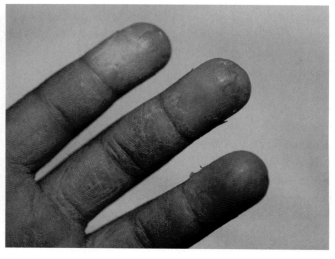

FIGURE 5.39 ■ Desquamating Rash. Desquamation of the fingertips occurred as the scarlitiform rash began to fade. Desquamation also occurred in the groin and toes of this patient. (Photo contributor: Clay B. Smith, MD.)

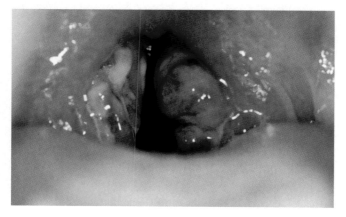

FIGURE 5.37 ■ Infectious Mononucleosis. Nearly kissing exudative tonsils in a patient with elevated liver transaminases and hepatosplenomegaly. (Photo contributor: Lawrence B. Stack, MD.)

Clinical Summary

Septal hematoma is an uncommon complication of direct nasal trauma, often associated with fracture of the nasal septum with or without concomitant nasal bone fracture. Other etiologies include septal surgery or rhinoplasty. Bleeding from submucosal blood vessels leads to an accumulation of blood between the mucoperichondrium and the septal cartilage, which may lead to ischemic avascular necrosis of the underlying cartilage, destruction of the cartilage and saddle deformity (see Figure 1.11b, Saddle Nose Deformity) of the distal nose. The hematoma and any necrotic cartilage may then serve as a nidus for infection, resulting in a septal abscess.

Septal hematoma may lead to cosmetic nasal deformity, chronic sinus infections, recurrent epistaxis, and sleep disturbances. Rarely, it can result in more serious complications such as cavernous sinus thrombosis and meningitis. Since the original trauma is often minor, patients may present days to weeks after the injury. Young children and infants may present with poor feeding, fever, and rhinorrhea. Older children and adults may note bleeding, headache, and more focal pain.

Examination reveals a large, red, round swelling originating off the septum and occluding most of the nasal cavity. The mass is tender to palpation and may cause the outer aspects of the nose to be tender as well. Septal abscesses tend to be more painful and larger than uncomplicated hematomas. Fever is frequently present. *Staphylococcus aureus,* group A β-hemolytic streptococcus, *Haemophilus influenzae,* and *Streptococcus pneumoniae* are the organisms most commonly isolated in septal abscesses.

Emergency Department Treatment and Disposition

Suspicion and recognition are essential in diagnosing septal hematomas. Prompt referral to an otolaryngologist is mandatory for incision of the hematoma and drainage through the mucosal surface. Purulent drainage should be sent for microbiology and culture.

Many authors recommend packing of the nasal cavity to prevent further accumulation. Some surgeons use temporary drains, such as a Penrose, while others place dissolvable sutures in the mucoperichondrium to prevent hematoma reaccumulation.

Pearls

1. Intranasal examination for septal hematoma in all patients with a history of nasal trauma regardless of severity is crucial.

2. Antibiotics are required in septal hematomas with a clinical suspicion for a secondary infection or abscess.

3. The physician must explore the possibility of child abuse in young children and infants with a septal hematoma and abscess.

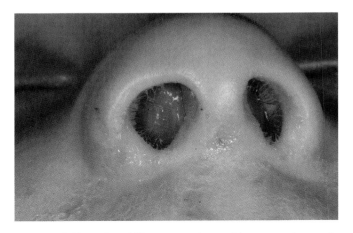

FIGURE 5.40 ■ Septal Hematoma. A septal hematoma is seen in both nares 1 week after blunt nasal trauma. (Photo contributor: Lawrence B. Stack, MD.)

Clinical Summary

Diphtheria is a highly contagious disease caused by the exotoxin-producing bacterium *Corynebacterium diphtheriae*. It is transmitted either by direct contact or through respiratory aerosolization. Many adults are now susceptible to diphtheria because their vaccine-induced immunity decreases over time or owing to decreased opportunity for naturally acquired immunity.

Diphtheria may involve any mucous membrane; but most commonly affects the mucosa of the upper respiratory tract. It typically produces an ulcerated pharyngeal mucosa with a white to gray inflammatory pseudomembrane, classically with a "wet mouse" odor. Patients present with symptoms, in order of frequency, of fever, sore throat, weakness, pain with swallowing, change in voice, loss of appetite, neck swelling, difficulty breathing, and nasal discharge.

While the organism remains localized to the mucosa, hematogenous spread of the exotoxin typically produces myocarditis or peripheral neuropathies. Deaths from diphtheria occur either from tracheobronchial obstruction by the pseudomembrane acutely or cardiac complications several weeks after the primary infection.

Emergency Department Treatment and Disposition

The diagnosis is initially made clinically and confirmed by successful isolation and toxigenicity testing of *C diphtheriae.*

Antitoxin, available from the CDC, is the mainstay of therapy and must be given before laboratory confirmation. Erythromycin or penicillin given promptly when diphtheria is suspected has been shown to decrease both exotoxin production and spread of the bacterium.

Patients require hospital admission for observation of airway obstruction, pulmonary support, and intravenous hydration and antibiotics. Strict isolation is essential.

Pearls

1. Outcome is improved with early treatment; thus the diagnosis of diphtheria must be made clinically and treatment begun empirically before bacteriologic confirmation.
2. Patients with a membranous pharyngitis need to be questioned regarding immunization, exposures, and recent travel.
3. All contacts should have a booster dose of vaccine (TD or Td, depending on age) while nonimmune contacts should also be given prophylactic antibiotics after a throat swab.
4. Myocarditis can be detected in up to two-thirds of cases.

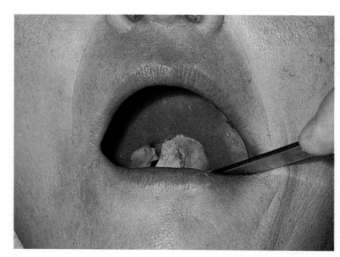

FIGURE 5.41 ■ Diphtheria Pharyngitis. An exudative pharyngitis with a gray pseudomembrane is seen in this patient with diphtheria. (Photo contributor: Peter Strebel, MBChB, MPH, and the *Journal of Infectious Diseases.*)

Clinical Summary

Peritonsillar abscess, or quinsy, is the most common deep neck infection. Although most occur in young adults, immune compromised and diabetic patients are at increased risk. Most abscesses develop as a complication of tonsillitis or pharyngitis, but they can also result from odontogenic spread, recent dental procedures, and local mucosal trauma. They recur in 10% to 15% of patients.

The pathogens involved are similar to those causing tonsillitis, especially streptococcal species, but many infections are polymicrobial and involve anaerobic bacteria. Patients present with a fever, severe sore throat that is often out of proportion to physical findings, localization of symptoms to one side of the throat, trismus, drooling, dysphagia, dysphonia, fetid breath, and ipsilateral ear pain.

During the early stages, the tonsil and anterior pillar are erythematous, appear full, and may be shifted medially. Later, the uvula and soft palate are shifted to the contralateral side. The tonsillar pillar may feel fluctuant and tender on palpation.

Emergency Department Treatment and Disposition

Most patients with signs of an abscess can have needle aspiration performed as the sole surgical drainage procedure and expect a satisfactory outcome. Alternative surgical drainage procedures—including incision and drainage and abscess tonsillectomy—can be performed by an otolaryngologist or oral surgeon. Most can be managed as outpatients on oral antibiotics following drainage. Patients who are immuno-compromised, have airway involvement, appear toxic, or cannot tolerate oral intake require admission for rehydration, parenteral antibiotics, and specialty consultation.

Although penicillin alone is arguably a good first choice, penicillin and metronidazole, amoxicillin with clavulanic acid, clindamycin, or third-generation cephalosporins are also suitable antibiotic choices.

Pearls

1. The value of culturing aspirates is questionable, with a review of several studies showing no clinical benefit from the cultures unless the patient is immunocompromised.

2. A peritonsillar phlegmon may appear similar to an early PTA but is differentiated by lack of fluctuance.

3. A contrasted CT scan of the neck will confirm the presence of a PTA if the diagnosis is uncertain.

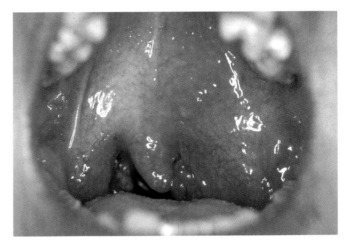

FIGURE 5.42 ■ Early Peritonsillar Abscess. Edema and marked erythema of the left tonsillar pillar in early peritonsillar abscess. (Photo contributor: Kevin J. Knoop, MD, MD)

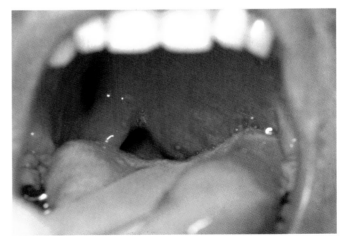

FIGURE 5.43 ■ Peritonsillar Abscess. Acute peritonsillar abscess showing medial displacement of the uvula, palatine tonsil, and anterior pillar. Some trismus is present, as demonstrated by patient's inability to open the mouth maximally. (Photo contributor: Kevin J. Knoop, MD, MS.)

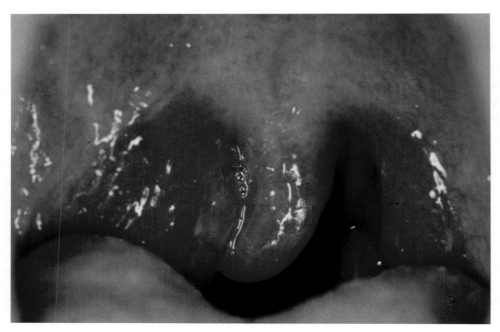

FIGURE 5.44 ■ Peritonsillar Phlegmon. Marked erythema of the tonsillar pillars is seen in this patient currently on oral penicillin. No swelling or fluctuance is present. (Photo contributor: Lawrence B. Stack, MD.)

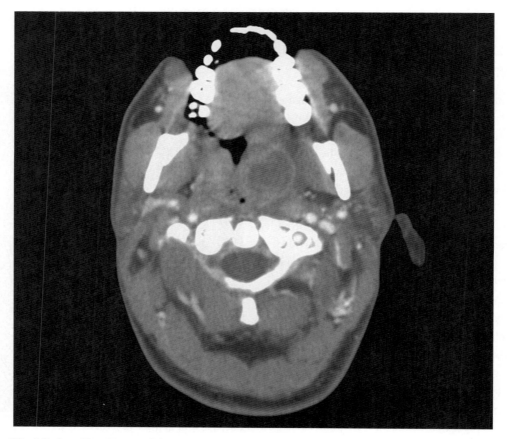

FIGURE 5.45 ■ CT of Peritonsillar Abscess. Ring-enhancing lesion with a hypodense core consistent with a left peritonsillar abscess. (Photo contributor: Lawrence B. Stack, MD.)

Clinical Summary

Epiglottitis or supraglottitis is an infection of the epiglottis and adjacent tissues. Bacterial epiglottitis, a rare but potentially fatal infection, is caused primarily by *Haemophilus influenzae,* but *Streptococcus pneumoniae, Staphylococcus aureus,* and β-hemolytic streptococcus have also been isolated. The advent of the *H influenzae* B vaccination for infants has changed what used to be a disease primarily of children, with a peak age range from 2 to 6 years, to one occurring increasingly in adults. Bacterial epiglottitis occurs most commonly in the winter and spring.

Patients, especially children, with acute epiglottitis appear quite ill. They present with sore throat, fever, drooling, severe dysphagia, dyspnea, muffled or hoarse voice, and occasionally inspiratory stridor. Patients with severe respiratory distress assume the "tripod" position: sitting upright with the neck extended, arms supporting the trunk, and the jaw thrust forward. This position maximizes airway patency and caliber. Adults typically have an indolent course with a prodromal viral illness, but many children have a sudden onset and rapid progression to respiratory distress.

Emergency Department Treatment and Disposition

Airway management is paramount. Even prior to diagnosis, children should be calmed, comforted by a parent, and allowed to assume whatever position they feel is most comfortable. Anesthesiology and ENT should be consulted immediately. Indications for intubation are clinical, but severe stridor and respiratory distress are clear reasons to intervene. Nasotracheal intubation in children is preferred but not when performed blindly. Needle cricothyrotomy can provide temporary oxygenation until a surgical airway is provided.

Radiographs of the neck may reveal the classic "thumb" sign, a thickened epiglottis on the lateral soft-tissue neck radiograph. Visualization of the epiglottis is possible in the stable adult patient via direct and indirect laryngoscopy and fiberoptic nasopharyngoscopy. In children, the top of the swollen epiglottis may be visualized on careful oral examination, whereas pharyngoscopy is typically reserved for an experienced anesthesiologist or otolaryngologist in a controlled setting.

The mainstay of epiglottitis treatment is antibiotics. Third-generation parenteral cephalosporins, ampicillin with sulbactam or trimethoprim-sulfamethoxazole, have proven efficacy in treating epiglottitis. Steroids or epinephrine, either nebulized or subcutaneous, may provide some improvement in edema.

In addition to airway compromise, complications of epiglottitis include epiglottic abscesses, meningitis, pulmonary edema, pneumonia, and empyema (associated with *H influenzae*).

Pearls

1. Transport of patients with suspected epiglottitis must be done by an experienced transport team. The airway must be secured before transport of all but the most stable patients.
2. During intubation, pushing on the patient's chest may cause a bubble to form at the airway orifice, guiding placement of the tube.
3. In areas with a significant prevalence of infection with community-associated methicillin-resistant *S aureus* (MRSA), clindamycin should be considered as part of the empiric choice for gram-positive coverage.
4. Failure to intervene prior to loss of the airway carries a six-fold increase in mortality.
5. If intubation fails, bagging the child may provide adequate oxygenation until a surgical airway can be obtained.

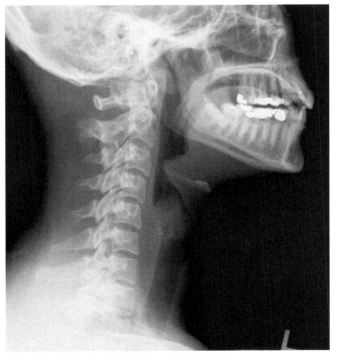

FIGURE 5.46 ■ Adult Epiglottitis. Soft-tissue lateral neck radiograph of an adult with epiglottitis demonstrating the classic "thumb" sign of a swollen epiglottis. (Photo contributor: Kevin J. Knoop, MD, MS.)

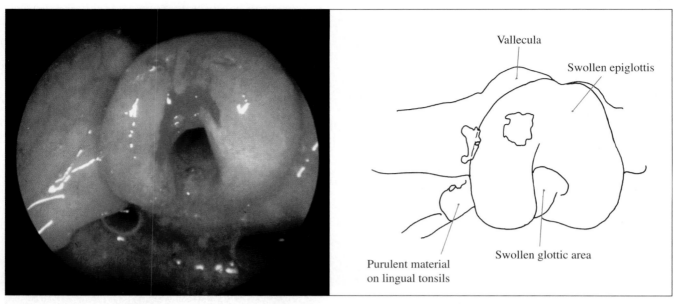

FIGURE 5.47 ■ Adult Epiglottitis. Fiberoptic laryngoscopy showing an edematous epiglottis and glottic area with marked airway compromise in an adult with epiglottitis. (Photo contributor: Edward C. Jauch, MD.)

Clinical Summary

The uvula is the fleshy midline extension of the posterior soft palate. Except for idiopathic, the two most common causes of uvular enlargement are infections and angioedema. Most patients complain of a sore throat, a gagging sensation, or a foreign-body sensation in the back of the mouth.

The infectious etiologies of uvulitis are bacterial, including *Haemophilus influenzae* and streptococci; fungal, such as *Candida albicans*; and viral. Infections are typically extensions from adjacent infections, such as epiglottitis, tonsillitis, peritonsillar abscesses, and pharyngitis. Patients note fever, odynophagia, trismus, facial pain, hoarseness, neck pain, and headache. On examination the uvula is red, firm, swollen, and very tender to palpation.

Angioedema of the uvula, known as the Quincke disease, can be hereditary, acquired, or idiopathic. Medications, allergens, thermal stimuli, pressure, and iatrogenic or accidental trauma can initiate angioedema. In addition to the swollen uvula, patients may note pruritus, urticaria, and wheezing. With uvular edema, the angioedema may involve the face, tongue, and oropharynx. Airway compromise is more common in angioedema of the uvula which appears pale, boggy, and edematous, resembling a large white grape (uvular hydrops).

Emergency Department Treatment and Disposition

Most cases of uvulitis are benign and self-limited. Angioedematous uvulitis is treated with steroids, antihistamines, and epinephrine in severe cases, either subcutaneously or nebulized. For infectious uvulitis, antibiotic coverage is dictated by the primary source of infection. For odontogenic infections, pharyngitis, or tonsillitis with uvulitis, penicillin, clindamycin, or amoxicillin with clavulanate are effective. Epiglottitis associated with uvulitis requires potent *H influenzae* coverage, such as third-generation cephalosporins. Admission is based on severity of airway compromise and accompanying infections.

Pearls

1. Any airway symptom dictates an evaluation of the hypopharynx, either by soft tissue lateral neck radiograph, fiber-optic nasopharyngoscope, or direct laryngoscopy.
2. If the uvula itself is causing enough airway compromise, uvular decompression by longitudinal incisions or a partial uvulectomy can be performed.

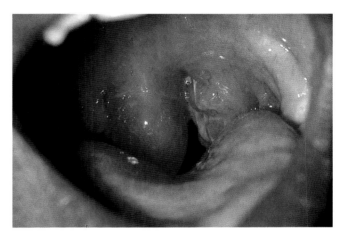

FIGURE 5.48 ■ Uvulitis. Angioedema of the uvula, known as the Quincke's disease. (Photo contributor: Robin T. Cotton, MD.)

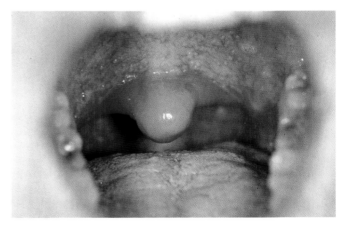

FIGURE 5.49 ■ Uvulitis. Isolated edema of the uvula in a patient who presents with a foreign body sensation of the throat. (Photo contributor: Lawrence B. Stack, MD.)

Clinical Summary

Ranulas are mucoceles (mucous retention cysts) that develop in the floor of the mouth, arising from obstructed sublingual or submandibular ducts or smaller minor salivary glands. Initially the cysts are small and barely noticeable, but over time they can expand outward or deeper into the neck (plunging ranula). Large cysts can displace the tongue forward and upward, making the patient uncomfortable. Unlike those with sialolithiasis, patients with ranulas may not always notice an increase in swelling associated with eating. Physical examination reveals a soft, minimally tender, translucent cyst with dilated veins running over its surface. Unlike carcinomas, no ulceration is noted with ranulas, and they are generally softer.

Emergency Department Treatment and Disposition

Recognition by the physician is essential for proper referral. Definitive treatment is excision or marsupialization, although needle aspiration of the cyst can provide temporary relief. Unless there is a secondary infection, no antibiotic coverage is required.

Pearls

1. Most ranulas are painless and are incidental findings on routine examinations.
2. Ranulas often recur, requiring total excision of the offending salivary gland.

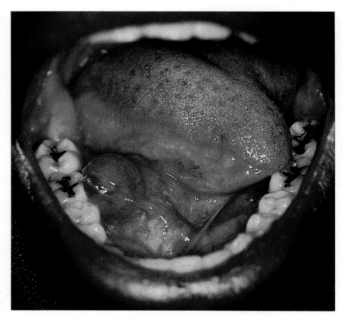

FIGURE 5.50 ■ Ranula. Sublingual ranula, or mucocele, lateral to Wharton duct. The patient was asymptomatic except for being aware of the lesion. (Photo contributor: Kevin J. Knoop, MD, MS.)

Clinical Summary

Sialoadenitis is a general term describing inflammation of any salivary gland. The three major salivary gland pairs are the parotid, submandibular, and sublingual. There are also numerous smaller salivary glands that empty into the oral cavity and all are capable of becoming inflamed. Salivary gland disorders have a broad spectrum of causes, including acute and chronic infections; metabolic, systemic, and endocrine disorders; infiltrative processes; obstructions; allergic inflammation; and neoplastic diseases. Key features in the history are the duration and course of the symptoms, complaints of pain, and unilateral or bilateral location.

Both viral and bacterial infections of the salivary gland can lead to enlarged, swollen, painful masses. Suppurative sialoadenitis is most commonly caused by *Staphylococcus aureus* and is found in patients who are elderly, diabetic, or have poor oral hygiene. It may also follow episodes of dehydration, such as those due to surgery or debilitation. Viral sialoadenitis, such as mumps parotitis, is the most common cause. It occurs with a concomitant viral illness and is usually bilateral, whereas bacterial infections are primarily unilateral.

Obstructive sialoadenitis occurs from a stone or calculus in the salivary gland or duct, most commonly in the submandibular gland. The flow of saliva is obstructed, causing swelling, pain, and firmness. Patients with sialolithiasis note general xerostomia and recurrent worsening of swelling and pain during mealtime.

A thorough head and neck examination is essential, especially a bimanual examination of the major salivary glands. In suppurative sialoadenitis, purulent drainage may be expressed from the submandibular duct (Wharton) or parotid duct (Stensen) and the glands are very tender and painful to examination. Sialolithiasis can manifest as enlargement of the ducts with minimal saliva expressed on stripping and, rarely, a palpable or visible stone or duct thickening. Facial radiographs are of limited utility. Ultrasound or CT may be useful to detect abscesses.

Emergency Department Treatment and Disposition

Treatment of suppurative sialoadenitis requires antibiotics with coverage of *Staphylococcus* and oral flora, rehydration, proper oral hygiene, sialogogues, local heat, and occasionally surgical irrigation and drainage of abscesses. Obstructive sialoadenitis is rarely an emergency. Most salivary stones pass spontaneously without complication, and patients can be discharged home on lozenges to stimulate salivary secretions and expel the stone. Prompt follow-up of sialoadenitis is essential to prevent possible morbidity and mortality associated with infections or neoplasms.

Pearls

1. Examine secretions of both mouth and eyes and elicit any history of dry eyes, keratoconjunctivitis, cutaneous lesions, or rheumatoid arthritis to establish the diagnosis of a systemic disorder.
2. Medications such as antihistamines, psychotropic drugs, and those possessing atropine-like side effects can cause xerostomia.
3. Lack of improvement on antibiotics suggests an abscess or multiple loculated abscesses that require drainage.

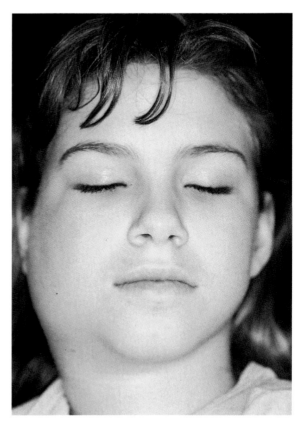

FIGURE 5.51 ■ Suppurative Parotid Sialoadenitis. Painful swelling over the right parotid initially had clear saliva from Stensen duct. (Photo contributor: Kevin J. Knoop, MD, MS.)

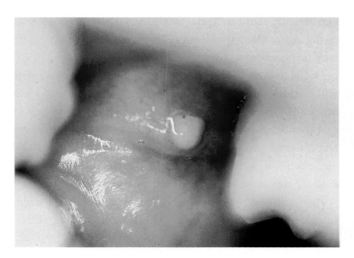

FIGURE 5.52 ■ Suppurative Parotid Sialoadenitis. After applying firm pressure on the cheek, purulent discharge is seen coming from Stensen duct. (Photo contributor: Kevin J. Knoop, MD, MS.)

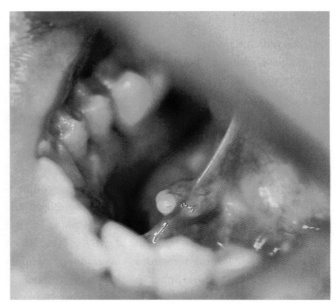

FIGURE 5.54 ■ Suppurative Submandibular Sialoadenitis. After applying firm pressure, purulent discharge is seen coming from Wharton duct. (Photo contributor: Jeffery D. Bondesson, MD.)

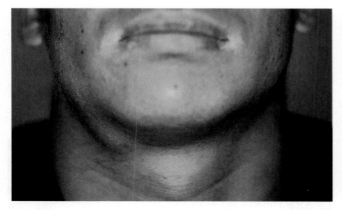

FIGURE 5.53 ■ Suppurative Submandibular Sialoadenitis. Unilateral submandibular swelling. (Photo contributor: Jeffery D. Bondesson, MD.)

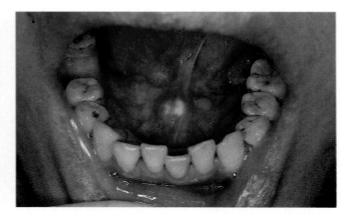

FIGURE 5.55 ■ Sialolithiasis. A stone is seen at the orifice of Wharton duct. (Photo contributor: David P. Kretzschmar, DDS, MS.)

Clinical Summary

Sinusitis is an inflammation of the mucous membranes lining the paranasal sinuses. Sinusitis can be classified as acute, subacute, or chronic; purulent or sterile; and allergic or nonallergic. All share an impairment of mucus clearance. Most cases of bacterial sinusitis are associated with antecedent viral upper respiratory tract infection.

Maxillary sinusitis is the most common form of sinusitis and is associated with paranasal facial pain, maxillary dental pain, purulent rhinorrhea, retroocular pain, and conjunctivitis. Ethmoid sinusitis is more common in children and produces a low-grade fever and periorbital pain. Frontal sinusitis can cause a severe headache above the eyes, which is exacerbated by leaning forward; a low-grade fever; upper lid edema; and rhinorrhea. Sphenoid sinusitis is fortunately rare and patients classically complain of a vertex headache and retroocular pain. Owing to its intracranial location, sphenoid sinusitis can involve several cranial nerves, the pituitary gland, and the cavernous sinus. Involvement of all sinus cavities is referred to as pansinusitis. Important complications of sinusitis include periorbital and orbital cellulitis, cavernous sinus thrombosis, and intracranial abscess.

Patients with the Pott puffy tumor (a rare osteomyelitis of the cranium from direct extension of a frontal sinusitis) present with a boggy, tender swelling above the eye.

Imaging modalities include transillumination of the maxillary sinuses, plain radiographs, CT, and MRI. CT is the most sensitive and specific technique and allows for better delineation of the sphenoid and ethmoid sinuses.

Common bacterial isolates are *Haemophilus influenzae*, *Streptococcus pneumoniae* (together representing 60% to 70% of all bacterial causes), *Streptococcus pyogenes*, *Staphylococcus aureus*, and *Moraxella catarrhalis*. Immunocompromised patients are susceptible to fungal infections, including *Aspergillus* and *Mucor* species.

Emergency Department Treatment and Disposition

Initial treatment is with decongestants and analgesics in most patients unless severely ill. If the patient remains symptomatic after 7 days, consider antibiotics.

For acute bacterial sinusitis, amoxicillin, macrolides, and trimethoprim-sulfamethoxazole are appropriate agents. Refractory cases or immunocompromised patients require broader-spectrum antibiotics such as amoxicillin with clavulanate, clarithromycin, third-generation cephalosporins, or the newer fluoroquinolones. Treatment for up to 3 weeks may be necessary.

Decongestants reduce local edema, increase air movement within the sinuses, and decrease local secretions. A short course of topical oxymetazoline or phenylephrine as well as oral pseudoephedrine for up to 10 days can help minimize secretions and assist in maintaining ostia patency. Humidified air, steam, or saline nasal sprays also facilitate drainage. Patients should be strongly encouraged to stop smoking.

Parenteral steroids are not used in acute or recurrent sinusitis. Intranasal steroids may have a role in allergic and chronic sinusitis.

Referral or follow-up by an otolaryngologist or primary care provider should be made for all patients within 3 weeks for routine cases. Patients with comorbid illnesses or more complicated sinusitis should be admitted for parenteral antibiotic therapy and supportive care.

Pearls

1. Chronic sinusitis may be due to mucoid retention cysts, deviated septum, or polyps, which are often visible on plain radiographs. Refer these patients for possible surgery.
2. Physicians must consider fungal etiologies in patients with comorbid illnesses.

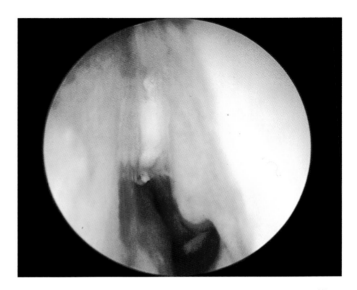

FIGURE 5.56 ■ Sinusitis. Purulent drainage from the maxillary sinus ostium in a patient with maxillary sinusitis. Drainage may not always be apparent, since the ostium may be occluded from swelling and inflammation. (Photo contributor: Robin T. Cotton, MD.)

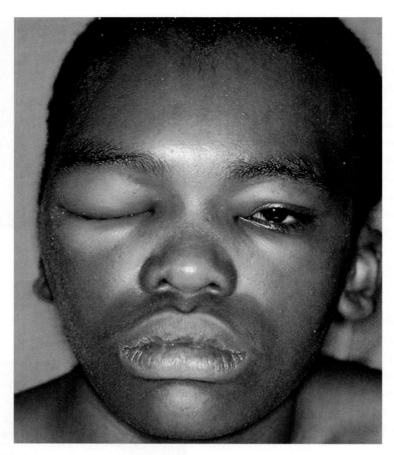

FIGURE 5.57 ■ Sinusitis. Adolescent with pansinusitis complicated by periorbital cellulitis. The patient was also found to have osteomyelitis of the frontal cortex (Pott's puffy tumor). (Photo contributor: Robin T. Cotton, MD.)

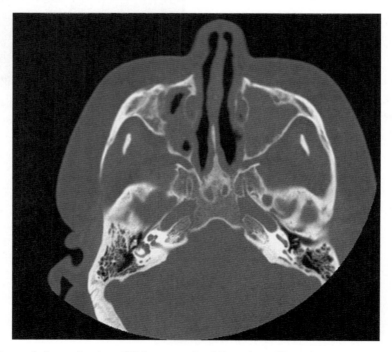

FIGURE 5.58 ■ Sinusitis. Bone windows of a sinus CT demonstrating bilateral maxillary sinus disease. (Photo contributor: Lawrence B. Stack, MD.)

Clinical Summary

Nasal cellulitis is an infection of the skin and subcutaneous tissues and does not include nasal cartilage. It is most common at the extremes of age. Bacterial invasion due to disruption of the skin is the usual cause. *Streptococcus pyogenes* and *Streptococcus aureus* cause most infections. Risk factors include nasal surgery, instrumentation, diabetes, immuno-compromise, and nasal piercing. Clinical features include pain, redness, swelling of the nasal tissues. Headache, fever, and malaise suggest complicated disease. Complications of nasal cellulitis include abscess, cavernous sinus thrombosis, chondritis of the nasal cartilage, bacteremia, and sepsis.

Emergency Department Treatment and Disposition

The diagnosis of nasal cellulitis is clinical. However, evaluation may include CBC, blood and tissue cultures, contrasted CT if abscess is suspected, and CT-V if a cavernous sinus thrombosis is suspected. Remove any foreign body that might be a nidus of infection. Amoxicillin-clavulanate or amoxicillin-sulbactam are first-line antibiotics. Clindamycin, vancomycin, trimethoprim-sulfamethoxazole, and first-generation cephalosporins are other options. Patients should be hospitalized if they have systemic symptoms, are immunocompromised, have diabetes or a suspected abscess, or have retained foreign bodies. Patients at extremes of age should be strongly considered for admission.

Pearls

1. Threshold for hospital admission for patients with nasal cellulitis should be low.
2. In children, consider *H influenza* and *S pneumoniae* as causative organisms of facial cellulitis.

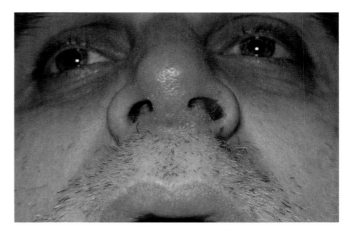

FIGURE 5.59 ■ Nasal Cellulitis. Swelling and erythema of the nose in a middle-aged man. A contrasted CT was done to exclude abscess because of the marked swelling of the nasal septum. (Photo contributor: Lawrence B. Stack, MD.)

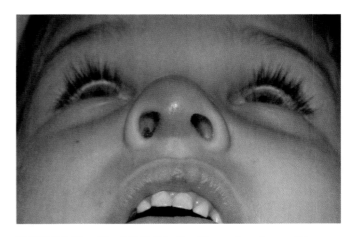

FIGURE 5.60 ■ Nasal Cellulitis. Swelling and erythema of the nose of a 2-year-old child, suggesting nasal cellulitis. (Photo contributor: Lawrence B. Stack, MD.)

MOUTH

Edward C. Jauch
Brent E. Gottesman

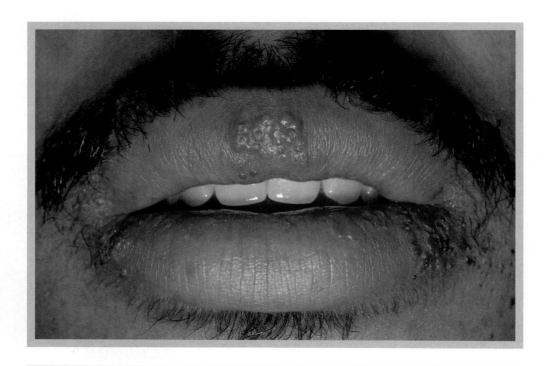

The authors acknowledge Edwin D. Turner, MD and Sara-Jo Gahm, MD for portions of this chapter
written for the previous editions of this book.

Clinical Summary

Tooth subluxation refers to the loosening of a tooth in its alveolar socket. Traumatic oral injury is the most common etiology; however, infection and periodontal disease may also produce loosening of teeth. Gingival lacerations and alveolar fractures are commonly associated with dental subluxations. Subluxated teeth are diagnosed by applying gentle pressure to the teeth with a tongue blade or fingertip. Movement, mild displacement, or blood along the crevice of the gingiva are signs of subluxation. Dental impaction and alveolar ridge fracture should be considered and ruled out clinically and radiographically.

Emergency Department Treatment and Disposition

1. *Primary teeth*: If the subluxated tooth is forced into close proximity to the underlying permanent tooth, extraction by a dentist or oral surgeon is indicated. Otherwise, the patient should be instructed to follow a soft diet for 1 to 2 weeks, allowing the tooth to reimplant spontaneously.
2. *Permanent teeth*: Unstable teeth should be temporarily immobilized using gauze packing, a figure-eight suture around the tooth and an adjacent tooth, aluminium foil, or a special periodontal dressing (Coe-Pak), and the patient should be referred for dental follow-up.

Pearls

1. Any evidence of tooth mobility following trauma is a subluxation by definition.
2. Always consider an associated underlying alveolar or occult root fracture.

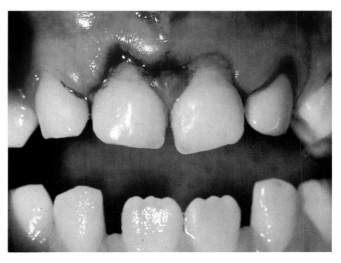

FIGURE 6.1 ■ Tooth Subluxation. Note the presence of blood along the crevice of the gingival margin of both central incisors—an indication of subluxation following trauma. Mild displacement of the subluxated teeth is noted. (Photo contributor: James F. Steiner, DDS.)

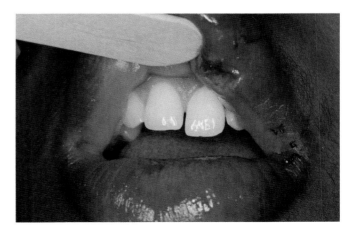

FIGURE 6.2 ■ Tooth Subluxation. Tooth subluxations can be quite subtle, as in this case of a slightly subluxed tooth #9 missed on initial examination. A careful dental examination is essential in patients with oral trauma. (Photo contributor: Kevin J. Knoop, MD, MS.)

Clinical Summary

Impacted or intruded teeth result when a tooth is forced deeper into the alveolar socket or surrounding tissues as a result of trauma. The tooth appears shorter than its contralateral partner. An impacted tooth may be partially visible or completely hidden by the gingiva and buried in the alveolar process. Completely impacted teeth may erroneously be considered avulsed until a radiograph demonstrates the intruded position. The apex of a completely impacted permanent central incisor may be driven through the alveolar bone into the floor of the nares, causing epistaxis. Associated injuries may include alveolar fractures, dental crown or root fractures, and oral mucosal or gingival lacerations. Dental pulp necrosis occurs in 15% to 50% of cases.

Emergency Department Treatment and Disposition

Primary teeth that are impacted usually re-erupt and reposition spontaneously within 1 to 3 months. Any intruded primary tooth whose apex is displaced toward or impacts on the follicle of its permanent successor should be extracted. These patients should have dental follow-up and be monitored clinically and radiographically for 1 year. Permanent teeth do not re-erupt. Surgical reduction is indicated to prevent complications such as external root resorption and loss of supporting bone. Orthodontic repositioning and splinting is generally carried out over 3 to 4 weeks. Follow-up for a minimum of 1 year is recommended.

Pearls

1. An undiagnosed impacted tooth is predisposed to infection and can have a poor cosmetic result.
2. The maxillary incisors are the most commonly impacted teeth.

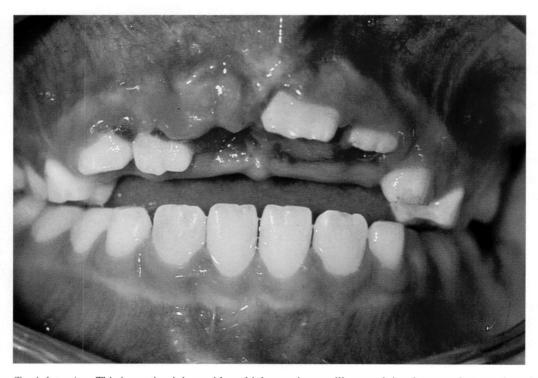

FIGURE 6.3 ■ Tooth Intrusion. This impaction injury with multiple anterior maxillary tooth involvement shows various degrees of tooth impaction. Also note the complete absence of a central incisor. This may indicate a complete intrusion into the alveolar socket or an avulsion of the tooth. Radiographic studies are required when a tooth's location is in question. (Photo contributor: James F. Steiner, DDS.)

Clinical Summary

Avulsion is the total displacement of a tooth from its socket. There is usually a history of trauma; however, infectious etiologies may result in complete disruption of the periodontal ligament from the affected tooth, causing an avulsion. Various degrees of bleeding from the socket and surrounding gingiva may be noted. There may be an associated underlying alveolar fracture depending on the mechanism of injury. Prompt inquiry into the location of any unaccountable tooth is indicated. Radiographic evaluation to rule out aspiration, soft tissue entrapment, impaction, or dentoalveolar fracture is indicated when the tooth's location is in question.

Emergency Department Treatment and Disposition

A successful reimplantation decreases by 1% for every minute the tooth is out of its socket. Permanent teeth should be replaced in their sockets as soon as possible. The tooth should first be rinsed with saline but not scrubbed, and the root should not be handled. Successful reimplantation depends on the survival of periodontal ligament fibers. The tooth should be placed in the socket and emergent dental consultation obtained. Tetanus prophylaxis and antibiotics targeting mouth flora (penicillin, clindamycin) should be administered. If not replaced, the avulsed tooth should be stored in the mouth of the patient or parent or in a container of milk. Normal saline or commercial preservatives (Hanks solution) are available, but tap water should not be used. Reimplantation of primary avulsed teeth may interfere with eruptions of permanent teeth because of ankylosing and fusion to the bone. Thus, primary teeth are not reimplanted, but follow-up should be obtained as a procedure may be needed to maintain tooth spacing until the permanent tooth erupts.

Pearls

1. Primary teeth should not be reimplanted.
2. Successful reimplantation of an avulsed tooth occurs best within the first 30 minutes.
3. Storage and transport media in decreasing order for preserving tooth viability include Hanks balanced salt solution or a tissue culture medium (Save-A-Tooth), cool low-fat or skim milk, saline, and saliva.

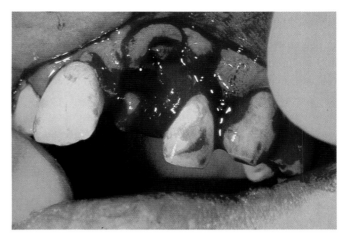

FIGURE 6.4 ■ Tooth Avulsion. Avulsion injury with angulation and displacement of teeth from the alveolar socket. (Photo contributor: James F. Steiner, DDS.)

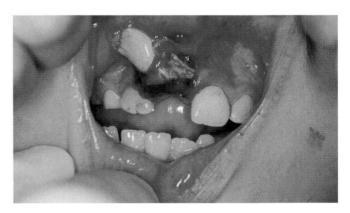

FIGURE 6.5 ■ Tooth Avulsion. Significant avulsion injury of tooth #8 in a patient with direct oral trauma. (Photo contributor: Lawrence B. Stack, MD.)

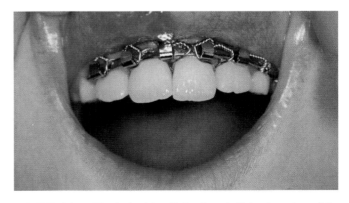

FIGURE 6.6 ■ Tooth Avulsion Reimplanted. Reimplantation of the avulsed tooth in Fig. 6.5 was performed by an oral surgeon with the use of an arch bar to secure the tooth. (Photo contributor: Lawrence B. Stack, MD.)

Clinical Summary

Anatomically, each tooth has crown and root portions. Externally, the crown is covered with white enamel and the root portion with cementum. The cementoenamel junction (cervical line) is where the crown and root meet. The yellow-to-tan dentin is the second innermost layer and comprises the bulk of the tooth. The red-to-pink pulp tissue is located in the center of the tooth and includes the neurovascular supply to the tooth. The Ellis classification system, while considered by some as inadequate, is still commonly used to describe tooth fractures above the cervical line in anterior teeth:

Ellis class I: Involves the enamel only.
Ellis class II: Involves the enamel plus exposure of the dentin. The patient may complain of temperature sensitivity.
Ellis class III: Fracture extends into the pulp. A pink or bloody discoloration on the fracture surface is diagnostic of this type of fracture. The patient may have severe pain but may also have no pain due to loss of nerve function.

Tooth fractures may also occur below the cementoenamel junction. These dental root fractures are commonly missed on initial evaluation. Bleeding may be observed at the gingival crevice with associated tooth tenderness on percussion. Radiographic evaluation will aid in differentiating these conditions if required.

Emergency Department Treatment and Disposition

Ellis class I: Pain control may be required. Rough tooth edges may be referred within 24 hours when soft tissue injury is caused by sharp pieces of the tooth.

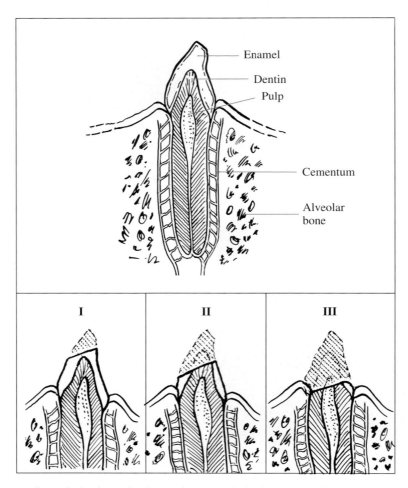

FIGURE 6.7 ■ Tooth Fractures. Enamel, dentin, and pulp are the anatomic landmarks used in the Ellis classification of tooth fractures.

Ellis class II: Patients under 12 years of age have less dentin than older patients and are at risk for pulp infection. They should have a calcium hydroxide dressing placed, covered with gauze or aluminum foil, and seen by a dentist within 24 hours. Older patients should see a dentist within 24 to 48 hours.

Ellis class III: This is considered a dental emergency, and dental consultation within 24 to 48 hours is indicated. Delay in treatment may result in abscess formation.

Root fractures: Early reduction, immobilization, and splinting are indicated; a commercial stabilizing compound (Coe-Pak) is available for this purpose. Dental referral is advised within 24 to 48 hours. Most teeth sustaining root fractures maintain pulp viability.

Pearls

1. Check for tooth mobility on initial examination to aid in differentiating mobility involving the entire tooth from involvement of only the fractured segment.
2. Consider nonaccidental trauma when dental injuries occur in young children.

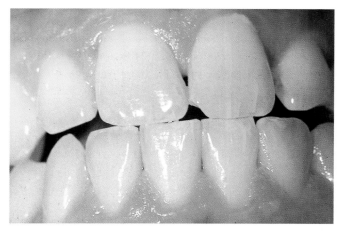

FIGURE 6.8 ■ Ellis Class I Tooth Fracture. Note the fracture of the left upper central incisor. The sole involvement of the enamel is consistent with an Ellis class I fracture. (Photo contributor: James F. Steiner, DDS.)

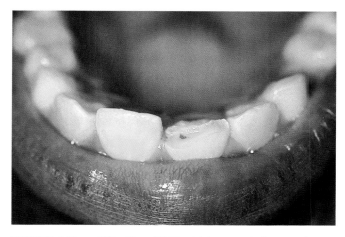

FIGURE 6.10 ■ Ellis Class III Tooth Fracture. A fracture demonstrating blood at the exposed dental pulp. This sign is pathognomonic for an Ellis class III fracture. (Photo contributor: Kevin J. Knoop, MD, MS.)

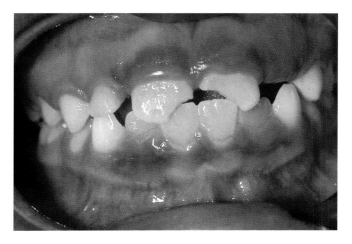

FIGURE 6.9 ■ Ellis Class II Tooth Fractures. Bilateral maxillary central incisor injuries with exposed enamel and dentin consistent with an Ellis class II fracture. (Photo contributor: James F. Steiner, DDS.)

Clinical Summary

The alveolus is the tooth-bearing segment of the mandible and maxilla. Fracture of the alveolar process tends to occur more often in the thinner maxilla than in the mandible. The anterior alveolar processes are at greatest risk for fracture due to more direct exposure to trauma. Both subluxation and avulsion of teeth may be associated with underlying alveolar fractures of the mandible or maxilla. Various degrees of tooth mobility and gingival bleeding may occur.

Emergency Department Treatment and Disposition

Significant cosmetic deformity may result from alveolar bone loss. Preservation of as much viable tissue as possible is important. The involved alveolar segment should have saline-soaked gauze applied with gentle direct pressure. Any avulsed teeth should also be preserved. The patient's tetanus status must be determined and antibiotic therapy with penicillin or clindamycin should be considered. Oral surgery consultation should be obtained for possible wire stabilization or arch bar fixation.

Pearls

1. Always consider the possibility of an associated cervical spine injury when evaluating patients with facial trauma.
2. Consider the possibility of avulsed tooth aspiration.

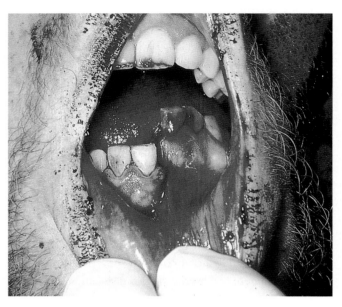

FIGURE 6.11 ■ Alveolar Ridge Fracture. Note the exposed alveolar bone segment and associated multiple teeth involvement. Attempts should be made to maximally preserve all viable tissue. (Photo contributor: Alan B. Storrow, MD.)

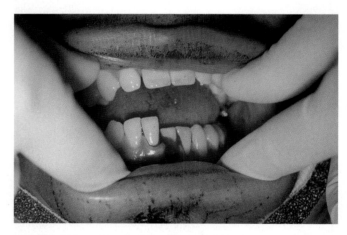

FIGURE 6.12 ■ Alveolar Ridge Fracture. This alveolar ridge fracture was caused by blunt trauma from a steering wheel in a frontal impact motor vehicle collision. (Photo contributor: R. Jason Thurman, MD.)

Clinical Summary

Temporal mandibular joint (TMJ) dislocation generally occurs in predisposed individuals after a vigorous yawn or seizure, or less commonly from direct trauma to the chin while the mouth is open. Acute dislocation occurs when the mandibular condyles displace forward and become locked anterior to the articular eminence. Masseter muscle spasm contributes to prevention of spontaneous relocation. Weakness of the temporomandibular ligament, an overstretched joint capsule, and a shallow articular eminence are predisposing factors. Patients usually present with an inability to close an open mouth. Other associated symptoms include pain, discomfort, and facial swelling near the temporomandibular joint. Difficulty speaking and swallowing is common. Anterior dislocations are most common; however, posterior dislocation may occur with significant trauma, often in association with a basilar skull fracture. Unilateral dislocation results in deviation of the mandible to the unaffected side. TMJ hemarthrosis and dystonic reactions may mimic the true process of TMJ dislocation. Mandibular fractures should be considered, particularly if there is a history of facial trauma.

Emergency Department Treatment and Disposition

Acute reduction of pain, muscle spasm, and anxiety is achieved using reassurance, analgesics, and benzodiazepine muscle relaxants. Panorex or TMJ x-ray films (pre- and postreduction) should be considered to exclude a fracture. While facing the sitting patient, the physician grasps the angles of the mandible with both hands. The thumbs are wrapped in

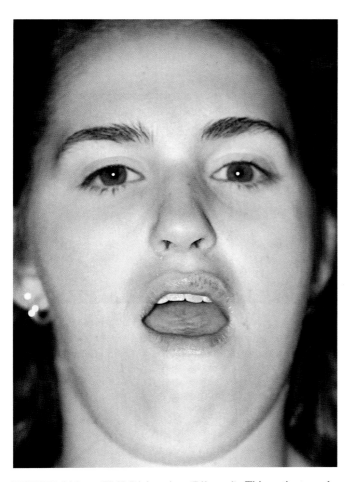

FIGURE 6.13 ■ TMJ Dislocation (Bilateral). This patient awoke from sleep with the inability to close her mouth. Note the dry lips and tongue secondary to prolonged exposure. (Photo contributor: Warren K. Russell, MD.)

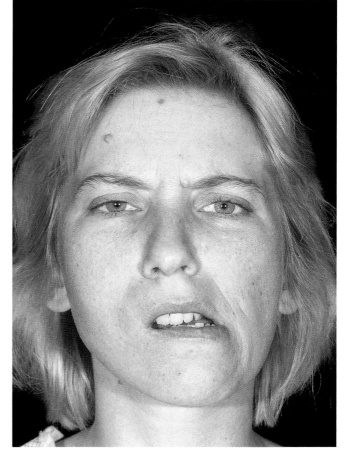

FIGURE 6.14 ■ TMJ Dislocation (Unilateral). Note the asymmetric jaw deviation toward the unaffected side. Always consider the possibility of an associated underlying fracture or cervical spine injury. (Photo contributor: Frank Birinyi, MD.)

gauze for protection and rest on the occlusive surfaces of the molars while downward and backward pressure is steadily applied until the condyle slides back into the articular eminence. Reduction may require some time to overcome muscle spasm. Following reduction, instruct the patient to avoid excessively wide mouth opening while eating and yawning for 3 to 4 weeks. Apply warm compresses to the TMJ areas. A soft diet for 1 week and the use of nonsteroidal anti-inflammatory drugs is advised. Dental/oral surgery follow-up should be arranged.

Pearls

1. TMJ dysfunction secondary to a neuroleptic or antipsychotic medication–related dystonic reaction is treated with diphenhydramine or benztropine.
2. When trauma is the cause of TMJ dislocation, maintain a high index of suspicion for mandible fractures and cervical spine injuries.
3. A Barton bandage to temporarily secure the mandible may be useful in patients who are unable to understand and comply with their aftercare instructions (developmentally delayed patients, etc).

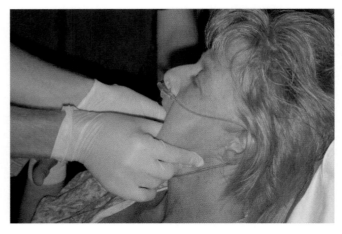

FIGURE 6.16 ■ TMJ Reduction Technique. Under sedation, the patient in Fig. 6.15 undergoes reduction with inferior-posterior force applied by the physician. The thumbs are not wrapped with gauze in this case as the patient is edentulous. (Photo contributor: R. Jason Thurman, MD.)

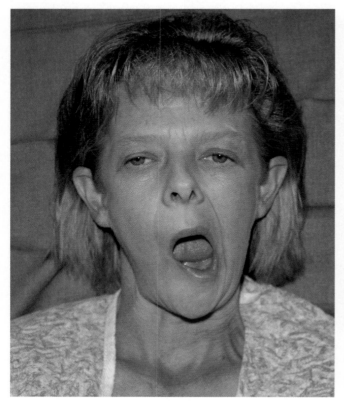

FIGURE 6.15 ■ TMJ Dislocation, Edentulous Patient (Unilateral). The mandible is deviated toward the unaffected side. (Photo contributor: R. Jason Thurman, MD.)

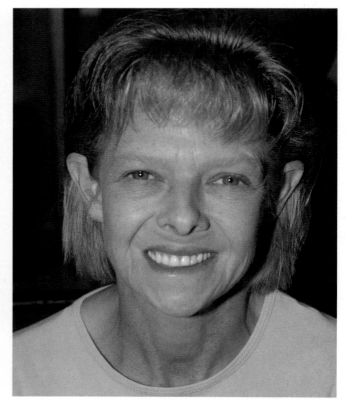

FIGURE 6.17 ■ TMJ Reduced. Improved anatomic alignment and a happy patient after reduction of her unilateral TMJ dislocation is accomplished. (Photo contributor: R. Jason Thurman, MD.)

Clinical Summary

Tongue lacerations are usually the result of obvious oral trauma and tongue biting. Injuries to the tongue or mouth floor can cause serious hemorrhage and potential airway compromise. Careful examination of the oral cavity for associated injuries is necessary. Specifically, injury to or absence of teeth should be ascertained by inspecting the wound for possibly entrapped dental elements. Dorsal surface tongue lacerations may be associated with a mandibular surface laceration.

Emergency Department Treatment and Disposition

Most lacerations to the tongue do not mandate surgical repair. An exception to this rule is lacerations involving the tip, where rapid healing may produce a "forked tongue." Lacerations greater than 1 cm in length that gape widely, actively bleed, or those involving a lateral margin are best stabilized by a few well-placed rapidly absorbable sutures. Place sutures using large bites to include both mucosa and muscle. Anesthesia of the anterior two-thirds of the tongue is obtained using an inferior alveolar nerve block (blocks the lingual nerve on the ipsilateral side). Local anesthesia, infiltrated at the site of the wound, may also be used.

Pearls

1. Extensive complex tongue lacerations are at risk for infection and should be prophylactically treated with antibiotics covering oropharyngeal flora.
2. Tongue lacerations involving the floor of the mouth or having persistent bleeding may result in tongue swelling and airway compromise. Consultation for admission with airway surveillance may be indicated.

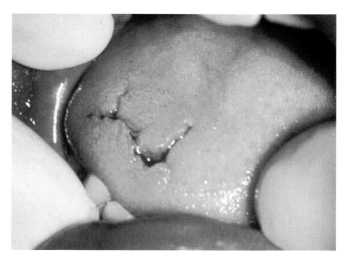

FIGURE 6.18 ■ Tongue Laceration. A stellate tongue laceration that does not require suturing is shown. The ventral aspect of the tongue should be examined for additional lacerations sustained from the mandibular teeth. (Photo contributor: James F. Steiner, DDS.)

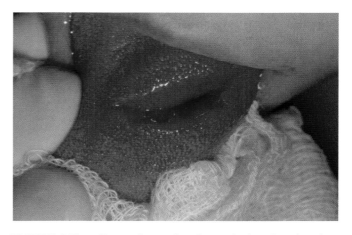

FIGURE 6.19 ■ Tongue Laceration. Due to its length and gaping, this tongue laceration was repaired with absorbable sutures. (Photo contributor: Lawrence B. Stack, MD.)

Clinical Summary

Anatomically, the vermilion border of the lips represents the transition area from mucosal tissue to skin. Lip lacerations involving the vermilion border present a unique clinical situation, since relatively minor malalignment after repair may cause an unacceptable cosmetic result. Marked tissue edema is frequently noted with most lip trauma, which may distort the anatomy. An associated underlying gingival or dental injury is a common finding.

Emergency Department Treatment and Disposition

Accurate vermilion margin reapproximation is the first goal of lip repairs. An unapproximated vermilion margin of 2 mm or greater results in a cosmetic deformity. A regional block of the mental or infraorbital nerve is recommended for anesthesia to avoid additional tissue edema and anatomic distortion produced by local infiltration. Deep or through-and-through lacerations involving the vermilion border should be closed in layers. After closure of the deeper tissue, the first skin suture is always placed at the vermilion border to reestablish the anatomic margin. Using 5-0 or 6-0 nylon, sutures should be placed along the vermilion surface until the moist mucous membrane is encountered. The deep muscular and dermal layer may be closed with 4-0 chromic or Vicryl sutures. Mucosal layers are loosely reapproximated with absorbable suture. The patient should be given wound care instructions. Follow-up for wound evaluation and possible suture removal in 3 to 7 days should be arranged.

Pearls

1. A vermilion border with as little as 2 mm of malalignment may produce a cosmetically noticed defect.
2. Always carefully place the first skin suture at the vermilion border in any lip laceration involving this area.

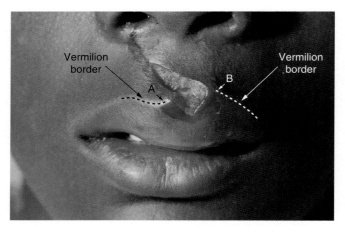

FIGURE 6.20 ■ Vermilion Border Lip Laceration. A lip laceration with disruption of the vermilion border. Wound repair begins at the vermilion-skin junction (precise approximation of A to B in this case) for a good cosmetic result. (Photo contributor: Kevin J. Knoop, MD, MS.)

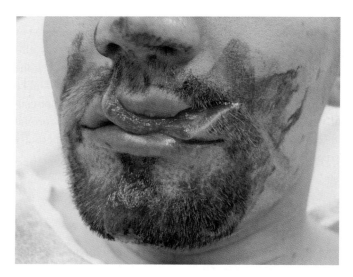

FIGURE 6.21 ■ Complex Vermilion Border Lip Lacerations. This patient suffered vermilion border lacerations in two areas from an assault with a broken bottle. Following shaving of the moustache, each vermilion-skin junction was repaired before remaining superficial wound closure was achieved. (Photo contributor: R. Jason Thurman, MD.)

Clinical Summary

Gingival abscesses tend to involve the marginal gingiva and result from entrapment of food and plaque debris in a gingival pocket. Subsequent staphylococcal, streptococcal, anaerobic, or mixed bacterial overgrowth leads to abscess formation. Localized swelling, erythema, tenderness, and possible fluctuance in the space between the tooth and the gingiva (the so-called pocket) ensue. There may be spontaneous purulent drainage from the gingival margin, or an area of pointing (purulent material seen through thin mucosa) may be seen. In cases of acute gingival abscess formation, pus may be expressed from the gingival margin by gentle digital pressure. When the gingival abscess involves the deeper supporting periodontal structures, it is referred to as a periodontal abscess. This may present as a fluctuant vestibular abscess or with a draining sinus that opens onto the gingival surface.

In contrast, periapical abscesses are deep and not obvious on inspection. They usually present as tenderness to percussion or pain with chewing over the involved tooth. A parulis may also simulate a gingival abscess; however, a parulis represents the cutaneous manifestation of a deeper periapical abscess. Unlike a parulis or periapical abscess, gingival abscesses are not usually associated with dental caries or fillings. Pericoronal abscesses tend to involve the gingiva overlying a partially erupted third molar.

Emergency Department Treatment and Disposition

The initial management is a small incision with drainage and warm saline irrigation. Oral antibiotic therapy with penicillin or clindamycin is recommended. Analgesics should be provided along with dental follow-up. The patient's tetanus status should be addressed.

Pearls

1. Patients with gingival abscesses are usually afebrile. Consider more extensive abscess formation and oral disease processes in the febrile toxic-appearing patient.
2. Patients with chronic, deep periodontal abscesses complain of dull, gnawing pain as well as a desire to bite down on and grind the tooth.

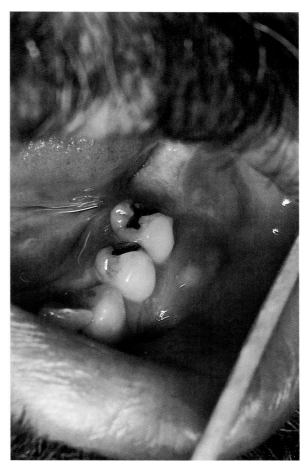

FIGURE 6.22 ■ Periodontal Abscess. Localized gingival swelling, erythema, and fluctuance are seen in this periodontal abscess with spontaneous purulent drainage. (Photo contributor: Kevin J. Knoop, MD, MS.)

Clinical Summary

Acute pain, swelling, and mild tooth elevation is characteristic of a periapical or dentoalveolar abscess. Exquisite sensitivity to percussion or chewing on the involved tooth is a common sign. The involved tooth may have had dental caries, a filling, or a root canal treatment. Periapical abscesses can enlarge over time and "point," either internally on the lingual or buccal mucosal surfaces or extraorally with swelling and redness of the overlying skin. Occasionally these lesions may track up to the alveolar periosteum and gingival surface to form a parulis. Radiographically, these abscesses appear as well-circumscribed areas of radiolucency at the dental apex or along the lateral aspect of the root. Early acute periapical abscesses may not demonstrate any radiographic changes. Both deep periodontal and periapical abscesses may have sinuses draining purulent material onto the gingival surface. If the infection is allowed to progress, it can erode through the nearest cortical bone, manifesting itself in a variety of locations. Panorex films, dental radiographs, or a CT scan may aid in the diagnosis.

Emergency Department Treatment and Disposition

Nonsteroidal anti-inflammatory drugs (NSAIDs) or oral narcotics for pain should be administered in conjunction with oropharyngeal antibiotic therapy. A regional nerve block may be performed for more immediate temporary relief. Administer tetanus toxoid as indicated. Dental consultation for follow-up in 1 to 2 days is recommended for endodontic evaluation or possible extraction of the involved tooth. Incision and drainage along with saline irrigation and prompt referral constitutes the initial treatment of a parulis.

Pearls

1. More than one tooth may be involved.
2. Exquisite tenderness and pain on tooth percussion is a key feature on physical examination and identifies the involved tooth.
3. Periapical abscesses are almost always associated with carious or nonviable teeth.

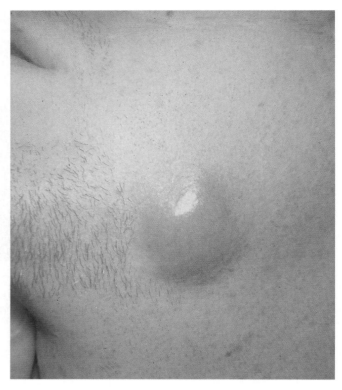

FIGURE 6.23 ■ Periapical Abscess. This periapical abscess points externally to the overlying skin. (Photo contributor: Robin Cotton, MD.)

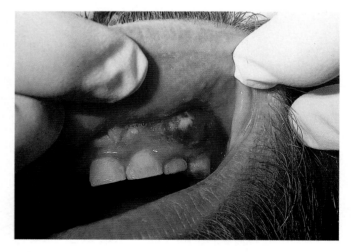

FIGURE 6.24 ■ "Gumboil" (Parulis). This lesion is a sinus tract extension of a periapical abscess. It is differentiated from a periodontal abscess by tenderness to tooth percussion. (Photo contributor: Alan B. Storrow, MD.)

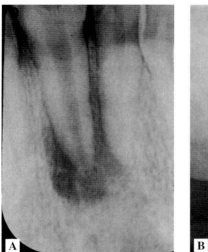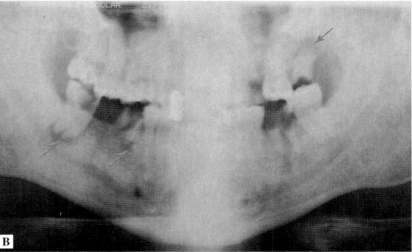

FIGURE 6.25 ■ *Periapical Abscess.* (**A**) Note the well-defined radiolucent area at the apex and lateral root of the tooth in this radiograph. (Photo contributor: James L. Kretzschmar, DDS, MS.) (**B**) This Panorex film shows lucencies consistent with periapical abscesses, most notably of the right inferior posterior molar tooth (see arrows). (Photo contributor: David P. Kretzschmar, DDS, MS.)

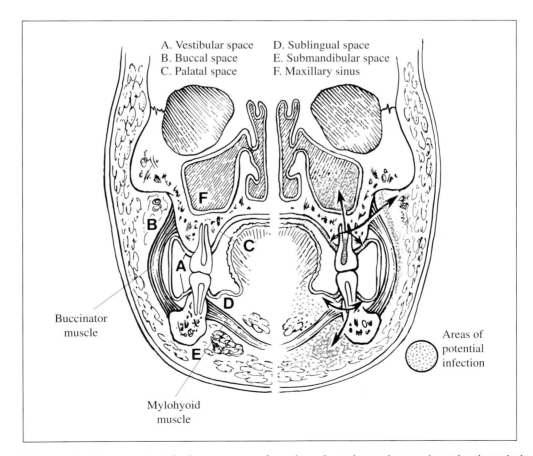

FIGURE 6.26 ■ *Odontogenic Abscesses.* As infection progresses from the pulp at the tooth apex, it erodes through the bone and can express itself in a variety of places. This illustration notes several possible locations or spaces. (Adapted with permission from Cummings C, Schuller D. (eds). *Otolaryngology Head and Neck Surgery.* Chicago: Mosby-Year Book; 1986.)

Clinical Summary

A partially erupted or impacted third molar (wisdom tooth) is the most common site of pericoronitis and pericoronal abscesses. The accumulation of food and debris between the overlying gingival flap and crown of the tooth sets up the foci for pericoronitis and subsequent abscess formation. The gingival flap becomes irritated and inflamed. The area is also repeatedly traumatized by the opposing molar tooth and may interfere with complete jaw closure as swelling and tenderness increase. The inflamed gingival process may eventually become infected and form a fluctuant abscess. Foul taste, inability to close the jaw, and fever may occur. Swelling of the cheek and angle of the jaw as well as localized lymphadenopathy are also characteristic. More advanced disease may spread posteriorly to the base of the tongue and oropharyngeal area. Potential spread into the deep cervical spaces with resulting Ludwig angina and peritonsillar abscesses are also an important concern.

Emergency Department Treatment and Disposition

Superficial incision and drainage with warm saline irrigation may be performed initially in the emergency department. Adequate analgesia and antibiotic coverage should be provided. Consultation or referral to an oral maxillofacial surgeon for follow-up is indicated for possible extraction of the involved teeth.

Pearls

1. Pericoronitis and abscess formation rarely occur in the pediatric population and tend to be late adolescent and adult processes.
2. The mandibular third molar is the most commonly involved tooth.
3. Airway compromise is a potential complication with posterior extension of a pericoronal abscess.

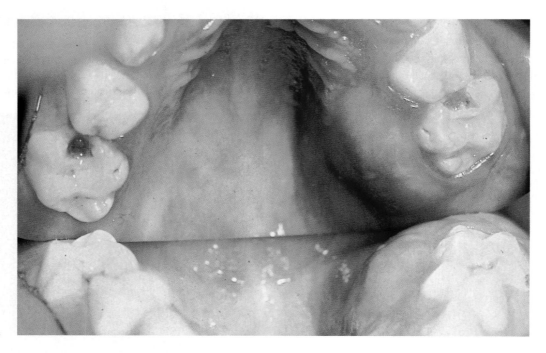

FIGURE 6.27 ■ Pericoronal Abscess. Note the inflamed fluctuant gingival tissue approximating the incompletely erupted third molar. (Photo contributor: James F. Steiner, DDS.)

Clinical Summary

The buccal space lies between the buccinator muscle and the overlying superficial fascia and skin. The maxillary second and third molars are the usual nidus of disease. Infection from the involved teeth erodes either superiorly through the maxillary alveolar bone, or rarely, inferiorly from the third mandibular molar through the mandibular alveolar bone into the buccal space. These patients present with unilateral facial swelling, redness, and tenderness of the cheek. Trismus is generally not present. Parotid gland enlargement due to mumps and suppurative bacterial parotitis should also be considered. The former lacks erythema and warmth of the overlying skin, while the latter is accompanied by trismus and purulent drainage from the Stensen duct. Inspection of all the maxillary and third mandibular molar teeth is essential to help make the diagnosis. CT scan can aid in localizing the infection.

Emergency Department Treatment and Disposition

Parenteral antibiotic therapy with penicillin, clindamycin, or a third-generation cephalosporin is recommended. Antibiotic coverage for anaerobic organisms may be added to the treatment regimen. NSAIDs or oral narcotic analgesics should be provided as indicated. Dental or oral surgical consultation is necessary for endodontic therapy, abscess drainage, and/or extraction.

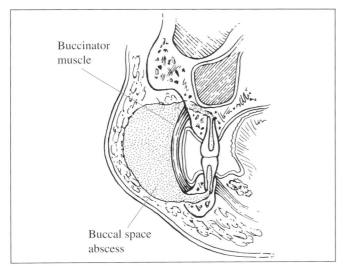

FIGURE 6.28 ■ Buccal Space Anatomy. The buccal space lies between the buccinator muscle and the overlying skin and superficial fascia. This potential space may become involved secondary to maxillary or mandibular molar infections. (Adapted with permission from Cummings C, Schuller D (eds). *Otolaryngology Head and Neck Surgery*. 2nd ed. Chicago: Mosby-Year Book; 1993.)

144

Pearls

1. Odontogenic infections of the second or third maxillary molars are the most common source for buccal space abscesses.
2. Ovoid cheek swelling with sparing of the nasolabial fold helps to differentiate this from a canine space abscess.

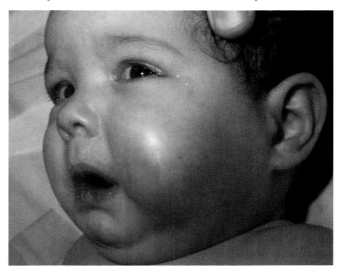

FIGURE 6.29 ■ Buccal Space Abscess. Note the ovoid cheek swelling with sparing of the nasolabial fold. This finding, along with accompanying redness and tenderness, helps to identify buccal space abscess formation. (Photo contributor: Michael J. Nowicki, MD.)

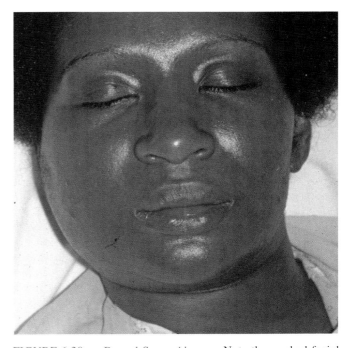

FIGURE 6.30 ■ Buccal Space Abscess. Note the marked facial asymmetry in this adult patient presenting with a buccal space abscess. (Photo contributor: David Effron, MD.)

Clinical Summary

The canine space lies between the anterior surface of the maxilla and levator labii superioris muscle of the face. Erosion of maxillary tooth infection through the alveolar bone into the canine space leads to abscess formation, although cutaneous infections from the upper lip and nose are a rare source. The origin of these abscesses can be from maxillary incisor teeth and bicuspids, although it is almost exclusively from the maxillary canine tooth. Unilateral facial redness, pain, and swelling lateral to the nose with obliteration of the nasolabial fold are characteristic. Severe upper lip and lower eyelid swelling may cause drooling at the corner of the mouth or eye closure. Maxillofacial CT scan may aid in differentiating these lesions.

Emergency Department Treatment and Disposition

Parenteral antibiotic therapy including anaerobic coverage is indicated. Dental or oral surgical consultation for incision and drainage is the most definitive treatment for canine space abscesses. Extraction or endodontic treatment of the involved anterior maxillary teeth is usually necessary.

Pearls

1. Loss of the nasolabial fold is characteristic of canine space abscesses.
2. The maxillary canine (cuspid) teeth are the most common source for canine space abscesses.
3. Although these patients may drool when significant upper lip swelling is present, they typically do not have trismus, dysphagia, or odynophagia.

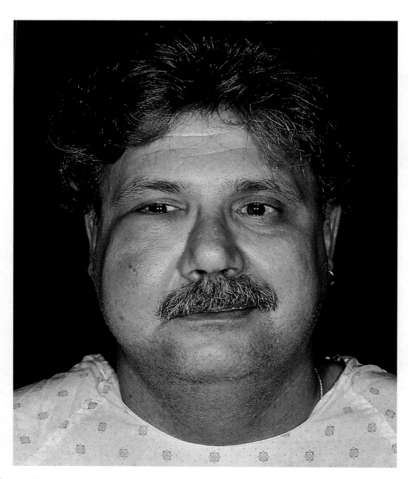

FIGURE 6.31 ■ Canine Space Abscess. Unilateral facial swelling lateral to the nose with associated redness and the typical loss of the nasolabial fold is shown. The maxillary canine tooth is usually the source of this process. (Photo contributor: Frank Birinyi, MD.)

Clinical Summary

Ludwig angina is defined as bilateral cellulitis of the submandibular and sublingual spaces with associated tongue elevation. A characteristic painful, brawny induration is present in the involved tissue. The posterior mandibular molars are the usual odontogenic origin for the infection. *Streptococcus, Staphylococcus,* and *Bacteroides* species are the most common pathogens. Affected individuals are typically 20 to 60 years old, with a male predominance. Patients are usually febrile and may demonstrate impressive trismus, dysphonia, and odynophagia. Dysphagia and drooling are secondary to tongue displacement and oropharyngeal swelling. Potential airway compromise or spread of infection to the deep cervical layers and the mediastinum is possible. The presence of dyspnea or cyanosis is a late and ominous sign indicating impending airway closure.

Emergency Department Treatment and Disposition

Acute laryngospasm with airway compromise is a potentially life-threatening complication and concern with Ludwig angina; therefore plans for definitive airway management should be prepared. Up to one-third of patients require definitive airway placement. Parenteral antibiotic therapy should be initiated with penicillin or a third-generation cephalosporin in combination with clindamycin or metronidazole for anaerobic coverage. The role of steroids for potential airway edema is controversial and ill defined in this setting. Analgesia should be given as needed. CT or MRI can be used to identify abscess location, but great care should be taken to ensure the patient can tolerate the imaging process. Definitive treatment requires operative surgical drainage of the abscess by an oral or maxillofacial surgeon. Admission to the intensive care unit is indicated for airway surveillance and management.

Pearls

1. Brawny submandibular induration and tongue elevation are common and characteristic clinical findings.
2. The second mandibular molar is the most common site of origin for Ludwig angina.
3. Acute laryngospasm with sudden total airway obstruction may be precipitated by attempts at oral or nasotracheal intubation.

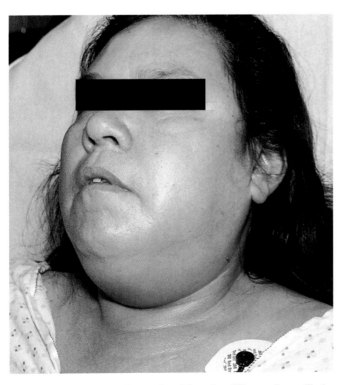

FIGURE 6.32 ■ Ludwig Angina. Note the diffuse submandibular swelling and fullness. Direct palpation of this area would reveal a characteristic brawny induration. Potential airway compromise is a key concern in all patients with Ludwig angina. (Photo contributor: Jeffrey Finkelstein, MD.)

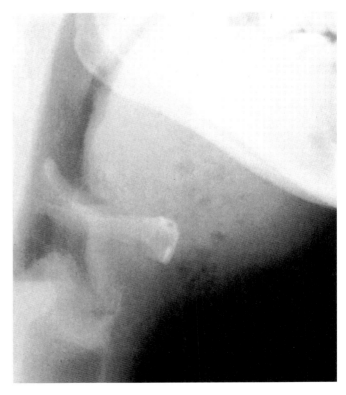

FIGURE 6.33 ■ Ludwig Angina. Note the presence of subcutaneous gas in the abscessed submandibular area on this radiograph of a patient with Ludwig angina. (Photo contributor: Edward C. Jauch, MD, MS.)

Clinical Summary

The parapharyngeal space is also known as the lateral pharyngeal or pharyngomaxillary space. Anatomically it is a pyramid-shaped space with its apex at the hyoid bone and base at the base of the skull. Laterally it is bound by the internal pterygoid muscle and the parotid gland with the superior pharyngeal constrictor muscle acting as the medial border. The posterior aspect of this space is in close proximity with the carotid sheath and cranial nerves IX through XII. Presenting symptoms of parapharyngeal space abscesses include fever, dysphagia, odynophagia, drooling, and ipsilateral otalgia. Unilateral neck and jaw angle facial swelling in association with rigidity and limited neck motion is common. Potentially disastrous complications associated with infections of this space include cranial neuropathies, jugular vein septic thrombophlebitis, and erosion into the carotid artery. The origin of parapharyngeal abscesses may be from bacterial pharyngitis, sinuses, dental, or lymphatic spread. A CT scan aids in making the diagnosis.

Emergency Department Treatment and Disposition

Preparations for definitive airway management via endotracheal intubation or surgery are vital. Early recognition and anticipation of other potentially disastrous complications should be considered and managed appropriately. Broad-spectrum antibiotic coverage for mixed aerobic and anaerobic infections should be initiated. Radiologic modalities used to assess parapharyngeal and other deep space neck infections include contrast-enhanced CT, ultrasound, plain radiography, and MRI. Otolaryngologic or oral surgical consultation is warranted for definitive intraoperative incision and drainage of the abscess.

Pearl

1. Suspected oropharyngeal abscesses in association with cranial nerves IX through XII involvement is pathognomonic of parapharyngeal abscesses.

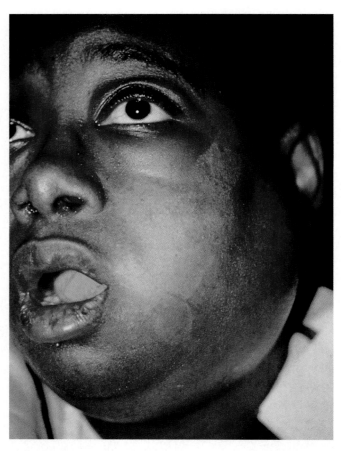

FIGURE 6.34 ■ Parapharyngeal Space Abscess. Unilateral facial, jaw angle, and neck swelling is seen in this patient. Nuchal rigidity may also be present. (Photo contributor: Sara-Jo Gahm, MD.)

Clinical Summary

Painful severely edematous interdental papillae are characteristic of trench mouth, or acute necrotizing ulcerative gingivitis (ANUG). Other associated features include the presence of ulcers with an overlying grayish pseudomembrane and a "punched out" appearance. The inflamed gingival tissue is friable, necrotic, and represents an acute destructive disease process of the periodontium. Fever, malaise, and regional lymphadenopathy are commonly associated signs. Patients may also complain of foul breath and a strong metallic taste. Poor oral hygiene, emotional stress, smoking, and immunocompromised states (eg, HIV, steroid use, diabetes) all predispose for ANUG. Anaerobic *Fusobacterium* and spirochetes are the predominant bacterial organisms involved. The anterior incisor and posterior molar gingival regions are the most commonly affected oral tissue. Acute herpetic, gonococcal, or streptococcal gingivostomatitis, aphthous stomatitis, desquamative gingivitis, and chronic periodontal disease may mimic ANUG.

Emergency Department Treatment and Disposition

Initial management includes warm saline irrigation, systemic analgesics, topical anesthetics, and antibiotic treatment with oropharyngeal coverage. Hydrogen peroxide or chlorhexidine oral rinses are also helpful. Follow-up with a dentist or periodontist in 1 to 2 days is recommended. Patients with more advanced disease may require admission and oral surgical consultation.

Pearls

1. Dramatic relief of symptoms within 24 hours of initiating antibiotics and supportive treatment is characteristic.
2. Periodontal abscesses and underlying alveolar bone destruction are common complications of ANUG and require dental follow-up.
3. Gingivitis is a nontender inflammatory disorder and is not synonymous with ANUG.
4. Consider HIV testing in patients with ANUG.

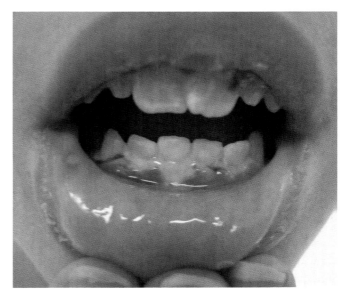

FIGURE 6.36 ■ Acute Necrotizing Ulcerative Gingivitis. Excessive purulent drainage was associated with this patient's ANUG. (Photo contributor: R. Jason Thurman, MD.)

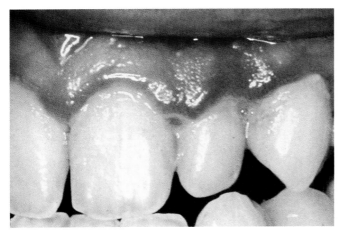

FIGURE 6.35 ■ Acute Necrotizing Ulcerative Gingivitis. Note the inflamed, friable, and necrotic gingival tissue. An overlying grayish pseudomembrane or punched out ulcerations of the interdental papillae are pathognomonic. (Photo contributor: David P. Kretzschmar, DDS, MS.)

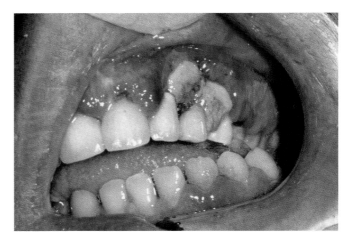

FIGURE 6.37 ■ Severe Acute Necrotizing Ulcerative Gingivitis. Note the extensive gingival necrosis in this advanced case of trench mouth. (Photo contributor: David Effron, MD.)

Clinical Summary

Bulimia nervosa is an eating disorder with significant associated physical complications. It is characterized by binge eating with self-induced vomiting, laxative use, dieting, and exercise to prevent weight gain. Patients with bulimia are at risk for damage to the dental enamel and dentin as a result of repeated episodes of vomiting with chronic exposure to regurgitated acidic gastric contents. The lingual dental surfaces are most commonly affected. In severe cases, all surfaces of the teeth may be affected. Buccal dental surface erosions may be noted as a result of excessive consumption of fruit (ie, lemons) and juices by some bulimic patients. Trauma to the oral and esophageal mucosa may also result from induced vomiting. The quantity, buffering capacity, and pH of both the resting and stimulated saliva are found to be reduced. Salivary gland enlargement, most commonly the parotid, may occur as well.

Included in the differential diagnosis of acid tooth erosion are conditions that involve recurrent vomiting. Xerostomia is a condition of excessive mouth dryness (associated with Sjögren syndrome) which can also accelerate the process of enamel loss. Tooth abrasions and erosions may be brought about by the use of chewing tobacco, eating betel nuts (Indian *paan*), dentifrice, bruxism, abnormal swallowing, and clenching.

Emergency Department Treatment and Disposition

The initial emergency department management of patients with bulimia should address any medical complication of the disorder (hypokalemia, metabolic acidosis, etc). Hospitalization to stabilize medical complications and provide nutritional support may be indicated. Dental treatment should begin with vigorous oral hygiene to prevent further destruction of tooth structures. Besides pain treatment, regular professional fluoride treatments to cover exposed dentin should be instituted. With the exception of temporary cosmetic procedures, definitive dental treatment should be deferred until the patient is adequately stabilized psychologically. A multidisciplinary team approach is necessary and should involve psychiatry, internal medicine, and dental consultation as needed.

Pearls

1. The lingual surfaces of the teeth are the most commonly involved tooth surfaces.
2. Bruxism tends to cause enamel loss from occlusal and incisal dental surfaces.
3. The labial and buccal surfaces of the teeth tend to show enamel loss from repeat or prolonged chemical contact (eg, lemon sucking or tobacco products).

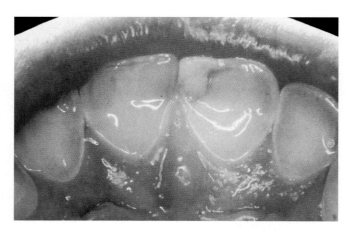

FIGURE 6.38 ■ Acid Tooth Erosion (Bulimia). Erosive dentin exposure of the maxillary teeth secondary to chronic vomiting. The involvement of the lingual dental surfaces is characteristic of bulimia. (Photo contributor: David P. Kretzschmar, DDS, MS.)

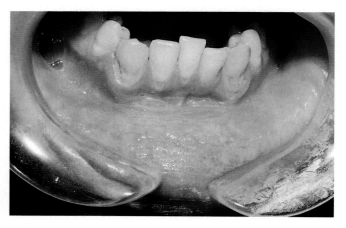

FIGURE 6.39 ■ Acid Tooth Erosion (Snuff User). Note the typical dentin exposure on the buccal dental surfaces resulting from prolonged snuff use and its accompanying acid erosion. (Photo contributor: David P. Kretzschmar, DDS, MS.)

Clinical Summary

White, flaky, curd-like plaques covering the tongue and buccal mucosa with an erythematous base are typical of thrush. These lesions tend to be painless; however, painful inflammatory erosions or ulcers may be noted, particularly in adults. Predisposing factors include antibiotic use, inhaled and oral corticosteroids, radiation to the head and neck, extremes of ages, patients with immunologic deficiencies, and chronic irritation (eg, denture use and xerostomia). Colonization of surface epithelium by *Candida* occurs as a result of an altered oral microflora. Hairy leukoplakia, lingual lichen planus, flecks of milk or food debris, and liquid antacid adhering to the tongue may be confused with candidiasis. Hairy leukoplakia cannot be removed with a tongue depressor (Fig. 20.3). This helps differentiate this process from thrush or residue from ingested materials. Microscopic examination of the removed specimen for the presence of hyphae in potassium hydroxide mount will aid in the identification of *Candida*.

Emergency Department Treatment and Disposition

Nystatin oral tablets, nystatin swish and swallow suspension, fluconazole, or clotrimazole oral troches are usually adequate therapy. Topical analgesic cocktails may also provide comfort for patients (eg, liquid antacid with diphenhydramine, viscous lidocaine).

Pearls

1. Thrush is most common in premature infants and immunosuppressed patients.
2. In young adults, thrush may be the first sign of AIDS; a history of HIV risk factors should be elicited.
3. Failure of oral candidiasis to respond to topical antifungal agents may suggest an immune deficiency.

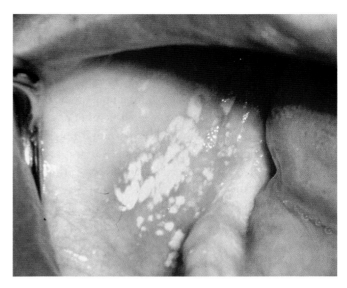

FIGURE 6.40 ■ Oral Candidiasis (Thrush). Whitish plaques are seen here on the buccal mucosa. These plaques are easily removed with a tongue blade, differentiating them from lichen planus or leukoplakia. (Photo contributor: James F. Steiner, DDS.)

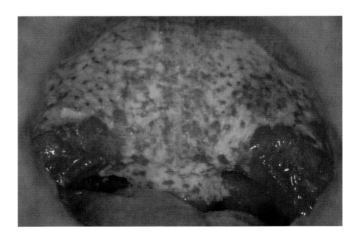

FIGURE 6.41 ■ Oral Candidiasis (Thrush). Extensive thrush is seen on the hard and soft palate of this immunocompromised patient. (Photo contributor: Lawrence B. Stack, MD.)

Clinical Summary

Oral herpes simplex may present acutely as a primary gingivostomatitis or as a recurrence. Painful vesicular eruptions on the oral mucosa, tongue, palate, vermilion borders, and gingiva are highly characteristic. A 2- to 3-day prodromal period of malaise, fever, and cervical adenopathy is common. The vesicular lesions rupture to form a tender ulcer with yellow crusting and an erythematous margin. Pain may be severe enough to cause drooling and odynophagia, which can discourage eating and drinking, particularly in children. The disease tends to run its course in a 7- to 10-day period with nonscarring resolution of the lesions. Recurrent herpes labialis may present with an aura of burning, itching, or tingling prior to vesicle formation. Oral trauma, sunburn, stress, and any variety of febrile illnesses can precipitate this condition. Oral erythema multiforme or Stevens-Johnson syndrome, aphthous lesions, oral pemphigus, and hand-foot-mouth (HFM) syndrome are in the differential diagnosis. It should be noted that aphthous ulcers tend to occur on movable oral mucosa and rarely on immovable mucosa (ie, hard palate and gingiva). The vermilion border is a characteristic location for herpes labialis as opposed to aphthous lesions. Posterior oropharyngeal ulcerations with associated hand and foot lesions help to define HFM syndrome.

Emergency Department Treatment and Disposition

Supportive care with rehydration and pain control are the mainstays of therapy. Temporary pain relief may be achieved with topical analgesics. Viscous lidocaine, 2%, may be used as an oral rinse, 5 mL every 3 to 4 hours. Oral antiviral agents may be useful in adults with primary infections. Secondary infection of herpetic lesions should be treated with oral penicillin or clindamycin.

Pearls

1. Fatal viremia and systemic involvement may occur in infants and children with herpetic gingivostomatitis.
2. Primary acute oral herpetic infection occurs most commonly in children and young adults.
3. Corticosteroid use is contraindicated in herpetic gingivostomatitis.
4. Initiation of suppressive therapy with acyclovir should be considered in the emergency department.

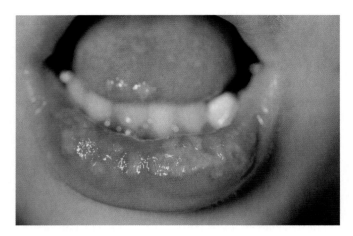

FIGURE 6.42 ■ Herpes Simplex Virus (HSV) Stomatitis. Note the extensive painful ulcerations on the patient's lower lip. A prodromal period of fever, malaise, and cervical adenopathy may herald the onset of these painful ulcerations. (Photo contributor: Lawrence B. Stack, MD.)

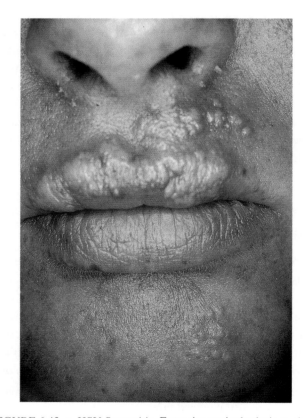

FIGURE 6.43 ■ HSV Stomatitis. Extensive vesicular lesions along the vermilion border and surrounding tissues are consistent with HSV infection. (Photo contributor: Frank Birinyi, MD.)

151

Clinical Summary

Aphthous ulcers are shallow painful mucosal ulcers of 1 to 15 mm. A prodromal burning sensation may be noted 2 to 48 hours before an ulcer is noted. The initial lesion is a small white papule that ulcerates and enlarges over 48 to 72 hours. Lesions are typically round or ovoid with a raised yellow border and surrounding erythema. Multiple aphthous ulcers may occur on the lips, tongue, buccal mucosa, floor of the mouth, or soft palate. Spontaneous healing occurs in 7 to 10 days without scarring. The exact etiology is unknown. Deficiencies of vitamin B_{12}, folic acid, and iron as well as viruses have been implicated. Stress, local trauma, and immunocompromised states have all been cited as possible precipitators.

Primary or recurrent herpetic oral lesions may present with an almost identical prodrome and similar appearance. Herpetic lesions, unlike aphthous ones, tend to occur on the gingiva, hard palate, and vermilion border. Oral erythema multiforme may also present similarly to aphthous stomatitis; however, like oral herpes, it may tend to present with multiple vesicles in the early stages. Stevens-Johnson syndrome represents a severe form of erythema multiforme characterized by hemorrhagic anogenital and conjunctival lesions as well as oral lesions. Herpangina results from Coxsackie and echoviruses with oral ulcerations typically involving the posterior pharynx. Oral pemphigus should also be considered. Behçet syndrome can present with recurrent oral lesions, genital ulcers, and uveitis.

Emergency Department Treatment and Disposition

Supportive care, rehydration, and pain control constitute the focus of therapy. A topical anesthetic agent such as 2% viscous lidocaine or liquid antihistamine/antacid mix as an oral rinse every 3 to 4 hours is palliative. Use of oral antimicrobial rinses containing 0.12% chlorhexidine or tetracycline promotes healing. Protective dental paste may be applied every 6 hours to prevent irritation of lesions. Triamcinolone acetonide in an emollient dental paste three to four times daily may reduce pain and promote healing.

Pearls

1. Aphthous ulcers may be associated with Crohn disease.
2. Topical anesthetics may be used as a temporary adjunct in pain relief. Care must be taken to avoid overdose or complications such as methemoglobinemia from overuse.
3. The first aphthous episode occurs most commonly in the second decade of life.
4. Aphthous ulcers almost never occur on gums or hard palate.

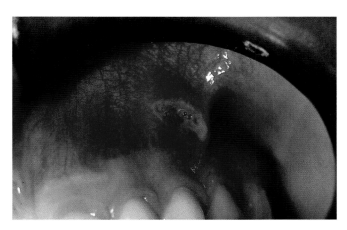

FIGURE 6.44 ■ Aphthous Ulcer (Single Lesion). Raised yellow borders with surrounding erythema are typical of aphthous ulcers. (Photo contributor: James F. Steiner, DDS.)

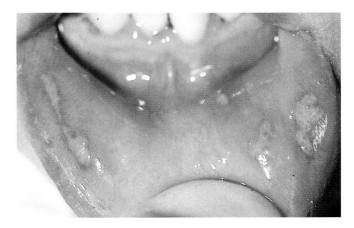

FIGURE 6.45 ■ Aphthous Ulcerations. Note the multiple ulcers of various sizes located on the lip and gingival mucosa. These lesions rarely occur on the immobile oral mucosa of the gingiva or hard palate. (Photo contributor: James F. Steiner, DDS.)

Clinical Summary

Reddened hypertrophied lingual papillae, called strawberry tongue, are associated primarily with scarlet fever caused by group A streptococcal enterotoxin. The tongue initially appears white with the erythematous papillae sticking through the white exudate. After several days, the white coating is lost and the tongue appears bright red. Other signs of group A streptococcal infection include fever, an exudative pharyngitis, a scarlatiniform rash, and the presence of Pastia lines (petechial linear rash in the skin folds). Kawasaki syndrome may also present with an injected pharynx and an erythematous strawberry-like tongue. It is essential to make the distinction between streptococcal infection and Kawasaki syndrome, since the latter is associated with a high incidence of coronary artery aneurysm if left untreated. Also consider toxic shock syndrome (TSS), in which one-half to three-fourths of patients have pharyngitis with a strawberry-red tongue.

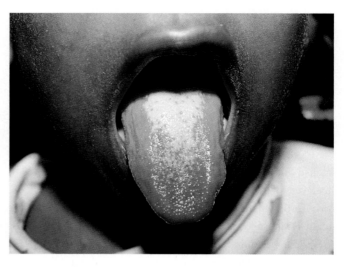

FIGURE 6.46 ■ Strawberry Tongue. Note the white exudate with bulging red papillae. The white coating is eventually lost after several days, and the tongue then appears bright red. (Photo contributor: Michael J. Nowicki, MD.)

Emergency Department Treatment and Disposition

Penicillin is the drug of choice for group A streptococcus. Pharyngeal cultures are useful for confirming the diagnosis. Antistreptolysin O (ASO) titers can be used for confirmation in the convalescent stage if the diagnosis is in question. Rapid streptococcal immunoassay testing may help expedite the diagnosis.

Pearls

1. Strawberry tongue initially appears white in color, with prominent red papillae bulging through the white exudate. After several days, the tongue becomes completely beefy red.
2. A coarse, palpable, sandpaper-like rash of the skin is highly characteristic of associated scarlet fever.

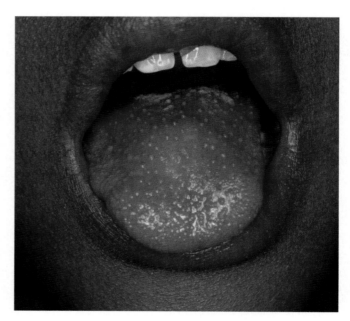

FIGURE 6.47 ■ Strawberry Tongue. This patient with scarlet fever demonstrates the bright red appearance of strawberry tongue after most of the white exudate is lost. (Photo contributor: Kevin J. Knoop, MD, MS.)

Clinical Summary

Tori are benign nodular overgrowths of cortical bone. Although their physical appearance can be somewhat alarming to those unfamiliar with this entity, there is generally no need for concern. These bony protuberances occur in the midline of the palate where the maxilla fuses. Tori may also be located on the mandible, typically on the lingual aspect of the molar teeth. Tori are covered by a thin epithelium, which is easily traumatized and ulcerated. These ulcerations tend to heal very slowly because of the poor vascularization of the tori. Torus palatinus, in particular, is slow growing and may occur at any age; however, it is most commonly noted prior to age 30 in adults. Torus palatinus affects women twice as frequently as men. There are a variety of oral conditions that may be confused with mandibular or palatal tori. Gingival fibromatosis, fibroma formation secondary to irritation, granulomas, abscesses, and oral neurofibromatosis located on the palate may resemble torus palatinus. Nodular bony enlargement in the oral cavity may also result from fibrous dysplasia, osteomas, and Paget disease. Oral malignancies may manifest themselves on the palate as primary lesions, though these are rare. Oral radiographs, CT scans, and biopsy may aid in differentiating these conditions.

Emergency Department Treatment and Disposition

Tori are normal structural variants and do not represent an inflammatory or neoplastic process. They require no treatment unless associated with a complication. Tori may enlarge enough to interfere with eating or speaking, and impair proper fitting of dental prostheses. For some patients, the mere presence of torus palatinus may be bothersome and undesirable. Oral and maxillofacial consultation is indicated for suspected malignancies or lesions of questionable origin.

Pearl

1. Torus palatinus and torus mandibularis are nontender and otherwise asymptomatic.

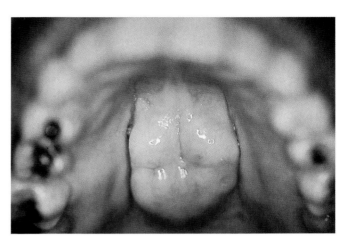

FIGURE 6.48 ■ Torus Palatinus. Note the nodular appearance and characteristic central palatal location. (Photo contributor: Kevin J. Knoop, MD, MS.)

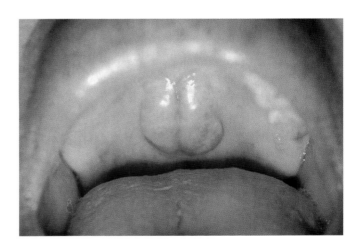

FIGURE 6.49 ■ Torus Palatinus. Due to location, abrasions and ulcerations can occur on the thin overlying epithelium secondary to trauma. (Photo contributor: R. Jason Thurman, MD.)

Clinical Summary

Black hairy tongue (BHT) represents a benign reactive process characterized by hyperplasia and dark pigmentation of the tongue's filiform papillae. The elongated filiform papillae may reach up to 2 cm in length and vary in actual degree of pigmentation from light tan to black. Predisposing factors may include excessive smoking, gastroesophageal reflux, poor oral hygiene, chemotherapy, and the use of broad-spectrum oral antibiotics. Pigment from consumed food, beverages, and tobacco products stains the entrapped food debris and desquamated papillary keratin. Some antibiotics may alter normal oral microflora and promote the growth of chromogenic organisms, also contributing to the tongue's discoloration. The darkly pigmented filament-like papillae give the tongue a black, hairy appearance. Males are more often affected than females; this condition very rarely occurs in children. Alteration of taste perception and fetid breath may be a consequence of BHT.

Geographic tongue and orolingual candidiasis may resemble more lightly pigmented forms of BHT. Similarly, dark discoloration of normal tongue papillae may also mimic BHT. This exogenous pigmentation of normal papillae may come from ingested food dyes and certain medications, such as bismuth-containing compounds, ketoconazole, and azidothymidine. The lack of hyperplastic filiform papillae with additional pigmentation of other oral mucosal surfaces may aid in distinguishing these conditions.

Emergency Department Treatment and Disposition

Improved oral hygiene with gentle tongue brushing and a reduction in the ingestion of exogenous pigment-containing substance represent the cornerstone of treatment. Removal of other predisposing factors (eg, antibiotic withdrawal and smoking cessation) will also promote resolution of this condition. The use of topically applied retinoid preparations and antifungal agents has been advocated for more refractory instances.

Pearls

1. BHT involves the superior aspect of the tongue.
2. The tongue is not always black and can be a tan or yellow color.

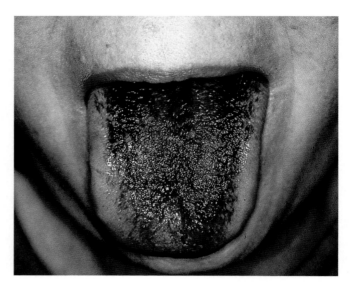

FIGURE 6.50 ■ Black Hairy Tongue. Hyperplasia of the filiform papillae on the dorsum of the tongue accompanied by deposition of dark pigment is characteristic of black hairy tongue. (Photo contributor: Department of Dermatology, National Naval Medical Center, Bethesda, MD.)

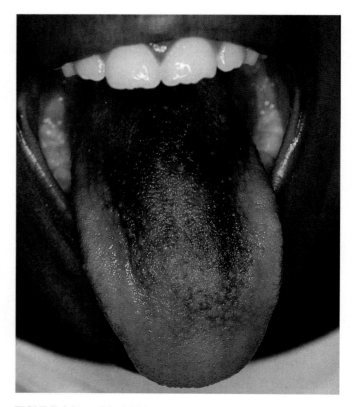

FIGURE 6.51 ■ Black Hairy Tongue. Deposition of black pigment secondary to bismuth ingestion. This patient ingested Pepto-Bismol. (Photo contributor: Kevin J. Knoop, MD, MS.)

Clinical Summary

Facial piercings are common. While external piercings such as ear and eyebrow rings are visibly apparent, intra- and extra-oral piercing may not be readily visible on initial inspection. An awareness and suspicion for recent lip or tongue piercings should be performed in any trauma patients as they may cause intraoral damage, interfere with CT scan quality if not removed, and obstruct the airway view during intubation. Common non-traumatic complications of intraoral include peri-piercing cellulitis, abscess formation, hemorrhage, penetrating wounds, and granuloma formation around a stud. Though infrequent, systemic infection may result. If the ball comes off the post, it may be swallowed, or rarely, aspirated. Playing with tongue rings may result in lingual surface tooth abrasion, erosion, chipping, fracture, and gingival resorption.

Emergency Department Treatment and Disposition

Piercing should be removed prior to any CT scan if possible. For localized hemorrhage after a recent piercing, direct pressure should be applied. If bleeding persists, consider removal of the piercing. Any infection surrounding a piercing warrants removal of the stud as it will serve as a nidus for continued infection. Consideration should be given to oral antibiotic therapy. Chest radiographs are required to evaluate for stud aspiration. Advise patients with chipped teeth to remove the bar or shorten the post.

Pearls

1. Remove piercings prior to cross-sectional imaging.
2. Piercings will act as a nidus for ongoing infection if not removed.
3. Ensure the prompt identification and removal of intraoral and extraoral piercings in any trauma patient potentially requiring emergent airway management, as the presence of jewelry can be a hindrance to successful intubation.

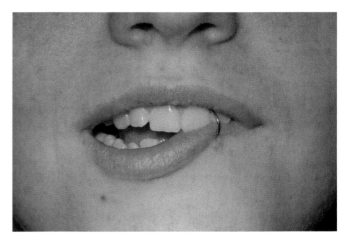

FIGURE 6.53 ■ Oral Piercing Complication. This patient suffered a painful injury when the stud of her lip ring came off, resulting in the penetration of her gingiva and inability to open her mouth. (Photo contributor: Lawrence B. Stack, MD.)

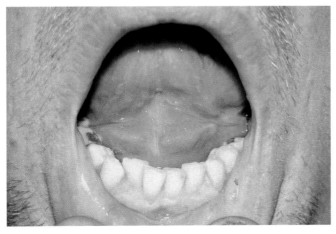

FIGURE 6.52 ■ Tongue Piercing Cellulitis. This patient presented with fever and tongue pain surrounding his piercing site. Note the erythema and swelling of the tongue and sublingual areas extending from the piercing site (central bubble). (Photo contributor: David Effron, MD.)

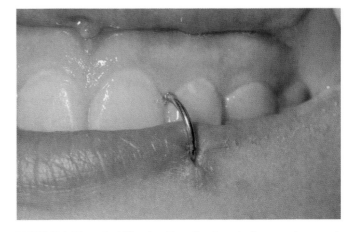

FIGURE 6.54 ■ Oral Piercing Complication. A close-up photograph of the oral piercing complication seen in Fig. 6.53. (Photo contributor: Lawrence B. Stack, MD.)

Chapter 7

CHEST AND ABDOMEN

Stephen W. Corbett
Lawrence B. Stack
Kevin J. Knoop

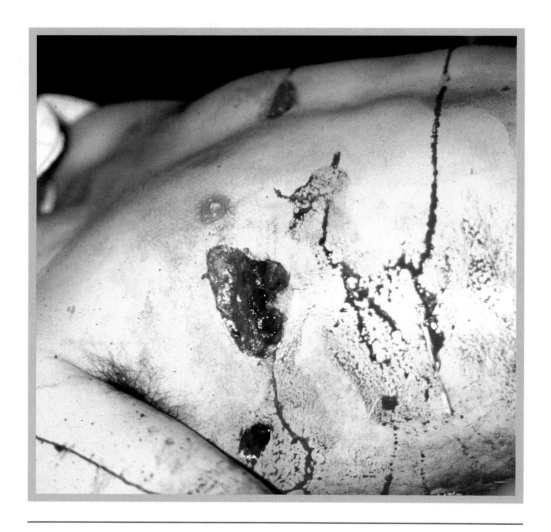

Clinical Summary

The clinical findings of traumatic asphyxia are due to a sudden increase in intrathoracic pressure against a closed glottis. The elevated pressure is transmitted to the veins, venules, and capillaries of the head, neck, extremities, and upper torso, resulting in capillary rupture. Strangulation and hanging are common mechanisms. Survivors demonstrate plethora, ecchymoses, petechiae, and subconjunctival hemorrhages. Severe cases may produce CNS injury with seizures, posturing, and paraplegia.

Emergency Department Treatment and Disposition

Treatment is supportive, with attention to other concurrent injuries. Long-term morbidity is related to the associated injuries.

Pearls

1. Facial petechiae are known as Tardieu spots.
2. One should be alert for associated rib and vertebral fractures.

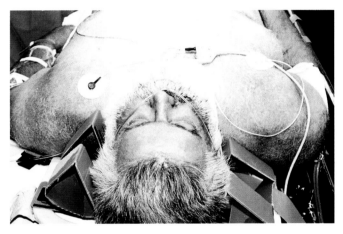

FIGURE 7.1 ■ Traumatic Asphyxia. This 45-year-old male was pinned when the truck he was working under fell on his chest. He was unable to breathe for 3 to 4 minutes until his coworkers rescued him. The violaceous coloration of the shoulders, face, and upper chest is apparent. (Photo contributor: Stephen W. Corbett, MD.)

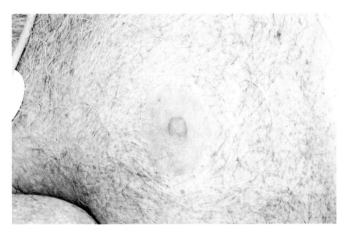

FIGURE 7.2 ■ Traumatic Asphyxia. A closer view showing the petechial nature of this rash. The patient was observed in the hospital overnight and recovered completely. (Photo contributor: Stephen W. Corbett, MD.)

Clinical Summary

A flail chest occurs when a segment of the thoracic cage is detached from the rest of the chest wall, resulting in suboptimal ventilation and oxygenation. Typically, several ribs are broken in one or more places. This creates a segment of the chest wall (a flail segment) that does not move in unison with the rest of the thorax. When the diaphragm produces negative inspiratory pressure, the flail segment, no longer anchored to the rib cage, tends to move inward, reducing ventilatory capacity. Pulmonary contusion, hemothorax, pneumothorax, and great vessel injuries frequently accompany a flail chest.

Emergency Department Treatment and Disposition

Pain control and pulmonary toilet are initial standard therapy. Mechanical ventilation is reserved for those with respiratory insufficiency or failure in spite of standard therapy. Treatment of underlying pulmonary injuries and intensive care unit admission is required for these critically ill patients.

Pearls

1. Intercostal nerve blocks may help provide adequate analgesia so that pain does not prevent the patient from ventilating adequately.
2. Positive end expiratory pressure (PEEP) may be helpful in patients that require mechanical ventilation.
3. Paradoxical movement of the flail segment is seen during the respiratory cycle in flail chest. As the rib cage expands with inspiration, the flail segment sinks into the chest. As it contracts in expiration, it balloons outward.

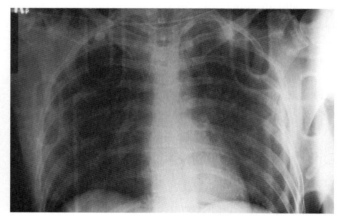

FIGURE 7.4 ■ Flail Chest: Trauma Chest X-Ray. Fractures in two places of ribs 3 and 4 result in a flail segment. Ribs 2 and 5 have single fractures. (Photo contributor: Lawrence B. Stack, MD.)

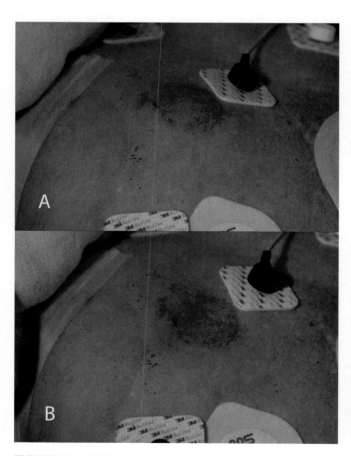

FIGURE 7.3 ■ Flail Chest. Localized blunt trauma to the left anterior chest 4 cm inferior to the mid-clavicle, with resultant flail segment. Positive intrathoracic pressure (panel A) and negative intrathoracic pressure (panel B) demonstrate the paradoxical movement of the flail segment. (Photo contributor: Lawrence B. Stack, MD.)

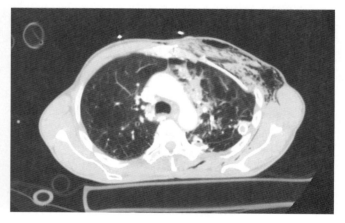

FIGURE 7.5 ■ Flail Chest: Chest CT Scan. A flail segment is seen of the left anterior chest on an axial cut of this chest CT scan. A chest tube is seen in the left pleural space. Subcutaneous emphysema is seen in the area of the fractures and tracking posteriorly. (Photo contributor: Lawrence B. Stack, MD.)

Clinical Summary

Dislocations of the sternoclavicular joint (SCJ) are uncommon due to the strength of the supporting ligaments. Anterior dislocations are nine times more frequent than posterior dislocations. Posterior dislocations are clinically more important due to the potential for injury to underlying structures. SCJ dislocations typically occur from motor vehicle crashes and sports injuries. Posterior dislocations may occur from a direct force to the proximal clavicle or from an indirect force to the shoulder with the shoulder rolled forward. Anterior dislocations occur from and indirect force to the shoulder with the shoulder rolled backward. Examination findings of an anterior SCJ dislocation include tenderness and prominence of the proximal clavicle from the sternum. The arm is often held in adduction. Movement of the arm typically causes pain. Posterior SCJ dislocations may be more difficult to identify as frequently they are associated with multiple injures. Pain and depression of the medial clavicle relative to the sternum may be seen. Superior and inferior dislocations may also be seen. CT scan through the SCJ is the best diagnostic study to evaluate this injury.

Emergency Department Treatment and Disposition

Orthopedic follow up is required. Closed reduction of anterior SCJ dislocations is preformed by placing the patient supine with a sandbag between their shoulders and placing downward pressure directly over the clavicle. A figure-of-eight clavicle harness is applied. Recurrence is common. Closed reduction of posterior SCJ dislocations may be attempted by an orthopaedic surgeon by placing a towel clip around the medial clavicle and pulling the clavicle forward. Open reduction is often necessary.

Pearls

1. SCJ dislocations account for less than 3% of shoulder girdle dislocations.
2. While typically it requires a tremendous force to cause an SCJ dislocation, spontaneous dislocations have been reported.
3. Plain films will not adequately demonstrate SCJ dislocations.
4. Posterior SCJ dislocations may result in underlying vascular injury.

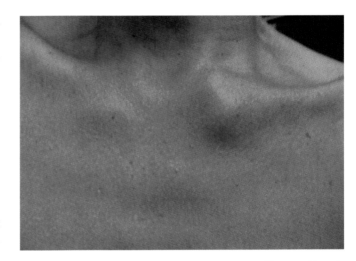

FIGURE 7.6 ■ Sternoclavicular Dislocation. A 43-year-old male complains of left sternoclavicular pain after direct trauma to the shoulder. Prominent proximal clavicle is seen prompting CT scan confirmation. (Photo contributor: R. Jason Thurman, MD.)

Clinical Summary

A tension pneumothorax results when air enters but does not exit the pleural space. Air in the pleural space accumulates and compresses the ipsilateral lung and vena cava, with a rapid decrease in cardiac output. The contralateral lung may suffer ventilation/perfusion mismatch. Subcutaneous air, tracheal deviation, jugular venous distention (JVD), and diminished or hyperresonant ipsilateral breath sounds can be clues. Subcutaneous emphysema may be visible on the neck and chest radiographs and is easily diagnosed by palpation. The released air from a tension pneumothorax can be heard escaping from a needle thoracostomy.

Emergency Department Treatment and Disposition

Treatment requires rapid recognition of the tension pneumothorax, frequently without benefit of chest radiographs. A 14-gauge needle or larger should be placed over the superior rib surface of the second interspace in the midclavicular line. A rush of air with improvement of vital signs confirms the diagnosis. If there is no immediate improvement, do not hesitate to place a second needle in the next interspace. A chest tube should be placed immediately.

Pearls

1. Do not overventilate patients with obstructive pulmonary disease. "Stacking" breaths traps air in the lungs and predispose to bleb rupture and pneumothorax. The pathophysiology of this disease requires a prolonged expiratory phase.
2. The diagnosis of a tension pneumothorax should be made clinically and should be treated immediately with needle thoracostomy and tube thoracostomy.
3. The radiographic "deep-sulcus sign" is seen in supine patients with a tension pneumothorax as air collects anteriorly and basally.

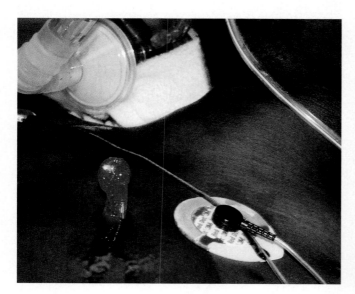

FIGURE 7.7 ■ Tension Pneumothorax. A 35-year-old male with severe asthma suffered respiratory arrest during transport by ambulance. He was intubated on arrival but soon became hard to ventilate and developed subcutaneous emphysema followed by hypotension. Needle thoracostomy produced a rush of air and bubbling from the needle with stabilization of vital signs. (Photo contributor: Stephen W. Corbett, MD.)

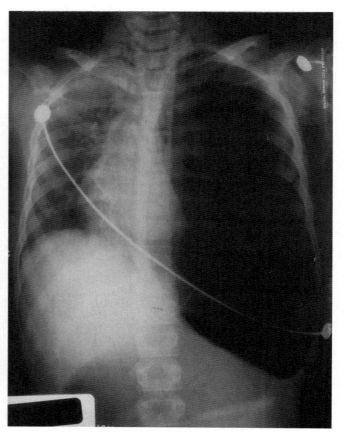

FIGURE 7.8 ■ Deep Sulcus Sign. Marked deepening of the left costophrenic angle is seen. Left to right mediastinal shift and mediastinal emphysema is also seen. (Photo contributor: Lawrence B. Stack, MD.)

Clinical Summary

The Beck triad of acute cardiac tamponade includes jugular venous distention (JVD) from an elevated central venous pressure (CVP), hypotension, and muffled heart sounds. In trauma, only one-third of patients with cardiac tamponade demonstrate this classic triad, although 90% have at least one of the signs. The simultaneous appearance of all three physical signs is a late manifestation of tamponade and usually seen just prior to cardiac arrest. Other symptoms include shortness of breath, orthopnea, dyspnea on exertion, syncope, and symptoms of inadequate perfusion.

Emergency Department Treatment and Disposition

The clinical diagnosis of tamponade requires suspicion and a careful evaluation of the signs and, when available, imaging techniques. Bedside ultrasonography provides rapid diagnosis and facilitates pericardiocentesis. Emergency department pericardiocentesis is a diagnostic and resuscitative procedure in patients with suspected cardiac tamponade. Goals of emergency department pericardiocentesis include identification of pericardial effusion and removal of blood from the pericardial space to relieve the tamponade.

Pearls

1. Electrical alternans seen on a 12-lead ECG suggests pericardial effusion.
2. The Beck triad for acute cardiac tamponade is a late manifestation and is seen in only 30% of trauma patients.
3. Ultrasonographic identification of pericardial fluid in patients with penetration chest trauma may lead to life-saving pericardiocentesis.

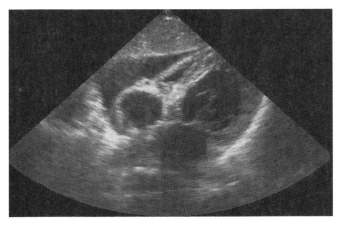

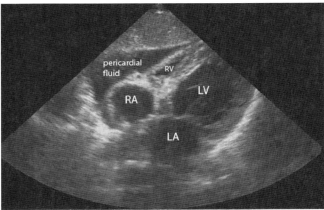

FIGURE 7.9 ■ Ultrasound of Cardiac Tamponade. This subxyphoid view of the heart reveals a large pericardial fluid collection and compression of the right ventricle (RV) suggesting tamponade physiology. (Photo contributor: Department of Emergency Medicine, Ultrasound Section, Vanderbilt University.)

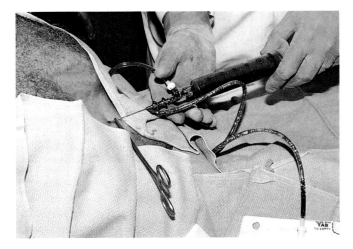

FIGURE 7.10 ■ Emergency Department Pericardiocentesis. A positive pericardiocentesis in a patient with a sudden onset of shortness of breath and electrical alternans. (Photo contributor: Lawrence B. Stack, MD.)

Clinical Summary

Emergency department thoracotomy is a resuscitative procedure performed in patients with penetrating chest trauma, who have lost signs of life in the presence of prehospital or emergency department personnel. Thoracotomy in the emergency department has specific goals once the chest is opened: relief of cardiac tamponade, support of cardiac function (internal cardiac compressions, cross-clamping the aorta to improve coronary perfusion, and internal defibrillation), and control of hemorrhage from the heart, pulmonary vessels, thoracic wall, and great vessels.

Emergency Department Treatment and Disposition

Patients with penetrating thoracic trauma who lose their vital signs on arrival, or shortly before arriving to the emergency department, should receive an immediate thoracotomy in the emergency department. Patients with penetrating thoracic trauma whose blood pressure cannot be maintained above 70 mm Hg with aggressive fluid and blood management should be considered for emergency department thoracotomy. Patients with blunt trauma who lose their vital signs en route to the emergency department should not undergo an emergency department thoracotomy, since they rarely survive. Surgical support should be notified as soon as possible.

Pearls

1. Injuries potentially responsive to emergency department thoracotomy include cardiac tamponade, pulmonary parenchymal and tracheobronchial injuries, large-vessel injuries, air embolism, and penetrating heart injuries.

2. Emergency department thoracotomy should be performed immediately once the indications have been met, since the likelihood of survival is greater when this is performed earlier in the resuscitation.

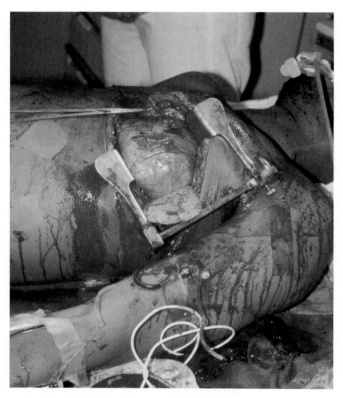

FIGURE 7.11 ■ Emergency Department Thoracotomy. An unsuccessful resuscitative emergency department thoracotomy with pericardiotomy in a patient with penetrating chest trauma who lost signs of life in the field after the paramedics arrived at the scene. (Photo contributor: Lawrence B. Stack, MD.)

Clinical Summary

Diagnostic peritoneal lavage (DPL) is a simple, fast, and reliable technique to identify hemoperitoneum in patients with blunt and penetrating abdominal trauma. A catheter is placed into the peritoneum and aspiration for gross blood is preformed. The aspiration is considered positive if 10 mL of blood is obtained. If the aspiration is negative, 1000 mL of crystalloid is instilled into the abdomen. The lavage fluid is then withdrawn and white and red cell blood counts are obtained. Interpretation of the results is based on the type of trauma. A DPL is considered positive in blunt abdominal trauma when greater than 100,000 RBC/mm^3 or greater than 500 WBC/mm^3 are present in the lavage fluid. In penetrating abdominal trauma, the procedure is considered positive when greater than 10,000 RBC/mm^3 are present (up to 100,000 RBC/mm^3 is used by some). Lavage fluid containing intestinal contents is evidence of perforating bowel injury.

Injuries that may not be diagnosed with DPL include subcapsular liver or spleen hematomas, injury to a hollow viscus, ruptured diaphragm, and ruptured bladder. Retroperitoneal injuries (pancreatic, duodenal, and partial colon) are not diagnosed with DPL.

FAST has replaced the DPL in many trauma centers. The FAST examination is more rapid, noninvasive, provides additional information about fluid in the chest, but does not detect small amounts (10 cc) of hemorrhage that may be seen in penetrating trauma.

Emergency Department Treatment and Disposition

A positive DPL is an indication for celiotomy. Patients with a negative DPL may require additional diagnostic imaging or observation.

Pearls

1. Thirty milliliters of intraperitoneal blood will typically give a DPL result of greater than or equal to 100,000 RBC/mm^3.
2. Controversy exists over the positive cell count in penetrating abdominal trauma, since the range for a positive result can vary between centers from 1000 to 100,000 RBC/mm^3.
3. If transfer is indicated, a sample of DPL fluid should accompany the patient.

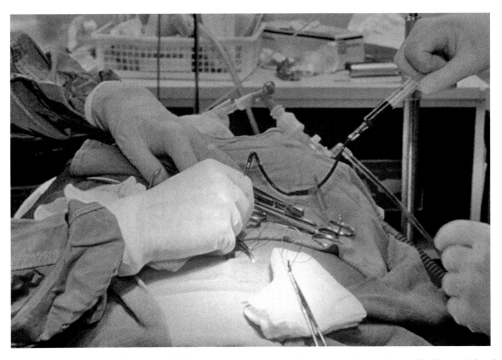

FIGURE 7.12 ■ Positive DPL Aspirate. A positive DPL aspirate is seen in this hypotensive patient with blunt abdominal trauma. (Photo contributor: David Effron, MD.)

Clinical Summary

Two- and three-point seat belt restraints have reduced mortality and the severity of trauma due to motor vehicle crashes; however, they occasionally produce injury. Abrasions to the neck, chest, and abdomen occur in less than 20% of patients, but are associated with a four-fold risk of intrathoracic and an eight-fold risk of intra-abdominal injury. Neck abrasions are associated with carotid artery injury, laryngeal fracture, and cervical spine injury. Chest abrasions are associated with fractures of the sternum, ribs and clavicles, and injuries to the aorta and heart. Abrasions to the abdomen include mesenteric injury, bowel perforation and hematoma, injuries to the abdominal aorta, and Chance fractures.

Emergency Department Treatment and Disposition

Patients with a mechanism for significant trauma or with other injuries requiring admission need to undergo a careful search for related injures. Patients discharged home from the emergency department should be given appropriate precautions to monitor for a delayed injury presentation.

Pearls

1. Thirty percent of patients involved in a motor vehicle crash who have a seat belt abrasion have a significant internal injury.
2. Children, who are more likely to be lap-belt only, rear-seat passengers are more likely to have Chance fractures and small bowel injury if they have an abdominal seat belt abrasion after a motor vehicle crash.

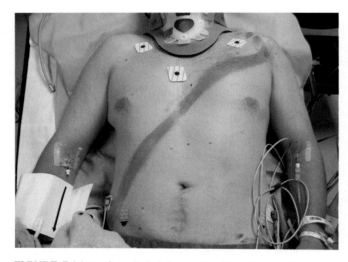

FIGURE 7.14 ■ Seat Belt Injury. Abrasions from a three-point restraint causing rib fractures and a pneumothorax. (Photo contributor: Brad Russell, MD.)

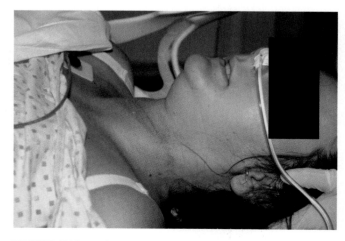

FIGURE 7.15 ■ Seat Belt Injury. Neck abrasions from at three-point restraint in a patient involved in a head-on motor vehicle crash. (Photo contributor: David Effron, MD.)

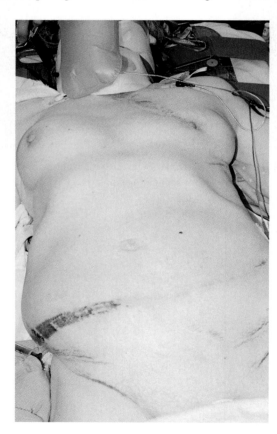

FIGURE 7.13 ■ Seat Belt Injury. Ecchymosis from the three-point seat belt is clearly seen. The injuries identified are multiple rib fractures and multiple hematomas of the small bowel wall. (Photo contributor: Stephen W. Corbett, MD.)

Clinical Summary

Bluish to purplish periumbilical discoloration (Cullen sign) and flank discoloration (Grey Turner sign) represent retroperitoneal hemorrhage that has dissected through fascial planes to the skin. Retroperitoneal blood may also extravasate into the perineum, causing a scrotal hematoma or inguinal mass. This hemorrhage may represent a hemodynamically significant bleed.

Cullen sign and Grey Turner sign are most frequently associated with hemorrhagic pancreatitis and are seen in 1% to 2% of cases, and typically are seen 2 to 3 days after onset. These signs may also be seen in ruptured ectopic pregnancy, severe trauma, leaking or ruptured abdominal aortic aneurysm, coagulopathy, or any other condition associated with bleeding into the retroperitoneum.

Emergency Department Treatment and Disposition

Treatment of patients with Grey Turner sign or Cullen sign depends on the etiology. Because the hemorrhage may represent a hemodynamically significant bleed, cardiovascular stabilization after airway stabilization is of the utmost importance. Once the patient has been stabilized, the source of bleeding can be elicited by selected laboratory (complete blood cell count, amylase, lipase, human chorionic gonadotropin and diagnostic studies [ultrasound, computed tomography]). Because of the severity of diseases associated with Grey Turner and Cullen signs, these patients are usually admitted to the hospital.

Pearls

1. Grey Turner sign (flank discoloration) and Cullen sign (periumbilical discoloration) are due to retroperitoneal bleeding that has dissected through fascial planes.
2. These signs are typically seen 2 to 3 days after the acute event.
3. These signs are seen in only 1% to 2% of patients with hemorrhagic pancreatitis.

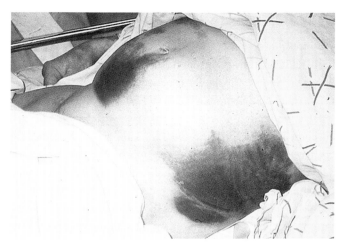

FIGURE 7.16 ■ Grey Turner and Cullen Signs. This patient displays both flank and periumbilical ecchymoses characteristic of Grey Turner and Cullen signs. (Photo contributor: Michael Ritter, MD.)

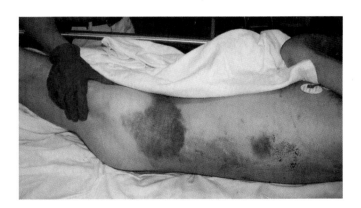

FIGURE 7.17 ■ Grey Turner Sign. A 68-year-old man with flank ecchymosis due to hemorrhagic pancreatitis. (Photo contributor: Stephen W. Corbett, MD.)

Clinical Summary

Stab wounds cause injury to tissue in their path. Stab wounds to the chest, in addition to causing pneumo- or hemothorax, may also cause life-threatening injuries to the heart and major blood vessels. One-third of stab wounds to the abdomen penetrate the peritoneal cavity. Half of the injuries that penetrate the peritoneum require surgical intervention. The path of the stab wound is difficult to determine if the inflicting object has been removed. The size of the external wound frequently underestimates the internal injury. Impaled foreign bodies to the chest or abdomen pose a complex problem. The object inflicting the injury may also be preventing significant blood loss and therefore should be removed by the trauma surgeon in the operating room.

Whether the impaled object has violated the peritoneum or if injury to a significant structure has occurred can be determined by local wound exploration, diagnostic peritoneal lavage (DPL), or focused assessment with sonography for trauma, depending on the stability of the patient and location of the wound.

Emergency Department Treatment and Disposition

Initial stabilization of the patient (intravenous fluid resuscitation, oxygen, and monitoring), obtaining appropriate laboratory studies including blood type and cross-matching, and resource mobilization (trauma team) are important steps in the initial management of penetrating chest or abdominal trauma. Prior to surgical evaluation, stabilization of the impaled foreign object should be performed to prevent further injury.

Pearl

1. Impaled chest or abdominal foreign bodies should be removed only by a trauma surgeon in a controlled setting.

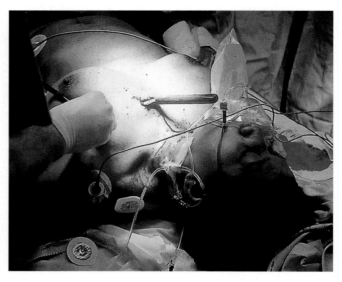

FIGURE 7.18 ■ Impaled Chest Wound. This patient was stabbed in the chest with a butcher knife in a family dispute. The knife was stabilized by EMS providers at the scene and removed in the operating room. Injury was isolated to the right atrium. (Photo contributor: Kevin J. Knoop, MD, MS.)

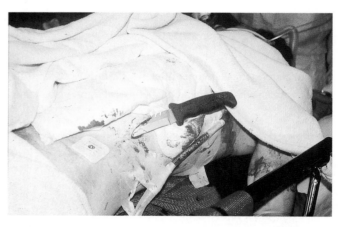

FIGURE 7.19 ■ Impaled Abdominal Foreign Body. Impaled knife to the left abdomen after a domestic argument. (Photo contributor: Ian D. Jones, MD.)

Clinical Summary

Evisceration of abdominal contents usually occurs after a stab or slash wound to the abdomen. It is an indication for celiotomy (laparotomy). Other indications for celiotomy in penetrating abdominal trauma include peritoneal penetration; unexplained shock; evidence of blood in the stomach, bladder, or rectum; and loss of bowel sounds.

Consideration of the anatomic boundaries of the abdomen is important in differentiating abdominal injuries from penetrating chest or retroperitoneal injuries.

Emergency Department Treatment and Disposition

Initial stabilization (intravenous fluid resuscitation, oxygen, and monitoring), obtaining appropriate laboratory studies including a blood type and cross-matching, and resource mobilization (notifying surgical team, operating room, and anesthesiology) are important steps in the initial management of penetrating abdominal trauma. In most cases, definitive treatment is celiotomy.

Pearls

1. Indications for celiotomy after penetrating wounds to the abdomen include evisceration; peritoneal signs; unexplained hypotension; blood in the stomach, bladder, or rectum; and loss of bowel sounds.

2. Selected patients with stab wounds to the abdomen and peritoneal penetration may be conservatively observed for delayed complications. Some centers are using a nonoperative approach for patients with gunshot wounds to the abdomen as well.

3. As many as 20% of patients with stab wounds to the abdomen can be discharged from the emergency department based on a negative wound exploration.

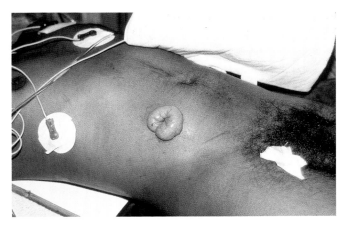

FIGURE 7.21 ■ Abdominal Evisceration. Evisceration of small bowel after assault and stab wound to the right lower abdomen. (Photo contributor: Frank Birinyi, MD.)

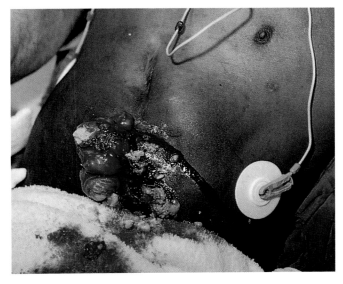

FIGURE 7.20 ■ Abdominal Evisceration. Self-induced evisceration with bowel perforation and spillage of food particles is clearly seen in this photograph. This patient went directly to the operating room. (Photo contributor: Lawrence B. Stack, MD.)

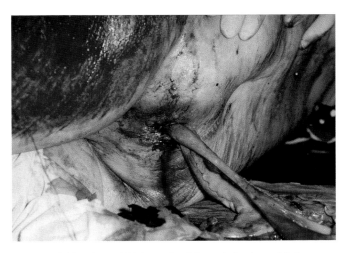

FIGURE 7.22 ■ Bowel Evisceration Through the Anus. High energy blunt abdominal trauma to this elderly man resulted in evisceration of small bowel and omentum through his anus. (Photo contributor: Alan B. Storrow, MD.)

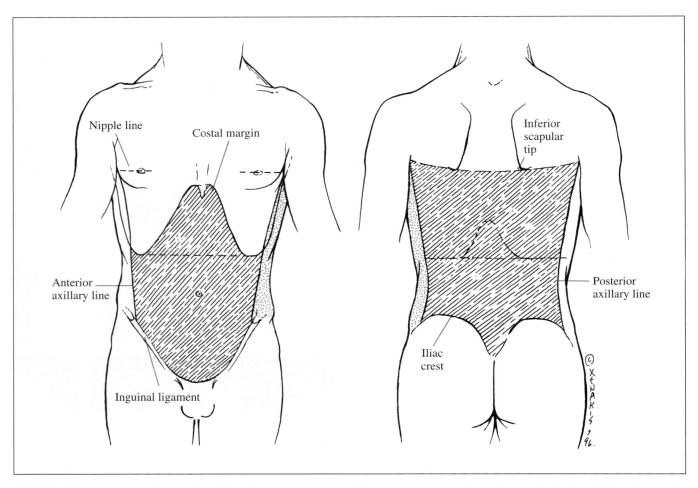

FIGURE 7.23 ■ Anatomic Boundaries of the Abdomen. *Anterior abdomen*: Anterior costal margins superiorly, laterally by the anterior axillary lines, and inferiorly by the inguinal ligaments. *Low chest*: Nipple line (fourth intercostal space) anteriorly and inferior scapular tip (seventh intercostal space) to inferior costal margins. *Flank*: (Shaded blue) Anterior axillary line anteriorly, posteriorly by the posterior axillary line, inferiorly by the iliac crest, and superiorly by the inferior scapular tip. The back is bounded laterally by the posterior axillary lines. *Back*: Inferior scapular tip to iliac crest and posterior axillary lines.

Clinical Summary

Blunt traumatic abdominal hernia is defined as herniation through disrupted musculature and fascia associated with adequate trauma, without skin penetration, and no evidence of a prior hernial defect at the site of injury. This occurs when a considerable blunt force is distributed over a surface area large enough to prevent skin penetration but small enough to cause a focal defect in the underlying fascia or muscle wall. Most of these injuries are due to seat belt injures in motor vehicle crashes; handlebar injuries are the second most common cause.

Abdominal computed tomography (CT) with contrast is the diagnostic procedure of choice in the evaluation of abdominal trauma. Ultrasound may play a limited role in the diagnosis of abdominal wall hernia.

Emergency Department Treatment and Disposition

Identification and treatment of life-threatening associated injuries takes priority over the hernia. The hernial defect should be repaired after the patient has been stabilized.

Pearls

1. Abdominal hernia due to blunt trauma is a rare injury, most frequently due to seat belt injuries in motor vehicle crashes.
2. CT scan is the diagnostic procedure of choice for abdominal wall hernia.

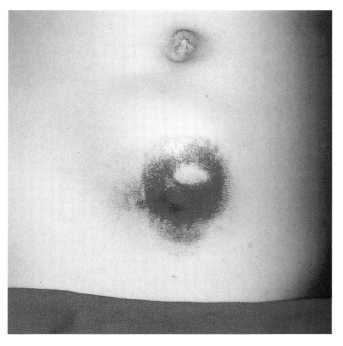

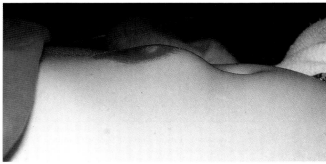

FIGURE 7.24 ■ Traumatic Abdominal Wall Hernia. This 5-year-old boy suffered a traumatic hernia from a handlebar injury. (Photo contributor: Lawrence B. Stack, MD.)

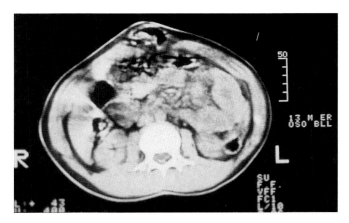

FIGURE 7.25 ■ CT Scan, Abdominal Wall Hernia. Abdominal contents are seen extruding through a fascial defect. (Photo contributor: Lawrence B. Stack, MD.)

Clinical Summary

Pelvic fractures are often the result of motor vehicle crashes or falls and are fraught with associated complications. The pelvis should be regarded as a ring; identification of one fracture or dislocation should prompt surveillance for another. The purpose of the pelvis is to bear weight and to protect the visceral organs; consequently, a fracture of the pelvis will often compromise these functions. Pain is the most common complaint; however, patients with pelvic fractures may present unconscious so a careful physical examination is necessary. Trauma to the genitourinary tract is suggested by blood at the urethral meatus, a high-riding prostate, gross hematuria, or scrotal hematoma. Spinal nerves, the lumbosacral plexus, sacral plexus, and the major lower extremity peripheral nerves such as the sciatic, femoral, obturator, and pudendal nerves, are found in close proximity to the pelvis. A neurologic examination of the lower extremities should include a rectal examination to assess tone and temperature sensation. The iliac arteries, veins, and their branches are also enveloped by the bony architecture of the pelvis and severe hemorrhage is a common complication. While ecchymosis of the anterior abdominal wall, flank, sacral, or gluteal region suggests hemorrhage, there may be no outward signs of a severe hemorrhage. Blood found during rectal examination may indicate that a fracture punctured the rectal wall.

Pelvic fracture classification is complicated. The emergency department physician should ascertain if the fracture transects the pelvic ring; involves the ischium, ilium, sacrum, or pubis; if the pubic symphysis is widened; if the sacroiliac joints are involved; or if the fracture is displaced.

Emergency Department Treatment and Disposition

All patients with a suspected pelvic fracture should undergo a radiographic evaluation with an AP x-ray of the pelvis. If a fracture is identified, more detailed films can be obtained. A CT scan is often necessary to identify associated injuries. A retrograde urethrogram may also be necessary if a GU injury is suspected. Angiography with selective embolization should be performed to control arterial bleeding. In the face of a widened pubic symphysis or "open book" pelvic fracture and continued hemodynamic instability, orthopedic consultation for emergent external fixation can help to reduce blood vessel tension and reduce hemorrhage.

Pearls

1. MAST (medical antishock trousers), a pelvic binder, or a sheet tied around the pelvis may be used to temporarily stabilize pelvic fractures.
2. Posterior pelvic fractures are more likely to result in neurovascular injuries while anterior pelvic fractures are more likely to cause urogenital injuries.
3. Displacement of pelvic ring fractures is usually associated with fracture or dislocation of another ring element.

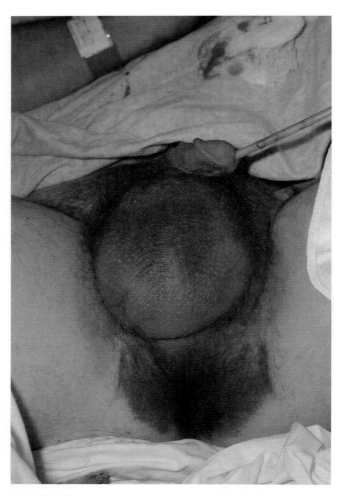

FIGURE 7.26. ■ Pelvic Fracture. Scrotal and perianal ecchymosis is seen in this patient with a vertical shear pelvic fracture due to a fall. (Photo contributor: Lawrence B. Stack, MD.)

Clinical Summary

Increased respiratory effort may be manifested by increased respiratory rate, increased chest wall excursion, and retractions of the less rigid structures of the thorax. Retractions of the sternum, suprasternal notch, and intercostal retractions reflect increased respiratory effort. This may be due to obstructive disease such as asthma or upper airway obstruction, pneumonia, or restrictive disease. The presence of stridor, wheezing, or rhonchi will help distinguish the cause.

Emergency Department Treatment and Disposition

An aggressive search for the cause of the retractions is required to direct therapy. Rapid evaluation of the airway for patency and breathing for oxygenation should be done immediately on presentation. High-flow oxygen by face mask is appropriate for patients in respiratory distress. Preparations for securing an airway should be underway for those patients in severe distress or respiratory failure. Routine measures for the mildly symptomatic patient depend on the cause of the retractions. For asthma or exacerbations of chronic obstructive pulmonary disease (COPD), nebulized β₂ agonists and steroid therapy may be appropriate. Patients with croup may require nebulized normal saline and possibly epinephrine or dexamethasone as initial therapy. Foreign-body aspiration requires imaging and consultation for confirmation of the suspected diagnosis and removal.

Pearls

1. Retractions are best observed with the patient at rest and the chest exposed.
2. Retractions from obstructive airway disease can be intercostal and supraclavicular and are usually accompanied by nasal flaring, increased expiratory phase, and increased respiratory rate.

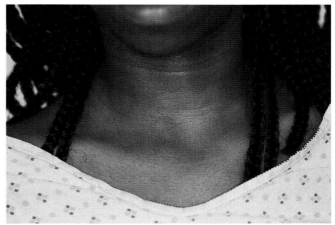

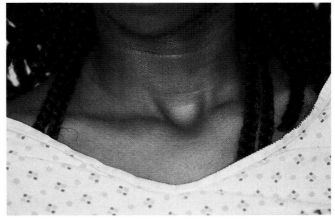

FIGURE 7.28 ■ Suprasternal Retractions. Suprasternal retractions in an adolescent with severe asthma. (Photo contributor: Kevin J. Knoop, MD, MS.)

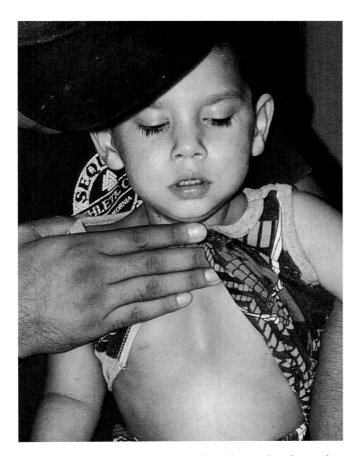

FIGURE 7.27 ■ Sternal Retractions. Sternal retractions in a patient with croup. (Photo contributor: Stephen W. Corbett, MD.)

Clinical Summary

This symptom complex develops from obstruction of venous drainage from the upper body, resulting in increased venous pressure, which leads to dilation of the collateral circulation. Superior vena cava (SVC) syndrome is most commonly caused by malignant mediastinal tumors. Dyspnea; swelling of the face, upper extremities, and trunk; chest pain, cough, or headache may be present. Physical findings include dilation of collateral veins of the trunk and upper extremities, facial edema and erythema (plethora), cyanosis, and tachypnea.

Emergency Department Treatment and Disposition

Radiation therapy is the treatment of choice for most malignant mediastinal tumors causing SVC syndrome. Administration of corticosteroids and diuretics initiated in the emergency department may provide temporary relief pending definitive therapy.

Pearls

1. SVC syndrome is most commonly caused by malignant mediastinal tumors.
2. Treatment of most mediastinal tumors causing SVC syndrome is radiation therapy.
3. CT scan of the chest is the diagnostic modality of choice for patients with SVC syndrome.

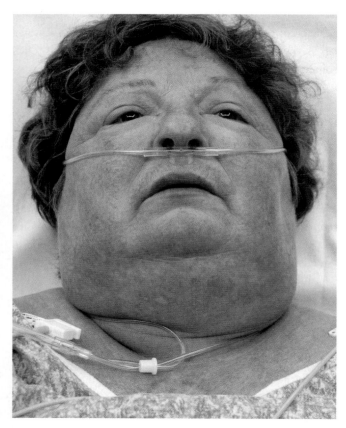

FIGURE 7.30 ■ Facial Plethora. A 53-year-old woman presents with shortness of breath and facial plethora. She has SVC syndrome due to lung cancer. (Photo contributor: R. Jason Thurman, MD.)

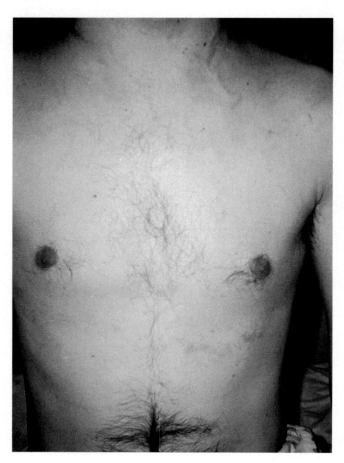

FIGURE 7.29 ■ Superior Vena Cava Syndrome. A 27-year-old man with SVC syndrome. Note the prominent collateral veins of the chest and neck. (Photo contributor: William K. Mallon, MD.)

Clinical Summary

Situs inversus (SI), a congenital condition of complete mirror-image reversal of the thoracic and abdominal organs, is present in 0.01% of the US population. Most patients lead a normal life, however 20% have Kartagener syndrome, characterized by ciliary dyskinesia, resulting in recurrent sinus and pulmonary infections. Diagnosis of SI often incidentally occurs during the evaluation of a thoracic or abdominal complaint. Angles of the mainstem bronchi appear reversed. Abdominal CT reveals liver, appendix, and biliary system on the left, and spleen and stomach on the right. ECG findings include inverted P wave, largely negative QRS, and inverted T wave in lead I. QRS complexes are negative in precordial leads. QRS patterns of AVR and AVL appear reversed.

Emergency Department Treatment and Disposition

Recognition of SI is important for prevention of medical errors due to seemingly atypical presentation of common conditions, such as appendicitis or cholecystitis that would have symptoms on the left abdomen, rather than the right. Documentation in the medical record and informing the patient so that future health-care givers are informed, may help prevent future medical errors.

Pearls

1. SI with dextrocardia has a 3% to 5% incidence of congenital heart disease.
2. Patients with Kartagener syndrome may have impaired sense of smell, nasal polyps, recurrent otitis media, chronic lung disease, and chronic respiratory infections.

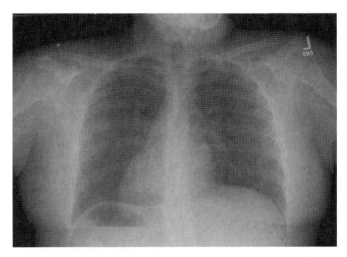

FIGURE 7.31 ■ Situs Inversus Chest X-Ray. A 26-year-old female complains of chest pain. Her evaluation was negative except of situs inversus. CXR shows a right-sided cardiac apex, aortic knob, gastric bubble. The angles of the mainstem bronchi suggest situs inversus. (Photo contributor: Katie Johnson, MD.)

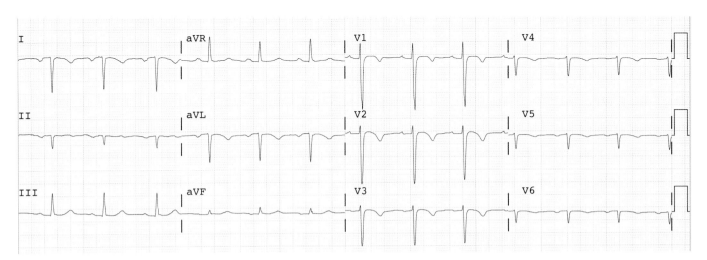

FIGURE 7.32 ■ Dextrocardia ECG. Characteristic ECG findings of dextrocardia are seen: inverted P wave, largely negative QRS complex, and inverted T wave in lead I. Precordial lead QRS complexes are negative. (Photo contributor: Katie Johnson, MD.)

Clinical Summary

Pancoast tumor involves the apical lung and may affect contiguous structures such as the brachial plexus, sympathetic ganglion, vertebrae, ribs, superior vena cava, and recurrent laryngeal nerve (more common for left-sided tumors). Horner syndrome, extremity edema, nerve deficits, hoarseness, and superior vena cava syndrome may result. Erosion of tumor through the chest wall can cause compression of venous outflow, with resultant jugulovenous distention (JVD). Virchow node of abdominal carcinoma, lymphoma, vascular abnormalities, and tuberculosis should also be considered.

Emergency Department Treatment and Disposition

Treatment depends on the staging and type of tumor. The superior vena cava syndrome can be treated acutely with radiation and diuretics. Thrombolytic therapy has been used successfully in some cases of acute vena caval thrombosis.

Pearls

1. Thrombosis may cause acute decompensation with edema, plethora, and airway collapse.
2. Prompt radiation therapy can be lifesaving in cases of vena caval obstruction.

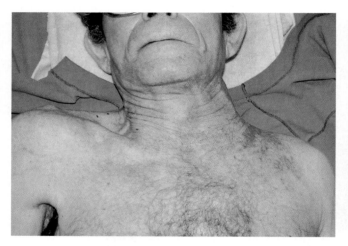

FIGURE 7.33 ■ Apical Lung Mass. This 68-year-old male cigarette smoker complained of cough and weight loss. A chest radiograph shows a left apical tumor. There is erosion of the tumor into the chest wall, with an indurated supraclavicular and infraclavicular mass. Moderate JVD is apparent, suggesting venous outflow obstruction. (Photo contributor: Stephen W. Corbett, MD.)

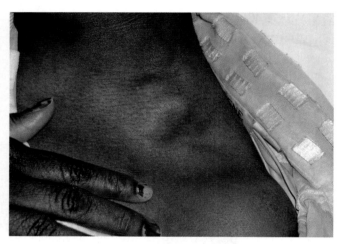

FIGURE 7.34 ■ Virchow Node. This middle-aged woman presents with multiple complaints including lateral neck swelling. She was diagnosed with lymphoma. (Photo contributor: David Effron, MD.)

JUGULOVENOUS DISTENSION

Clinical Summary

Central venous (right atrial) pressure is reflected by distention of the internal or external jugular veins. Normal pressure is less than 3 cm of distention above the sternal angle of Louis. Distention greater than 4 cm should be considered abnormal. Evaluation begins by raising the head of the supine patient 30° to 60°. The highest point of venous pulsation at the end of normal expiration is measured from the sternal angle of Louis. The presence of jugulovenous distention (JVD) should prompt an immediate search for possible pulmonary or cardiac pathology. The presence of crackles, murmurs, rubs, percussed hyperresonance, or crepitus may help disclose the etiology.

Causes of JVD include right ventricular failure, left ventricular failure, biventricular failure, parenchymal lung disease, pulmonary hypertension, pulmonic stenosis, restrictive pericarditis, pericardial tamponade, superior vena cava syndrome, pulmonary embolus, valvular disease, tension pneumothorax, increased circulating blood volume, and atrial myxoma. Temporary venous engorgement may result from Valsalva maneuver, positive pressure ventilation, and Trendelenburg position.

Emergency Department Treatment and Disposition

Treatment varies depending on the cause. Preload reduction may help in cases of congestive heart disease. Reversal of a traumatic etiology with needle thoracostomy or pericardiocentesis may be required.

Pearls

1. Right-sided myocardial infarction may produce JVD with clear lung fields.
2. JVD may be absent in the presence of the above-listed causes if hypovolemia is present.

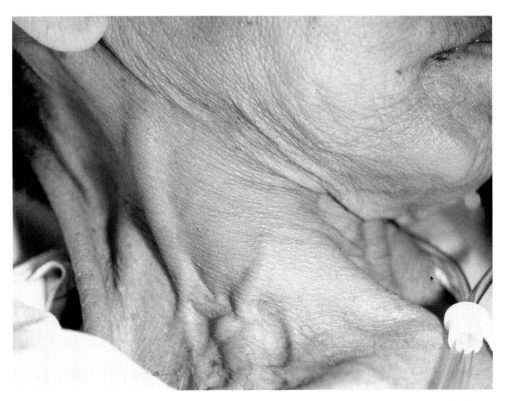

FIGURE 7.35 ■ Jugulovenous Distension. An engorged external jugular vein is noted as it crosses the sternocleidomastoid muscle into the posterior triangle of the neck and disappears beneath the clavicle to join the brachiocephalic vein and the superior vena cava. This patient has severe congestive heart failure requiring intubation. (Photo contributor: Alan B. Storrow, MD.)

Clinical Summary

Veins of the abdomen normally are scarcely visible within the abdominal wall. Engorged veins, however, are often visible through the normal abdominal wall. Engorged veins forming a knot in the area of the umbilicus are described as caput medusae. The extent of associated findings depends on the underlying etiology. It is usually secondary to liver cirrhosis, with subsequent portal hypertension and development of circulation circumventing the liver.

Emergency Department Treatment and Disposition

Treatment is directed at the underlying cause. This finding by itself does not require acute treatment.

Pearl

1. Caput medusae has the same clinical significance as the more common pattern of venous engorgement.

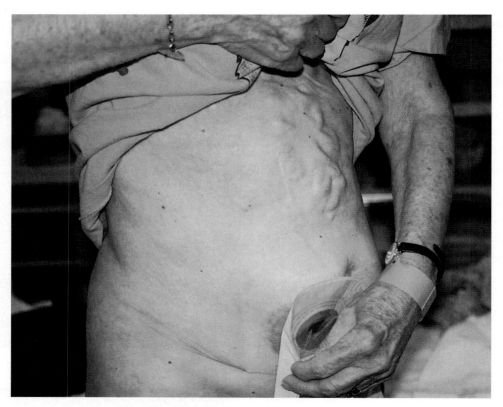

FIGURE 7.36 ■ Caput Medusae. This elderly female with alcoholic cirrhosis has engorged abdominal veins in the knotted appearance consistent with caput medusae. (Photo contributor: Gary Schwartz, MD.)

Clinical Summary

A hernia is a tissue protrusion through an abnormal body cavity opening. Most abdominal wall hernias occur at the groin and umbilicus. Incarceration is defined as the inability to reduce the protruding tissue to its normal position. Strangulation occurs when the blood supply of the hernia's contents is obstructed and tissue necrosis ensues. An *incisional* hernia may manifest clinically as a mass or palpable defect adjacent to a surgical incision and can be reproduced by having the patient perform the Valsalva maneuver. Obesity and wound infection, which interfere with wound healing, predispose to the formation of incisional hernias. The defect of an *indirect* inguinal hernia is the internal (abdominal) inguinal ring and may be manifest in either sex by a bulge over the midpoint of the inguinal ligament that increases in size with Valsalva maneuver. A fingertip placed into the external ring through the inguinal canal may palpate the defect. A *direct* hernia may be manifested by a bulge midway adjacent to the pubic tubercle and may be felt by the pad of the finger placed in the inguinal canal. The defect is in the posterior wall of the inguinal canal. Direct inguinal hernias are usually painless and occur in males. Femoral canal hernias are more common in women and are prone to both strangulation and incarceration.

Nausea and vomiting may be present if incarceration with bowel obstruction occurs. Strangulation can lead to fever, peritonitis, and sepsis.

Emergency Department Treatment and Disposition

When patients present without clinical evidence of strangulation (fever, leukocytosis, systemic signs of toxicity), reduction should be attempted. In the presence of these signs, prompt surgical consultation is warranted for surgical reduction. Reduction in the emergency department is facilitated with systemic analgesia (as most patients present with significant pain), placing the patient in the supine position, and applying a cold pack to the hernia. Routine consultation for operative repair is indicated in asymptomatic patients with reducible hernias.

Pearls

1.   Acutely strangulated or incarcerated hernias require immediate surgical evaluation.
2.   Direct inguinal hernias are usually painless.
3.   Evaluation and treatment of concomitant exacerbating conditions (cough, constipation, vomiting) prevent recurrences.

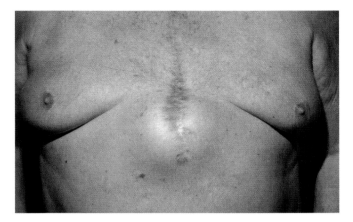

FIGURE 7.37A ■ Incisional Hernia. An asymptomatic incisional hernia in an obese male which developed after coronary artery bypass graft. The CT demonstrates a loop of bowel protruding through the abdominal wall defect. (Photo contributor: Lawrence B. Stack, MD.)

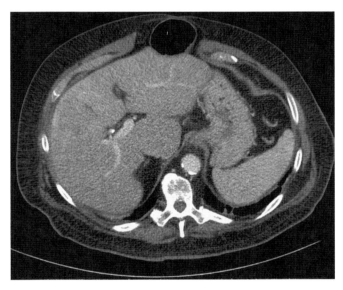

FIGURE 7.37B ■ Incisional Hernia CT Scan.

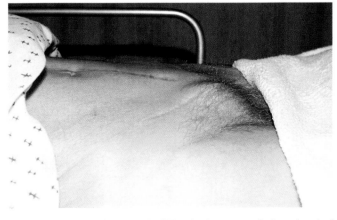

FIGURE 7.38 ■ Indirect Inguinal Hernia. A recurrent indirect inguinal hernia in a female patient. (Photo contributor: Frank Birinyi, MD.)

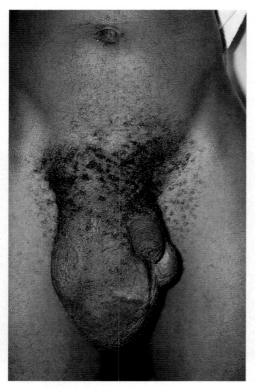

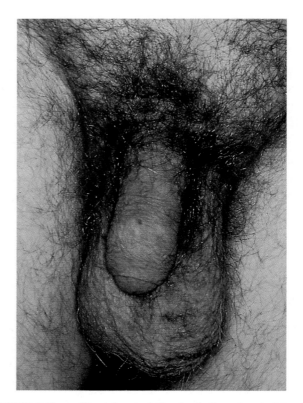

FIGURE 7.40 ■ Direct Inguinal Hernia. A direct inguinal hernia. Note the bulge adjacent to the left pubic tubercle. (Photo contributor: Daniel L. Savitt, MD.)

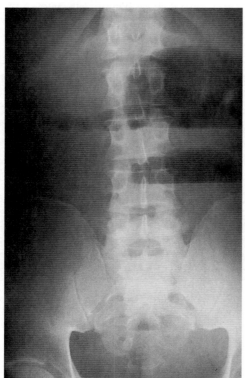

FIGURE 7.39 ■ Indirect Inguinal Hernia. This 35-year-old man has an incarcerated indirect inguinal hernia with small bowel obstruction seen on the upright abdominal film. (Photo contributor: Lawrence B. Stack, MD.)

Clinical Summary

The umbilicus is a common site of abdominal hernias. Predisposing conditions in adults most commonly include ascites and prior abdominal surgery. The size of the defect determines the symptomatology and incidence of incarceration, with smaller defects resulting in more pronounced symptoms and an increased incidence of incarceration. Pain is located in the area of the fascial defect. Contents of the hernia may be palpable and tender. Symptoms of obstruction (nausea, vomiting, and abdominal distention) may be present. If the hernia becomes strangulated, erythema of the overlying skin with fever and hypotension may occur.

Emergency Department Treatment and Disposition

Reduction is attempted in the stable patient without clinical evidence of strangulation. Treatment of any predisposing conditions (ie, abdominal paracentesis in the patient with tense ascites) may cause spontaneous reduction and avoid progression of the hernia to strangulation. Routine consultation for elective repair is indicated in asymptomatic patients with reducible hernias.

Pearls

1. Umbilical hernias in children usually resolve without treatment.
2. Umbilical hernias in adults usually become worse and require elective repair.

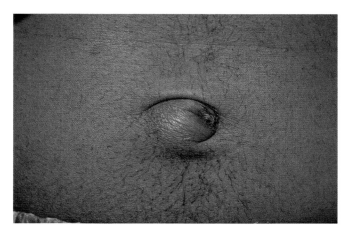

FIGURE 7.42A ■ Umbilical Hernia. A 53-year-old male with umbilical pain and swelling. (Photo contributor: Lawrence B. Stack, MD.)

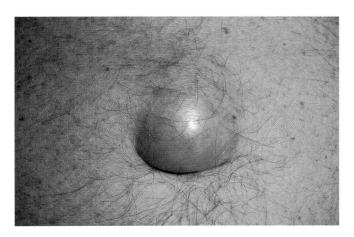

FIGURE 7.41 ■ Strangulated Umbilical Hernia. The skin overlying a strangulated umbilical hernia is erythematous and tender. (Photo contributor: Lawrence B. Stack, MD.)

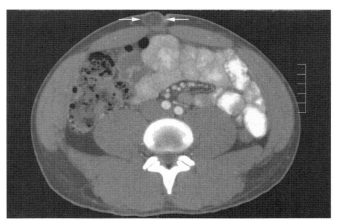

FIGURE 7.42B ■ Umbilical Hernia CT Scan. CT reveals omentum in the umbilical hernia defect (arrows).

Clinical Summary

When the vestigial urachal duct is not obliterated during development, drainage can occur from the bladder to the umbilicus. Cysts can often be palpated between the umbilicus and pubis. Besides drainage and pain, infection of the duct or cyst may occur. Rarely, adenocarcinoma may form in these remnants.

Emergency Department Treatment and Disposition

Acute treatment is usually not required unless an infection is evident. Routine urologic consultation for surgical revision is indicated. A retrograde study with radiopaque dye will outline the patent duct.

Pearl

1. This finding should prompt a careful search for other urogenital anomalies.

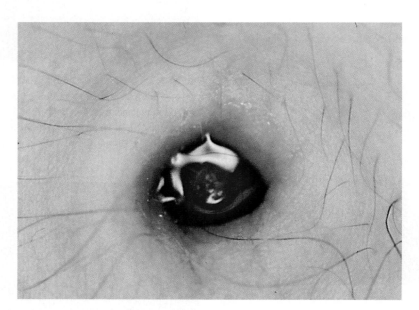

FIGURE 7.43 ■ Patent Urachal Duct. This 19-year-old man presented to the emergency department with clear fluid (urine) draining from the umbilicus, suggestive of a patent urachal duct. (Photo contributor: Kevin J. Knoop, MD, MS.)

Clinical Summary

A Sister Mary Joseph node is a metastasis manifesting as a periumbilical nodule secondary to abdominal or pelvic cancers. Cancers of the colon may cause pain, change in bowel habits, anemia, and obstruction. In general, left-sided cancers cause obstruction, whereas right-sided tumors may have significant metastases before they create signs and symptoms. These metastases typically involve peritoneal and omental spread with distant metastases to the liver. Spread to the umbilicus is colloquially known as the Sister Mary Joseph node.

Emergency Department Treatment and Disposition

Prompt referral for staging and treatment of the tumor is indicated. Other signs and symptoms (from obstruction, blood loss, malnutrition, and pain) should be addressed and treated.

Pearls

1. Virchow node, presenting as a supraclavicular mass, also heralds bowel carcinoma.
2. A Sister Mary Joseph node is commonly due to gastric carcinoma.

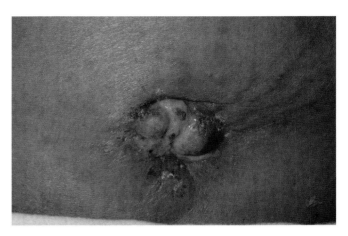

FIGURE 7.45A ■ Sister Mary Joseph Node. This 63-year-old woman presents with abdominal swelling and ascites. She was diagnosed with ovarian cancer. Axial CT scan of the abdomen at the level of the umbilicus demonstrates ascitic fluid and the umbilical nodularity (arrows). (Photo contributor: R. Jason Thurman, MD.)

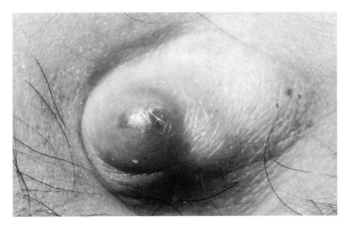

FIGURE 7.44 ■ Sister Mary Joseph Node. Sister Mary Joseph nodule of patient with gastric carcinoma. (Photo contributor: Department of Dermatology, Naval Medical Center, Portsmouth, VA.)

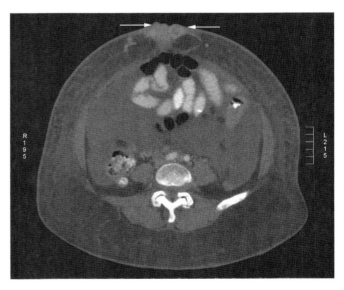

FIGURE 7.45B ■ Sister Mary Joseph Node. (Photo contributor: R. Jason Thurman, MD.)

Clinical Summary

Abdominal distension may be a symptom—often described by the patient as the feeling of being bloated—or a sign, an obvious protuberance of the patient's abdomen that may or may not be out of proportion to the rest of the body. Obesity, ascites, pregnancy, neoplasms, aneurysm, tympanites (excess gas), organomegaly, and constipation are important etiologies to consider in the differential.

In obesity, the abdomen is uniformly rounded while an increase in girth and fat concurrently accumulates in other parts of the body.

In patients with ascites, there may be shifting dullness, a fluid wave, bulging flanks, or hepatomegaly. The profile of the fluid-filled abdomen of ascites is a single curve from the xiphoid process to the pubic symphysis. The umbilicus may be everted, and there may be prominent superficial abdominal veins. Other physical findings suggestive of ascites include shifting dullness and a fluid wave.

In patients with neoplasms, there may be a palpable mass.

In gravid patients, fetal heart tones may be present and fetal motion may be felt. The pregnant abdomen profile shows the outward curve to be more prominent in the lower half of the abdomen. The umbilicus may be everted in the last trimester of pregnancy. Prominent abdominal wall veins may also be seen. In patients with excess gas from bowel obstruction, there may be absent or high-pitched bowel sounds and absence of bowel movements or flatus. Excess abdominal air can be located in the lumen of the stomach or intestines or free in the peritoneum. This abdominal profile is a single curve from the xiphoid process to the pubic symphysis. Nausea, vomiting, decreased bowel sounds, and colicky pain are present in a small bowel obstruction. Large bowel obstruction may be accompanied by feculent vomiting and absent production of flatus.

The abdominal profile of a patient with a leaking abdominal aortic aneurysm shows a mottled abdominal wall reflective of hypoperfusion of this structure. There may be a curve of the midabdomen to either side of the aorta, more often on the left. Palpation of a pulsatile mass supports the diagnosis. Ultrasound or computed tomography (CT) of the abdomen will confirm the diagnosis.

Emergency Department Treatment and Disposition

Treatment varies widely depending on the cause; thus emergent management is directed at determining the etiology. Life-threatening causes (aneurysm, obstruction, neoplasms) require stabilization and referral for definitive treatment.

Pearl

1. The "six f's" can categorize conditions causing abdominal distention: fat, flatus, fetus, fluid, feces, and fatal growth.

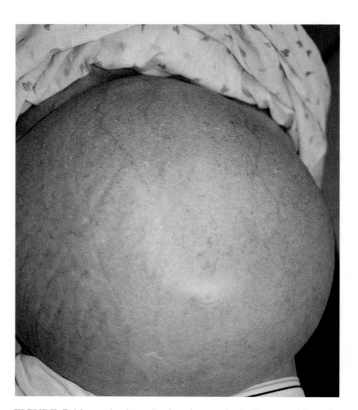

FIGURE 7.46 ■ Ascites. Ascites in an alcoholic man. Note the everted umbilicus and prominent superficial abdominal veins. (Photo contributor: Alan B. Storrow, MD.)

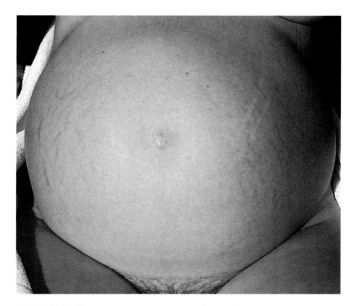

FIGURE 7.47 ■ Gravid Abdomen. The abdomen of a woman at 39 weeks' gestation. Note the abdominal wall striae, everted umbilicus, and prominent superficial abdominal wall veins. (Photo contributor: Stephen W. Corbett, MD.)

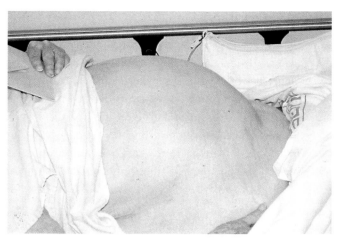

FIGURE 7.49 ■ Pseudoobstruction. An 85-year-old woman was brought from a nursing home with a complaint of abdominal distention and pain for 1 to 2 days. An eventual diagnosis of Ogilvie syndrome, or pseudoobstruction of the large bowel, was made. This is usually seen in debilitated patients and can be treated with decompression. (Photo contributor: Stephen W. Corbett, MD.)

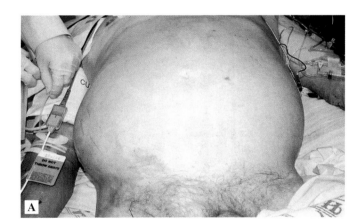

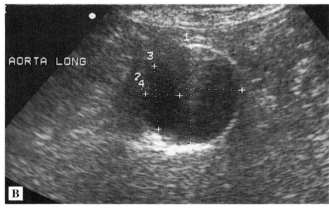

FIGURE 7.48 ■ Abdominal Aortic Aneurysm. (A) The abdomen of a patient with a leaking abdominal aortic aneurysm. Note the mottled abdominal wall and the prominent curvature of the right side of the abdomen. (Photo contributor: Stephen W. Corbett, MD.) (B) Abdominal aortic aneurysm seen on ultrasound in another patient. (Photo contributor: Sally A. Santen, MD.)

Clinical Summary

Mild trauma may produce hematomas of the rectus sheath. This injury results in intense abdominal pain, which can mimic an acute abdomen. The diagnosis is made by physical examination, since the ecchymosis is not always visible. Palpation of the abdominal wall reveals a tender mass that is accentuated by contraction of the rectus. Ultrasound and computed tomography (CT) may confirm the diagnosis.

Emergency Department Treatment and Disposition

Assuming that there is no underlying blood dyscrasia or coagulopathy, hematomas of the rectus sheath usually resolve in 1 to 2 weeks.

Pearl

1. Fothergill sign is enhancement of a rectus sheath hematoma when the abdominal wall is tensed. The mass should not cross the midline and should be easier to palpate with abdominal muscle contractions. Intra-abdominal masses are more difficult to palpate with such contractions.

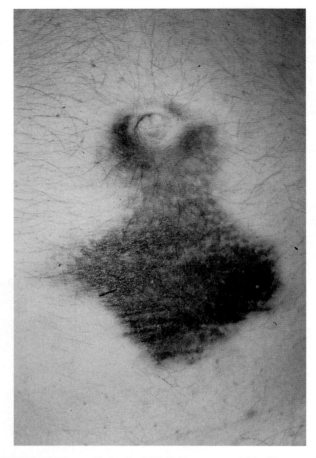

FIGURE 7.50 ■ Abdominal Wall Hematoma. This 50-year-old man with chronic obstructive pulmonary disease developed right-lower-quadrant pain after an episode of coughing. A repeat examination on the second visit showed clearly visible ecchymosis. There was no coagulopathy and amylase was normal. A CT scan revealed a 10- by 8-cm hematoma in the right rectus abdominis sheath. (Photo contributor: Stephen W. Corbett, MD.)

Clinical Summary

Pectus excavatum is a common developmental deformity of the anterior chest wall present in 0.25% of births. The cause is not well understood and may be related to intrauterine growth effects or muscle and connective tissue abnormalities within the thorax. In many cases there is a family history of the condition.

The defect is a concavity of the anterior chest wall. Although the condition is occasionally associated with Marfan, scoliosis, and congenital heart disease, most patients are asymptomatic. In some, there is slightly decreased exercise tolerance, felt to be the effect of the consequence of the increased work of breathing caused by the chest wall mechanics.

Emergency Department Treatment and Disposition

No definite treatment is needed, although cosmetic repairs of the anterior chest wall are sometimes recommended.

Pearl

1. Congential heart disease and Marfan syndrome are present in 1.5% of patients with pectus excavatum.

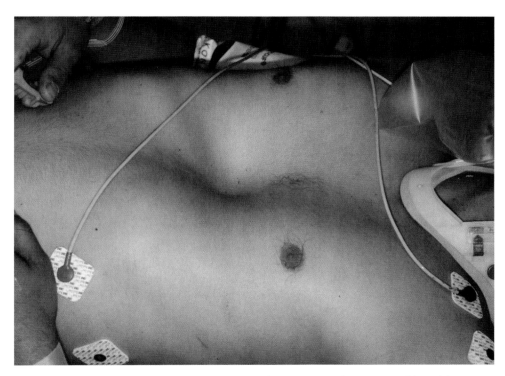

FIGURE 7.51 ■ Pectus Excavatum. A 26-year-old man presents to the emergency department with multisystem trauma after a motor vehicle crash. A long-standing pectus deformity is seen here. (Photo contributor: Lawrence B. Stack, MD.)

Clinical Summary

When a stoma prolapses, bowel telescopes out on itself, lengthening the stoma. A stoma of the ileum may prolapse in 3% to 11% of patients over a lifetime. Causes of stomal prolapse include stomal construction difficulties, abdominal wall abnormalities such as obesity, increased intra-abdominal pressure, and weak abdominal musculature. Clinical findings of stomal prolapse include increase in size and length of the stoma; edema of the mucosa; bleeding, and if ischemic may be dusky, cyanotic, or purple in color.

Emergency Department Treatment and Disposition

Emergent surgical consultation should occur in patients with a gangrenous stoma or if the prolapse is not reducible.

To reduce a prolapsed stoma have the patient lie supine or in slight Trendelenburg to decrease intra-abdominal pressure. Apply continuous gentle pressure on the prolapsed stomal tissues, into the abdominal cavity. If the bowel is edematous, a cold compress or osmotic therapy using table sugar applied for 15 minutes before reduction attempt may reduce the edema. If stomal prolapse reduction is successful, general surgery follow up should be arranged as soon as possible.

Pearls

1. Oral or intravenous diazepam may help facilitate prolapse reduction.
2. Your hospital stoma nurse may be a great resource to assist with management of stoma complications.

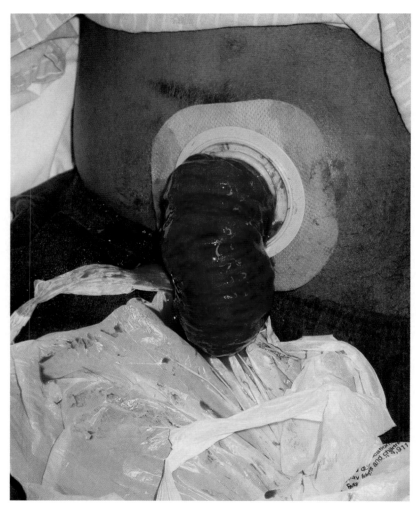

FIGURE 7.52 ■ Prolapsed Stoma. A 32-year-old male with inflammatory bowel disease and ileostomy presents with a prolapsed stoma. Note the bleeding, edema, and dusky appearance of the ileal mucosa. (Photo contributor: Lawrence B. Stack, MD.)

Chapter 8

UROLOGIC
CONDITIONS

Jeffery D. Bondesson

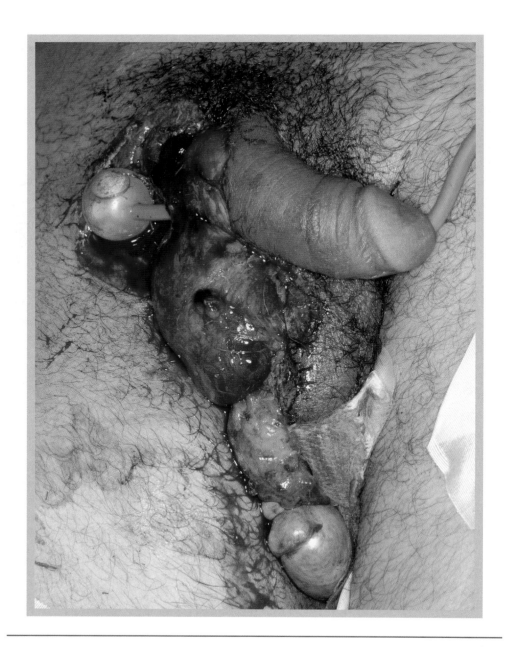

Clinical Summary

These patients are most often young men (average age 16 to 17.5 years) who present complaining of the sudden onset of pain in one testicle. The pain is then followed by swelling of the affected testicle, reddening of the overlying scrotal skin, lower abdominal pain, nausea, and vomiting. An examination reveals a swollen, tender, retracted testicle that often lies in the horizontal plane (bell-clapper deformity). The spermatic cord is frequently swollen on the affected side. In delayed presentations, the entire hemiscrotum may be swollen, tender, and firm. The urine is usually clear with a normal urinalysis. In one-third of cases there is a peripheral leukocytosis.

Emergency Department Treatment and Disposition

Urologic consultation should be obtained immediately and preparations made to go to the operating room without delay. Doppler ultrasound or technetium scanning may be helpful if these procedures will not delay surgery. In the interim, detorsion may be attempted if the patient is seen within a few hours of onset: the affected testicle should initially be opened like a book, that is, the right testicle turned counterclockwise when viewed from below and the left testicle turned clockwise when viewed from below. Pain relief should be immediate. Decreased pain should prompt additional turns (as many as three) to complete detorsion; increased pain should prompt detorsion in the opposite direction. Ancillary studies should not delay operative intervention, since testicular infarction will occur within 6 to 12 hours after torsion.

Pearls

1. The cremasteric reflex is almost always absent in testicular torsion.
2. Patients may report similar, less severe episodes that spontaneously resolved in the recent past.
3. Half of all torsions occur during sleep.
4. Abdominal or inguinal pain is sometimes present without pain to the scrotum.
5. The age of presentation has a bimodal pattern, since torsion is also more prevalent during infancy and adolescence.

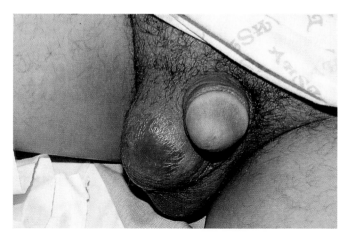

FIGURE 8.1 ■ Testicular Torsion. Swollen, tender hemiscrotum, with erythema of scrotal skin and retracted testicle. (Photo contributor: Stephen W. Corbett, MD.)

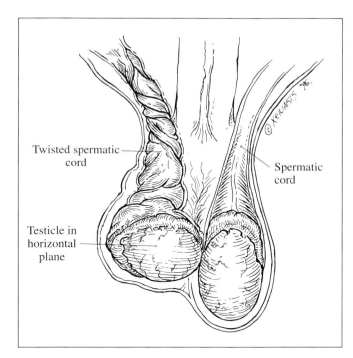

FIGURE 8.2 ■ Bell-Clapper Deformity. A bell-clapper deformity in testicular torsion results from the twisting of the spermatic cord and causes the testis to be elevated, with a horizontal lie. The lack of fixation of the tunica vaginalis to the posterior scrotum predisposes the freely movable testis to rotation and subsequent torsion. An elevated testis with a horizontal lie may be seen in asymptomatic patients at risk for torsion.

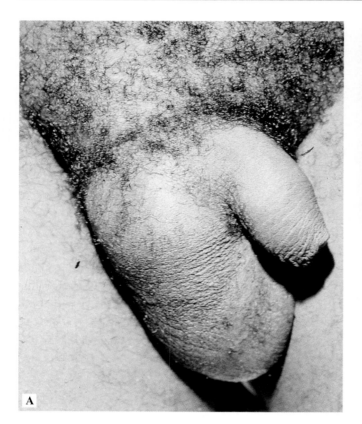

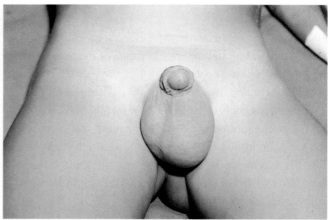

FIGURE 8.4 ■ Testicular Torsion. Swollen, tender scrotal mass. (Photo contributor: Patrick McKenna, MD.)

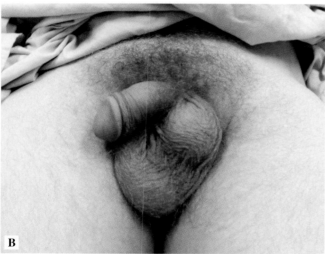

FIGURE 8.3 ■ A and B Testicular Torsion. A retracted testicle consistent with early testicular torsion (minimal edema) is seen in both of these patients. A. (Photo contributor: David W. Munter, MD, MBA.) B. (Photo contributor: The Emergency Medicine Department, Naval Medical Center Portsmouth.)

Clinical Summary

Small vestigial remnants in the embryology of the scrotum are often found on the superior portions of the testicle or the epididymis. These appendages, which have no known function, are occasionally on a stalk that is subject to torsion. This most commonly occurs in boys up to 16 years of age but has been reported in adults. The patient will complain of sudden pain around the superior pole of the testicle or epididymis as the appendix undergoes necrosis and inflammation. Early in the course, palpation of a firm, tender nodule in this area will confirm the diagnosis.

Emergency Department Treatment and Disposition

Urologic consultation should be obtained immediately. Differentiating from the more emergent testicular torsion is the key responsibility. Ancillary studies are generally not helpful in making this diagnosis unless it presents very early in its course. A urinalysis is generally normal. The characteristic physical signs of a small, tender, upper-pole nodule along with a color Doppler ultrasound showing good flow to the testicle may mitigate the need for emergent surgery. With later presentations or an equivocal ultrasound, the diagnosis may not be made with confidence before surgery. Necrotic appendices are excised if found during an exploration to rule out testicular torsion. If surgery is not deemed necessary by the urologic consultant, analgesics and rest are all that is required. The appendix will involute and calcify in 1 to 2 weeks.

Pearls

1. Stretching of the scrotal skin across the necrotic nodule will occasionally reveal a bluish discoloration of the nodule, called the "blue-dot sign." This is pathognomonic for torsion of the appendix.
2. A reactive hydrocele may accompany appendiceal torsion. When the hydrocele is transilluminated, the blue-dot sign may be revealed.

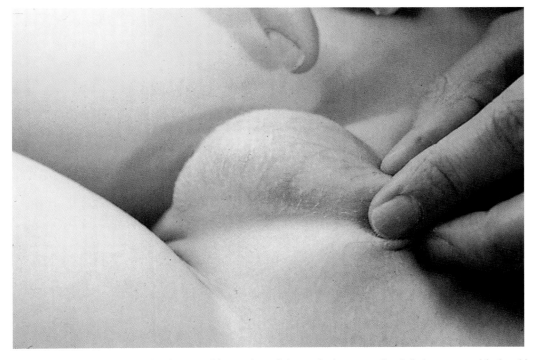

FIGURE 8.5 ■ Blue-Dot Sign. A blue-dot sign is caused by torsion of the testicular appendix. It is best seen with the skin held taut over the testicular appendix. (Photo contributor: Javier A. Gonzalez del Rey, MD.)

Clinical Summary

The onset of scrotal pain typically occurs over hours and is often referred to the ipsilateral inguinal canal or lower abdominal quadrant. Recent urinary tract instrumentation or urinary tract infection is a risk factor. Early in the course, a tender, indurated, edematous epididymis can be palpated separately from the nontender testicle. Late presentations will have generalized scrotal swelling and tenderness making examination and differentiation more difficult. The urinalysis will reveal pyuria or bacteriuria half of the time and the peripheral white blood cell count is frequently elevated. Patients can present with fever and signs of sepsis.

Emergency Department Treatment and Disposition

Outpatient treatment of younger men (<35 years) should be directed at sexually transmitted organisms. Older men tend to have infections caused by organisms in common with urinary tract infection. Adolescents and children should be referred for urological evaluation to rule out congenital anomalies, which are common in nongonococcal infections in this age group. Febrile patients should be considered for admission and IV antibiotics.

Pearls

1. Elevation of the affected hemiscrotum while supine may provide relief of symptoms (Prehn sign).
2. Older men should be evaluated for urinary retention, as this is a frequent cause of epididymitis.
3. Testicular tumors are most frequently misdiagnosed as epididymitis.
4. The absence of pyuria or bacteriuria does not exclude the diagnosis.
5. Referred pain to the lower quadrants can mimic appendicitis or diverticulitis.

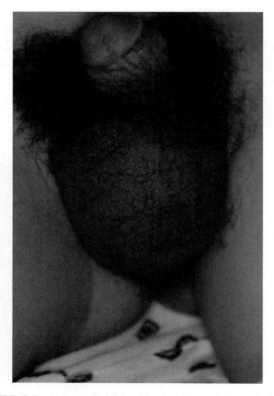

FIGURE 8.6 ■ Acute Epididymitis. Swelling of the right hemiscrotum and tenderness of the inferior posterior portion of the testicle. (Photo contributor: Adam R. Saperston, MD, MS.)

Clinical Summary

Orchitis has a variable onset and may be just mildly uncomfortable or severely painful. It is most frequently a complication of mumps infection and more rarely other viruses. Bacterial orchitis is rarer still and associated with concurrent epididymitis. Mumps orchitis occurs 4 to 7 days after parotid symptoms with testicular pain and swelling. It is unilateral 70% of the time with a contralateral infection developing later 30% of the time. The testicle is swollen and tender, sparing the epididymis. The overlying scrotal skin can be edematous and erythematous. Constitutional symptoms of malaise, headache, myalgias, and fever are common.

Emergency Department Treatment and Disposition

Supportive care with analgesics, hot or cold packs, and scrotal elevation is sufficient for mumps orchitis. Bacterial orchitis is treated the same as epididymitis.

Pearls

1. Pain and swelling from mumps orchitis can mimic testicular torsion mandating Doppler ultrasonography to differentiate.
2. An enlarged, tender epididymis or boggy, tender prostate supports bacterial orchitis.
3. Preceding or concurrent parotid swelling supports mumps orchitis.

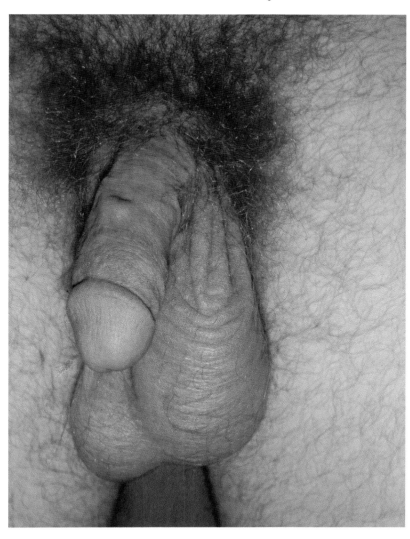

FIGURE 8.7 ■ Orchitis. Unilateral testicular pain, swelling, scrotal erythema, and edema is seen in this patient with parotitis. (Photo contributor: Lawrence B. Stack, MD.)

194

Clinical Summary

Most hydroceles occur in older patients and develop gradually without any significant symptoms. A hydrocele generally presents as a soft, pear-shaped, fluid-filled cystic mass anterior to the testicle and epididymis that will transilluminate. However, it can be tense and firm and will transilluminate poorly if the tunica vaginalis is thickened. Almost all hydroceles in children are communicating, resulting from the same mechanism that causes inguinal hernia. A persistent narrow processus vaginalis acts like a one-way valve, thus permitting the accumulation of dependent peritoneal fluid in the scrotum. Acute symptomatic hydroceles are rarer and can occur in association with epididymitis, trauma, or tumor.

Emergency Department Treatment and Disposition

In an acute hydrocele, treatment must be directed at discovering a possible underlying cause. A positive urinalysis may point toward an infectious etiology. Transillumination helps demonstrate whether the mass is cystic or solid. Ultrasound can be very helpful in imaging the scrotal contents and delineating the composition of the mass. Acute hydroceles should not be considered benign and require referral to a urologist to rule out tumor or infection. Chronic accumulations are referred to a urologist on a more routine basis for elective drainage.

Pearls

1. Ten percent of testicular tumors have a reactive hydrocele as the presenting complaint.
2. An inguinal hernia with a loop of bowel in it may emit bowel sounds.
3. Hydroceles are almost never symptomatic.
4. Acute reactive hydroceles may be caused by infection, trauma, or torsion.

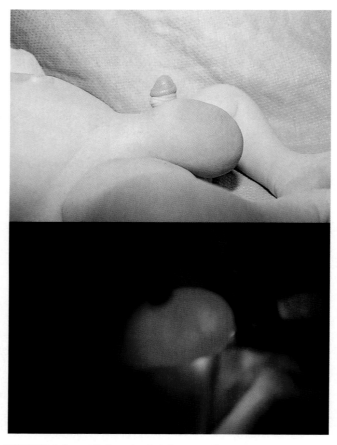

FIGURE 8.8 ■ Hydrocele. Painless swelling in the scrotum of a young boy (*top*). Transillumination of the swelling (*bottom*) identifies the hydrocele. (Photo contributor: Michael J. Nowicki, MD.)

Clinical Summary

In testicular tumor, a painless, firm testicular mass is palpated, with the patient often complaining of a "heaviness" of his testicle. If the patient presents early, the mass will be distinct from the testis, whereas later presentations will have generalized testicular or scrotal swelling. These lesions occasionally present with pain due to infarction of the tumor.

Emergency Department Treatment and Disposition

Patients should be promptly referred to a urologist for surgical exploration.

Pearls

1. Acute hydroceles and hematoceles should prompt the physician to consider a tumor as the cause.
2. Pain from tumor infarction is usually not as severe as pain due to torsion or epididymitis.
3. Findings of an unexplained supraclavicular lymph node, abdominal mass, or chronic nonproductive cough resistant to conventional therapy should prompt a testicular examination for tumor.

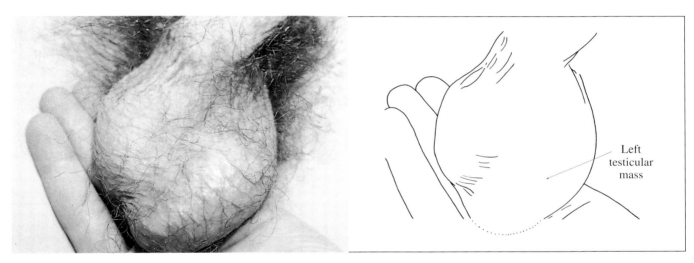

FIGURE 8.9 ■ Testicular Tumor. This painless left testicular mass is highly suspicious for tumor, as proved to be the case in this patient. (Photo contributor: Patrick McKenna, MD.)

Clinical Summary

A scrotal abscess is a suppurative mass with surrounding erythema involving the superficial layers of the scrotal wall. The usual history is of progressive swelling of a small pustule or papule followed by increasing pain and induration or fluctuance. Constitutional symptoms and fever are generally absent.

Emergency Department Treatment and Disposition

Using local anesthesia, simply make a stab incision and drain the abscess. The patient is then instructed to use a sitz bath and to change the dressing frequently. An alternative method of treatment is to unroof the abscess by circumferential excision. This ensures that there is adequate wound drainage. Immunocompromised patients may require intravenous antibiotics and admission.

Pearl

1. If the patient appears ill out of proportion to the superficial appearance, suspect that this mass is the point of a deep scrotal abscess.

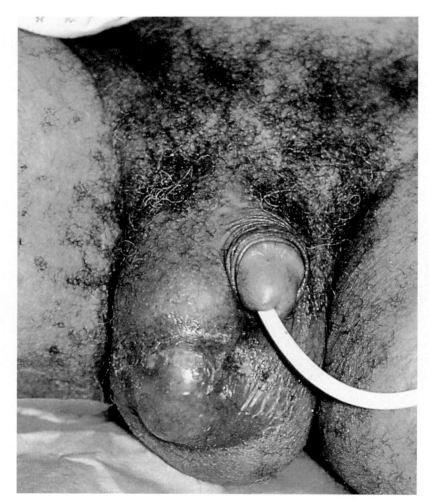

FIGURE 8.10 ■ Scrotal Abscess. Suppurative mass on the scrotum. (Photo contributor: David Effron, MD.)

Clinical Summary

Fournier gangrene most frequently occurs in a middle-aged diabetic male who presents with swelling, erythema, and severe pain of the entire scrotum, but it is also known to occur in females. In males, the scrotal contents often cannot be palpated because of the marked inflammation. The patient has constitutional symptoms with fever and frequently is in shock. There is often a history of recent urethral instrumentation, an indwelling Foley catheter, or perirectal disease. A localized area of fluctuance cannot be appreciated.

Emergency Department Treatment and Disposition

These patients require aggressive fluid resuscitation and early surgical consultation for immediate debridement and surgical drainage. Broad-spectrum antibiotics effective against gram-positive, gram-negative, and anaerobic organisms should be given as soon as possible in the emergency department. There is anecdotal experience that treatment is enhanced by hyperbaric oxygen.

Pearls

1. Pain out of proportion to the clinical findings may represent an early presentation of Fournier gangrene.
2. A plain pelvic radiograph may reveal subcutaneous air.
3. Fournier gangrene is usually quite painful but has been known to present with only a mildly uncomfortable necrosis of the scrotal wall and exposed testis.

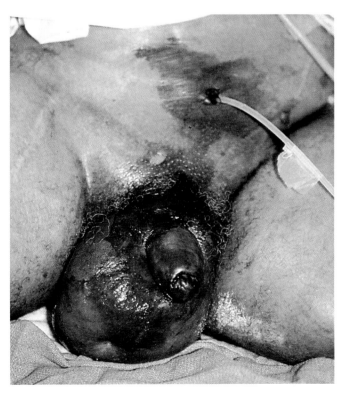

FIGURE 8.11 ■ Fournier Gangrene. Markedly swollen, necrotic, tender scrotum, perineum, and adjacent thighs are seen. (Photo contributor: David Effron, MD.)

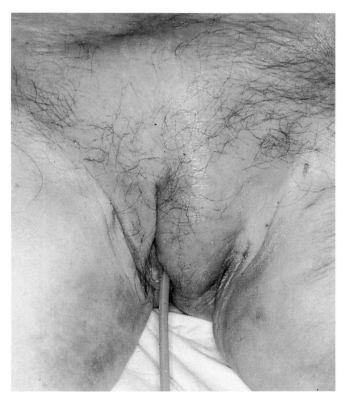

FIGURE 8.12 ■ Fournier Gangrene. Swollen, tender, erythematous labia, perineum, and inner thighs in a female patient with Fournier gangrene. (Photo contributor: Daniel L. Savitt, MD.)

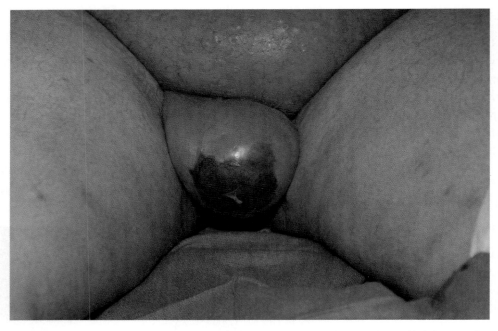

FIGURE 8.13 ■ Fournier Gangrene. Necrosis of overlying scrotal skin along with swelling, erythema, high fever, and severe pain was noted in this diabetic patient with Fournier gangrene. (Photo contributor: R. Jason Thurman, MD.)

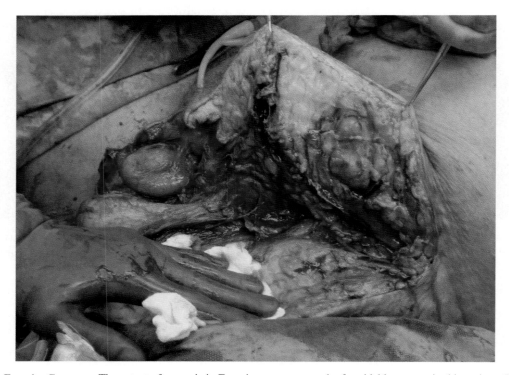

FIGURE 8.14 ■ Fournier Gangrene. The extent of necrosis in Fournier gangrene can be formidable as seen in this patient. (Photo contributor: R. Jason Thurman, MD.)

Clinical Summary

Paraphimosis is the entrapment of a retracted foreskin that cannot be reduced behind the coronal sulcus. Pain, swelling, and erythema are common. If severe, the constriction causes edema and venous engorgement of the glans, which can lead to arterial compromise with subsequent tissue necrosis. In contrast to paraphimosis, phimosis is the inability to retract the foreskin.

Emergency Department Treatment and Disposition

Squeezing the glans firmly for 5 minutes to reduce the swelling can lead to successful reduction of the foreskin. Local infiltration of anesthesia with vertical incision of the constricting band should be performed by a urologist if manual reduction fails.

Pearls

1. In the presence of arterial compromise, if a urologist is not immediately available, the emergency physician should incise the constricting band.
2. The patient should be referred to a urologist for circumcision if successfully reduced.
3. Phimosis is "physiologic" in young males (generally <5 to 6 years old).
4. Phimosis, if "reduced" (retracted proximally over the glans), can cause a paraphimosis—a true emergency.

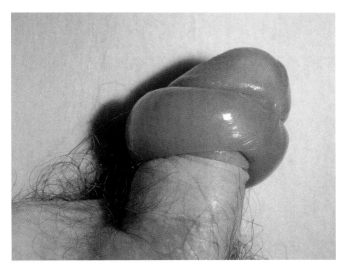

FIGURE 8.15 ■ Paraphimosis. Moderate edema of retracted foreskin, which is entrapped behind the coronal sulcus. (Photo contributor: Lawrence B. Stack, MD.)

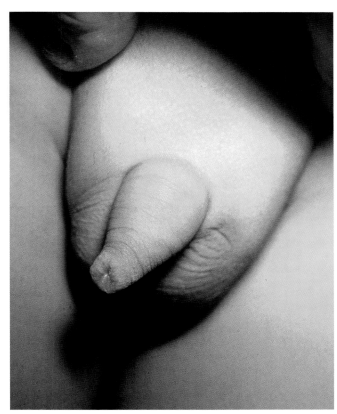

FIGURE 8.16 ■ Phimosis. Phimosis in a young patient is physiologic, but also may have obstruction from meatal stenosis and scarring. (Photo contributor: Alan B. Storrow, MD.)

Clinical Summary

These patients present with persistent, usually painful erection due to pathologic engorgement of the corpora cavernosa. Patients may present acutely or several days after their first symptoms. The glans penis and corpus spongiosum are not engorged and remain flaccid. The physiology is either arterial, which is generally traumatic, or veno-occlusive. Reversible causes of veno-occlusive disease include sickle cell disease, direct injection of erectile agents, and leukemic infiltration. Nonreversible causes include idiopathic ones—the most common, spinal cord lesions, and medications.

Emergency Department Treatment and Disposition

Diseases that are associated with reversible priapism should be treated. Ice packs to the perineum are frequently unsuccessful. Terbutaline given orally or subcutaneously occasionally reverses priapism. Aspiration of blood from the corpus cavernosum can lead to detumescence and should be followed by a compressive dressing. Injectable erectile agents can be reversed by aspiration followed by intracavernous injection of α-adrenergic agents such as phenylephrine.

Urologic consultation should be obtained immediately for traumatic or persistent priapism despite initial treatment, with close urologic follow-up for those that are successfully reversed in the emergency department.

Pearls

1. Patients should be advised that impotence is a frequent complication of priapism, regardless of the length of the symptoms or the success of any treatment.
2. A prolonged erection with a flaccid glans and corpus spongiosum confirms priapism.
3. Urinary retention often accompanies priapism.

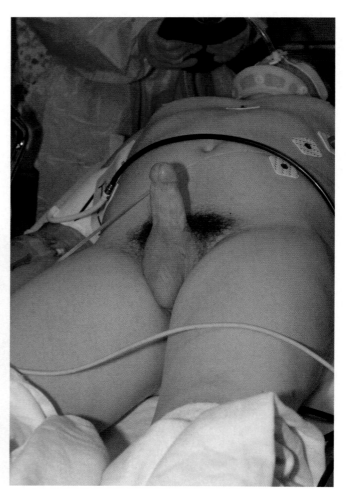

FIGURE 8.18 ■ Traumatic Priapism. A persistent erection is seen in this trauma victim who has sustained a cord injury. (Photo contributor: R. Jason Thurman, MD.)

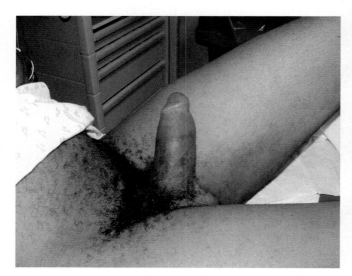

FIGURE 8.17 ■ Priapism. A painful persistent erection due to pathologic engorgement of the corpora cavernosa is seen in this patient with sickle cell disease. The glans penis and corpus spongiosum are not engorged. (Photo contributor: Kevin J. Knoop, MD, MS.)

Clinical Summary

Urethral injury is rarely an isolated event; it is often associated with multiple trauma. Anterior urethral injuries are most often the result of a straddle injury and may present late (many patients are still able to void), with a local infection or sepsis from extravasated urine. Posterior urethral injuries occur in motor vehicle and motorcycle accidents and are usually the result of pelvic fractures. Patients have blood at the urethral meatus, cannot void, and have perineal bruising. In males, the prostate is often boggy or free-floating or may not be palpable at all if there is a retroperitoneal hematoma between the prostate and the rectum.

Emergency Department Treatment and Disposition

Urethral instrumentation such as Foley catheterization should not occur prior to a retrograde urethrogram with highly concentrated water-soluble contrast. If there is only a partial anterior tear, a gentle attempt at catheterization can be made if it is abandoned at the first sign of resistance. If catheterization is unsuccessful and whenever there is a posterior tear, a suprapubic catheter should be placed in the emergency department with a trocar if relief of bladder distention is required prior to operative repair.

Pearls

1. Foley catheter insertion is contraindicated in patients with a suspected urethral injury prior to a retrograde urethrogram.
2. Urethral injury should be suspected in the multiple-trauma patient who is unable to void or has blood at the meatus, a high-riding prostate, or perineal trauma.
3. Vaginal lacerations due to trauma in females should prompt consideration of a urethral tear.
4. Occasionally urine from an anterior urethral tear will extravasate into the scrotum, causing marked swelling.
5. Posterior injuries are frequently associated with other intra-abdominal injury.

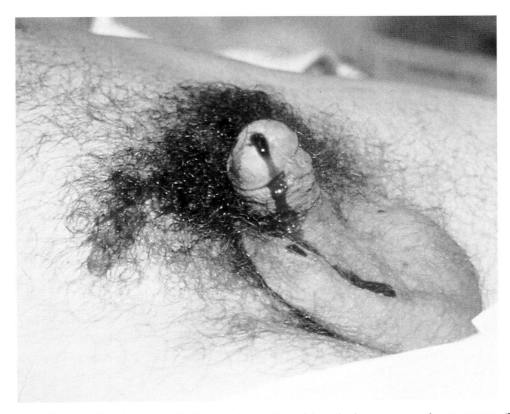

FIGURE 8.19 ■ Urethral Rupture. Blood at the urethral meatus in a patient with urethral rupture secondary to trauma. (Photo contributor: David Effron, MD.)

Clinical Summary

Patients usually present complaining of trauma during sexual arousal and often relate a sudden "snapping" sound or sensation, pain, and deformity, which is caused by a tearing of the tunica albuginea. The shaft of the penis is swollen and often angulated at the fracture site.

Emergency Department Treatment and Disposition

If the patient cannot urinate, a retrograde urethrogram may be required to rule out urethral injury. These patients require admission and referral to a urologist, who frequently takes them immediately to the operating room for repair.

Pearls

1. Patients sometimes concoct elaborate stories which are not sexually related surrounding the circumstances of injury, but penile fracture most commonly occurs during sexual arousal.

2. Penile implants are also subject to injury in a similar fashion.

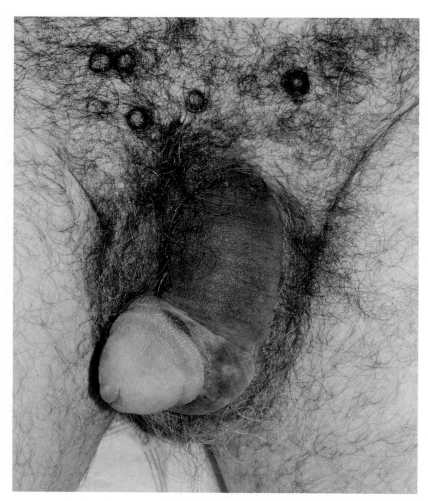

FIGURE 8.20 ■ Fractured Penis. Penile fracture with ecchymosis and angulation. (Photo contributor: Stephen W. Corbett, MD.)

Clinical Summary

A hair or filament that wraps around the penis can lead to a surgical emergency. The constricting band will impair distal venous and lymphatic drainage causing more edema and further impairing drainage in a vicious cycle. The ultimate sequela is arterial compromise and amputation. These are most commonly seen in young children although it has also been reported in men who use penile rings or constrictors.

Emergency Department Treatment and Disposition

Immediate release of the constriction generally gives relief and restores any impaired circulation. Care must be taken not to injure any underlying structures. If the edema is so great that the constricting band cannot be easily released, emergent urological consultation may be required.

Pearls

1. Edema may obscure the hair or filament and bury it subcutaneously.
2. Measures to decrease the swelling, such as direct pressure and ice packs, may facilitate visualization and incision of the tourniquet.
3. Clitoral tourniquets have been described.
4. Penile tourniquet should be considered when presented with a fussy infant.

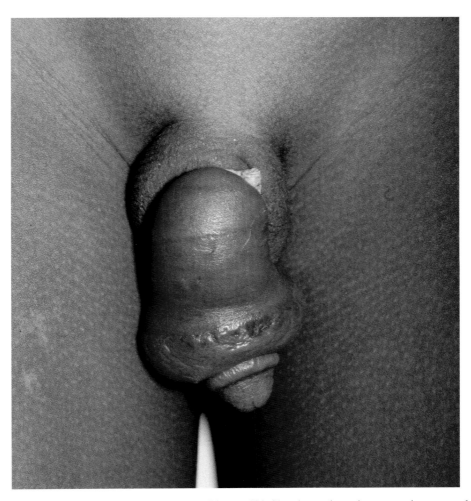

FIGURE 8.21 ■ Penile Hair Tourniquet. Penile engorgement due to self-inflicted tourniquet in a pre-pubescent male. (Photo contributor: Lawrence B. Stack, MD.)

Clinical Summary

In straddle injury, the patient has pain, swelling, contusion, and hematoma of the perineum or scrotum following direct blunt trauma. This injury is commonly caused by a fall onto a bicycle frame cross-tube, playground equipment, or a toilet seat. Swelling can be severe enough to interfere with urination. Scrotal contents can also be contused or crushed with this injury.

Emergency Department Treatment and Disposition

Treatment is supportive and includes cold packs, elevation, rest, and analgesics. If unable to void, the patient may require catheterization.

Pearls

1. Perineal laceration can be obscured by swelling if a careful examination is not performed.
2. Pelvic radiographs should be obtained in all perineal injuries.

3. Males and females are at high risk for urethral injuries with this type of injury.
4. Straddle injury is differentiated from abuse with a good history from a reliable caregiver that matches the injury.

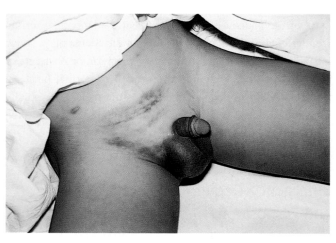

FIGURE 8.23 ■ Straddle Injury. Contusion of the scrotum and lower abdomen in a young boy consistent with a straddle injury. (Photo contributor: David W. Munter, MD.)

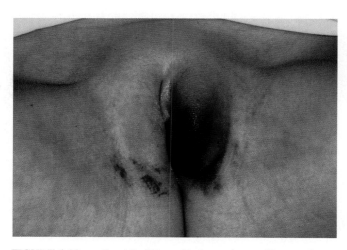

FIGURE 8.22 ■ Straddle Injury. Ecchymosis, swelling, and contusion of the perineum in a 3-year-old female who tripped and fell on a large plastic toy. (Photo contributor: James Mensching, MD.)

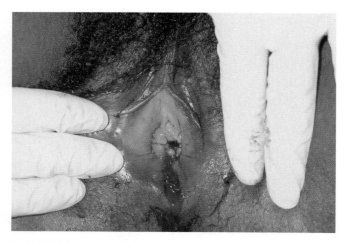

FIGURE 8.24 ■ Straddle Injury. This unfortunate patient suffered a vaginal tear as a result of slipping forward off the seat of her bicycle and landing on its top tube. (Photo contributor: R. Jason Thurman, MD.)

Clinical Summary

Balanoposthitis is an infection and inflammation of the glans penis that also involves the overlying foreskin (prepuce). *Balanitis* is isolated to the glans, whereas *posthitis* involves only the prepuce. Pain, erythema, and edema of the affected parts of the penis are typically present. Patients may refrain from urination secondary to dysuria, or the edema may induce meatal occlusion, leading to urinary retention or obstruction. Common etiologies include overgrowth of normal bacterial flora secondary to poor hygiene (pediatric patients), sexually transmitted diseases (adolescents and adults), and candidal infections (the elderly or immunocompromised).

Emergency Department Treatment and Disposition

Treatment is directed at the suspected etiology. Warm soaks and topical antibiotics (bacitracin) are the mainstay of therapy for infectious etiologies owing to poor hygiene. Parents should be counseled about proper cleansing and handling of the prepuce.

Oral or intravenous antibiotics may be indicated if there is an accompanying cellulitis. If urinary obstruction is present, catheterization may be attempted using a small catheter. If catheterization is unsuccessful, urologic consultation for emergent surgical correction of the prepuce is required. Candidal infections are treated with meticulous hygiene and topical antifungal agents. Routine urologic referral is indicated for suspected lichen sclerosus et atrophicus and squamous cell carcinoma.

Pearls

1. The inability to retract the foreskin completely is normal in young males up to age 4 or 5. Attempting to do so could cause a paraphimosis, a true emergency.
2. Placing the child in a bathtub with warm water will help alleviate difficulty with micturition assuming that no obstruction is present.
3. Candidal balanitis or balanoposthitis may be indicative of an undiagnosed immunocompromised state.
4. Suspected sexually transmitted diseases require treatment for the partners as well.

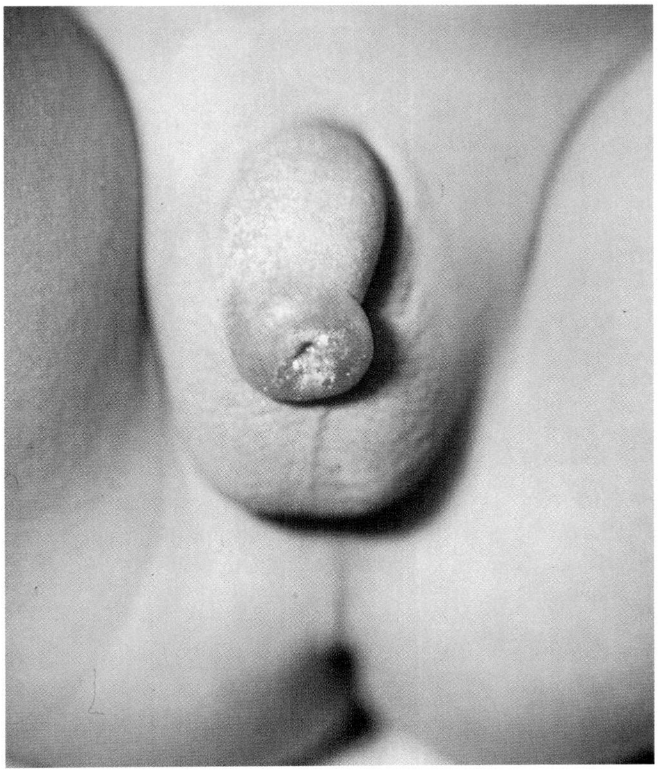

FIGURE 8.25 ■ Balanoposthitis. Note the erythema, localized edema, and significantly constricted preputial orifice of the distal penis. (Photo contributor: Lawrence B. Stack, MD.)

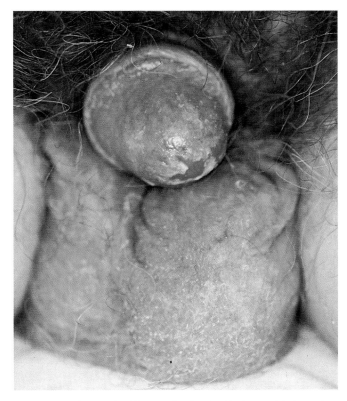

FIGURE 8.26 ■ Balanitis. Candidal balanitis in an elderly patient with no other complaints. New-onset diabetes was diagnosed. (Photo contributor: Kevin J. Knoop, MD, MS.)

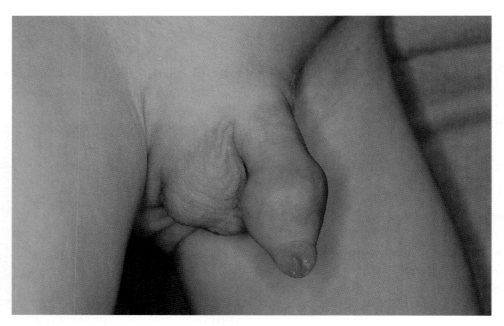

FIGURE 8.27 ▪ Balanoposthitis. This toddler presented with physiologic phimosis, inflamed distal foreskin, dysuria, and swelling of the glans. (Photo contributor: James Palma, MD.)

Clinical Summary

Zipper injury is usually seen in young children. The foreskin becomes entrapped in the teeth of the zipper or between the fastener and the zipper teeth as the zipper is being opened (downward). Accessibility to the median bar of the zipper facilitates removal.

Emergency Department Treatment and Disposition

Treatment is directed at removing the zipper and freeing the entrapped penile foreskin or prepuce while minimizing trauma and pain. A penile block with local injection at the base of the penis eases removal, but might not be necessary if the child is cooperative and removal can be effected atraumatically. Several methods are described depending on the mechanism.

Pearls

1. Zipper entrapment of the penis is one of the most common genital injuries in prepubertal boys.
2. When tissue is entrapped by the zipper teeth only, release can be effected by cutting the cloth of the zipper either between the teeth or below the point of entrapment.
3. Cutting the median bar with a bone cutter allows the whole zipper to fall apart and release the entrapped skin.
4. Lateral compression of the distal zipper fastener with pliers may immediately release the tissue without need for anesthesia. This method requires application of equal pressure to both the anterior and posterior fastener plates simultaneously.
5. After removal, ensure that the urethra is patent and the child can void.

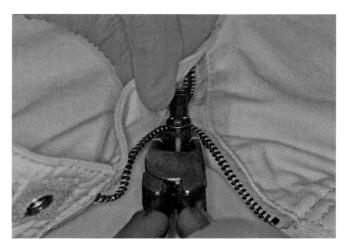

FIGURE 8.29 ■ Penile Zipper Injury. Separation of the zipper by cutting the median bar of the zipper with a bone cutter allows release. (Photo contributor: Kevin J. Knoop, MD, MS.)

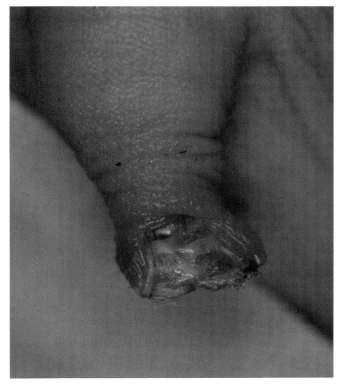

FIGURE 8.30 ■ Penile Zipper Injury. Crushed tissue after zipper removal did not obstruct urine flow in this patient. (Photo contributor: Kevin J. Knoop, MD, MS.)

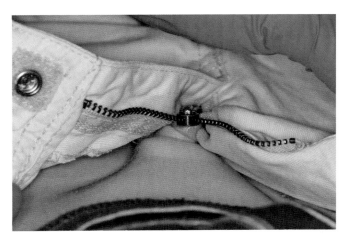

FIGURE 8.28 ■ Penile Zipper Injury. Entrapment of the foreskin between the fastener and the zipper teeth is seen. The median bar is exposed and easily accessible for cutting. (Photo contributor: Kevin J. Knoop, MD, MS.)

Chapter 9

SEXUALLY TRANSMITTED INFECTIONS AND ANORECTAL CONDITIONS

Diane M. Birnbaumer
Lynn K. Flowers

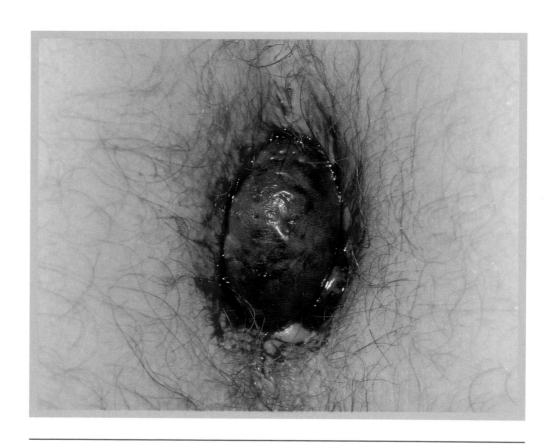

Clinical Summary

Lesions of primary syphilis generally appear after an incubation period of 2 to 6 weeks, but they may appear up to 3 months after exposure. The patient usually presents with a solitary, round-to-oval, painless genital ulcer. However, the ulcer may be slightly painful, and several lesions are sometimes seen. The base of the genital ulcer is dry in males, moist in females; purulent fluid in the base is uncommon. The borders of the ulcer are often indurated. Patients may develop ulcers at any site of inoculation on the body. Bilateral, nontender, nonfluctuant adenopathy is common. Lesions resolve spontaneously in 3 to 12 weeks without treatment as the infection progresses to the secondary stage. Patients with primary syphilis are at risk for concurrent infection with other sexually transmitted diseases.

Emergency Department Treatment and Disposition

Treat with benzathine penicillin G, 2.4 million units intramuscularly once. Penicillin-allergic patients should be given doxycycline, 100 mg orally twice a day for 2 weeks or tetracycline, 500 mg orally four times a day for 2 weeks. An RPR or VDRL should be checked as well a test for HIV. Testing for other sexually transmitted infections such as gonorrhea and *Chlamydia* is recommended. Partners within the last 90 days should be treated presumptively; partners over the last 90 days should be treated on the basis of their serologic testing results. This is a reportable disease, and appropriate paperwork should be filed.

Pearls

1. Lesions are usually painless and solitary, but they may be slightly painful; two or three lesions may also be seen.
2. Consider dark-field examination of the lesion to rapidly confirm the diagnosis.
3. Chancres of primary syphilis can occur anywhere on the body at the site of inoculation.
4. Evaluate patients with primary syphilis for concurrent sexually transmitted diseases and treat accordingly.

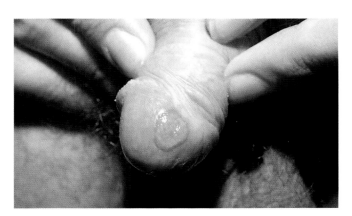

FIGURE 9.1 ■ Primary Chancre—Male. This dry-based, painless ulcer with indurated borders is typical for a primary chancre in a male patient. (Reproduced with permission from A. Wisdom. *Sexually Transmitted Diseases.* London: Mosby-Wolfe; 1992.)

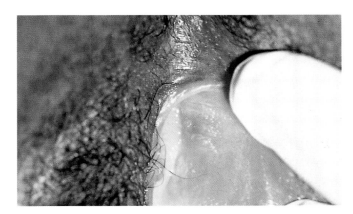

FIGURE 9.2 ■ Primary Chancre—Female. A solitary, painless genital chancre with a clean base in a patient with primary syphilis. (Photo contributor: Department of Dermatology, Naval Medical Center, Portsmouth, VA.)

Clinical Summary

The rash of secondary syphilis occurs 2 to 10 weeks after resolution of the primary lesions. It begins as a nonpruritic macular rash that evolves into a papulosquamous rash involving primarily the trunk, palms, and soles. The rash is often annular in shape. Diffuse, painless lymphadenopathy is also seen at this stage. Mucous patches represent mucous membrane involvement of the tongue and buccal mucosa. Condyloma lata can be seen during this stage, as can patchy alopecia. The manifestations of this stage resolve without treatment in several months.

Emergency Department Treatment and Disposition

Benzathine penicillin G, 2.4 million units intramuscularly once; penicillin-allergic patients should receive doxycycline, 100 mg orally twice daily for 2 weeks or tetracycline, 500 mg orally four times a day for 2 weeks. Testing for RPR or VDRL should be sent and titers followed to determine adequate response to therapy. Patients should also be tested for other sexually transmitted infections including HIV, gonorrhea, and *Chlamydia*. Suspected and confirmed cases of syphilis must be reported to public health officials.

Pearls

1. Lesions of secondary syphilis are very infectious. It is prudent to always wear gloves when examining a patient with a rash that may be due to secondary syphilis.
2. Consider using dark-field examination of scrapings of the rash, mucous patches, and condyloma lata to make a rapid diagnosis.
3. Patients should be warned about the potential development of the Jarish-Herxheimer reaction after they are treated. This syndrome, characterized by fever, headache, malaise, and myalgias, occurs within 24 hours of treatment and is caused by massive release of pyrogens by the dying spirochetes.

FIGURE 9.3 ■ Secondary Syphilis—Trunk. Rash on trunk in secondary syphilis. (Reproduced with permission from A. Wisdom. *Sexually Transmitted Diseases*. London: Mosby-Wolfe; 1992.)

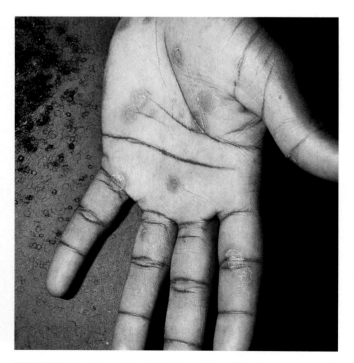

FIGURE 9.4 ■ Secondary Syphilis—Palms. Papulosquamous rash of secondary syphilis. Note the annular appearance of the palmar rash. (Photo contributor: H. Hunter Handsfield. *Atlas of Sexually Transmitted Diseases*. New York: McGraw-Hill; 1992.)

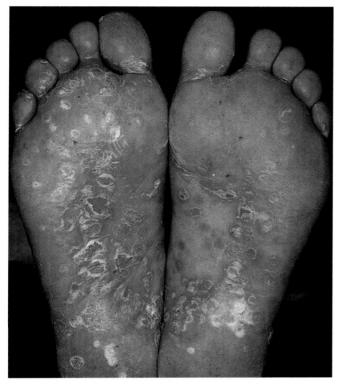

FIGURE 9.5 ■ Secondary Syphilis—Soles. Hyperkeratotic plantar rash in a patient with secondary syphilis. (Photo contributor: H. Hunter Handsfield. *Atlas of Sexually Transmitted Diseases.* New York: McGraw-Hill; 1992.)

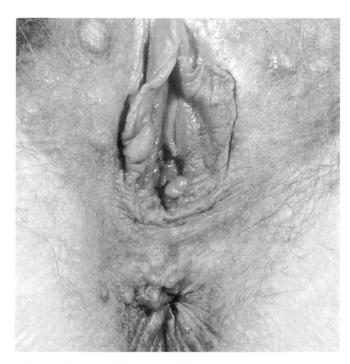

FIGURE 9.7 ■ Condyloma Lata. Typical appearance of the verrucous, heaped up lesions of condyloma lata, a manifestation of secondary syphilis. (Photo contributor: H. Hunter Handsfield. *Atlas of Sexually Transmitted Diseases.* New York: McGraw-Hill; 1992.)

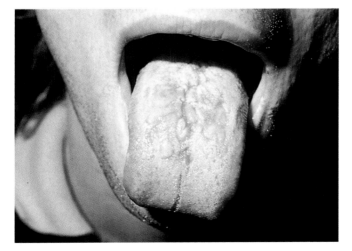

FIGURE 9.6 ■ Mucous Patches. Oral involvement in secondary syphilis manifested by mucous patches. These lesions are very infectious, and dark-field examination is often positive for spirochetes. (Reproduced with permission from Morse, Moreland, Thompson. *Atlas of Sexually Transmitted Diseases.* London: Mosby-Wolfe; 1990.)

Clinical Summary

Gonorrhea has an incubation period of 2 to 7 days. In men, the most common manifestation is urethritis, characterized by purulent, usually copious urethral discharge with dysuria; however, up to 10% of men are asymptomatic. Women may also develop urethritis and complain of dysuria. More commonly, however, women develop cervicitis, which is often asymptomatic. If symptomatic, women may complain of increased vaginal discharge or vaginal spotting, particularly after intercourse. On speculum examination, the cervix is friable, often with a mucopurulent endocervical exudate. Patients with gonococcal conjunctivitis have chemosis and copious purulent exudate; untreated, these patients can develop endophthalmitis and perforation of the globe. Untreated gonorrhea may disseminate and more commonly does so in women. Disseminated gonococcal infection (DGI) typically presents with a monoarticular septic arthritis usually involving the knees, ankles, elbows, or wrists. Skin lesions are necrotic pustules on an erythematous base; they may ulcerate and are more commonly found on the distal extremities.

Emergency Department Treatment and Disposition

Treatment is dependent on the site of infection:

Urethritis and cervicitis: Ceftriaxone, 125 mg intramuscularly once, or cefixime, 400 mg orally once. Due to rapidly emerging resistance to fluoroquinolones, these agents are no longer recommended for treating gonorrhea.

Conjunctivitis: Ceftriaxone 1 g intramuscularly once; eye irrigation with normal saline as needed.

DGI: The primary regimen is ceftriaxone, 1 g intravenously or intramuscularly daily for 7 to 10 days. Alternative agents for parenteral treatment are: cefotaxime 1 g intravenously every 8 hours, or ceftizoxime 1 g intravenously every 8 hours, or spectinomycin 2 g intramuscularly every 12 hours. Parenteral treatment should continue until 24 to 48 hours after improvement, and then should be changed to cefixime, 400 mg orally twice a day, or cefpodoxime 400 mg orally twice a day, to complete a total of a 7- to 10-day course. Sexual partners should be notified and treated. Gonorrhea is a reportable disease.

Pearls

1. Patients with gonorrhea need to be treated for concurrent infection with *Chlamydia*. Coinfection with these organisms is seen in 30% of men with urethritis and 50% of women with cervicitis.

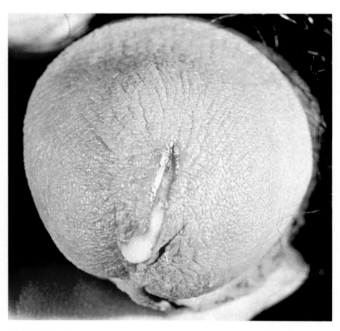

FIGURE 9.8 ■ Male Urethritis. Purulent, copious urethral discharge in a patient with gonococcal urethritis. (Photo contributor: H. Hunter Handsfield. *Atlas of Sexually Transmitted Diseases*. New York: McGraw-Hill; 1992.)

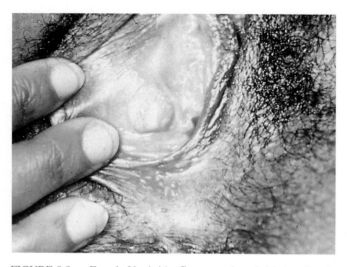

FIGURE 9.9 ■ Female Urethritis. Gonococcal urethritis in a female patient. Note the purulent urethral discharge. (Reproduced with permission from Morse, Moreland, Thompson. *Atlas of Sexually Transmitted Diseases*. London: Mosby-Wolfe; 1990.)

2. Gonococcal arthritis is the most common cause of mono-articular arthritis in young, sexually active patients.

3. Suspect gonococcal conjunctivitis in patients with copious eye discharge and chemosis.

4. Cultures are the gold standard for confirming the diagnosis of DGI. Selective media should be used when specimens are obtained from the cervix, pharynx, urethra, or rectum. Nonselective medium (blood agar) should be used in culturing joint fluid, blood, or cerebrospinal fluid.

5. Fluoroquinolones are no longer recommended for the treatment of gonococcal infections due to the rapid emergence of resistance to these agents.

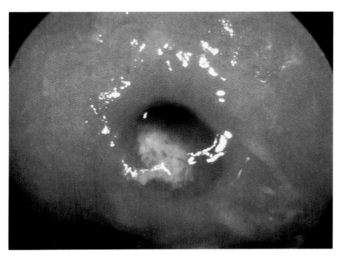

FIGURE 9.10 ■ Cervicitis. Endocervical purulent exudate in an asymptomatic patient with gonococcal cervicitis. The cervix is very friable. (Photo contributor: King K. Holmes, MD, from H. Hunter Handsfield. *Atlas of Sexually Transmitted Diseases.* New York: McGraw-Hill; 1992.)

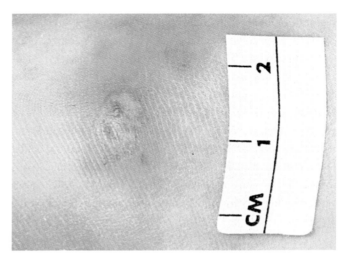

FIGURE 9.12 ■ Skin Lesions. Small pustules with hemorrhage suggestive of the skin lesions of disseminated gonococcal infection. (Photo contributor: H. Hunter Handsfield. *Atlas of Sexually Transmitted Diseases.* New York: McGraw-Hill; 1992.)

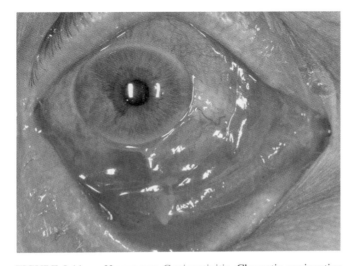

FIGURE 9.11 ■ Hyperacute Conjunctivitis. Chemotic conjunctiva and copious purulent exudate in a patient with gonococcal conjunctivitis. (Photo contributor: Lawrence B. Stack, MD.)

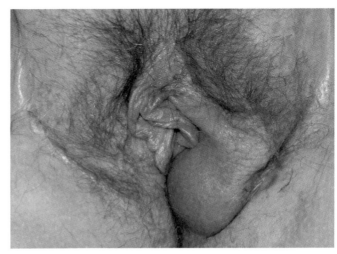

FIGURE 9.13 ■ Bartholin Abscess. Enlarged, fluctuant, tender Bartholin abscess of the labia, usually but not always a result of gonorrhea. (Photo contributor: Lawrence B. Stack, MD.)

Clinical Summary

After an incubation period of 1 to 3 weeks, males with chlamydial urethritis may present with a thin, often clear urethral discharge and/or dysuria. Up to 10% of these men may be asymptomatic. Women may also develop urethritis, which may only cause dysuria with pyuria but not bacteruria and can be misdiagnosed as a urinary tract infection. Chlamydial cervicitis in women is almost always asymptomatic. Women may develop pelvic inflammatory disease with upper genital tract infection. Men may develop epididymitis.

Emergency Department Treatment and Disposition

The preferred treatment consists of azithromycin, 1 g orally once; erythromycin 500 mg orally four times a day for 7 days; or doxycycline 100 mg orally twice a day for 7 days. Alternatives include ofloxacin, 300 mg orally twice a day for 7 days, levofloxacin 500 mg orally once daily for 7 days, or erythromycin ethylsuccinate 800 mg orally four times a day for 7 days. Partners should be examined and treated appropriately.

Pearls

1. Chlamydial infection often accompanies gonococcal infection, and patients being treated for gonorrhea should also be treated for chlamydial infection.
2. Women with chlamydial infections may be completely asymptomatic for long periods of time.
3. Consider syphilis serologic testing and HIV testing in patients presenting with sexually transmitted diseases.

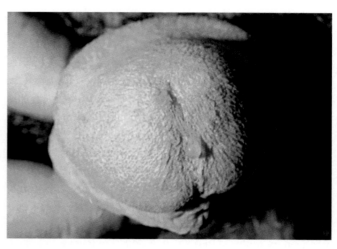

FIGURE 9.14 ■ Male Urethritis. Thin urethral discharge of chlamydial urethritis. (Photo contributor: Walter Stamm, MD, from H. Hunter Handsfield. *Atlas of Sexually Transmitted Diseases.* New York: McGraw-Hill; 1992.)

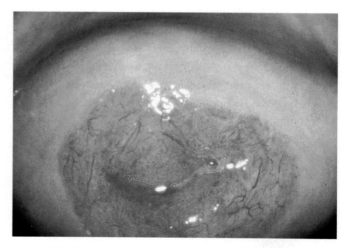

FIGURE 9.15 ■ Cervicitis. Mucopurulent cervicitis from chlamydial infection. (Photo contributor: H. Hunter Handsfield. *Atlas of Sexually Transmitted Diseases.* New York: McGraw-Hill; 1992.)

Clinical Summary

Herpes genitalis presents in several ways: symptomatic primary infection, first-episode nonprimary infection, and recurrent infection. Symptomatic primary infection occurs when the patient develops symptoms upon first acquiring the virus. These symptoms can range from asymptomatic infection to a more prolonged and sometimes serious course. Patients initially infected asymptomatically may present at a later time with their first symptomatic episode of nonprimary genital herpes. Patients with either symptomatic primary infection or first-episode nonprimary infection may develop recurrences.

Symptomatic primary infection with genital herpes is characterized by multiple vesicles that quickly ulcerate into shallow, painful ulcers which may coalesce, particularly in women. The development of the lesions may be preceded by a viral syndrome with low-grade fever and myalgias. Up to 10% of patients may develop aseptic meningitis. Women may develop sacral autonomic dysfunction and require urinary catheterization because of urinary retention. The lesions last up to 3 weeks and heal without scarring.

The clinical presentation of first-episode nonprimary genital herpes and recurrent genital herpes is less dramatic. Patients with first-episode nonprimary genital herpes do not have systemic symptoms, have solitary to several painful lesions, and resolve their symptoms in 1 to 2 weeks. Recurrences of genital herpes are often heralded by a warning prodrome of tingling or numbness in the perineal area. Vesicles and their subsequent ulcers are often solitary or may be only a few lesions. The duration of symptoms is often several days and usually less than a week.

Emergency Department Treatment and Disposition

Primary genital herpes: Acyclovir, 400 mg orally three times daily, or 200 mg orally five times daily, for a total duration of 7 to 10 days or until symptoms resolve. Alternatives include famciclovir 250 mg orally three times daily or valacyclovir 1 g orally twice a day for the 7- to 10-day course.

Recurrent genital herpes: Choices include acyclovir, 200 mg orally five times daily; acyclovir 400 mg orally three times a day; acyclovir 800 mg orally twice a day; famciclovir 125 mg orally twice a day; or valacyclovir 500 mg orally. All courses are 5 days in duration, with the exception of valacyclovir, which can be for 3 to 5 days.

Pearls

1. Women with genital herpes must be counseled to inform their obstetrician of this history of herpes when they become pregnant.
2. Genital herpes is the most common cause of ulcerating genital lesions in the developed world.

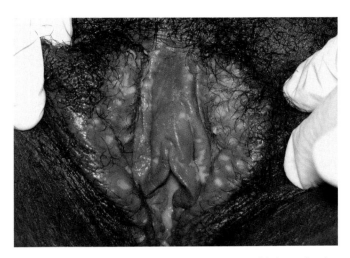

FIGURE 9.16 ■ Primary Lesions—Female. Multiple coalescing superficial ulcerations of primary genital herpes. (Photo contributor: Lawrence B. Stack, MD.)

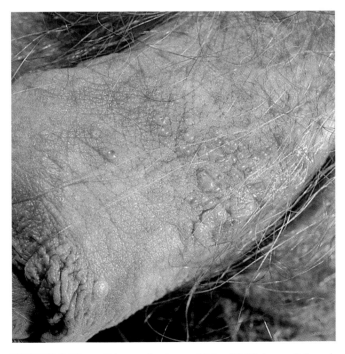

FIGURE 9.17 ■ Primary Lesions—Male. Multiple genital vesicles of primary genital herpes. (Photo contributor: H. Hunter Handsfield. *Atlas of Sexually Transmitted Diseases.* New York: McGraw-Hill; 1992.)

3. Patients may initially present with full-blown primary genital herpes symptoms or may have their first clinical presentation as a recurrence of an asymptomatically acquired infection.

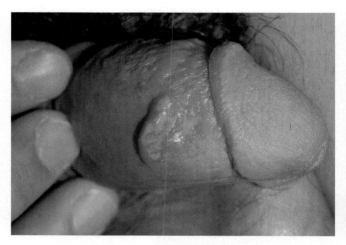

FIGURE 9.18 ▪ Primary Lesions—Male. Confluence of ulcerations on an erythematous base in a patient with primary herpes simplex type II. (Photo contributor: Lawrence B. Stack, MD.)

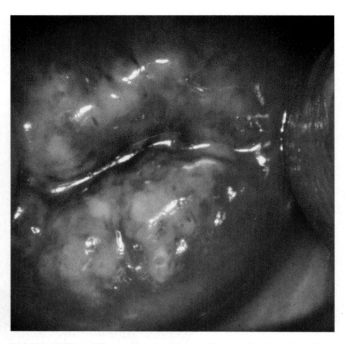

FIGURE 9.20 ▪ Herpes Simplex Virus—Cervix. Erosive ulcerations of the cervix in a patient with genital herpes infection. This patient may be completely asymptomatic and may transmit the disease. (Reproduced with permission from A. Wisdom. *Sexually Transmitted Diseases.* London: Mosby-Wolfe; 1992.)

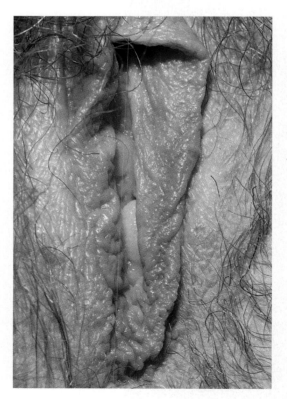

FIGURE 9.19 ▪ Recurrent Lesions—Female. Solitary, minimally painful lesion of recurrent genital herpes. (Photo contributor: H. Hunter Handsfield. *Atlas of Sexually Transmitted Diseases.* New York: McGraw-Hill; 1992.)

Clinical Summary

Lymphogranuloma venereum (LGV) is caused by a serotype of *Chlamydia trachomatis* and is primarily a disease of lymphatic tissue. Initially, LGV causes a painless genital ulceration that is not noticed by the patient more than 90% of the time. Patients usually present with painful, nonfluctuant inguinal adenopathy, which is often but not always unilateral. Lymphadenopathy may lie above and below the inguinal ligament, causing the "groove sign" suggestive of this diagnosis. The enlarged lymph nodes may spontaneously open into draining sinus tracts to the skin.

Emergency Department Treatment and Disposition

Treatment is doxycycline, 100 mg orally twice a day for 3 weeks. Rarely, patients may need needle aspiration of the lymph nodes if they become fluctuant. Serologic testing is needed to confirm the diagnosis.

Pearls

1. Patients rarely notice the evanescent ulcer associated with LGV.
2. The lymphadenopathy of LGV progresses over several weeks.
3. Treatment for LGV requires 3 weeks of therapy for a cure.

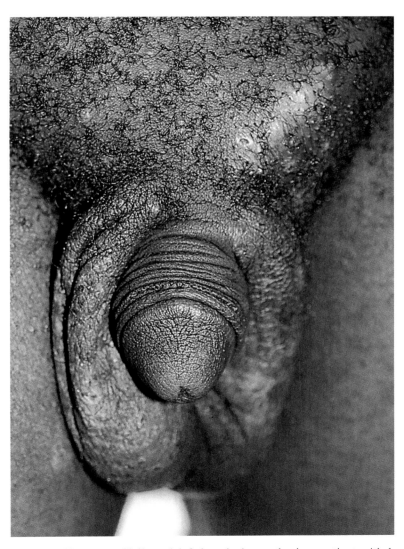

FIGURE 9.21 ■ Lymphogranuloma Venereum. Unilateral left lymphadenopathy in a patient with lymphogranuloma venereum. (Photo contributor: Lawrence B. Stack, MD.)

Clinical Summary

Chancroid is caused by *Haemophilus ducreyi*. After an incubation period of 2 to 10 days, this disease presents with multiple, painful, nonindurated genital ulcerations that are often deep and undermined and may have a purulent base. Inguinal adenopathy may develop and becomes fluctuant, large, and painful. Infected lymph nodes may rupture spontaneously. Systemic symptoms are uncommon.

Emergency Department Treatment and Disposition

Ceftriaxone, 250 mg intramuscularly once, or azithromycin, 1 g orally once. Alternatives include ciprofloxacin, 500 mg orally twice a day for 3 days or erythromycin base 500 mg orally four times a day for 7 days. Large, fluctuant nodes should be aspirated to prevent rupture; incision and drainage should be avoided to prevent development of chronic draining sinus tracts. Partners should be notified of exposure to the disease.

Pearls

1. Chancroid is usually found in high-risk populations, including illicit drug users, and in developed countries it is usually seen in localized isolated outbreaks.
2. Chancroid is a diagnosis of exclusion, as culturing *H ducreyi* requires a special medium not readily available. Genital herpes and syphilis must be ruled out.
3. The lymphadenopathy of chancroid is often very tender and fluctuant.
4. The ulcerative lesions of chancroid are very tender and usually multiple.

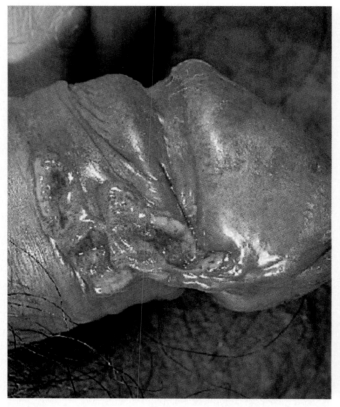

FIGURE 9.22 ■ Chancroid Lesions. Multiple painful, deep ulcerations of chancroid. (Photo contributor: H. Hunter Handsfield. *Atlas of Sexually Transmitted Diseases.* New York: McGraw-Hill; 1992.)

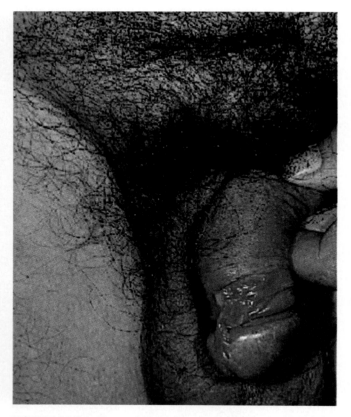

FIGURE 9.23 ■ Chancroid Lesions and Inguinal Nodes. Chancroid lesions with an enlarged lymph node. On examination, this node is tender and fluctuant. (Photo contributor: H. Hunter Handsfield. *Atlas of Sexually Transmitted Diseases.* New York: McGraw-Hill; 1992.)

CONDYLOMA ACUMINATA (GENITAL WARTS)

Clinical Summary

Caused by human papillomavirus (HPV), these flesh-colored lesions may be flat, sessile, or pedunculated. They often have a cauliflower-like appearance and are usually asymptomatic, but may be seen or felt by patients or their sexual partners. They range in size from 1 to 4 mm to masses that may be several centimeters large.

Emergency Department Treatment and Disposition

Local caustic agents (eg, podophyllin) are used to treat the lesions; multiple treatment is often needed, and recurrence is common. Other therapies include cryotherapy, electrocautery, and trichloracetic acid. Laser therapy or surgery may be needed in cases of giant warts.

Pearls

1. Evidence suggests that HPV is linked with increased risk of cervical cancer.
2. Women with genital warts need to have a Pap smear to rule out coexisting carcinoma in situ.

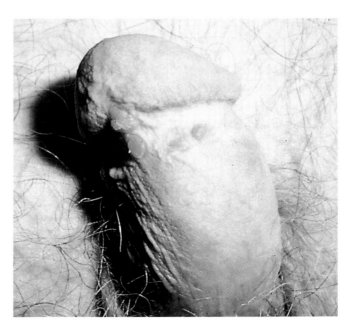

FIGURE 9.25 ■ Genital Warts—Male. Typical appearance of condyloma acuminata of the glans penis. (Reproduced with permission from Morse, Moreland, Thompson. *Atlas of Sexually Transmitted Diseases.* London: Mosby-Wolfe; 1990.)

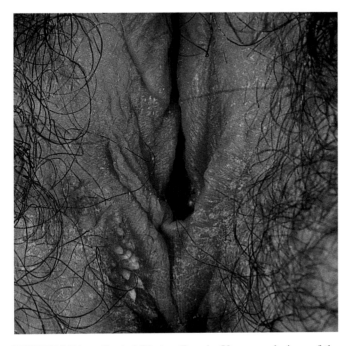

FIGURE 9.24 ■ Genital Warts—Female. Verrucous lesions of the posterior fourchette in a patient with condyloma acuminata. (Used with permission from H. Hunter Handsfield. *Atlas of Sexually Transmitted Diseases.* New York: McGraw-Hill; 1992.)

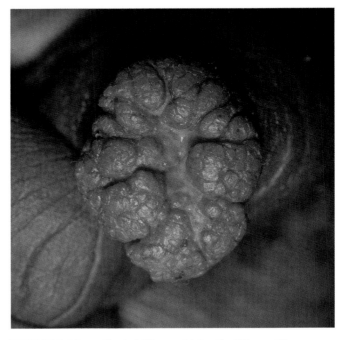

FIGURE 9.26 ■ Genital Warts—Male. Cauliflower-like appearance of condyloma acuminata of the foreskin of this uncircumcised male. (Photo contributor: Lawrence B. Stack, MD.)

3. Large lesions should be biopsied to rule out cancer.
4. Patients should be advised that it may take several or many visits to completely eradicate the condyloma.
5. In cases where the diagnosis is not obvious, rule out condyloma lata (secondary syphilis) by sending serologic studies.

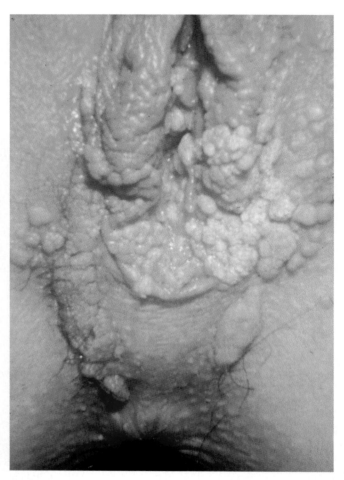

FIGURE 9.28 ■ Giant Warts—Female. Giant warts of a female patient with extensive condyloma acuminata. (Reproduced with permission from Morse, Moreland, Thompson. *Atlas of Sexually Transmitted Diseases.* London: Mosby-Wolfe; 1990.)

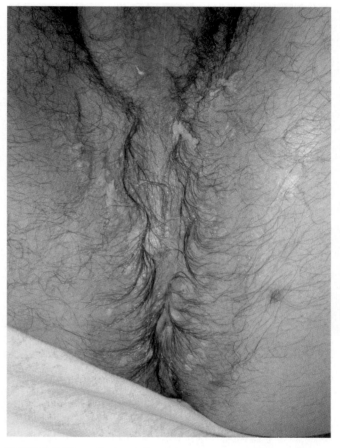

FIGURE 9.27 ■ Perianal Condyloma Acuminata. Multiple perianal warts are seen in this patient with HIV. (Photo contributor: Lawrence B. Stack, MD.)

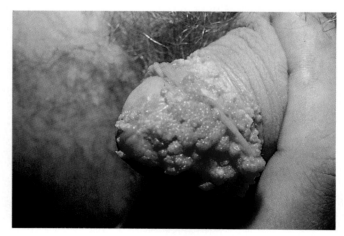

FIGURE 9.29 ■ Giant Warts—Male. Giant warts in a male patient with extensive condyloma acuminata. (Reproduced with permission from A. Wisdom. *Sexually Transmitted Diseases.* London: Mosby-Wolfe; 1992.)

Clinical Summary

Pediculosis can be caused by either the body louse or the crab louse. Body lice are not sexually transmitted and tend to cluster around the waist, shoulders, axillae, neck, and head. They are extremely itchy; patients may present with excoriations and intense pruritus. The lice are very small and may not be easily seen. The larval form of the louse, the nit, may be mistaken for dandruff in the hair. Unlike dandruff, however, the nits are extremely adherent to the hair shaft and cannot be brushed out of the hair. The adult lice and their eggs are often found in the seams of clothing.

Pubic infestation is caused by *Phthirus pubis,* the crab louse. Patients may present with intense itching in the pubic area; however, as many as half of patients with this infestation may be asymptomatic. Patients may notice the lice or may note tiny rust-colored spots on their underwear, which represent bleeding from the sites of louse bites. Nits may be found at the base of pubic hairs and hatch in 5 to 10 days.

Emergency Department Treatment and Disposition

Lindane shampoo should be lathered into the pubic, perineal, and perianal hair or lindane lotion applied in the affected areas and left on for 10 minutes and rinsed off. Synergized pyrethrins (RID), or synthetic pyrethrins, may also be used. Since lindane may be toxic, pyrethrins are preferred in pregnant women and children. Treatment should be repeated in 1 week to treat any nits that may have hatched. Clothing worn or linen used in the preceding 24 hours should be washed. Mechanical removal of nits attached to hairs should be attempted. Petroleum jelly or any bland ophthalmic ointment can be applied to the eyelashes twice daily for a week to treat infestation of the eyelashes. Sexual contacts should be examined.

Pearls

1. Nits are easier to find on examination than are mature lice; the average number of lice in an infestation is only 10.

2. Patients with pediculosis pubis should be considered at risk for other sexually transmitted diseases and examined.

3. Lindane shampoo or lotion should not be used in infants under 1 year of age or in pregnant women.

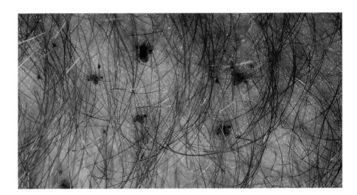

FIGURE 9.30 ■ Pediculosis Pubis—On Hairs. *Phthirus pubis,* or the crab louse, in the pubic hair of a patient complaining of itching. Note also the nits attached to the hairs. (Reproduced with permission from Morse, Moreland, Thompson. *Atlas of Sexually Transmitted Diseases.* London: Mosby-Wolfe; 1990.)

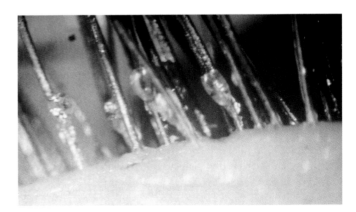

FIGURE 9.31 ■ Pediculosis Pubis—On Eyelashes. *Phthirus pubis* lice noted in the eyelashes. (Reproduced with permission from Spalton, Hitchings, Hunter. *Atlas of Clinical Ophthalmology.* 2nd ed. London: Mosby—Year Book Europe; 1994.)

Clinical Summary

An anal fissure is a longitudinal tear of the skin of the anal canal and extends from the dentate line to the anal verge. Fissures are thought to be caused by the passage of hard or large stools with constipation, but may also be seen with diarrhea. The fissures are typically a few millimeters wide and occur in the posterior midline, but may occur elsewhere. An anal fissure that is off the midline may have a secondary cause, such as inflammatory bowel disease or sexually transmitted infection. Although often seen in infants, this condition is found mostly in young and middle-aged adults. Patients present with intense sharp, burning pain during and after bowel movements. They may see bright red blood at the time or shortly after the passage of stool. Gentle examination with separation of the buttocks usually provides good visualization. The diagnosis of inflammatory bowel disease, ulcerative colitis, or Crohn disease should be considered in the differential, particularly if the fissure is atypical. Anal fissures may result from *Chlamydia*, gonorrhea, herpes, and syphilis. Tuberculosis, anal neoplasms, and sickle cell disease can also present as an anal fissure.

Emergency Department Treatment and Disposition

Acute treatment of anal fissures consists of anal hygiene, bulk fiber diet supplements to soften stools, warm sitz baths, and topical anesthetics. Oral pain medication and muscle relaxants such as diazepam may be required in certain patients.

Pearls

1. Pain and involuntary sphincter spasm may preclude a routine digital or anoscopic examination and require an examination under anesthesia.
2. A proctoscopic examination should be done at some point to rule out secondary causes.
3. Most anal fissures heal spontaneously, but refractory cases may require surgical repair.

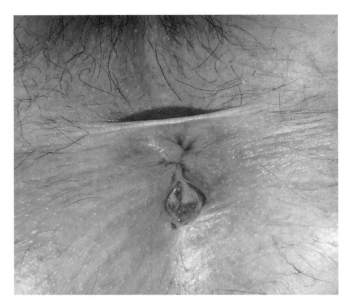

FIGURE 9.32 ■ Anal Fissure. A typical anal fissure located in the posterior midline. (Photo contributor: Paul J. Kovalcik, MD.)

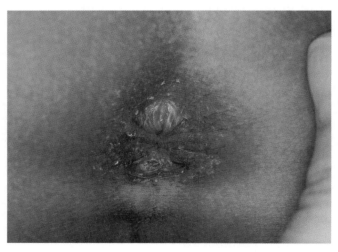

FIGURE 9.33 ■ Anal Fissure. An anal fissure is seen at the superior midline in a patient with 2 weeks of constipation. (Photo contributor: Kevin J. Knoop, MD, MS.)

Clinical Summary

The perianal abscess is the most common anorectal abscess. Symptoms include pain in the anal area worsened by bowel movements, straining, coughing, or palpation. Examination findings include a fluctuant and possibly erythematous mass found at the perianal region. Perianal abscesses are usually fairly superficial and easy to drain with local anesthesia. The patient may notice swelling or a pressure sensation. Perirectal abscesses tend to be more complex and are named according to the involved space: ischiorectal, intersphincteric, or supralevator. These are fluctuant masses that are usually palpable along the rectal wall. Patients may complain of pain, fever, and mucous or bloody discharge with bowel movement. Crohn disease should be considered, because 36% of Crohn patients have a perianal abscess at the presentation of their disease. An underlying process may also exist, such as diabetes mellitus, leukemia, or other malignancy.

Emergency Department Treatment and Disposition

Incision and drainage of perianal abscesses should be performed with a small radial or cruciate incision lateral to the external sphincter. For an uncomplicated abscess, this can be accomplished under local anesthesia. The cavity should be cleared of loculations and then loosely packed with iodoform gauze, which should be removed in 24 to 48 hours. All patients require outpatient follow-up. Antibiotic therapy is not indicated unless there is underlying disease affecting the patient's immunologic function or the patient appears septic. Surgical consultation should be obtained for treatment of perirectal abscesses under anesthesia.

Pearls

1. Surgical consultation and treatment may be required in the patient with a large or complicated anorectal abscess or where adequate analgesia cannot be obtained.
2. Consider admission for debilitated, elderly, febrile, obese, or otherwise ill-appearing patients.
3. All patients warrant follow-up referral due to the high incidence of fistulae with anorectal abscesses.

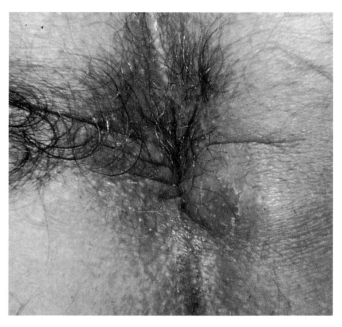

FIGURE 9.34 ■ Perianal Abscess. Swelling and erythema around the anus consistent with a perianal abscess. (Photo contributor: The American Society of Colon and Rectal Surgeons.)

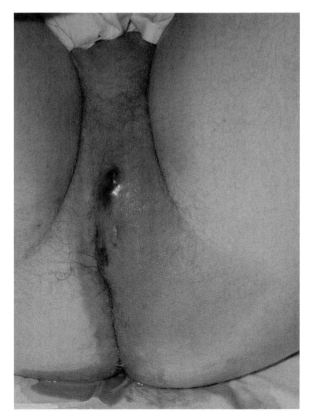

FIGURE 9.35 ■ Perirectal Abscess. This large, spontaneously draining perirectal abscess required further surgical debridement in the operating room. (Photo contributor: Lawrence B. Stack, MD.)

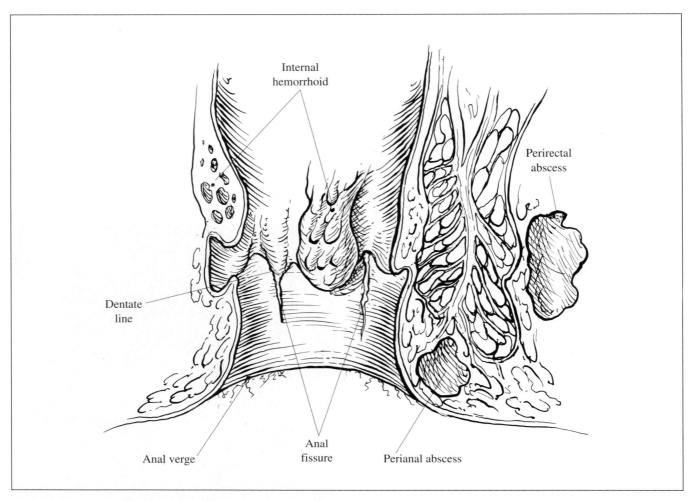

FIGURE 9.36 ■ Perianal-Perirectal Abscesses. The anatomy of perianal and perirectal abscesses is illustrated. Also shown are anal fissure and internal and external hemorrhoids.

Clinical Summary

External hemorrhoids result from the dilatation of the venules of the inferior hemorrhoidal plexus below the dentate line. They have a covering of skin, or anoderm, versus internal hemorrhoids, which have a mucosal covering. Hemorrhoids commonly present with an episode of rectal bleeding of bright red blood after defecation. This results from the passage of the fecal mass over the thin-walled venules, causing abrasions and bleeding. Symptoms from external hemorrhoids include swelling, burning, pruritus, and wetness of the anal area. Contributing factors include constipation, family history, pregnancy, portal hypertension, and increased intra-abdominal pressure. Hemorrhoids are commonly found at three anatomic locations: right anterior, right posterior, and left lateral positions. A thrombosed external hemorrhoid contains intravascular clots and causes exquisite pain the first 48 hours.

Internal hemorrhoids present with painless rectal bleeding or the sensation of prolapse. Other diagnoses to consider include infection, perianal or perirectal abscess, inflammatory bowel disease, malignancy, local trauma, herpes or other sexually transmitted infection, rectal polyp, or rectal prolapse.

Emergency Department Treatment and Disposition

In the case of severe bleeding, fluid resuscitation would need to be instituted and the bleeding vessel located, clamped, and ligated. Treatment for less severe cases includes increased dietary fiber, increased fluid intake, hot sitz baths, bed rest, and nonnarcotic pain medication. Advanced cases may require surgical consultation and treatment. Emergency department treatment of thrombosed external hemorrhoids includes an elliptical excision and extrusion of the clot under local anesthesia.

Pearls

1. Patients with serious anorectal problems complain of "hemorrhoids." Therefore, careful examination and consideration of the differential diagnosis should be undertaken with each patient.

2. Having the patient strain during the examination may reveal bleeding or prolapse that might otherwise go unnoticed.

3. Internal hemorrhoids are not typically painful, whereas external hemorrhoids do cause pain.

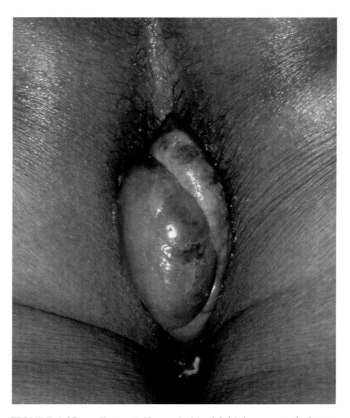

FIGURE 9.37 ■ External Hemorrhoids. Multiple engorged, thrombosed external hemorrhoids are seen in this patient. (Photo contributor: Lawrence B. Stack, MD.)

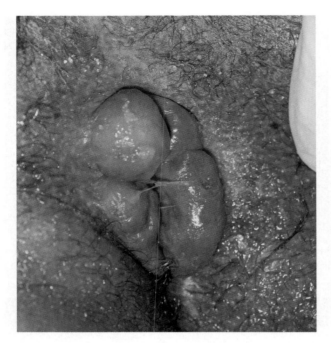

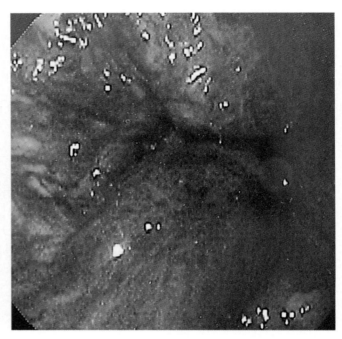

FIGURE 9.38 ▪ External Thrombosed Hemorrhoids. Typical appearance of acute thrombosed hemorrhoids. (Photo contributor: Lawrence B. Stack, MD.)

FIGURE 9.39 ▪ Internal Hemorrhoids. Internal hemorrhoids are seen in this endoscopic view of the rectum. (Photo contributor: Virender K. Sharman, MD.)

Clinical Summary

Rectal prolapse occurs when anorectal tissue slides through the anal orifice. Prolapse may be partial, involving only the mucosa (prolapse is <2 cm), or complete, involving in full thickness extrusion of the rectal wall. Prolapse may result from laxity of the pelvic floor, weak anal sphincters, and/or lack of mesorectal fixation. Patients complain of bleeding, mucous discharge, rectal pressure, or a mass. Problems with fecal incontinence, constipation, and rectal ulceration are common as well. Prolapse may be associated with an increased familial incidence, chronic cough, dysentery, or parasitic infection. Other diagnoses to consider include foreign body, tumor, perianal or perirectal abscess, rectal polyp, or engorged external hemorrhoids.

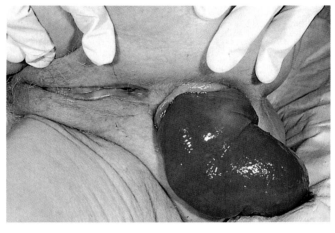

FIGURE 9.40 ■ Prolapsed Rectum. The rectum is completely prolapsed in this elderly patient. (Photo contributor: Alan B. Storrow, MD.)

Emergency Department Treatment and Disposition

Reduction is usually accomplished with gentle manual pressure. If manual reductions fail, surgical consultation and operative reduction are needed. Surgical treatment is also indicated with a complete prolapse. All patients should undergo an anoscopic and sigmoidoscopic examination at some point; if rectal bleeding is a problem, full colonic evaluation should be completed.

Pearls

1. This is commonly seen in children with cystic fibrosis (22%); therefore, all children with rectal prolapse should have a sweat chloride test.
2. Examination of rectal prolapse reveals concentric mucosal rings and a sulcus between the anal canal and the rectum, whereas prolapsed hemorrhoids are separated by radial grooves and the sulcus is absent.
3. To confirm the diagnosis, prolapse may be reproduced by having the patient bear down.

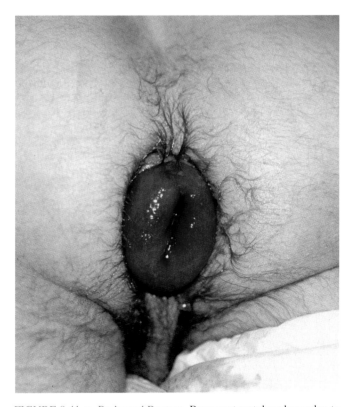

FIGURE 9.41 ■ Prolapsed Rectum. Recurrent rectal prolapse due to chronic constipation. (Photo contributor: Lawrence B. Stack, MD.)

Clinical Summary

Pilonidal abscesses are typically seen at or just superior to the gluteal fold and are more common in teenage and young adult males. Patients complain of localized pain, swelling, and drainage but usually do not have systemic symptoms. The abscess begins with the formation of a small opening in the skin that develops into a cystic structure involving surrounding hairs. This opening is occluded by hair or keratin, creating a closed space that does not allow drainage. The acute abscess contains mixed organisms including *Staphylococcus aureus* and *Streptococcus,* but anaerobes and gram-negative organisms may also be present. Evidence of cellulitis in the sacrococcygeal area may result from a simple abscess or furuncle. However, other causes should be considered, such as anal fistulae, hidradenitis, inflammatory bowel disease, or tuberculosis.

Emergency Department Treatment and Disposition

An acutely fluctuant abscess requires incision and drainage under local anesthesia with removal of pus and debris. The patient should be instructed on meticulous wound care and sitz baths. Antibiotic therapy is not indicated unless the patient is immunocompromised. Surgical referral is given, particularly with a chronic or recurrent cyst, which may require surgical excision and closure.

Pearls

1. Pilonidal abscesses almost always occur in the midline but can have sinus tracts extending off the midline.
2. Pilonidal disease is three times more common in men than in women.

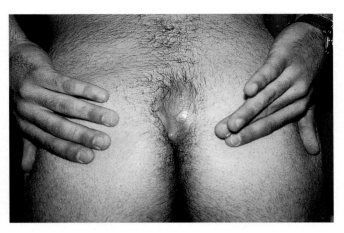

FIGURE 9.42 ■ Pilonidal Abscess. Redness, fluctuance, and tenderness in the gluteal cleft seen with a pilonidal abscess. (Photo contributor: Louis La Vopa, MD.)

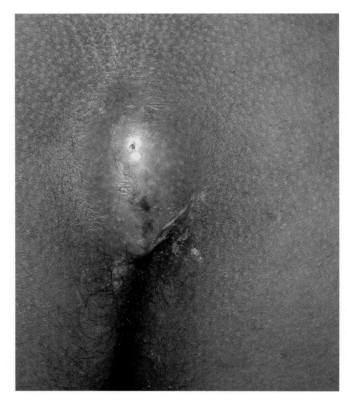

FIGURE 9.43 ■ Pilonidal Abscess. Close-up of the cutaneous manifestations of a large pilonidal abscess. (Photo contributor: Lawrence B. Stack, MD.)

Clinical Summary

The diagnosis of rectal foreign body is usually made by history and confirmed by digital examination. Most often the foreign body is inserted, but it is possible to have an ingested foreign body trapped in the rectum. The most serious complication of a rectal foreign body is perforation of the rectum or distal colon. The patient must be carefully evaluated for evidence of perforation with x-rays demonstrating free air and clinically for the presentation of an acute abdomen. Perforation above the peritoneal reflection is associated with free air in the abdominal cavity and peritoneal signs. Perforation below the peritoneal reflection presents with more insidious signs of pain and infection in the perianal or perineal region. It is important to determine the size, shape, and number of objects to assess the risk of perforation. In children, rectal foreign bodies usually present as rectal bleeding. Depending on the clinical scenario, the diagnoses of sexual assault or child abuse should be considered.

Emergency Department Treatment and Disposition

Removal can often take place in the emergency department with sedation of the patient and local anesthesia of the anal sphincter. If the risk of perforation appears high or adequate relaxation and anesthesia cannot be obtained, then the patient is prepared for surgery. After removal, proctoscopic or sigmoidoscopic examination is recommended to rule out perforation or laceration.

Pearls

1. A Foley catheter or an endotracheal tube may be used to release the vacuum effect of some foreign bodies, and the balloon can be inflated and aid in the removal.
2. A rectal foreign body in a child should raise the suspicion of abuse.

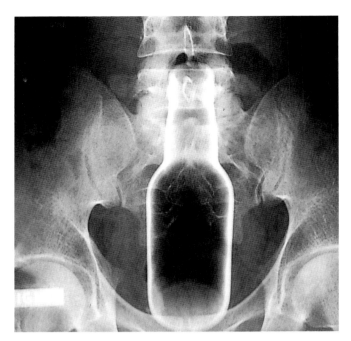

FIGURE 9.44 ■ Rectal Foreign Body. This foreign body (a 7-oz beer bottle) required removal in the operating room. (Photo contributor: Kevin J. Knoop, MD, MS.)

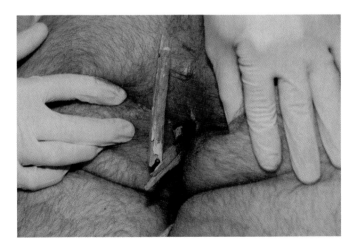

FIGURE 9.45 ■ Rectal Foreign Body. This victim of assault had a stick forced into his rectum. After removal, sigmoidoscopy revealed a retained small broken stick. (Photo contributor: R. Jason Thurman, MD.)

Clinical Summary

Gastrointestinal bleeding commonly presents with the alteration of stool color. By definition, melena is the passage of dark, pitchlike stools stained with blood pigments. Generally, but not always, melena results from bleeding into the upper gastrointestinal tract proximal to the ligament of Treitz. Black stools have been seen with as little as 60 mL of blood in the upper gastrointestinal tract, but melena typically does not develop until 100 to 200 mL is present. Melena can be found in lower bleeds with decreased transit time, as with an obstruction distal to the site of bleeding. Melenic stools may occur from swallowed blood, as from epistaxis or other oropharyngeal bleeding. Dark or black stools can also be seen with the ingestion of bismuth salicylate, food coloring, and iron supplements.

Emergency Department Treatment and Disposition

Patients with melenic stools should be evaluated in a monitored setting and undergo assessment for signs and symptoms of hypovolemia and treated accordingly. One or more large-bore intravenous line should be placed and saline infused. Depending on the patient's stability, type-specific packed red blood cells or other blood products may be required. Abdominal radiographs are done to look for free air in the peritoneum, and gastric aspiration should be done to assess for active gastric bleeding. Stable patients who present with melena may be admitted to the ward. Evidence of unstable vital signs, continued bleeding, severe anemia, or comorbid disease warrants admission to the intensive care unit. Consultation with a gastroenterologist should be sought unless patients require more than two units of blood for resuscitation, which would call for surgical intervention.

Pearls

1. Melena is the most common presenting symptom of bleeding from peptic ulcer disease.
2. Melena represents approximately 200 mL of blood loss in the gastrointestinal tract.

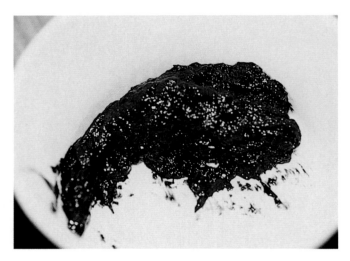

FIGURE 9.46 ■ Melena. The black, tarry appearance of melena in a patient with a duodenal ulcer. (Photo contributor: Alan B. Storrow, MD.)

Chapter 10

GYNECOLOGIC AND OBSTETRIC CONDITIONS

Robert G. Buckley
Kevin J. Knoop

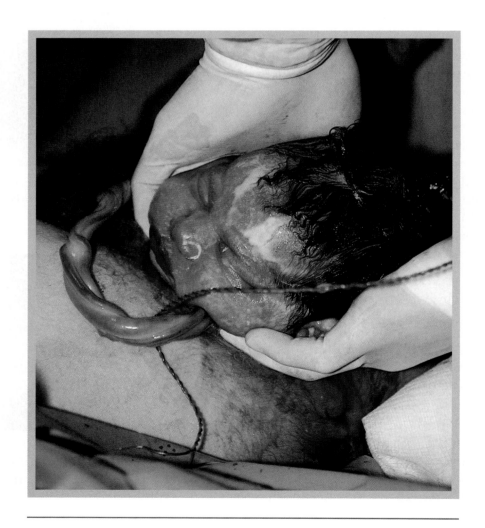

Clinical Summary

Candidal vaginitis is characterized by a thick, curdy, white discharge and vulvar discomfort. Intense vulvar erythema, pruritus, or burning is often present. A microscopic slide prepared with 10% potassium hydroxide yielding characteristic branch chain hyphae and spores establishes the diagnosis (Fig. 25.13). The pH of the discharge is less than 4.5. Predisposing factors that should be considered include oral contraceptive, antibiotic, or corticosteroid use; pregnancy; and diabetes. Sexually transmitted diseases are not usually associated with isolated candidal vaginitis.

Trichomonas vaginitis presents as a persistent, thin, copious discharge that is often frothy, green, or foul-smelling. The pH of these secretions is greater than 4.5. The amount of vaginal and cervical erythema and inflammation varies considerably; thus the diagnosis depends on the presence of motile flagellates on normal saline wet-mount microscopy. Occasionally, multiple petechiae on the vaginal wall (strawberry spots) or cervix (strawberry cervix) are seen.

Bacterial vaginosis (previously termed *Haemophilus* or *Gardnerella* vaginitis) is characterized by a malodorous, homogeneous discharge with a pH greater than 4.5 and a transient amine (fishy) odor when mixed with a drop of KOH solution (positive sniff test). The presence of clue cells on normal saline wet mount establishes the diagnosis (Fig. 25.14). Other associated vaginal or abdominal complaints are minimal and, if significant, may represent another disease process.

Vaginal foreign bodies, particularly in children, atrophic vaginitis, and contact dermatitis, should all be considered in the differential diagnosis.

Emergency Department Treatment and Disposition

For candidal vaginitis, various regimens of topical antifungal agents are the mainstay of treatment (clotrimazole 1% cream, one applicatorful inserted high into the vaginal vault for 7 nights, clotrimazole, two 100-mg vaginal tablets for 3 nights, or one 500-mg vaginal tablet for single-dose treatment). Oral fluconazole (Diflucan, 150 mg as a single dose) is also effective.

For Trichomonas vaginitis, a single, one-time dose of metronidazole (2 g) is generally curative but is contraindicated in pregnancy and is associated with an Antabuse-like reaction when taken with alcohol. For the pregnant patient, clotrimazole (100-mg vaginal suppositories daily for 7 to 14 days) may provide symptomatic relief.

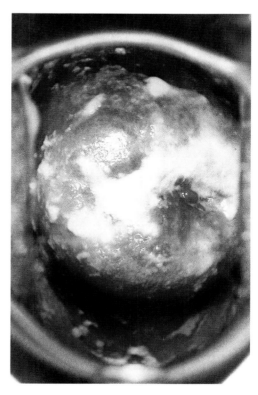

FIGURE 10.1 ■ Candidal Vaginitis. Thick, curdy white discharge secondary to candidal vaginitis. (Photo contributor: Kevin J. Knoop, MD, MS.)

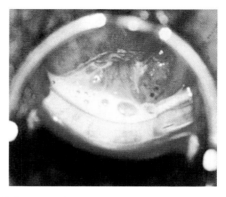

FIGURE 10.2 ■ *Trichomonas* Vaginitis. Thin vaginal discharge suggestive of *Trichomonas* vaginitis. (Photo contributor: H. Hunter Handsfield. *Atlas of Sexually Transmitted Diseases.* New York: McGraw-Hill; 1992.)

For *bacterial vaginosis*, metronidazole (500 mg twice daily for 7 days) is recommended in the nonpregnant patient. Treatment for asymptomatic infection or for male sexual partners is not generally recommended.

Pearls

1. Diabetes mellitus or immunosuppression should be considered in refractory or recurrent cases of candidal vaginitis.
2. A history of balanitis in the sexual partner should be sought and treated if present.
3. *Trichomonas* should be considered a sexually transmitted disease. It is therefore generally recommended that concomitant culturing for gonorrhea and *Chlamydia* be performed, as well as serologic testing for syphilis, HIV, and hepatitis B should be considered for both patient and partner.

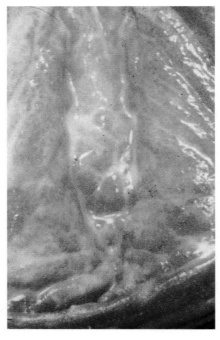

FIGURE 10.3 ■ *Gardnerella* Vaginitis. Thin, milky white discharge suggestive of *Gardnerella* vaginitis. (Photo contributor: Curatek Pharmaceuticals.)

Clinical Summary

The patient's chief complaint is often a purulent vaginal discharge. Speculum examination reveals a purulent, viscous discharge emanating from the cervical os. Otherwise, a purulent discharge may be seen on a cervical swab. A Gram stain may reveal either gram-negative intracellular diplococcus consistent with *Neisseria gonorrhoeae* (Fig. 25.11) or be nonspecific, consistent with *Chlamydia trachomatis*, a coinfectant with the gonococcus about 50% of the time. The diagnosis of pelvic inflammatory disease should be considered, when accompanied by symptoms of lower abdominal pain and signs of pelvic peritonitis such as cervical motion and adnexal tenderness.

Emergency Department Treatment and Disposition

Cultures for *C trachomatis* and *N gonorrhoeae* should be obtained prior to initiation of therapy. Ceftriaxone (125 mg as a single intramuscular dose) provides coverage for *N gonorrhoeae*. Single-dose oral quinolones (ciprofloxacin, 500 mg, or ofloxacin, 400 mg) can be used in penicillin-allergic patients. Doxycycline (100 mg) or ofloxacin (300 mg) twice a day for 7 days or a single 1-g dose of azithromycin provides coverage for *Chlamydia*.

Pearls

1. Mucopurulent cervicitis is almost always secondary to a sexually transmitted disease; thus sexual partners should be treated as well.
2. Refer all patients for formal gynecologic follow-up after culture and treatment, since early cervical neoplasia may have a similar appearance.

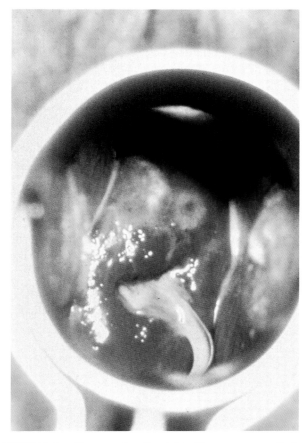

FIGURE 10.4 ■ Mucopurulent Cervicitis. Viscous, opaque discharge emanating from the cervical os, consistent with mucopurulent cervicitis. The string from an intrauterine device is seen descending through the os in this patient. (Photo contributor: Sue Rist, FNP.)

Clinical Summary

Cervical polyps are friable fleshy fingerlike growths that emanate from the cervical os or endocervical canal. They are typically asymptomatic, but may bleed with minimal trauma such as intercourse or douching. The etiology is variable and is thought to be either from infection, chronic inflammation, or hormonal (estrogen) increase. Single polyps are more common, but multiple polyps can occur.

Emergency Department Treatment and Disposition

No specific treatment is offered in the emergency department. If found during evaluation for vaginal bleeding, infection and pregnancy should be treated/excluded. Incidental diagnosis may be referred for ligation and histologic evaluation.

Pearls

1. Almost all cervical polyps are benign, but all should be evaluated.
2. Cervical polyps are the most common benign neoplasm of the cervix.

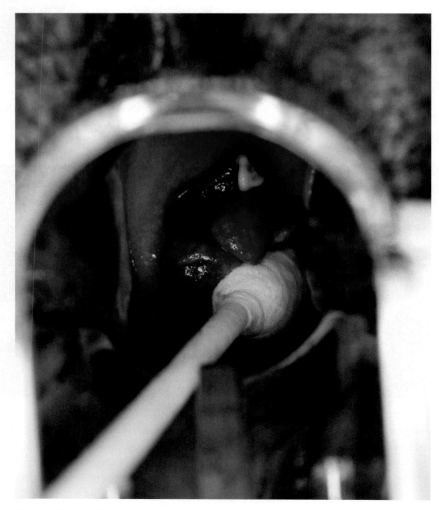

FIGURE 10.5 ■ Cervical Polyps. Several fleshy fingerlike growths are seen protruding from the cervical os. (Photo contributor: Kevin J. Knoop, MD, MS.)

Clinical Summary

Bartholin glands and ducts are located over the lower third of the introitus near the labia minora. A cyst or abscess can result from an obstructed duct, which usually occurs secondary to scarring from trauma, delivery, or episiotomy. Infection of the cyst is usually with mixed vaginal or fecal flora (*Escherichia coli*) but may also contain *Neisseria gonorrhoeae* and *Chlamydia trachomatis*. Progressive enlargement and infection lead to increasing pain, swelling, and dyspareunia. A tender, fluctuant cystic mass with surrounding labial edema is easily appreciated on examination. Epidermal inclusion cysts and sebaceous cysts of the labia majora, hidradenitis suppurativa, vulvar hematomas, leiomyomas, lipomas, and fibromas may be confused with a noninfected Bartholin cyst.

Emergency Department Treatment and Disposition

Simple incision and drainage followed by sitz baths provide the most effective and expeditious relief on an emergency basis. Reocclusion and reaccumulation of cystic swelling are common.

Pearls

1. Antibiotics are usually not required.
2. Placement of a Word catheter into the cyst cavity decreases the incidence of reocclusion, but it must be allowed to remain in place for up to 6 weeks to ensure epithelialization of the drainage tract.

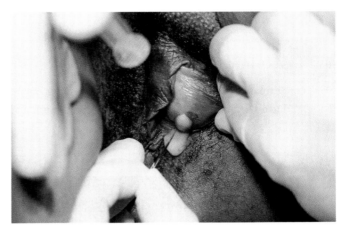

FIGURE 10.7 ■ Bartholin Gland Abscess. Medial incision of the cyst yielding purulent fluid, consistent with a Bartholin gland abscess. (Photo contributor: Medical Photography Department, Naval Medical Center, San Diego, CA.)

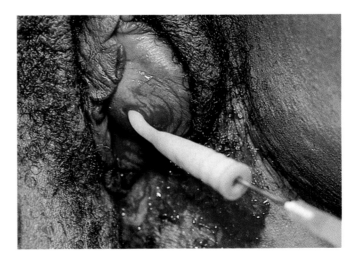

FIGURE 10.6 ■ Bartholin Gland Abscess. Bartholin gland abscess with the labial fluctuance pointing medially. (Photo contributor: Medical Photography Department, Naval Medical Center, San Diego, CA.)

FIGURE 10.8 ■ Bartholin Gland Abscess. Insertion and inflation of a Word catheter into the cyst cavity. The free end of the catheter can be tucked into the vagina for long-term placement, allowing for epithelialization of the incision site. (Photo contributor: Medical Photography Department, Naval Medical Center, San Diego, CA.)

Clinical Summary

Spontaneous abortion is associated with vaginal bleeding and abdominal discomfort. Severe pain, heavy bleeding with the passage of clots or tissue, and hypotension may also be present. *Threatened abortion* is diagnosed when mild cramping and vaginal bleeding are not accompanied by tissue extrusion, cervical dilation, or ectopic pregnancy. Uterine cramping with progressive cervical dilation indicates an *inevitable abortion.* In *incomplete abortion,* some of the products of conception (POC) have passed, yet retained intrauterine tissue leads to ongoing symptoms. Ectopic pregnancy should always be ruled out by ultrasound, close clinical follow-up, and serial hCG testing. The presence of frank tissue passage or cervical dilation generally excludes this diagnosis. However, large blood clots or an intrauterine decidual cast may be mistaken for POC. Therefore, gross inspection cannot rule out ectopic pregnancy.

Emergency Department Treatment and Disposition

Intravenous access, fluid resuscitation, cross-matching of blood, and urgent gynecologic consultation are implemented with severe pain, heavy bleeding, or hypovolemia. All tissue is sent to pathology for definitive identification. Anti-Rh immunoglobulin (RhoGAM) should be administered in all cases of vaginal bleeding where the mother is Rh-negative and the father is not confirmed to be Rh-negative.

Pearls

1. The passage of large clots usually indicates rapid heavy bleeding.
2. *Completed abortion* is characterized by the passage of tissue, followed by resolution of bleeding and closure of the cervical os.
3. Fever, leukocytosis, pelvic tenderness, and malodorous cervical discharge suggest *septic abortion.*

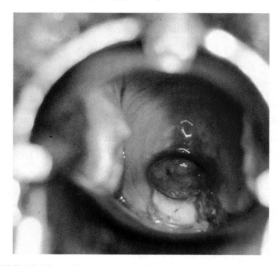

FIGURE 10.10 ■ Spontaneous Abortion. Dilation of the cervical os with partial extrusion of tissue in the setting of an inevitable abortion. (Photo contributor: Robert Buckley, MD.)

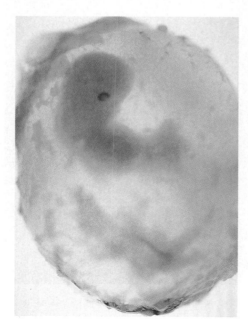

FIGURE 10.9 ■ Spontaneous Abortion. Passage of tissue in a spontaneous abortion at 4 weeks. (Photo contributor: Lawrence B. Stack, MD.)

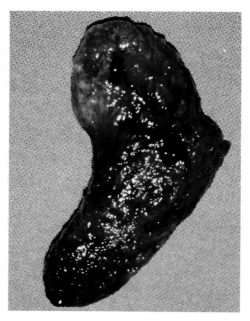

FIGURE 10.11 ■ Decidual Cast. A decidual cast or organized clot may occasionally be mistaken for products of conception. (Photo contributor: Medical Photography Department, Naval Medical Center, San Diego, CA.)

Clinical Summary

Patients who present for examination and treatment following an incident of sexual assault are ideally cared for by a multidisciplinary team capable of addressing the immediate medical and psychosocial needs of the patient in concert with forensic and legal requirements. A thorough general examination may reveal associated contusions and other soft tissue injuries. A meticulous inspection of the perineum, rectum, vaginal fornices, vagina, and cervix is required to identify inflicted injuries. Toluidine staining and colposcopy are often useful in enhancing less apparent injuries such as those to the posterior fourchette following sexual assault. These are most commonly found between the 3 and 9 o'clock distribution when the patient is examined in the dorsal lithotomy position. Perianal lacerations may also be seen as toluidine-enhanced linear tears. Examination of the cervix and posterior vaginal vault may reveal injuries to those structures. Perineal injuries from accidental trauma may be indistinguishable from those of sexual assault and should be interpreted in the context of the history.

Emergency Department Treatment and Disposition

Treatment is preceded by forensic evidence gathering, consisting of a Wood lamp examination to identify semen for collection, pubic hair sampling and combing, vaginal and cervical smears (air-dried), a cervical and vaginal wet mount to identify sperm, vaginal aspirate to test for acid phosphatase, and rectal or buccal swabs for sperm. A prepackaged kit with directions may be available to facilitate the collection of evidence.

Cervical cultures for *Chlamydia* and *Neisseria gonorrhoeae* should be obtained as well as serum testing for syphilis, hepatitis, and HIV. Empiric antibiotic coverage against sexually transmitted diseases should be provided and an oral contraceptive offered (after confirming a nonpregnant state) to prevent unwanted pregnancy.

Pearls

1. The medical care of the patient who has been sexually assaulted should ideally be performed by experienced supportive staff familiar with the details of forensic evidence gathering and colposcopic photography.
2. Normal findings on physical examination and no sperm on wet preparation do *not* exclude the possibility of assault.

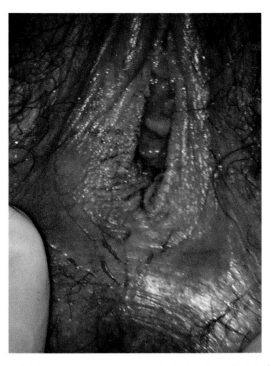

FIGURE 10.12 ■ Genital Trauma (Posterior Fourchette). Linear tears to the posterior fourchette—due to sexual assault—enhanced by toluidine staining. (Photo contributors: Hillary J. Larkin, PA-C, and Lauri A. Paolinetti, PA-C.)

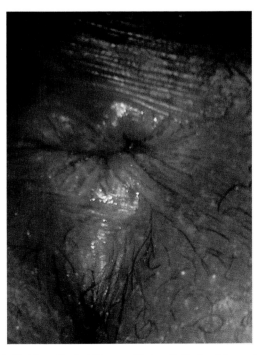

FIGURE 10.13 ■ Genital Trauma (Perianal). Perianal lacerations following sexual assault. (Photo contributors: Hillary J. Larkin, PA-C, and Lauri A. Paolinetti, PA-C.)

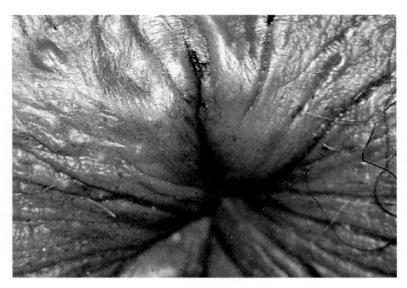

FIGURE 10.14 ▪ Genital Trauma (Toluidine Staining). Toluidine staining showing subtle perianal lacerations following forceful anal penetration. (Photo contributor: Aurora Mendez, RN.)

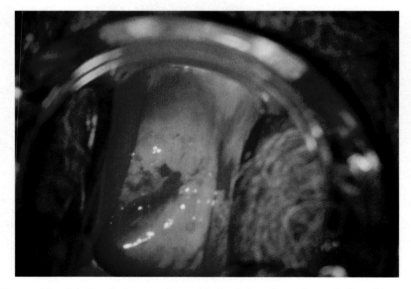

FIGURE 10.15 ▪ Genital Trauma (Cervix). Cervical trauma in an elderly victim of sexual assault. Petechiae and freshly bleeding abrasions are noted from 10 to 3 o'clock. (Photo contributors: Hillary J. Larkin, PA-C, and Lauri A. Paolinetti, PA-C.)

Clinical Summary

Uterine prolapse is defined as the propulsion of the uterus through the pelvic floor or vaginal introitus. In first-degree prolapse, the cervix descends into the lower third of the vagina; in second-degree prolapse, the cervix usually protrudes through the introitus; whereas in third-degree prolapse, or procidentia, the entire uterus is externalized with inversion of the vagina. Symptoms include a sensation of inguinal traction, low back pain, urinary incontinence, and the presence of a vaginal mass. Uterine prolapse can occasionally be confused with a cystocele (discussed below), enterocele, or soft tissue tumor.

Emergency Department Treatment and Disposition

Patients with first- or second-degree prolapse should be referred to a gynecologist for pessary placement or surgical correction. With procidentia, the uterus should be manually reduced into the vaginal vault and the patient placed at bed rest until evaluated by a gynecologic consultant.

Pearl

1. With procidentia, the exposed uterus is prone to abrasion and possible secondary infection.

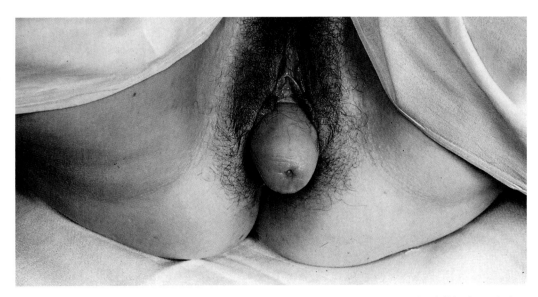

Figure 10.16 ■ Third-Degree Uterine Prolapse. Note the protrusion of the entire uterus with cervix visible through the vaginal introitus. (Photo contributor: Matthew Backer, Jr., MD.)

Clinical Summary

A cystocele occurs when there is relaxation and bulging of the posterior bladder wall and trigone into the vagina and is usually due to birth trauma. Patients complain of bulging or fullness over the introitus that is worsened with Valsalva and relieved with recumbency. It is often associated with urinary incontinence or symptoms of incomplete emptying. Enteroceles, rectoceles, uterine prolapse, and soft tissue tumors should also be considered.

Emergency Department Treatment and Disposition

Larger cystoceles or those associated with urinary symptomatology, pain, or bothersome bulging should be referred to a gynecologist for further evaluation.

Pearl

1. Most cystoceles are asymptomatic and are detected incidentally at the time of pelvic examination.

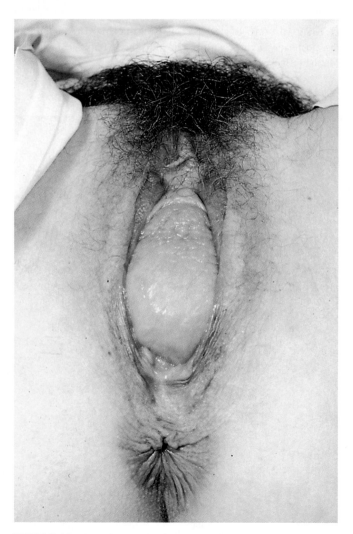

FIGURE 10.17 ■ Cystocele. Cystocele with bulging of the posterior bladder wall into the vagina. (Photo contributor: Matthew Backer, Jr., MD.)

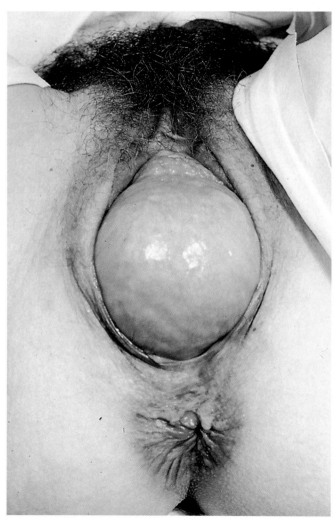

FIGURE 10.18 ■ Cystocele. Cystocele worsening with Valsalva. (Photo contributor: Matthew Backer, Jr., MD.)

Clinical Summary

Most small rectoceles are completely asymptomatic, though symptoms of introital bulging, constipation, and incomplete rectal evacuation may occur. Bulging of the introitus can be seen grossly on physical examination and can become worse with Valsalva. Rectovaginal examination reveals a thin-walled protrusion of the rectovaginal septum into the lower part of the vagina.

Emergency Department Treatment and Disposition

Supportive measures with hydration, laxatives, and stool softeners are generally all that is needed to relieve the patient's symptoms. Those patients with large symptomatic rectoceles who do not desire further childbearing are candidates for posterior colpoperineorrhaphy.

Pearl

1. A rectocele is the herniation of the rectovaginal wall and is usually due to childbirth.

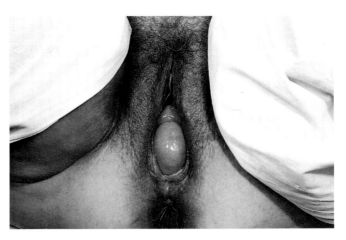

FIGURE 10.19 ■ Rectocele. This is characterized by bulging of the posterior vaginal wall at the introitus. (Photo contributor: Matthew Backer, Jr., MD.)

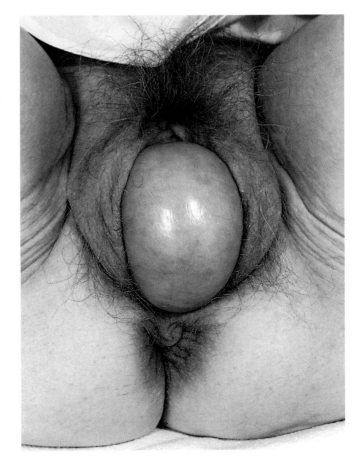

FIGURE 10.20 ■ Rectocele. Worsening of the rectocele with Valsalva. (Photo contributor: Matthew Backer, Jr., MD.)

Clinical Summary

The hymen is a membrane visible at the introitus that separates the vestibule externally from the vagina internally. The opening of the hymen can take on a variety of shapes—annular, semi-lunar, cribriform, and septate. The congenital absence of a hymenal orifice is called an imperforate hymen (IH). This condition may become evident in infants or young children as a smooth, glistening, protruding membrane due to the buildup of vaginal secretions known as a mucocolpos. More commonly, an imperforate hymen presents in adolescent girls with primary amenorrhea and recurrent abdominal pain. The buildup of menstrual blood and secretions behind the hymen is called hematocolpos and may become large enough to cause urinary retention by pressing on the bladder neck.

Physical examination reveals a smooth, dome-shaped, bluish-red bulging membrane. A large, smooth, cystic mass can often be palpated anteriorly on digital rectal examination.

Occasionally, the buildup of blood may spill over through the fallopian tubes into the peritoneal cavity, resulting in signs of pelvic or abdominal peritonitis.

Emergency Department Treatment and Disposition

Imperforate hymen as well as other abnormalities of the vaginal outlet should be referred to a gynecologist for definitive treatment. This includes incision of the hymen to allow drainage of the hematocolpos. Those instances detected in preadolescence should ideally be referred to a practitioner who specializes in pediatric cases.

Pearl

1. An imperforate hymen presents in adolescent girls with primary amenorrhea and recurrent abdominal pain.

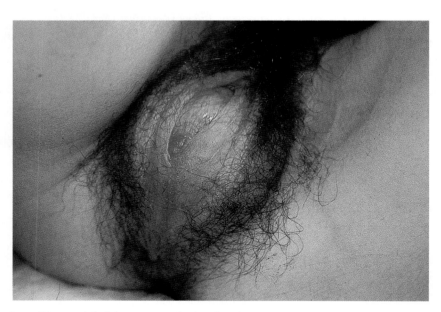

FIGURE 10.21 ■ Imperforate Hymen. A bulging mass at the introitus is seen in this patient with abdominal distention and amenorrhea. The imperforate hymen was diagnosed, with subsequent incision and drainage of the hematocolpos. (Photo contributor: Mark Eich, MD.)

Clinical Summary

Ectopic pregnancy is the leading cause of maternal obstetric morbidity in the first trimester of pregnancy. Presentations commonly include mild vaginal bleeding and lower abdominal pain, but patients can present in shock secondary to massive hemorrhage. The menstrual history, although often unreliable, may reveal a missed or recent abnormal menses. Pelvic examination may be normal or there may be frank cervical motion and adnexal tenderness.

The visualization of an intrauterine pregnancy (IUP) by ultrasound (US) essentially excludes the diagnosis of ectopic pregnancy, the exception being a rare dual pregnancy (IUP and ectopic). The appearance of a gestational sac at about 5 weeks is the first significant finding on US suggestive of an IUP; however, definitive diagnosis of IUP should be deferred until a yolk sac is present. A fetal pole develops next and can be seen on part of the yolk sac. The double decidual sac sign is evidence of a true gestational sac and should be differentiated from the pseudogestational sac formed from a decidual cast in ectopic pregnancy. When no gestational sac is visualized ("empty uterus"), ectopic pregnancy cannot be distinguished from an early IUP too small to be seen on US.

Differential diagnosis of ectopic pregnancy includes threatened or incomplete abortion, molar pregnancy, ruptured corpus luteum cyst, adnexal torsion, urinary tract infection, appendicitis, pelvic inflammatory disease, and ureteral calculi.

Emergency Department Treatment and Disposition

Unstable patients require aggressive resuscitation with fluid and blood followed by surgery. Stable patients with an ultrasound diagnosis consistent with ectopic pregnancy warrant immediate gynecologic consultation. Definitive therapeutic options range from observation in asymptomatic patients with declining hCG levels, traditional or laparoscopic surgery, to pharmacologic therapy with methotrexate. Despite the diminished diagnostic accuracy of ultrasound at lower levels (up to half of all ectopic pregnancies have a serum hCG level <2000 mIU/mL), if there is a strong clinical suspicion for ectopic pregnancy, gynecologic consultation should be considered. Those patients in whom a normal IUP is visualized can be safely discharged with early outpatient follow-up.

Pearls

1. Ectopic pregnancy should be considered in all women of reproductive age presenting with vaginal bleeding, abdominal pain or tenderness, or a missed menstrual period.

2. Failure to visualize an intrauterine pregnancy by transvaginal ultrasonography when the serum hCG level is **above** the discriminatory zone of the machine and examiner (typically between 1000 and 2000 mIU/mL) is highly suggestive of the diagnosis of ectopic pregnancy.

3. A decidual cast in the uterus of an ectopic pregnancy may resemble a gestational sac of an intrauterine pregnancy on ultrasound.

4. Consider ectopic pregnancy in any female of reproductive age presenting with syncope.

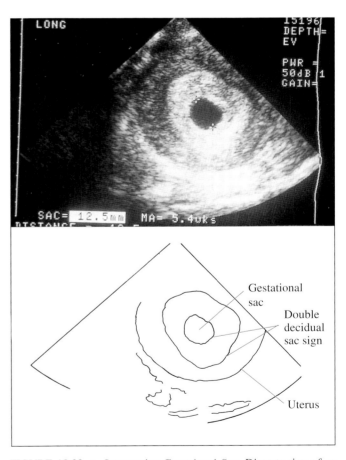

FIGURE 10.22 ■ Intrauterine Gestational Sac. Discrete ring of an intrauterine gestational sac seen on transvaginal ultrasound. No yolk sac is visualized. A double decidual sac sign is seen, however, lending evidence of a true gestational sac versus a pseudogestational sac formed from a decidual cast in ectopic pregnancy. A thorough look in the adnexa is important in diagnosing ectopic pregnancy when a gestational sac is the only finding. (Photo contributor: Janice Underwood.)

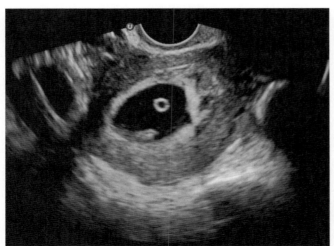

FIGURE 10.23 ■ Intrauterine Yolk Sac. Discrete ring of an intra-uterine yolk sac within the gestational sac seen on transvaginal ultra-sound. Definitive diagnosis of IUP should be deferred until a fetal pole is present in the sac. (Photo contributor: Geoffrey E. Hayden, MD.)

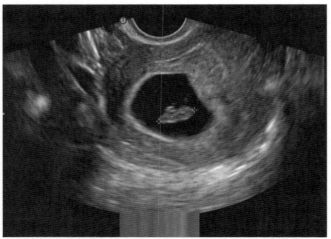

FIGURE 10.24 ■ Intrauterine Fetal Pole. Ultrasound image of an intrauterine pregnancy with a fetal pole consistent with a 7-week 4-day gestation. (Photo contributor: Geoffrey E. Hayden, MD.)

FIGURE 10.26 ■ Empty Uterus. Transvaginal ultrasound image of an apparently empty uterus. Ectopic pregnancy should be strongly suspected if a transvaginal ultrasound reveals an empty uterus in the setting of a serum quantitative hCG level above the institution's discriminatory zone. (Photo contributor: Janice Underwood.)

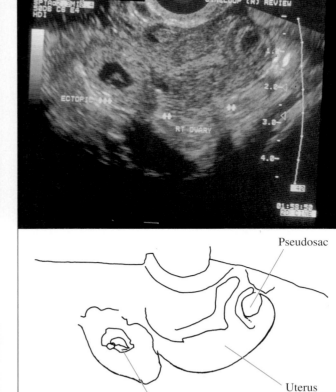

FIGURE 10.25 ■ Ectopic Pregnancy. Transvaginal ultrasound image of a right ectopic pregnancy with a decidual reaction in the uterus resembling a gestational sac, or "pseudosac." Visualization of a pseudo-gestational, or "single," sac sign could be consistent with an early gestational sac or an ectopic pregnancy with a uterine decidual cast. (Photo contributor: Janice Underwood.)

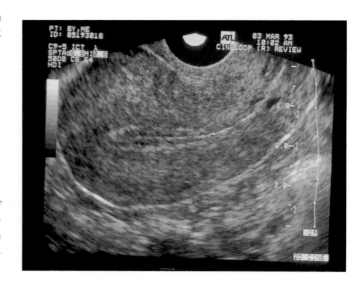

Clinical Summary

Molar pregnancy is part of a spectrum of gestational tro-phoblastic tumors that include benign hydatidiform moles, locally invasive moles, and choriocarcinoma. The classic clinical presentation is painless first- or early second-trimester vaginal bleeding with a uterine size larger than the estimated gestational age based on the last menstrual period. Signs of preeclampsia in the first trimester or early second trimester (hypertension, headache, proteinuria, and edema), are highly suggestive of this diagnosis. Hyperthyroidism can be found in roughly 5% of cases. Acute respiratory distress may occur owing to embolization of trophoblastic tissue into the pulmonary vasculature, thyrotoxicosis, or simply fluid overload.

Emergency Department Treatment and Disposition

Gynecologic consultation for dilatation and curettage should be obtained in all cases. Close outpatient monitoring of serum hCG levels is required to rule out the presence of malignant gestational trophoblastic disease.

Pearls

1. All patients with pregnancies of less than 20 weeks' gestation with clinical findings of preeclampsia should have gestational trophoblastic disease ruled out.
2. A "snowstorm" pattern on ultrasonography demonstrating multiple intrauterine echoes with no fetus coupled with a high hCG level is typical of molar pregnancy.
3. Moles commonly produce serum hCG levels greater than 100,000 mIU/mL.

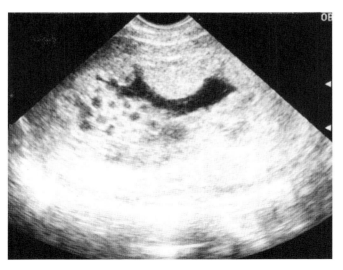

FIGURE 10.27 ■ Molar Pregnancy. "Snowstorm" pattern demonstrating multiple intrauterine echoes with no fetus is seen on transvaginal ultrasonography in a patient with a molar pregnancy. Serum β-hCG was greater than 180,000 mIU/mL. (Photo contributor: Robin Marshall, MD.)

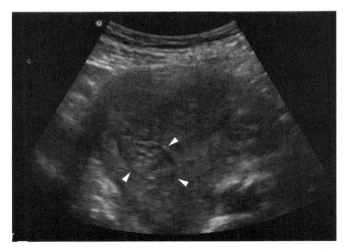

FIGURE 10.28 ■ Molar Pregnancy. Transabdominal study showing molar pregnancy. These are exceedingly difficult to identify and diagnose by ultrasound. They can be easily mistaken for non-specific intrauterine findings (eg, missed abortion, fibroid, etc). (Photo contributor: Geoffrey E. Hayden, MD.)

Clinical Summary

Trauma is a major cause of maternal and fetal mortality. In addition to the common injuries to a solid organ and/or hollow viscus associated with blunt abdominal trauma, special consideration should be given to the possibility of preterm labor, fetal-maternal hemorrhage, uterine rupture, and, most importantly, abruptio placentae. Abruptio placentae is defined as the premature separation of the placenta from the site of uterine implantation. It is found in up to 50% of major blunt trauma patients and up to 5% of those with apparent minor injuries. There are generally signs of uterine hyperactivity and fetal distress when significant placental detachment occurs. Most patients have vaginal bleeding, but the margins of detachment are above the cervical os in up to 20%, thus they have little or no bleeding. Laboratory evidence of a consumptive coagulopathy may be seen with significant abruption. Electronic fetal monitoring is indicated in all cases of significant trauma in patients beyond 20 weeks' gestation. As the pregnancy progresses toward term, a normal heart rate averages between 120 and 160 bpm. Rapid, frequent fluctuations in the baseline are characteristic of normal "reactivity." The loss of this reactivity can occur during a normal sleep cycle, following narcotic administration, or, most importantly, in the setting of fetal hypoxia or distress. Decelerations are transient reductions in the fetal heart rate. *Late decelerations* begin after the contraction begins and return to baseline well after it ends, with the nadir of the deceleration occurring after the peak of the uterine contraction. Late decelerations suggest fetal hypoxia, especially when they are accompanied by a loss of normal baseline beat-to-beat variability. *Variable decelerations* are characterized by deep, broad decreases in fetal heart rate, often falling below 100 bpm. They can occur slightly before, during, or after the onset of a uterine contraction. Variable decelerations are caused by the transient compression of the umbilical cord during a contraction and are rarely associated with significant hypoxia or acidosis unless they are frequent or prolonged. They are most commonly appreciated during the second stage of labor, when forceful uterine compression transiently occludes the umbilical cord as the infant is propelled through the birth canal.

Emergency Department Treatment and Disposition

An obstetrician should be consulted immediately in all trauma patients beyond 20 weeks' gestation. Blood for type- and cross-matching, complete blood count, prothrombin time (PT), partial thromboplastin time (PTT), fibrinogen, and fibrin degradation products or D-dimer should be obtained. It is generally recommended that patients undergo continuous toco fetal monitoring for a minimum of 4 hours to rule out preterm labor or fetal distress. Ultrasound is essential in visualizing placental abruption and differentiates this from placenta previa. Indications for emergency cesarean section include placental abruption, signs of ongoing fetal distress, or uncontrolled maternal hemorrhage.

Pearls

1. Ecchymotic markings imparted by a significant blunt force are not always present on a gravid abdomen; thus, a careful history of the mechanism of trauma and associated complaints is essential.
2. Anti-Rh immunoglobulin should be administered for all cases of significant third-trimester blunt abdominal trauma if the mother is Rh-negative and the father is Rh-positive.

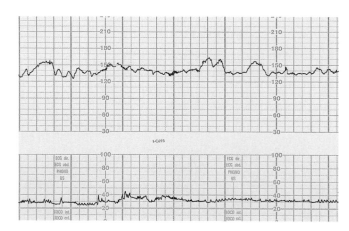

FIGURE 10.29 ■ Normal Beat-to-Beat Variability (BBV). A normal reactive fetal monitor strip showing a baseline heart rate between 120 and 160 with fluctuations in the short- and long-term heart rate. (Photo contributor: Timothy Jahn, MD.)

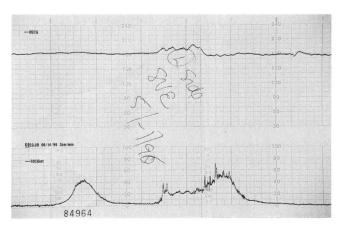

FIGURE 10.30 ■ Loss of BBV. Loss of beat-to-beat variability (BBV) in the fetal heart rate, which may forewarn of fetal distress. This same pattern may also be seen during a normal sleep cycle or following maternal narcotic administration. (Photo contributor: Gerard Van Houdt, MD.)

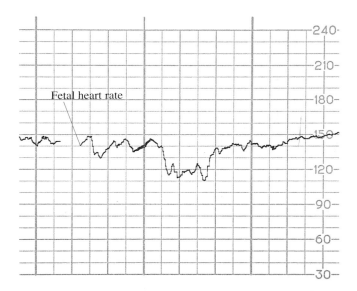

FIGURE 10.31 ■ Late Deceleration. The nadir of a late deceleration always follows the peak of the uterine contraction with the heart rate approaching the baseline after the completion of the uterine contraction; this is suggestive of hypoxia. (Photo contributor: James Palombaro, MD.)

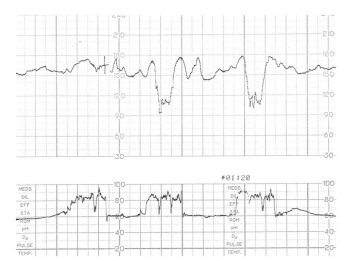

FIGURE 10.32 ■ Variable Deceleration. Variable decelerations are due to cord compression. They are characterized by a rapid onset and recovery and may occur slightly before, during, or after the onset of the contraction. (Photo contributor: John O'Boyle, MD.)

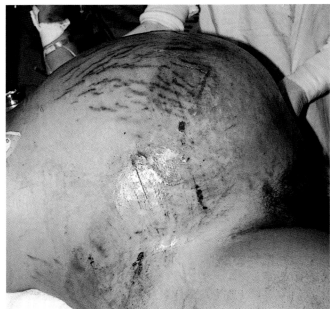

FIGURE 10.33 ■ Gravid Abdomen. A third-trimester gravid abdomen with ecchymotic markings imparted by a significant blunt force. Fetal assessment should occur simultaneously with maternal resuscitation. (Photo contributor: John Fildes, MD.)

Clinical Summary

The second stage of labor begins when the cervix is fully dilated, allowing for the gradual descent of the head toward the vaginal outlet. As the head approaches the perineum, the labia begin to separate with each contraction and then recede once the contraction subsides. *Crowning* is the term applied when the head separates the labial margins without receding at the end of the contraction.

Emergency Department Treatment and Disposition

The appearance of crowning heralds imminent vaginal delivery. Equipment for delivery and neonatal resuscitation should be brought to the bedside. Both the on-call obstetric consultant and pediatrician should be notified while preparations are being made for emergency department delivery.

Pearls

1. Primigravida patients may still require multiple sets of contractions and pushing to fully expel the head through the vaginal outlet.
2. If meconium secretions are detected well before delivery, continuous electronic toco fetal monitoring should be begun and the obstetric and pediatric consultants notified.

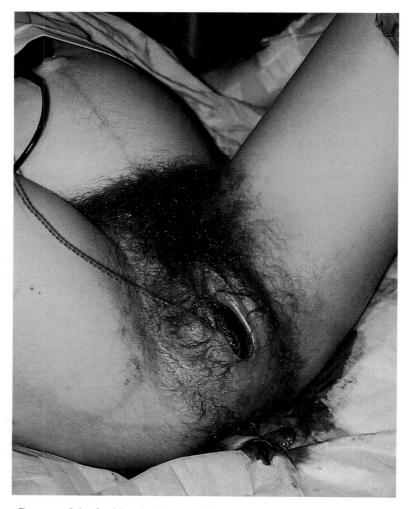

FIGURE 10.34 ■ Crowning. Descent of the fetal head with separation of the labia is known as crowning and heralds imminent vertex delivery. (Photo contributor: William Leninger, MD.)

Clinical Summary

A gravid female with regular forceful contractions and the urge to strain (push) can present without warning. Crowning may be present and heralds imminent vaginal delivery. Important historical questions include the number of previous pregnancies, a diagnosis of twin gestations, and whether there is a history of prenatal care or complications. The presence of greenish brown fetal stool, known as meconium, is associated with fetal hypoxia and is a clinical indicator of fetal distress. Fetal bradycardia or late decelerations (Fig. 10.31) may be present and are also evidence of fetal distress.

Emergency Department Treatment and Disposition

Intravenous access, oxygen, and equipment for delivery and neonatal resuscitation (suction, oxygen, warming light, etc) are immediately obtained as preparation for the impending delivery.

Delivery of the Head

As the vertex passes through the vaginal outlet, extension of the head occurs, followed by the appearance of the forehead and chin. Extension and delivery of the fetal head can be facilitated by applying gentle pressure upward on the chin through the perineum—known as the modified Ritgen maneuver. Simultaneously, the fingers of the other hand can be used to elevate the scalp to help extend the head. Once the head has been delivered, the occiput promptly rotates toward a left or right lateral position. At this stage, the nuchal region should be swept to detect the presence of a nuchal umbilical cord (Fig. 10.48). Before the delivery of the shoulders, the nasopharynx should be gently suctioned with a bulb syringe to clear away any blood or amniotic debris. If thick meconium is present, deeper and more thorough suctioning of the posterior pharynx and glottic region should be accomplished with a mechanical suction trap as aspiration of thick meconium can lead to pneumonitis and hypoxia.

Delivery of the Shoulders

Delivery of the shoulders generally occurs spontaneously with little manipulation. Occasionally, gentle downward traction applied by grasping the sides of the head with two hands eases the delivery of the anterior shoulder. The head can then be directed upward to permit the delivery of the posterior shoulder. Following delivery of both shoulders, the body and legs are easily delivered. Attention is then directed toward the immediate care of the newborn. The cord is doubly clamped and ligated and inspected for three vessels: two umbilical arteries and one umbilical vein. The pediatrician should be notified of a two-vessel umbilical cord. The newborn is immediately placed under a warming lamp for drying and gentle stimulation while being observed for signs of distress (heart rate <100, limp muscle tone, poor color, and weak cry).

Delivery of the Placenta

Following delivery, gentle traction can be placed on the cord while the opposite hand is used to massage the uterine fundus. The placenta is generally delivered within 20 minutes and should be grossly inspected for evidence of a missing segment or cotyledon. The obstetrician should be notified as retained placental fragments often warrant manual exploration of the uterus, especially in the context of persistent postpartum bleeding. Unusual placental vasculature, such as a velamentous placenta, should be communicated to obstetrician and pediatric consultants.

Pearls

1. Both obstetric and pediatric consultants should be alerted of a possible emergency department delivery.
2. A two-vessel cord (found in about 1 in 500 singleton deliveries) is associated with an increased incidence of congenital defects.
3. Retained placental fragments may be a cause of postpartum hemorrhage or endometritis.

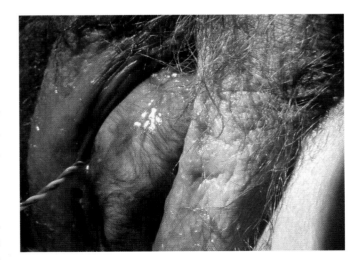

FIGURE 10.35 ■ Meconium. Meconium (greenish brown fetal stool), seen covering the scalp and perineum, is associated with fetal hypoxia and is a clinical indicator of fetal distress. Fetal bradycardia or late decelerations may be present and are also evidence of fetal distress. (Photo contributor: William Leninger, MD.)

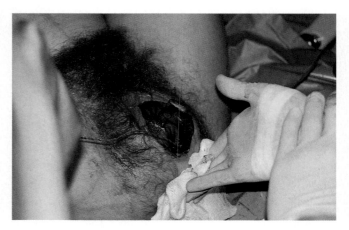

FIGURE 10.36 ■ Modified Ritgen Maneuver. Modified Ritgen maneuver: upward pressure is applied on the fetal chin through the perineum. (Photo contributor: William Leninger, MD.)

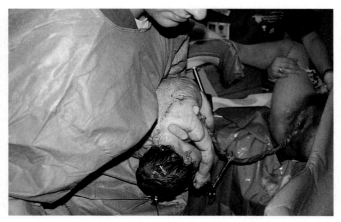

FIGURE 10.39 ■ Clamping the Cord. The cord is clamped immediately after delivery. (Photo contributor: William Leninger, MD.)

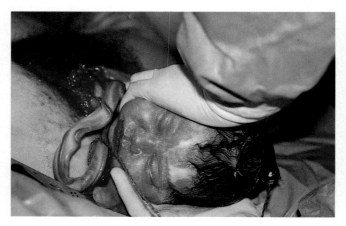

FIGURE 10.37 ■ Anterior Shoulder Delivery. Delivery of the anterior shoulder is facilitated with downward traction. (Photo contributor: William Leninger, MD.)

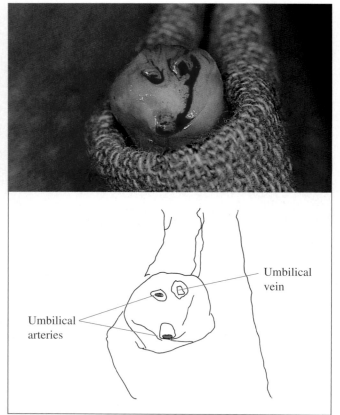

FIGURE 10.40 ■ Normal Umbilical Cord. Cross-sectional view of the two arteries and single vein of a normal three-vessel umbilical cord. (Photo contributor: Jennifer Jagoe, MD.)

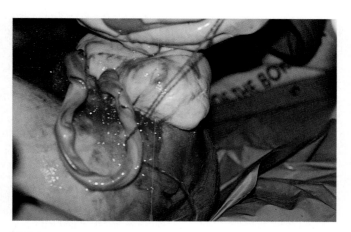

FIGURE 10.38 ■ Posterior Shoulder Delivery. Delivery of the posterior shoulder with upward traction. (Photo contributor: William Leninger, MD.)

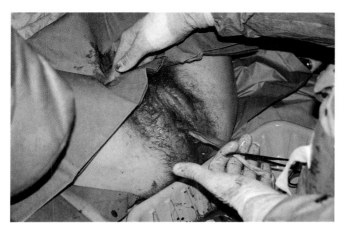

FIGURE 10.41 ■ Placenta Delivery. Gentle traction is applied to the cord while the opposite hand massages the uterus. (Photo contributor: William Leninger, MD.)

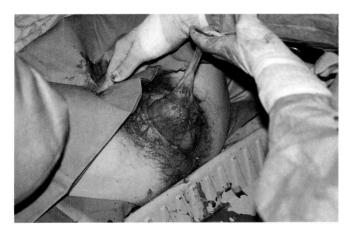

FIGURE 10.42 ■ Placenta Delivery. Delivery of the placenta. (Photo contributor: William Leninger, MD.)

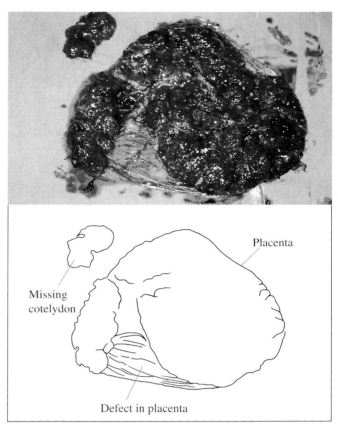

FIGURE 10.43 ■ Placenta. Placenta with a missing segment or cotyledon. The missing placental tissue can be seen in the upper left-hand corner of the photograph. (Photo contributor: John O'Boyle, MD.)

Clinical Summary

The incidence of singleton breech presentation is approximately 3% but rises to higher than 20% in preterm infants weighing less than 2000 g. In a frank breech, both hips are flexed and both knees extended. In a complete breech, both hips and knees are flexed, whereas a footling breech has one or both legs extended below the buttocks. Frank breech is most common in full-term deliveries, whereas footling presentation can be found in up to half of all preterm deliveries. Breech deliveries carry a much higher mortality rate than cephalic deliveries. Complications of breech delivery include umbilical cord prolapse, nuchal arm obstruction, and difficulty in delivery of the head.

Emergency Department Treatment and Disposition

The specific maneuvers for breech extraction are beyond the scope of this text. If breech delivery appears imminent, support and gentle traction should be applied as the various parts spontaneously pass through the vaginal outlet, keeping in mind that the biparietal diameter is greater than either the bitrochanteric or bisacromial diameter.

Pearl

1. Immediate obstetric consultation should be obtained in all breech deliveries.

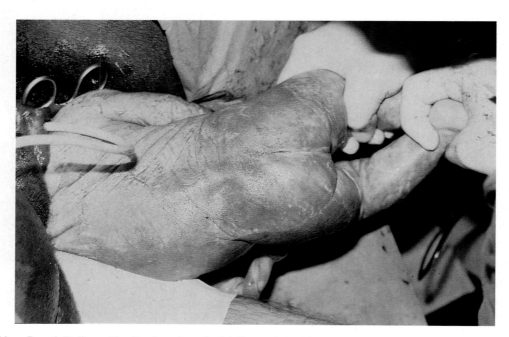

FIGURE 10.44 ■ Breech Delivery. Footling breech vaginal delivery of the following head. (Photo contributor: John O'Boyle, MD.)

Clinical Summary

In an overt cord prolapse, a loop of umbilical cord is visualized either at the introitus or on speculum examination following membrane rupture. Alternatively, a small loop of cord may be palpated at the cervical os. In a funic cord prolapse, a loop of umbilical cord is palpated directly through intact fetal membranes. Occult prolapse occurs when the umbilical cord descends between the presenting part and the lower uterine segment, but is not visible or directly palpable on examination. Intermittent compression of the umbilical cord with each uterine contraction may be detected by the presence of variable decelerations of the fetal monitor. The new onset of variable decelerations should always prompt immediate cervical examination to rule out an overt cord prolapse. Severe persistent bradycardia may ensue if cord compression is sustained beyond the duration of the contraction, which is often the case in an overt prolapse.

Emergency Department Treatment and Disposition

Prolapse of the umbilical cord presents an immediate threat to the fetal circulation and constitutes a true obstetrical emergency. If an overt prolapse is detected in the emergency department, the patient should immediately be placed in a knee-chest position and continuous upward pressure applied by the examining hand to relieve the pressure of the presenting part on the lower uterine segment. An obstetrician should be summoned immediately and the patient taken directly to the operating room for cesarean delivery. Continuous upward pressure should be applied to the presenting part of the fetus at all times during transport. Occasionally, precipitous vaginal delivery may ensue in the emergency department shortly after a cord prolapse is detected. Resuscitative equipment should be available in anticipation of a physiologically compromised infant. If a funic prolapse is appreciated in the emergency department, an obstetrician should be notified and the patient prepared for cesarean delivery. Under no circumstance should the membranes be broken. Occult prolapse is rarely appreciated in the emergency department.

Pearl

1. Pelvic examination to exclude umbilical cord prolapse should be performed immediately following rupture of membranes, the appearance of variable decelerations, or the detection of bradycardia.

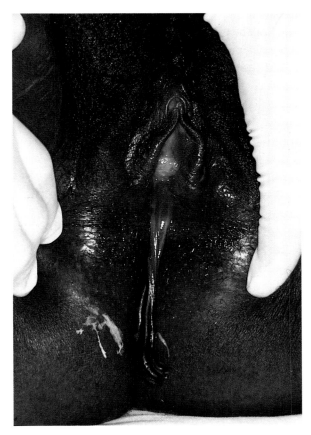

FIGURE 10.45 ■ Umbilical Cord Prolapse. Prolapsed umbilical cord visible at the vaginal introitus in a patient with twin gestations. (Photo contributor: Kevin J. Knoop, MD, MS.)

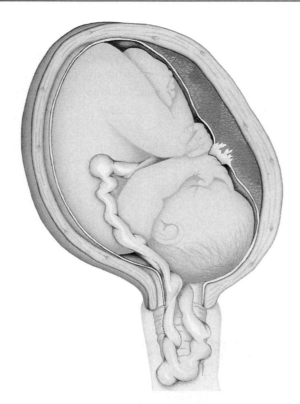

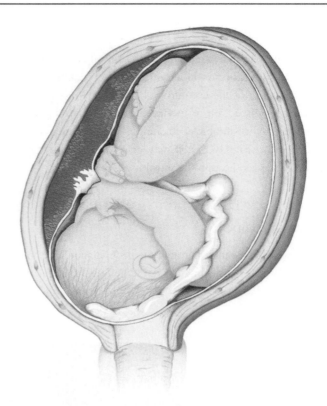

FIGURE 10.46 ■ Umbilical Cord Prolapse. Schematic drawing of an overt prolapse of the umbilical cord through a partially dilated cervical os. (Photo contributor: Judy Christensen.)

FIGURE 10.47 ■ Funic Cord Prolapse. Schematic drawing of a funic prolapse of the umbilical cord with intact membranes. (Photo contributor: Judy Christensen.)

Clinical Summary

The circumferential wrapping of the umbilical cord around the child's neck occurs in about 20% of all deliveries. Tight approximation of the cord around the infant's neck can lead to transient disruption of uterine blood flow during contractions, leading to variable decelerations noted on the fetal heart rate monitor (Fig. 10.32); it may also impede delivery once the head passes through the introitus.

Emergency Department Treatment and Disposition

Once a cord is identified around the neck, it should be slipped over the head using the index and middle fingers. Occasionally two coils are identified.

Pearl

1. A loosely applied cord should be pulled over the child's head. If the cord is wrapped too tightly, it can be clamped and ligated on the perineum, followed by the immediate delivery of the shoulders and body.

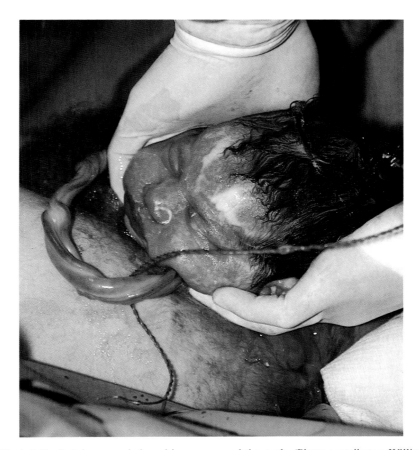

FIGURE 10.48 ■ Nuchal Cord. A loose nuchal cord is seen around the neck. (Photo contributor: William Leninger, MD.)

Clinical Summary

Shoulder dystocia is defined as failure to deliver the shoulders, following delivery of the head, because of impaction of the fetal shoulders against the pelvic outlet. Risk factors include gestational diabetes, prior delivery of large infants, and post-term delivery.

Emergency Department Treatment and Disposition

Shoulder dystocia is an acute obstetric emergency, with the immediate life threat being asphyxia from prolonged delivery. An obstetrician should be summoned immediately. Equipment for neonatal resuscitation should be set up and, ideally, a pediatric consultant should be summoned. In the absence of an obstetric consultant, a wide episiotomy should be performed. The least invasive maneuver is to forcefully flex the mother's knees toward her chest (McRoberts maneuver). This extreme dorsal lithotomy position occasionally allows for the appropriate engagement of the fetal shoulders. If this is unsuccessful, a Wood maneuver can be attempted by hooking two fingers behind the infant's posterior scapula and rotating the entire body in a screwlike manner. As the posterior shoulder rotates upward, it can generally be delivered past the symphysis pubis. If the Wood's maneuver fails to deliver the anterior shoulder, delivery of the posterior arm may be attempted by inserting two fingers into the sacral fossa and bringing down the entire posterior arm by flexing it at the elbow. The remaining anterior shoulder should then deliver, either spontaneously or else following rotation into the oblique position to facilitate its delivery.

Pearls

1. Shoulder dystocia is an acute obstetric emergency that requires quick action:
   Call for help.
   Cut a wide episiotomy.
   Perform McRoberts maneuver.
   Rotate the posterior shoulder.
2. After delivery, look for fracture of the clavicles or humerus and possible brachial plexus injury.

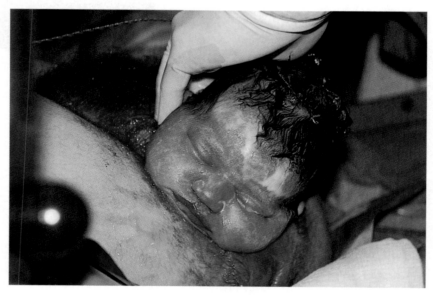

FIGURE 10.49. ■ Shoulder Dystocia. Firm approximation of the fetal head against the vaginal outlet consistent with shoulder dystocia. (Photo contributor: William Leninger, MD.)

Clinical Summary

Lacerations to the perineum occur commonly following a rapid, uncontrolled expulsion of the fetal head. Postpartum perineal lacerations range from minor to severe. Perineal lacerations due to birth trauma are categorized into four groups. First-degree lacerations are limited to the mucosa, skin, and superficial subcutaneous and submucosal tissues. Second-degree lacerations penetrate deeper into the superficial fascia and transverse perineal musculature. In addition to these structures, a third-degree laceration disrupts the anal sphincter, whereas a fourth-degree laceration extends into the rectal lumen.

Emergency Department Treatment and Disposition

In precipitous emergency department deliveries, the repair of the episiotomy and/or perineal lacerations can often be performed by the obstetric consultant, the details of repair being beyond the scope of this book.

Pearl

1. Perineal laceration repair fundamentally involves the sequential anatomic reapproximation, using absorbable suture material, of the rectal mucosa, anal sphincter, transverse perineal musculature, vaginal mucosa, and skin.

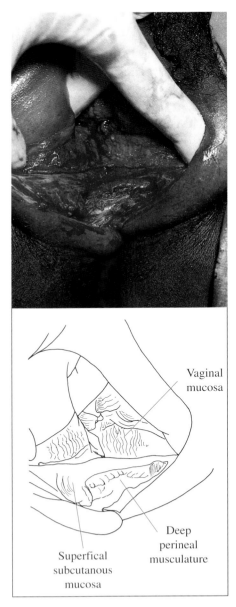

FIGURE 10.51 ■ Second-Degree Laceration. There is disruption of the hymenal ring and the deep perineal musculature, extending into the vaginal mucosa and transversalis fascia, but no involvement of the anal sphincter or mucosa. (Photo contributor: Pamela Ambroz, MD.)

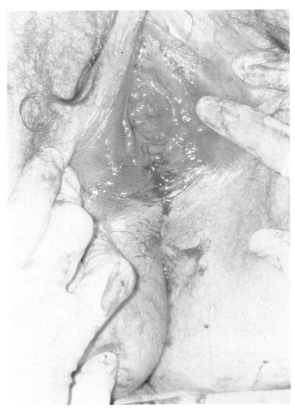

FIGURE 10.50 ■ First-Degree Laceration. First-degree laceration limited to the mucosa, skin, and superficial subcutaneous and submucosal tissues. There is no involvement of the underlying fascia and muscle. (Photo contributor: Jerry Van Houdt, MD.)

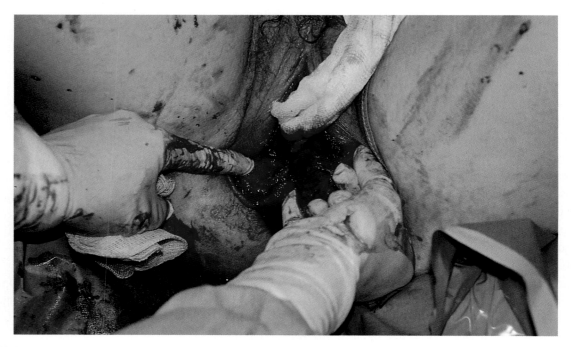

FIGURE 10.52 ■ Fourth-Degree Laceration. Fourth-degree perineal laceration revealing wide separation of the perineal fascia and anal sphincter. The examiner's small finger is in the rectal lumen, showing extension of the tear proximally. (Photo contributor: Timothy Jahn, MD.)

Clinical Summary

The timing of intrauterine fetal demise (IUFD) is important for the emergency department physician to appreciate for both consoling and advising the parents, as well as to know the likelihood of successful resuscitation after delivery. This tragic event may occur immediately before or during the birthing or in the prior weeks before delivery. The appearance of the fetus at delivery can be used to estimate that antepartum fetal demise has occurred and that resuscitative efforts are fruitless.

The process of tissue degeneration (maceration) is due to the effects of autolytic enzymes on the fetus in a sterile environment. Lysis occurs at the epidermal-dermal junction with subtle changes in the gross appearance of the fetus (skin desquamation, positive Nikolsky sign) seen as early as 6 hours. Further changes involve desquamation and bullae formation of the face, back, or abdomen by 12 hours, at least 5% of the body surface at 18 hours, and generalized skin desquamation at 24 hours. Sloughing of skin from a large area indicates a prolonged interval between death and delivery. Mummification occurs after approximately 2 weeks.

Emergency Department Treatment and Disposition

Anticipation of and preparation for a normal delivery should be made unless information of the condition of the fetus is known. Obstetric consultation should be made immediately as for any emergency delivery. If signs of maceration are present, no resuscitative efforts are indicated.

Pearl

1. Desquamation and/or sloughing of skin from large or numerous areas in an *unresponsive* fetus indicate antepartum IUFD.

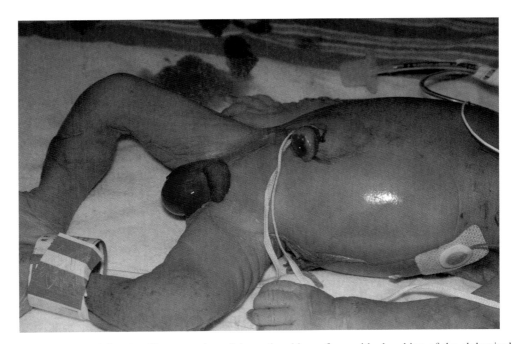

FIGURE 10.53 ■ Intrauterine Fetal Demise. Desquamation of the entire skin surface, with sloughing of the abdominal and scrotal skin, is seen in this IUFD. (Photo contributor: Lawrence B. Stack, MD).

Chapter 11

EXTREMITY TRAUMA

Neha P. Raukar
George J. Raukar
Daniel L. Savitt

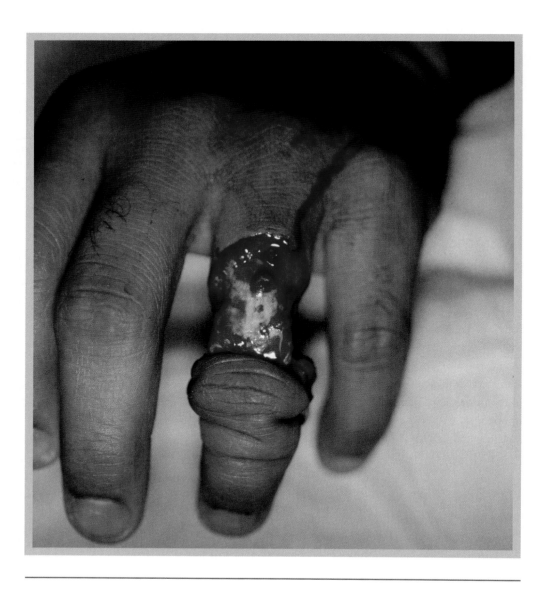

Clinical Summary

Injury to the acromioclavicular (AC) joint is a common finding in the emergency department, usually resulting directly from an impact on the superior aspect of the acromion. The classification system for AC joint includes six types. A type I injury is equivalent to a stretching of the acromioclavicular ligament. A type II injury consists of tearing of the AC ligaments and stretching of the coracoclavicular ligaments. Complete disruption of the AC and coracoclavicular ligaments is seen in types III to VI.

Patients complain of pain at the AC joint and will actively splint the injured shoulder. Ecchymosis may be present; however, an obvious deformity is not always seen. There is significant tenderness upon palpation of the AC joint.

Standard radiographs should include anteroposterior (AP) and axillary lateral views of the shoulder. Type I injuries will appear normal. Type II injuries may show 0% to 50% displacement at the AC joint but no increase in the coracoclavicular interval. Types III to VI will demonstrate displacement at the AC joint and the clavicle will appear to be displaced superiorly (the acromion actually is rotated inferiorly) 50% to greater than 100% its width when compared with the normal side.

Emergency Department Treatment and Disposition

Type I and type II injuries are treated with rest, ice, analgesics, and a simple sling until acute pain with movement is relieved. Treatment of type III injuries is controversial with the literature supporting both nonoperative and operative management. Types IV, V, and VI are treated operatively. Referral to a musculoskeletal specialist is essential for all AC joint injuries since many patients who initially appear to have minor injuries will have more obvious deformity after the swelling and pain have subsided.

Pearls

1. The early AC joint stress radiograph can be negative due to splinting of the shoulder girdle muscles.
2. Differentiating between types I and II versus types III to VI is the goal of the ED physician since the treatment is significantly different.

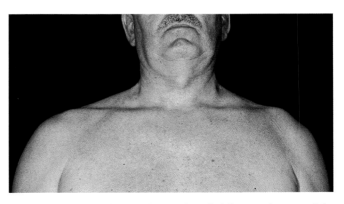

FIGURE 11.1 ■ AC Joint Separation. Subtle prominence of the left distal clavicle. The upward displacement of the clavicle is due to stretching or disruption of the suspending ligaments. (Photo contributor: Frank Birinyi, MD.)

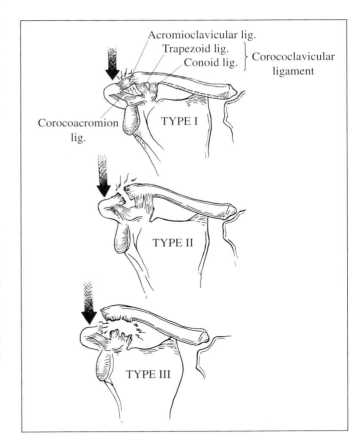

FIGURE 11.2 ■ Acromioclavicular Joint Injuries. Types of acromioclavicular joint injuries. Classification schemes may subdivide type III injuries into III through VI depending on the position of the clavicle.

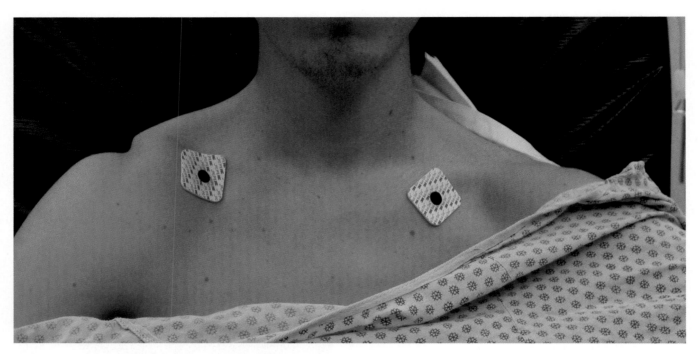

FIGURE 11.3 ▪ AC Joint Separation. Large deformity at the right distal clavicle suggesting complete ligament disruption. (Photo contributor: R. Jason Thurman, MD.)

Clinical Summary

Anterior shoulder dislocations are the most common dislocations seen in the emergency department. They are most frequently caused by falling with the arm externally rotated and abducted. Acutely, patients present with the affected extremity held in adduction and internal rotation. Often, the patient complains of shoulder pain, refuses to move the affected arm, and may support the dislocated shoulder with the other arm. The acromion becomes prominent and there is a loss of the rounded contour of the deltoid. A neurovascular examination of the upper extremity should be performed to rule out associated injury, most commonly of the axillary nerve (sensation over the deltoid), and of the musculocutaneous nerve (sensation on the anterolateral forearm). Standard radiographic examination to evaluate for associated fracture should include anteroposterior (AP) and either axillary lateral or scapular Y views.

Posterior shoulder dislocations are commonly missed because of subtle radiographic findings. The arm is held internally rotated and slightly abducted. Patients are unable to externally rotate their shoulder. On examination, a posterior prominence exists. Posterior dislocations can occur with a posterior directed force. They can also occur during grand mal seizures or electric shock.

The Hill-Sachs lesion (an impaction of the humeral head) can occur in up to 50% of patients. Neuropraxic injury of the axillary nerve (more common) or the musculocutaneous nerve can significantly delay recovery. Vascular injuries have rarely been reported to occur.

Emergency Department Treatment and Disposition

Closed reduction is the treatment of choice and should be completed as soon as possible to avoid avascular necrosis to the humeral head. Due to spasm of the shoulder girdle, conscious sedation is often required. There are many methods to reduce shoulder dislocations, including Stimson, Rockwood traction and countertraction, and Milch. Neurovascular and radiographic examination should occur before and after reduction. The patient should be placed in a sling after reduction and follow up with a musculoskeletal specialist should be recommended.

Pearls

1. An occult nondisplaced greater tuberosity fracture can easily occur with attempts at shoulder relocation. It is helpful to discuss this potential complication prior to attempts at shoulder reduction.

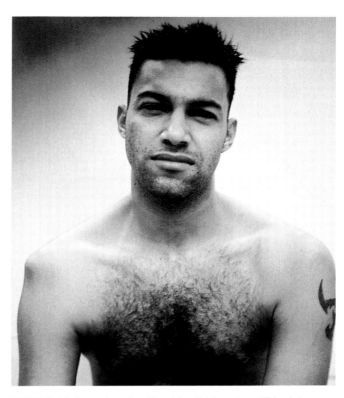

FIGURE 11.4 ■ Anterior Shoulder Dislocation. This right anterior shoulder dislocation occurred when the patient fell while playing basketball. There is an obvious contour deformity as well as prominence of the acromion. (Photo contributor: Kevin J. Knoop, MD, MS.)

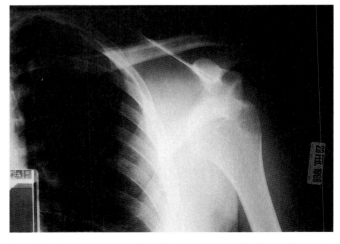

FIGURE 11.5 ■ Anterior Shoulder Dislocation. Radiographic evaluation demonstrates that the humeral head is not in the glenoid fossa but is located anterior and inferior to it. (Photo contributor: Kevin J. Knoop, MD, MS.)

2. Relaxation of the pectoral musculature is an excellent aid in shoulder reduction. This can be accomplished by manual massage of the muscle. Some patients can relax this muscle voluntarily when asked to do so (eg, weightlifters).

3. Luxatio erecta is inferior glenohumeral dislocation that is rarely encountered. The humeral head is forced below the inferior aspect of the glenoid fossa due to a hyperabduction of the arm. These patients present with the arm locked fully abducted and externally rotated. Axillary nerve injury is reported to occur up to 60% of the time. Vascular injury occurs most frequently with this type of dislocation. Reduction is accomplished with overhead traction.

4. Posterior shoulder dislocations can be bilateral and are often missed due to preserved symmetry on standard chest x-rays.

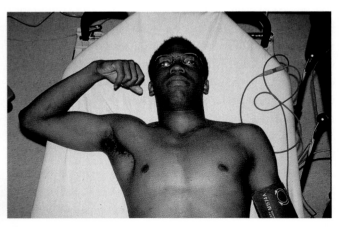

FIGURE 11.8 ■ Luxatio Erecta. Hyperabduction may cause the relatively rare inferior dislocation known as luxatio erecta. The patient presents with the arm held in elevation and the humeral head may be palpated along the lateral chest wall. (Photo contributor: Kevin J. Knoop, MD, MS.)

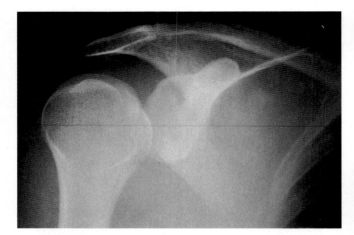

FIGURE 11.6 ■ Posterior Shoulder Dislocation. AP radiograph of this rare type of shoulder dislocation. Because of internal rotation of the greater tuberosity, the humeral head appears like a dip of ice cream on a cone, thus called the "ice cream cone sign." (Photo contributor: Alan B. Storrow, MD.)

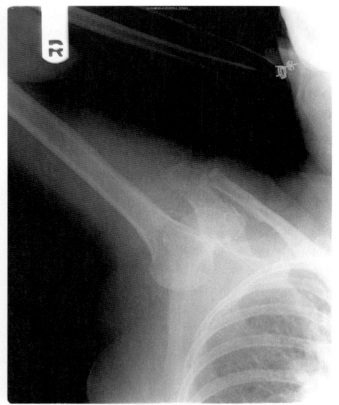

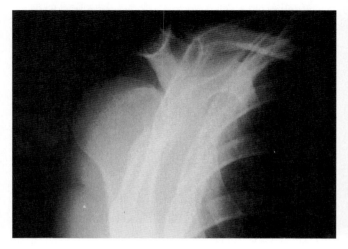

FIGURE 11.7 ■ Posterior Shoulder Dislocation. A scapular Y view of the same patient in Fig. 11.6 confirms the diagnosis. (Photo contributor: Alan B. Storrow, MD.)

FIGURE 11.9 ■ Luxatio Erecta. This radiograph demonstrates an inferior dislocation of the humeral head with the arm above consistent with luxatio erecta. (Photo contributor: Benjamin Milligan, MD.)

Clinical Summary

Direct trauma or fall on an outstretched hand may result in elbow fractures. The patient may be unable to extend the elbow and may have pain on supination/pronation. Anteroposterior (AP), lateral, and oblique views of the elbow should visualize most elbow fractures. The radial head should be aligned with the capitellum on all views. The anterior fat pad may be seen on normal radiographs but displacement anteriorly and superiorly (sail sign) suggests effusion or hemarthrosis. The posterior fat pad is not normally visualized and, if seen, is indicative of effusion or hemarthrosis and is associated with a radial head fracture in adults 76% of the time.

Supracondylar fractures often occur in pediatric patients. Neurovascular insult occurs in 7% of supracondylar fractures, with the anterior interosseous nerve most commonly injured. This can be checked by having the patient make an "ok" sign. This neuropraxia usually resolves in 6 months. Arterial injury to the brachial artery occurs approximately 5% of the time and arteriography is indicated if the radial pulse is decreased either before or after reduction.

Capitellum fractures represent less than 1% of adult elbow fractures and are difficult to diagnose radiographically; a CT scan my be required. This fracture is commonly associated with fractures of the radial head.

Emergency Department Treatment and Disposition

Treatment of supracondylar fractures is influenced by stability of the fracture pattern as well as associated neurovascular injuries. If neurovascular compromise exists, the emergency physician may need to apply forearm traction to reestablish distal pulses. If the pulse is not restored with traction, emergent operative intervention for brachial artery exploration or fasciotomy is indicated. In children, nondisplaced fractures can be splinted in 90 degrees of flexion. Angulated or displaced fractures often require operative intervention.

Fractures of the capitellum are treated with immobilization in a posterior long arm splint with the elbow in 90 degrees of flexion and the forearm in supination. Complications of displaced capitellum fractures include arthritis, avascular necrosis, and decreased range of motion.

Radial head fractures can be treated with a sling for comfort and patients should be told to discontinue the sling as early as possible. Fractures that are greater than 2 mm displaced, those

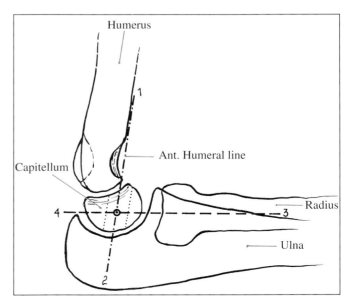

FIGURE 11.10 ■ Radiographic Elbow Relationships. In lateral views, the anterior humeral line (1-2) should bisect the middle third of the capitellum. The radiocapitellar line (drawn through the center of the radius, 3-4) should also pass through the center of the capitellum. Disruption of these relationships may indicate fracture.

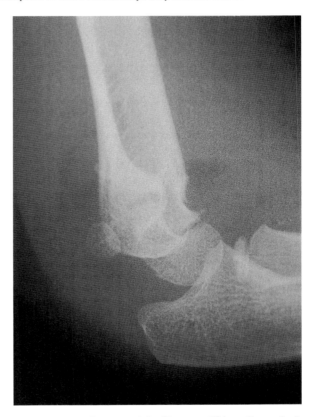

FIGURE 11.11 ■ Supracondylar Fracture. This radiograph shows both a pronounced anterior fat pad (sail sign) and posterior fat pad indicative of a supracondylar fracture. (Photo contributor: Alan B. Storrow, MD.)

that have greater than 20% of articular depression, or open fractures may need operative treatment and should follow up within a week with an orthopaedic surgeon.

Pearls

1. An intimal arterial injury may not be initially apparent and frequent radial artery checks are warranted in the pediatric population. Some practitioners opt to admit supracondylar fractures so these neurovascular checks can be done.
2. Capitellum and radial head fractures often occur together.
3. The presence of a joint effusion with a history of trauma is presumptive evidence of a fracture.

Clinical Summary

Elbow dislocations are the second most common major joint dislocation and usually occur posteriorly, although they can be anterior, medial, or lateral. All dislocations require immediate reduction to relieve pain and prevent neurovascular compromise, which occurs more commonly with open dislocations. Brachial artery function and ulnar, median, and radial nerve integrity must be evaluated when examining any patient with a suspected dislocation. Elbow dislocations are often associated with a radial head fracture. Patients with posterior dislocation present with their elbow held in flexion and examination reveals a swollen, tender, and deformed elbow with a prominent olecranon. Anterior dislocations, though rare, present with the elbow extended with the forearm supinated and elongated. The arm appears shortened.

Radiographic evaluation should include an anteroposterior (AP) and a lateral. The presence of fractures should be noted, as this may complicate reduction.

Emergency Department Treatment and Disposition

Most patients require conscious sedation prior to reduction. Posterior dislocations are accomplished by applying posterior pressure to the humerus while an assistant applies longitudinal traction to the forearm. Alternatively, the patient with a posterior dislocation is placed in the prone position so the humerus hangs perpendicular to the stretcher. A 5- to 10-lb weight is applied to the wrist or axial traction is applied to the wrist while the elbow at the humerus is stabilized. After a few minutes, the olecranon slips back into place. Neurologic and radiographic reexamination should occur after any attempt at reduction. It is possible to entrap the nerve while attempting reduction so neurovascular integrity must be checked before and after reduction. If this occurs, an orthopaedic surgeon should be consulted immediately. After reduction, the elbow should be immobilized in 90 degrees of flexion in a posterior splint and sling. Elbow dislocations with associated fractures may make closed reduction difficult and also leave the joint unstable. In these cases, consultation with an orthopedic surgeon is recommended prior to reduction attempts.

Pearls

1. The ulnar nerve is the most common nerve injured.
2. The olecranon should form a straight line with the two epicondyles when the elbow is extended. At 90 degrees of flexion, the olecranon and the two epicondyles should form a triangle. This relationship is disrupted in the dislocated elbow.

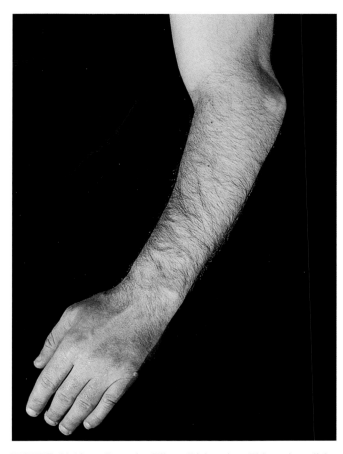

FIGURE 11.12 ■ Posterior Elbow Dislocation. This patient dislocated his elbow while playing basketball. Note the flexed position of the elbow and the prominence of the olecranon. (Photo contributor: Frank Birinyi, MD.)

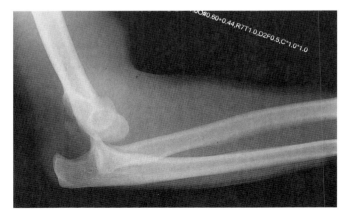

FIGURE 11.13 ■ Posterior Elbow Dislocation. Lateral radiograph demonstrating posterior elbow dislocation. (Photo contributor: Selim Suner, MD, MS.)

Clinical Summary

The biceps has two origins, crosses the shoulder and elbow joints, and inserts on the proximal radius. The long head of the biceps is more susceptible to injury and rupture of the biceps may occur anywhere along its route. Clinically, patients with proximal rupture present with pain along the anteromedial aspect of the shoulder. On inspection, ecchymosis is often acutely noted. The muscle may be noted to retract within the arm, creating a "Popeye" deformity. Due to the two proximal attachments, the short head of the biceps can allow for maintenance of forearm supination strength. Rupture may also occur at the tendon insertion into the radial tuberosity at the elbow. This diagnosis is made on the basis of a history of a painful, tearing sensation in the antecubital region. A snap or pop may also occur. The ability to palpate the tendon in the antecubital fossa may indicate partial tearing of the biceps tendon.

Emergency Department Treatment and Disposition

Proximal and distal biceps tendon ruptures can be discharged with a sling as needed for comfort. Treatment of proximal biceps tendon ruptures consists of anti-inflammatory medication, and physical therapy encouraging early range of motion. Distal biceps tendon ruptures require surgical management due to the significant loss of forearm supination strength. Partial proximal biceps tendon ruptures should also be referred to a specialist.

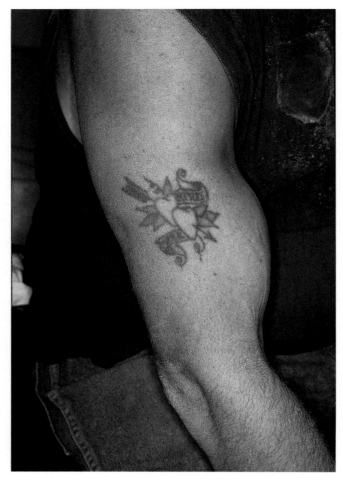

FIGURE 11.14 ■ Biceps Tendon Rupture. The biceps tendon is noted to contract within the arm after rupture. (Photo contributor: Daniel L. Savitt, MD.)

Pearls

1. Functional deficits from a long head rupture are usually temporary and are influenced by coexistent tears.
2. Biceps rupture occurs most commonly in the dominant extremity of men between 40 and 60 years of age when an unexpected extension force is applied to the flexed arm.

Clinical Summary

Fractures of the wrist and elbow usually involve a fall onto the outstretched arm, while fractures of the ulnar shaft are more commonly the result of a direct blow. Anteroposterior (AP) and lateral views of the wrist, forearm, and elbow are required when a forearm fracture is suspected. Functional deficits in the hand are important clues to identification of occult injury to forearm nerve and vascular structures that could require immediate surgical intervention. Monteggia fracture-dislocation is an ulna fracture (usually proximal third) with associated proximal dislocation of the radial head. This fracture is occasionally associated with radial nerve injury.

Galeazzi fracture-dislocation is a fracture of the distal one-third of the radius with dislocation of the distal radioulnar joint. It occurs three times more often than a Monteggia fracture. This fracture can be associated with an ulnar nerve injury.

Isolated fractures of the ulna's middle third may result from direct trauma, while the forearm is used to block the blow, and are called nightstick fractures. Fractures of the forearm may result in compartment syndrome.

Emergency Department Treatment and Disposition

Both Monteggia and Galeazzi fracture-dislocations require emergent orthopedic consultation and are treated with immobilization in a long-arm splint (with elbow flexed at 90 degrees). The forearm is placed in a neutral position for a Monteggia fracture and pronated for Galeazzi fracture. Treatment is usually surgical for both injuries, although children may be treated by reduction and casting.

Pearls

1. Any ulnar fracture with greater than 10 degrees of angulation or with a bony fragment displaced more than 50% of the bones' diameter is considered displaced and usually requires surgical correction.
2. Do not be satisfied with the diagnosis of an isolated proximal third ulnar shaft fracture. A line drawn through the radial shaft and head must align with the capitellum in all views to exclude dislocation.

3. A distal ulnar styloid fracture, if found, can be a clue to a Galeazzi fracture.
4. Since the radius and the ulna create a ring, injury to one of the bones of the forearm is often associated with fracture or dislocation of the other. Consequently, upon recognition of one fracture or dislocation, one must continue to seek out the other half of the injury by examining both the elbow and wrist joints.

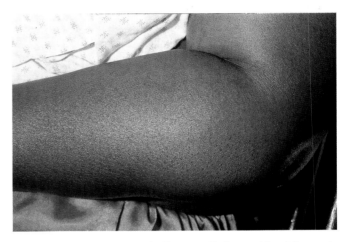

FIGURE 11.15 ■ Monteggia Fracture. Patients with a Monteggia fracture present with swelling and pain in the forearm, and often a palpable radial head in the antecubital fossa. (Photo contributor: Alan B. Storrow, MD.)

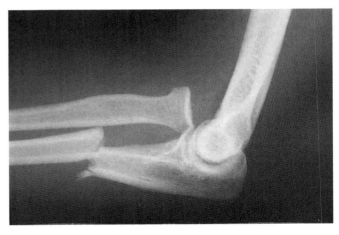

FIGURE 11.16 ■ Monteggia Fracture Radiograph. A Monteggia fracture is defined by a fracture of the proximal one-third of the ulna combined with dislocation of the radial head. (Photo contributor: Alan B. Storrow, MD.)

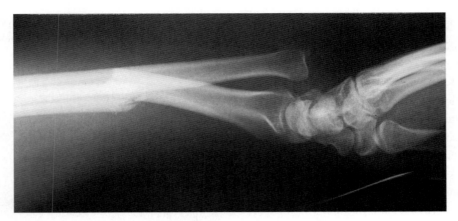

FIGURE 11.17 ■ Galeazzi Fracture. Note the fracture of the distal one-third of the radius and dislocation of the distal radioulnar joint. (Photo contributor: Lawrence B. Stack, MD.)

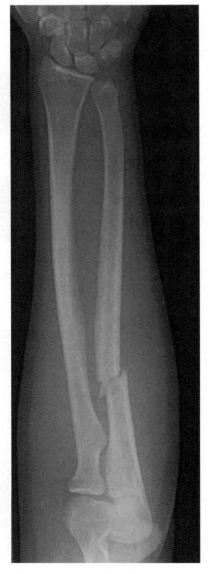

FIGURE 11.18 ■ Nightstick Fracture. Isolated fracture of the middle third of the ulna. (Photo contributor: Lawrence B. Stack, MD.)

Clinical Summary

Falls on an outstretched arm are common and, often, the radius is first to fracture. If there is a supinating component to the fall, the distal ulna may also fracture. Open fractures are common, and one must look closely for overlying soft tissue injury. In the elderly, these distal radius fractures are usually extraarticular metaphyseal fractures, whereas in younger patients they are usually intraarticular with displacement of the joint surface. There are four types of radial fractures, associated with commonly known eponyms: Colles fracture, Smith fracture, Barton fracture and Hutchinson (chauffeur's) fracture.

Colles fracture is the most common. There is dorsal displacement and apex palmer angulation of the distal fracture fragments; on physical examination, a "dinner fork" deformity is often described.

The Smith fracture is a fracture of the distal metaphysis with volar displacement and apex dorsal angulation. This usually results from a blow to the dorsum of the wrist or hand or a hyperflexion injury. Examination reveals a reverse dinner fork deformity. Barton fracture is a fracture of the dorsal or palmer rim of the distal radius. It may be associated with dislocation of the radiocarpal joint. A chauffeur's or Hutchinson fracture is a fracture due to a direct impact to or an avulsion of the radial styloid.

Emergency Department Treatment and Disposition

Evaluation of these fractures requires anteroposterior (AP), lateral, and oblique views. Orthopaedic attention is required for comminuted, displaced, unstable, or open fractures, and those with greater than 20 degrees of angulation or more than 1 cm of shortening. The patient can be immobilized in a sugar-tong splint. Stable fractures respond well to closed reduction and casting for 6 to 8 weeks. Detailed discharge instructions should be given regarding symptoms of median nerve impingement, including paresthesias and hand weakness, which should prompt return to the emergency department.

Pearls

1. All fractures of the distal radius must be evaluated for median nerve function before and after reduction.
2. Colles fractures warrant a high index of suspicion for intraarticular injury, especially when a radial styloid fracture is noted.

3. With a Hutchinson fracture, associated ligamentous injuries should be sought, especially scapholunate dissociation and perilunate or lunate dislocation.

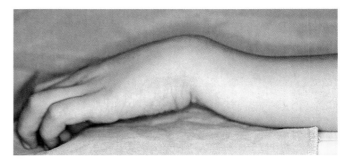

FIGURE 11.19 ■ Colles Fracture. The classic dinner-fork deformity is demonstrated in this photograph. The distal forearm is displaced dorsally. (Photo contributor: Cathleen M. Vossler, MD.)

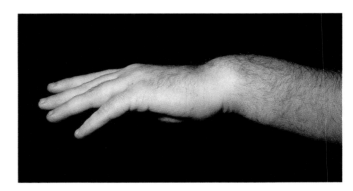

FIGURE 11.20 ■ Smith Fracture. A Smith fracture is sometimes described as a reverse Colles. (Photo contributor: Frank Birinyi, MD.)

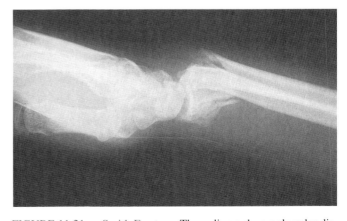

FIGURE 11.21 ■ Smith Fracture. The radiograph reveals volar displacement of the distal radial fragment together with the bones of the wrist and hand. (Photo contributor: Frank Birinyi, MD.)

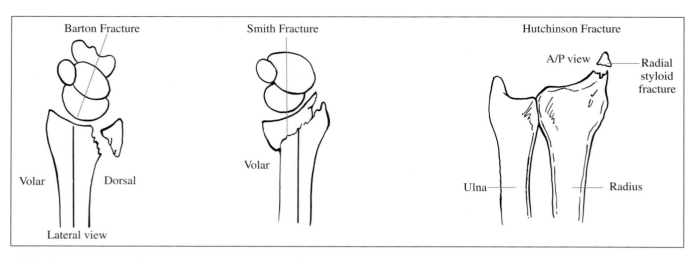

FIGURE 11.22 ■ Distal Forearm Fractures. These illustrations depict three different types of distal forearm fractures: Smith, Barton, and Hutchinson. (Adapted from Simon R. *Emergency Orthopedics: The Extremities*. Norwalk, CT: Appleton & Lange; 1987: pp 118-119.)

Clinical Summary

Carpal and carpometacarpal dislocations are serious wrist injuries usually occurring from hyperextension. Patients complain of decreased range of motion, pain, swelling, and ecchymosis.

Lunate dislocation can occur in a palmer or dorsal position with the lunate displaced relative to the other carpal bones. The normal lunoradial relationship is disrupted. The median nerve is commonly involved and should be evaluated.

If the lunoradial articulation is intact and the other carpal bones are dislocated relative to the lunate, it is termed a perilunate dislocation.

Another potentially serious injury is scapholunate dissociation, often mistakenly diagnosed as a sprained wrist. Although the physical examination may be unremarkable except for wrist pain, an anteroposterior (AP) radiograph reveals a widening of the scapholunate joint space. This space is normally less than 3 mm. A space of 4 mm or greater should prompt suspicion of disruption of the scapholunate ligament. The lateral radiograph may reveal an increase of the scapholunate angle to greater than 60 to 65 degrees (normal 45 to 50 degrees). All these injuries may present with concomitant fractures of the carpal bones or distal forearm.

A scaphoid fracture is particularly troublesome, since misdiagnosis of this problem can result in delayed healing or avascular necrosis. This is due to lack of a direct blood supply to the proximal portion of the bone. Tenderness on palpation of the anatomic snuffbox, or with axial loading, is a common finding. Negative radiographs do not rule out an occult scaphoid fracture.

Carpometacarpal dislocations of the index and long metacarpals are fortunately rare since functional loss is often marked. Thumb, ring, and small finger carpometacarpal dislocations are more common and frequently missed injuries.

Emergency Department Treatment and Disposition

Initial management includes adequate radiographic evaluation followed by ice, elevation, and splinting. Referral to a hand specialist is essential for adequate reduction and long-term care.

Pearls

1. A true lateral wrist radiograph best demonstrates a lunate dislocation by exhibiting the usual cup-shaped lunate bone as lying on its side and displaced either dorsally or palmerly.

2. On lateral wrist radiographs, the metacarpal, capitate, lunate, and radius should all be aligned so that a line drawn through the long axis will bisect all four bones including the lunate. If this is not found, then some element of dislocation, subluxation, or ligamentous instability exists.

3. Patients in whom there is a clinical suspicion of an occult scaphoid fracture (anatomic snuff-box tenderness or axial load tenderness of the thumb without radiologic evidence of fracture) should receive a thumb spica splint and a repeat examination in 7 to 10 days.

4. Carpometacarpal dislocations are frequently difficult to reduce and require open reduction and fixation approximately 50% of the time.

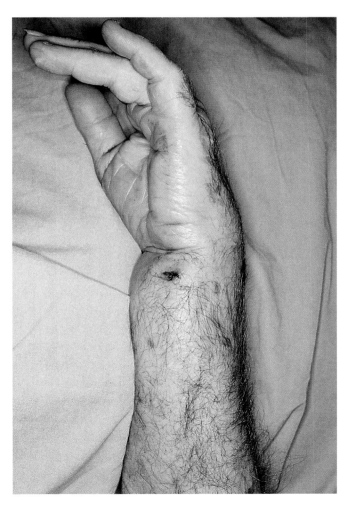

FIGURE 11.23 ■ Lunate Dislocation. This photograph demonstrates swelling associated with a volar lunate dislocation. (Photo contributor: Cathleen M. Vossler, MD.)

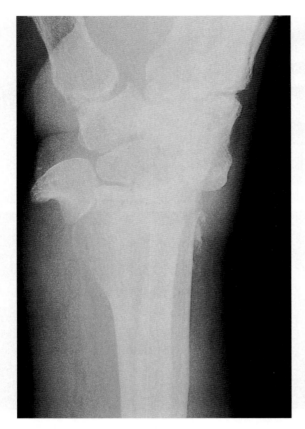

FIGURE 11.24 ■ Lunate Dislocation. Radiographic examination of a dorsal lunate dislocation. (Photo contributor: Cathleen M. Vossler, MD.)

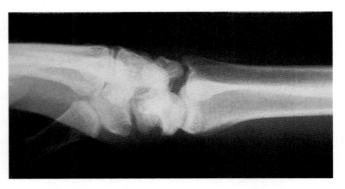

FIGURE 11.26 ■ Perilunate Dislocation. This slightly oblique radiograph of the patient in Fig. 11.25 reveals dorsal displacement of the carpal bones in relation to the lunate. (Photo contributor: Alan B. Storrow, MD.)

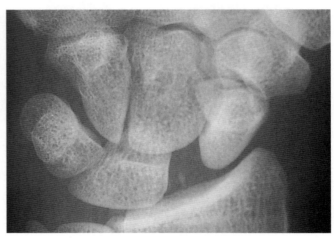

FIGURE 11.27 ■ Scapholunate Dissociation. Note the widened scapholunate joint space. This injury is often misdiagnosed as simple wrist sprain. (Photo contributor: Alan B. Storrow, MD.)

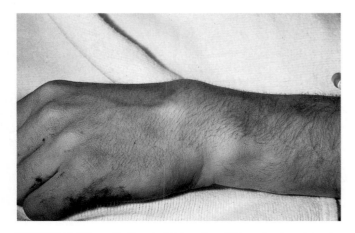

FIGURE 11.25 ■ Perilunate Dislocation. This patient sustained a fall on his outstretched hand. The force disrupted the lunate-capitate articulation, and the capitate and other carpal bones were driven posteriorly with respect to the lunate. (Photo contributor: Alan B. Storrow, MD.)

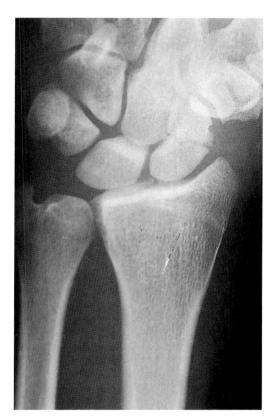

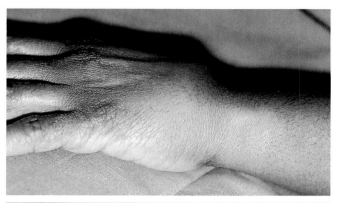

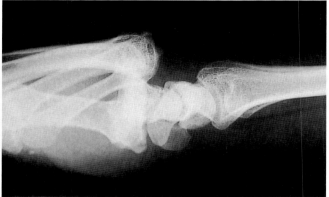

FIGURE 11.28 ■ Scaphoid Fracture. Fracture of the waist, or middle third, of the scaphoid. These injuries can be associated with delayed healing and avascular necrosis. (Photo contributor: Alan B. Storrow, MD.)

FIGURE 11.29 ■ Carpometacarpal Dislocation. Note the prominent deformity of the proximal metacarpals, II to IV, on the dorsal hand and the normal prominence of the ulnar styloid. Top, clinical; bottom, radiograph. (Photo contributor: Alan B. Storrow, MD.)

Clinical Summary

The clenched fist injury classically occurs during a fight when the metacarpophalangeal (MCP) joint contacts human teeth, resulting in a laceration. Many patients will not divulge the true circumstances surrounding the injury; therefore all wounds at the MCP joint must be considered a clenched fist injury until proven otherwise. These wounds occur most often in the dominant hand. Serious complications can result, including infection, loss of function, and amputation. Most wounds are polymicrobial. Patients who present initially may have little evidence of intraarticular injury on physical examination, whereas those who present more than 18 hours after injury are more likely to have evidence of infection, including pain, swelling, erythema, and purulent drainage.

Emergency Department Treatment and Disposition

All wounds should be irrigated, debrided, explored, elevated, and immobilized. Patients should receive antibiotics directed at both oral and skin flora. Tetanus prophylaxis is given if needed.

Radiographs should be obtained to evaluate for fractures and any foreign bodies remaining in the wound. These wounds should never be closed and should be allowed to heal by secondary intention. All patients require careful follow-up with a hand specialist and often require IV antibiotics. Reliable patients who present early, without evidence of infection or significant comorbidity, and no involvement of bone, joint, or tendon may be treated on an outpatient basis. They must follow-up in 24 hours for a wound check, sooner if any signs of infection develop. Any patient who does not meet these requirements must be hospitalized for intravenous antibiotics and wound care.

Pearls

1. Complications include cellulitis, lymphangitis, septic arthritis, abscess formation, osteomyelitis, and flexor tenosynovitis.
2. All wounds need to be examined in full flexion and extension so that tendon injuries are not missed. A tendon injury sustained with the fingers flexed may be missed if the hand is examined only in extension due to tendon retraction.

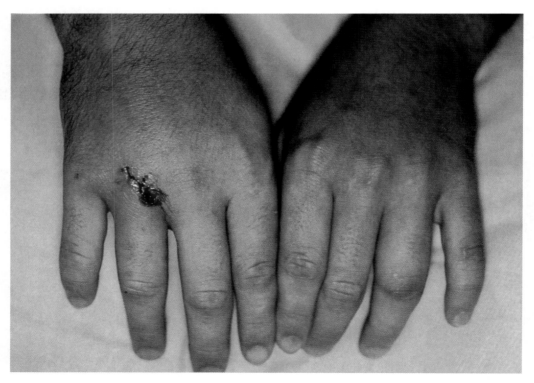

FIGURE 11.30 ■ Clenched Fist Injury. The lacerations in this photograph were sustained from teeth during a fight. Note the subtle black ink stamp across the proximal metacarpals possibly revealing a clue about the wound's etiology. (Photo contributor: Lawrence B. Stack, MD.)

Clinical Summary

A boxer's fracture is a metacarpal neck fracture of the fifth digit, which commonly occurs after a direct blow to the metacarpophalangeal (MCP) joints of the clenched fist. The apex of the fractured metacarpal bone is dorsal. On physical examination, the "knuckle" is flattened and can be palpated on the volar surface.

Examination should address neurovascular integrity and rotational deformity. Rotational deformity is evaluated by having the patient flex the digits at the proximal interphalangeal (PIP) and distal interphalangeal (DIP) joints; the four digits should point towards the scaphoid. If the involved digit overlaps another digit or does not point toward the scaphoid, a rotational deformity is present and needs to be reduced.

Emergency Department Treatment and Disposition

Radiographic evaluation is needed to determine the degree of angulation. Angular deformity of up to 40 degrees is acceptable for the 4th and 5th metacarpals, while 10 to 20 degrees is acceptable for the 2nd and 3rd metacarpals. Any more requires reduction. Closed reduction can be attempted in the emergency department under appropriate nerve block.

Treatment includes ice, elevation, and immobilization in a short arm gutter splint in the intrinsic plus position. For reduction, the MCP joint is held in 90 degrees of flexion and pressure exerted on the metacarpal head, directed dorsally. Simultaneously, the apex of the fracture is directed palmerly. Postreduction radiographs are needed to ensure adequate reduction. Early follow-up (within 7 days) with a hand specialist is essential, the

reduction can be lost with simple splinting. Higher degrees of angulation and fractures with any rotational deformity require follow-up for possible open reduction and fixation.

Pearls

1. Subtle malrotation can be recognized by looking at the alignment of the nail beds with the digits flexed.
2. Complications include collateral ligamentous damage, extensor injury damage, and malposition or clawing of the fingers secondary to incomplete reduction.

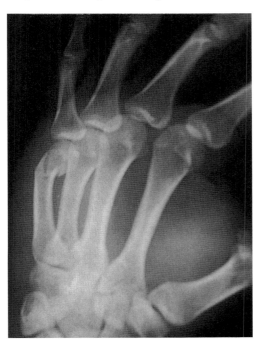

FIGURE 11.32 ■ Boxer's Fracture. Radiographic examination reveals a fracture through the neck of the metacarpal and volar displacement of the fractured segment. (Photo contributor: Cathleen M. Vossler, MD.)

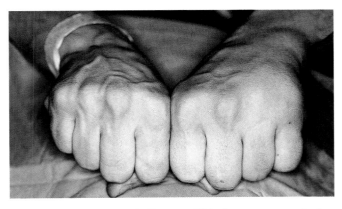

FIGURE 11.31 ■ Boxer's Fracture. This fracture occurred when the patient punched a wall. There is loss of the "knuckle" when the dorsum of the hand is examined, especially noticeable when the patient makes a fist. (Photo contributor: Cathleen M. Vossler, MD.)

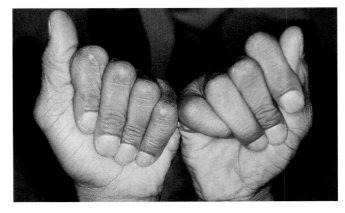

FIGURE 11.33 ■ Boxer's Fracture: Rotational Deformity. Malpositioning of the right fifth digit. Normally, all digits point toward a single spot on the scaphoid. (Photo contributor: Alexander T. Trott, MD.)

Clinical Summary

Chronic ulnar nerve injury results in the classic claw-hand (intrinsic minus) deformity because of the atrophy and contracture of the lumbrical and interosseus hand muscles. The deformity is formed by hyperextension of the metacarpophalangeal (MCP) joint and flexion at the proximal and distal interphalangeal joints of the fourth and fifth digits. There is wasting of the interosseous and hypothenar muscles, as well as the hypothenar eminence. The acutely injured patient is unable to abduct or adduct the digits.

Chronic median nerve damage also results in the claw-hand deformity, but to the second and third digits. Thenar eminence atrophy also occurs. Acute and chronic damage to the proximal portion of the median nerve results in weakness of wrist flexion, forearm pronation, thumb apposition, and flexion of the first three digits.

Wrist drop is the most common symptom seen with radial nerve damage, occurring in situations of acute compression. It is frequently referred to as Saturday night palsy (as when a person falls asleep on an arm, or with the arm over a chair, resulting in temporary radial nerve damage).

Sensory and two-point discrimination sense is lost in the distribution of any acutely or chronically injured nerve.

Emergency Department Treatment and Disposition

Treatment is aimed at recognizing the underlying cause of the nerve damage. Such causes include laceration of the nerve, compression from swelling, or hematoma formation. In the emergency department, splinting and appropriate referral is the treatment.

Pearl

1. Long-term nerve injury results in muscle wasting. Prior to any nerve damage, the thenar and hypothenar eminences have a full appearance. Initially, there is flattening of each eminence, followed by a concave or hollow appearance.

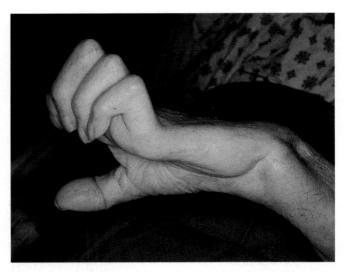

FIGURE 11.34 ■ Claw Hand. Claw-hand appearance resulting from median and ulnar nerve injury. Note metacarpophalangeal joint hyperextension. (Photo contributor: Daniel L. Savitt, MD.)

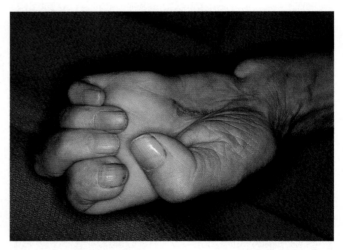

FIGURE 11.35 ■ Claw Hand. Atrophy of the thenar and hypothenar eminences also occurs as a result of damage to the median and ulnar nerves, respectively. Note the concavity to the hypothenar eminence. (Photo contributor: Cathleen M. Vossler, MD.)

Clinical Summary

These patients complain of pain, swelling, and decreased range of motion at the thumb carpometacarpal joint. Bennett fracture is an intraarticular fracture at the ulnar aspect of the base of the first metacarpal with radial displacement of the thumb metacarpal and subluxation or dislocation of the carpometacarpal joint. A Rolando fracture is an intraarticular comminuted fracture at the base of the first metacarpal, with radial and ulnar fragments resulting in a Y- or T-shaped intraarticular fragment.

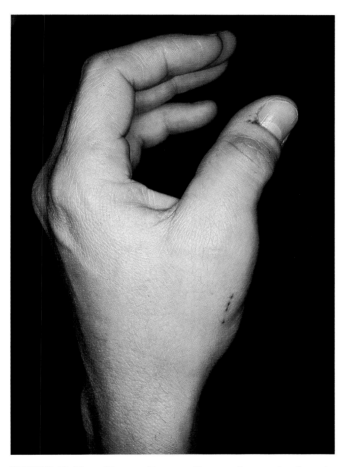

FIGURE 11.36 ■ Bennett Fracture. Bennett fracture involves the base of the first metacarpal. The digit is swollen and ecchymotic over the affected area. (Photo contributor: Daniel L. Savitt, MD.)

Emergency Department Treatment and Disposition

The treatment of these fractures in the emergency department consists of ice, elevation, immobilization in a thumb spica splint, and early referral to a hand specialist. These fractures generally require operative reduction and fixation.

Pearls

1. Osteoarthritis is a common long-term complication, even after optimal management.
2. Swelling can mask significant angulation.
3. Neurovascular and tendon injuries are not commonly associated with Bennett and Roland's fractures.

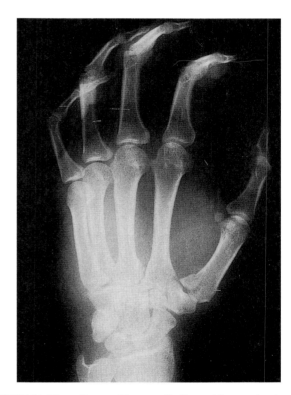

FIGURE 11.37 ■ Bennett Fracture. Radiographic examination of a Bennett fracture illustrates an intraarticular fracture at the base of the first metacarpal with the metacarpal displaced radially and proximally. (Photo contributor: Cathleen M. Vossler, MD.)

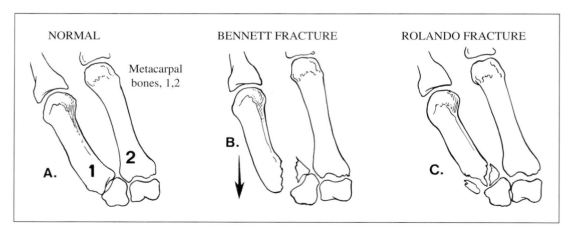

FIGURE 11.38 ■ Intraarticular Fractures of the First Metacarpal Base. A radial, intraarticular fracture at the base of the first metacarpal is a Bennett fracture (**B**). A comminuted intraarticular fracture at the base of the first metacarpal is a Rolando fracture (**C**). Normal anatomy (**A**).

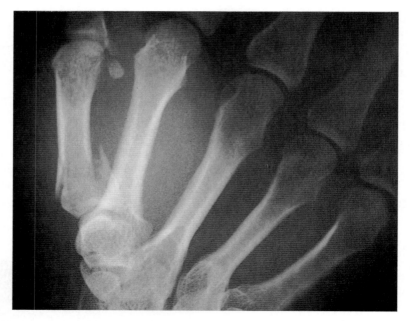

FIGURE 11.39 ■ Rolando Fracture. Note the comminuted intraarticular fracture at the base of the first metacarpal. (Photo contributor: Cathleen M. Vossler, MD.)

Clinical Summary

Fine control of the fingers is achieved by a delicate balance between the extensor, flexor, and intrinsic tendons in each finger. The boutonnière deformity is a result of injury to the central slip insertion of the extensor hood on the dorsal surface of the middle phalanx. After a tear of the central slip, the flexor tendon is unopposed at the proximal interphalangeal (PIP) and the lateral bands of the extensor tendon contract. With time, these displace palmerly resulting in additional flexion at the PIP joint and extension at the distal interphalangeal (DIP) joint. The central slip rupture is the result of a forceful flexion of the PIP joint during full extension, a laceration over the dorsal PIP joint, or a palmar PIP joint dislocation. The deformity may not be immediately apparent as it takes time for the lateral bands to slide down to create extension of the DIP joint. The patient will present with pain and swelling over the dorsal PIP joint, tenderness over the PIP central slip, inability to extend the PIP, and possible hyperextension of the DIP joint. Radiographically, a small fragment of bone may be visualized at the proximal portion of the dorsal aspect of the middle phalanx.

Swan-neck deformity occurs as a result of the contracture of intrinsic hand muscles secondary to systemic diseases such as rheumatoid arthritis. The digit is contorted with hyperextension of the PIP and flexion of the DIP and metacarpophalangeal (MCP) joints.

Emergency Department Treatment and Disposition

In dealing with a closed injury resulting in a boutonnière deformity, immobilization of the PIP joint in extension for 4 weeks is adequate after which active range of motion can start. Open injuries must be carefully explored and repaired. If the deformity is associated with a bony fragment, surgical repair may be necessary. Swan-neck deformities should be splinted and referred as an outpatient. Both deformities require outpatient referral to a hand specialist.

Pearls

1. Boutonnière deformity generally develops weeks after the initial injury as the lateral bands contract; therefore, it is frequently missed in the emergency department. Early diagnosis can be made with proper examination. The digit should be adequately anesthetized and then examined for range of motion and joint stability.

2. Any injury involving the dorsal PIP surface should be reexamined for development of a boutonnière deformity after 7 to 10 days.

3. Surgical repair may be required for patients when conservative therapy yields inadequate results.

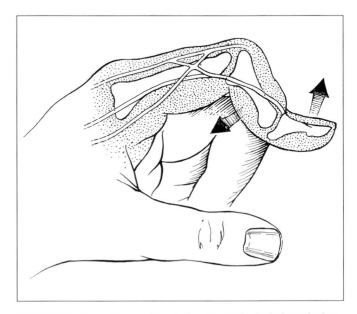

FIGURE 11.40 ■ Boutonnière Deformity. This depiction of a boutonnière deformity illustrates the rupture of the central slip and the resultant subluxation of the lateral bands. The subluxation exerts a pull on the middle phalanx resulting in the deformity.

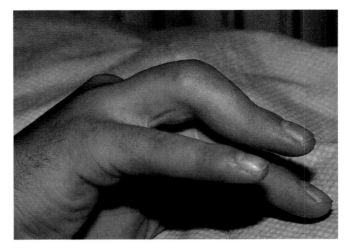

FIGURE 11.41 ■ Boutonnière Deformity. A boutonnière deformity of the fourth digit. Note the flexion of the PIP joint and the extension of the DIP joint. (Photo contributor: E. Lee Edstrom, MD.)

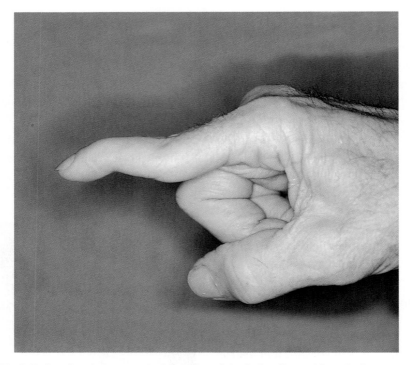

FIGURE 11.42 ■ Swan-Neck Deformity. A swan-neck deformity of the index finger. Note the hyperextension of the PIP joint and the flexion of the DIP joint. (Photo contributor: Cathleen M. Vossler, MD.)

Clinical Summary

A large number of commercial devices are able to deliver liquids and gases at pressures exceeding 5000 psi. Unfortunately, these devices may accidentally introduce these substances into the body, especially the upper extremities, leading to digital ischemia. This can result as a consequence of direct chemical irritation, venous outflow obstruction, arterial compression secondary to the volume of material, spasm, or edema. Soon after the injection, the injury can appear very innocuous. The injected material spreads along fascial planes, so the extent of injury can be quite misleading and is often subtle on initial presentation. A small puncture wound, or no apparent skin break, with minimal swelling may be found. Over time, swelling and pain increase.

Emergency Department Treatment and Disposition

Immediate operative debridement is the treatment of choice. Therefore, early consultation with a hand specialist is necessary. Radiographic examination to evaluate for fractures and to delineate the spread of the injected material can be considered. Tetanus, analgesia, and broad-spectrum antibiotics should be administered. The affected extremity should be elevated and splinted.

Pearls

1. Do not be misled by the "benign" appearance of the initial injury.
2. Delays in treatment can lead to compartment syndrome.
3. Digital blocks are contraindicated because of the potential for increased tissue pressure and compromise of tissue perfusion.

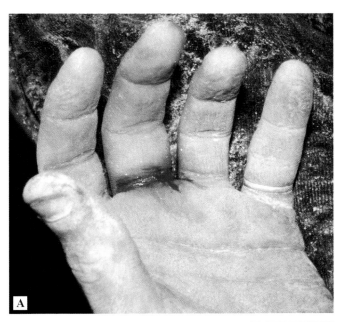

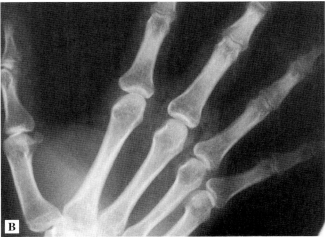

FIGURE 11.44 ■ High-Pressure Injection Injury. Industrial worker with initially benign appearing high-pressure injection injury at the base of his third finger (**A**). Note the spread along fascial planes demonstrated radiographically (**B**). (Photo contributor: Kevin J. Knoop, MD, MS.)

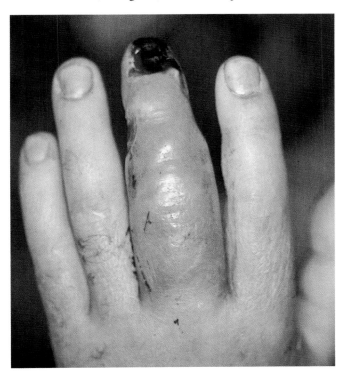

FIGURE 11.43 ■ High-Pressure Injection Injury. Injury incurred by a grease gun that accidentally discharged into a hand. Note the swelling and erythema. (Photo contributor: Richard Zienowicz, MD.)

Clinical Summary

Forced radial deviation (abduction) of the thumb can cause a rupture of the ulnar collateral ligament, also known as game-keeper's or skier's thumb. The tear usually occurs at the the proximal phalanx insertion and can be associated with volar plate and dorsal capsule injury. Pain and swelling are present over the ulnar aspect of the proximal phalanx and thumb metacarpal.

Radiographs may reveal a small avulsion fracture of the proximal phalanx. Abduction stress testing (stabilizing the metacarpal with one hand while applying radial stress on the proximal phalanx) may provide additional clinical information, especially in patients with normal radiographs. Classically, more than 30 to 40 degrees radial angulation indicates complete rupture. Stress testing should be done on both sides in extension and 30 degrees of flexion while feeling for a firm endpoint and excessive laxity.

Emergency Department Treatment and Disposition

Apply a thumb spica splint and appropriate analgesia. Patients with pincer function weakness, point tenderness at the volar-ulnar aspect of the thumb metacarpophalangeal (MCP), a bony fragment of greater than 15% of the articular surface, avulsed fragment displacement of greater than 5 mm, or significant angulation on stress testing should prompt hand surgery referral. Complete tears need repair within 1 week. A sprain without instability is commonly treated with thumb spica casting or splinting for 4 to 6 weeks followed by range of motion exercises.

Pearls

1. Radial collateral ligament rupture can also occur with forced adduction, but is uncommon.
2. Skier's thumb refers to an acute injury, while game-keeper's has classically been associated with repetitive trauma.
3. Thumb MP joint laxity is highly dysfunctional, painful, and may lead to late arthritis.

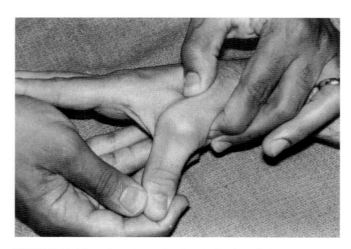

FIGURE 11.45 ■ Gamekeeper's Thumb. Laxity of 30 to 40 degrees more than the uninjured thumb measured in neutral and 30 degrees of flexion are strongly suggestive of a complete ulnar collateral ligament tear. There is no "endpoint" to the radial deviation of the phalanx. (Used with permission from Brunicardi FC, Anderson DK, Billar TR, et al. *Schwartz's Principles of Surgery*, 8th ed. © 2005 McGraw-Hill, New York, NY.)

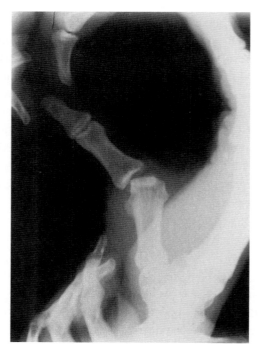

FIGURE 11.46 ■ Gamekeeper's Thumb. Stress x-ray of a thumb with a complete ulnar collateral ligament tear demonstrates marked instability of the ulnar side of the MP joint and radial deviation of the proximal phalanx. (Used with permission from Brunicardi FC, Anderson DK, Billar TR, et al. *Schwartz's Principles of Surgery*. 8th ed. © 2005 McGraw-Hill, New York, NY.)

Clinical Summary

Phalangeal dislocations are common and can occur at all three finger joints. Proximal interphalangeal (PIP) dislocations are especially common. These are generally dislocated dorsally, caused by hyperextension and axial compression, and may have associated damage to the volar plate. PIP volar dislocations can be irreducible secondary to rupture of the extensor tendon and herniation of the proximal phalanx through the extensor hood, requiring operative repair. Metacarpophalangeal (MCP) joint dorsal dislocations are often due to hyperextension. Distal interphalangeal (DIP) dislocations are the rarest but can occur when an axial force is applied to the distal phalanx. Gross deformity is noted on examination, with the distal phalanx generally displaced dorsally.

Emergency Department Treatment and Disposition

Digital nerve block is appropriate anesthesia for the PIP and DIP joints. Ulnar, median, or radial nerve blocks are necessary for the MCP joints. Reduction with splinting is the treatment of choice. Reduction of dorsal dislocations is accomplished via hyperextension of the joint with concurrent application of horizontal traction followed by joint flexion. Flexion at the MCP joint will facilitate reduction of interphalangeal joints. Postreduction radiographs are necessary to ensure adequate reduction. After closed reduction of a dorsal dislocation, the DIP joint should be splinted in slight flexion and the PIP joint in at least 20 degrees of flexion for 3 to 5 weeks, depending on the degree of ligamentous damage. Hand specialist follow-up is mandatory.

Pearls

1. All joints should be tested for instability after reduction, using a digital nerve block to facilitate testing.
2. PIP joint volar dislocation can be unstable, requiring open reduction and internal fixation.
3. Joint dislocations that have volar plate entrapment may be impossible to reduce and require surgical repair for successful reduction.

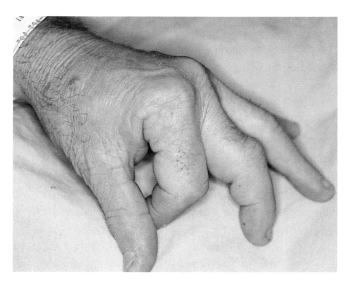

FIGURE 11.47 ■ Phalangeal Dislocation. This patient dislocated the long finger PIP joint during an altercation. The PIP joint is displaced dorsally with an obvious deformity. (Photo contributor: Cathleen M. Vossler, MD.)

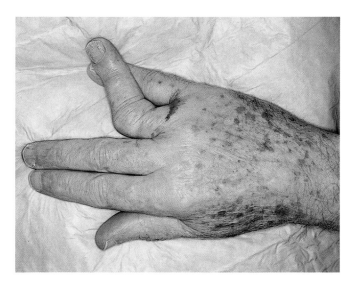

FIGURE 11.48 ■ Phalangeal Dislocation. Medial angulation of the ring finger suggests PIP dislocation. (Photo contributor: Daniel L. Savitt, MD.)

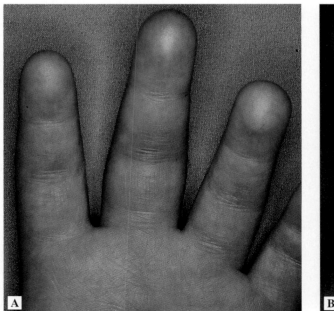 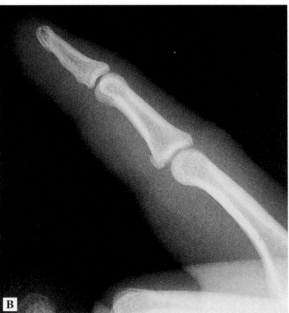

FIGURE 11.49 ■ Volar Plate Injury. Subtle PIP swelling and ecchymosis of the long digit seen with a volar plate injury (**A**). Radiographs of volar plate injuries often reveal a small fragment on the volar surface of the PIP joint (**B**). (Photo contributor: Cathleen M. Vossler, MD.)

Clinical Summary

Mallet finger commonly occurs after the distal interphalangeal (DIP) joint is forcibly flexed against an actively extended finger tearing the extensor mechanism as it inserts on the distal phalanx. This can occur after a sudden axial blow to the tip of the extended finger. The patient presents with an inability to actively extend the distal phalanx while maintaining a normal passive range of motion and the DIP joint remains passively flexed. On radiographic evaluation, there may be a small bony avulsion fragment on the dorsum at the distal phalanx.

A Jersey finger involves an avulsion of the flexor mechanism of the distal phalanx. The FDP tears as a result of forced extension of a fully flexed DIP, as would occur when someone grabs the jersey of an opponent while attempting to tackle them. Most commonly, the ring finger is involved. Clinically, the patient presents unable to actively flex the DIP joint while maintaining a full passive range of motion. Radiographically, a bony avulsion fragment may be present.

Emergency Department Treatment and Disposition

A closed mallet finger without involvement of the joint can be treated by splinting the DIP joint in extension; the proximal interphalangeal (PIP) joint should not be splinted. This splint should be worn continuously for at least 6 weeks. Operative treatment is not usually required.

Jersey finger often requires surgical repair so early referral is required. Prognosis worsens if treatment is delayed or severe tendon retraction is present.

Pearls

1. Avulsion of a significant portion of the articular surface of a mallet finger (more than one-third) may require open reduction with internal fixation.
2. The Jersey finger involves the flexor digitorum profundus tendon at the DIP joint. It may be tested by isolating the affected DIP (ie, holding the MCP and PIP joints in extension while the other fingers are in flexion) and asking the patient to flex the DIP joint.

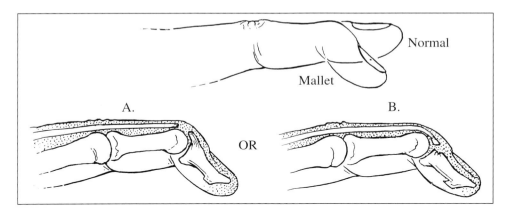

FIGURE 11.50 ■ Mallet Finger. This illustration demonstrates that the unopposed flexion of the DIP joint is secondary to the complete tear of the tendon (**A**), or an avulsion of a small chip fragment (**B**).

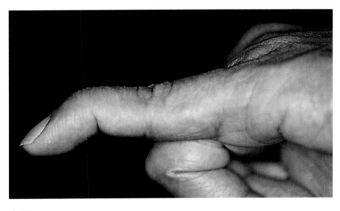

FIGURE 11.51 ■ Mallet Finger. The distal phalanx is held in flexion and the patient is unable to extend it. (Photo contributor: Kevin J. Knoop, MD, MS.)

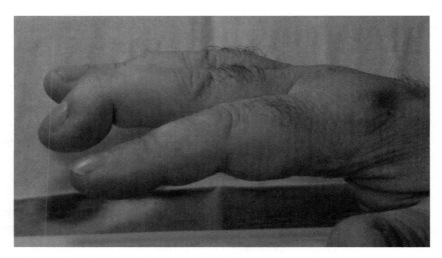

FIGURE 11.52 ■ Mallet Finger. Classic presentation of a mallet finger. The long finger remains flexed at the DIP joint while the patient is attempting to actively extend his fingers. (Photo contributor: Matthew Kopp, MD.)

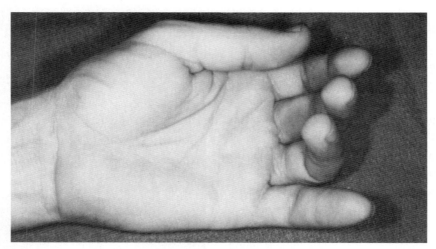

FIGURE 11.53 ■ Jersey Finger. The normal cascade of flexion is disrupted in the injured hand, consistent with a Jersey finger. (Used with permission from Brunicardi FC, Andersen DK, Billiar TR, et al. *Schwartz's Principles of Surgery*. 8th ed. © 2005 McGraw-Hill, New York, NY.)

Clinical Summary

Compartment syndrome develops when the pressure in the inelastic fascial space increases to a point where it causes compression and dysfunction of venous outflow. Major vascular and neural compromise lead to the classic five "Ps" that characterize late compartment syndrome: *pallor, paresthesias, poikilothermia, paralysis,* and *pulselessness.* Compartment syndrome may result from exertion, circumferential burns, frostbite, constrictive dressings, arterial bleeding, severe soft tissue injury, and fracture. It can occur anywhere in the body, most commonly in the anterior compartment of the leg.

The earliest symptom is severe pain out of proportion to the physical findings. The involved compartment is extremely firm. The pain is worsened with passive range of motion due to ischemic muscle fiber stretch. Consequently, the patient often holds the injured part in a position which relaxes the involved muscle groups.

Paresthesia is a later sign of nerve compromise, commonly with vibratory sensation lost first. Motor weakness, pallor, poikilothermia, and pulselessness are very late signs and only occur after irreversible muscle, nerve, and vascular damage have occurred. The goal of the emergency physician is to identify compartment syndrome before these late signs occur.

The diagnosis is confirmed by measuring the pressures of compartments in question using either the Stryker device or an arterial line setup. Pressures greater than 30 mm Hg are suggestive of compartment syndrome and should prompt surgical consultation for fasciotomy consideration.

A serious complication is Volkmann ischemic contracture, classically following a supracondylar fracture. Postischemic swelling, producing increased pressure within the enclosed osteofascial forearm compartment, reduces capillary blood perfusion below the level necessary for tissue viability. If not addressed, muscle and nerve necrosis, and eventual replacement by fibrotic tissue, produces a contracture. Refusal to open the hand, pain with passive extension of the fingers, and forearm tenderness are signs of impending Volkmann ischemia.

Emergency Department Treatment and Disposition

The initial treatment is removal of constrictive dressings and jewelry as well as frequent reevaluation. If there is no improvement, decompression via a fasciotomy should be considered. Aside from muscle and nerve damage, complications of compartment syndrome include myonecrosis which can cause myoglobinuria and renal failure.

Pearls

1. The diagnosis of compartment syndrome should be made early and be based on clinical evaluation and the mechanism of injury. Crush or compression injuries should heighten suspicion.

2. The most common areas of the extremities affected by compartment syndrome are the anterior compartment of the leg due to proximal tibial fractures and the volar compartment of the forearm secondary to fractures of the ulna or radius, as well as supracondylar fractures.

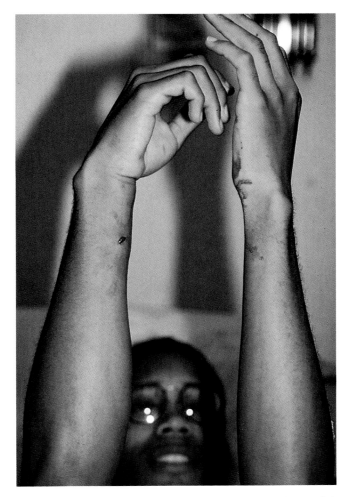

FIGURE 11.54 ■ Compartment Syndrome. A swollen and tense right forearm as a result of compartment syndrome. (Photo contributor: Lawrence B. Stack, MD.)

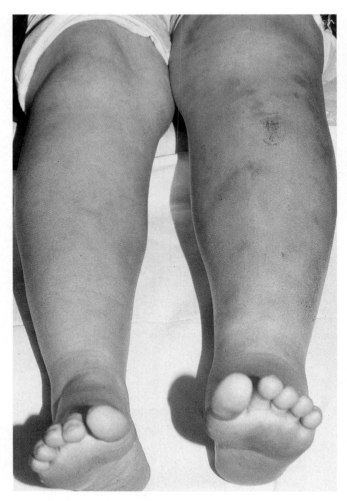

FIGURE 11.55 ■ Compartment Syndrome. Late anterior compartment syndrome of the left lower extremity is manifested by anterior tibial pain and tense "woody" swelling. (Photo contributor: Timothy Coakley, MD.)

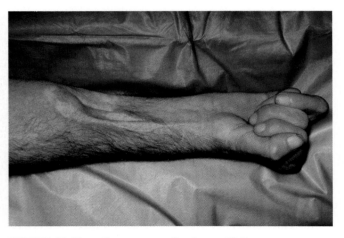

FIGURE 11.56 ■ Compartment Syndrome. Volkmann contracture is a serious late complication of unrelieved compartment syndrome. (Photo contributor: Lawrence B. Stack, MD.)

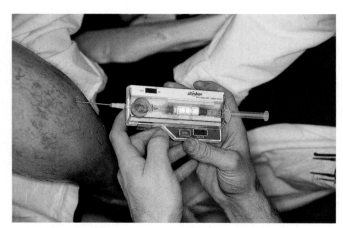

FIGURE 11.57 ■ Compartment Pressures. Intracompartmental pressure monitoring can be accomplished with commercially available devices. Normal tissue pressures should be less than 10 mm Hg; orthopaedic consultation is recommended when pressures exceed 30 mm Hg. (Photo contributor: Selim Suner, MD, MS.)

Clinical Summary

A subungual hematoma is a collection of blood underneath the nail, usually occurring secondary to distal digit trauma. Such patients usually present with throbbing pain secondary to pressure beneath the nail. Associated injuries include nail bed trauma and distal tuft fractures. When fractures are present, these are considered open.

Emergency Department Treatment and Disposition

A radiograph should be done to evaluate for possible fracture. Acutely, if the subungual hematoma involves less than 50% of the nail matrix, trephining the nail with a sterile needle or electrocautery is adequate to relieve pain by allowing drainage. A digital block may be required prior to trephination. The involved digit can be soaked in sterile water with peroxide after trephination to encourage drainage.

Management of larger hematomas is controversial. Some authors advocate nail removal for bed injury repair if the hematoma covers more than 50% of the nail, or if there is an associated fracture. A more recent conservative approach states that removal of the nail is best reserved for those injuries that damage the nail plate and surrounding tissues, regardless of the size of the hematoma or presence of a tuft fracture. After the nail is removed, the patient's clean nail, a piece of foil, or petroleum gauze should be placed between the eponychial nail fold and the germinal matrix.

The patient with a fracture should be discharged with a splint supporting the distal joint in extension and all dressings should be kept dry. Antibiotics are not required unless the area is contaminated.

Pearls

1. Subungual hematomas are a sign of nail bed injury.
2. Subungual hematomas with surrounding nail bed and nail fold injuries require nail removal and evaluation of the nail bed for injury and careful repair if needed.
3. A hand-held, high-temperature, portable cautery device is a good tool for drainage of a subungual hematoma.

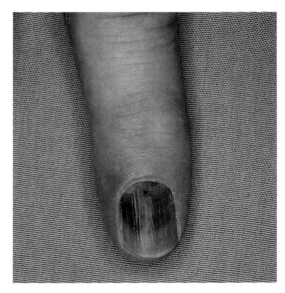

FIGURE 11.58 ■ Subungual Hematoma. This subungual hematoma occurred after the patient hit his finger with a hammer; it covers approximately 50% of the subungual area. (Photo contributor: Margaret P. Mueller, MD.)

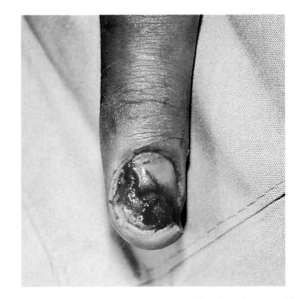

FIGURE 11.59 ■ Nail Bed Laceration. Bleeding from a nail bed laceration causes a subungual hematoma. This image depicts a nail bed laceration seen after removal of the nail. (Photo contributor: Alan B. Storrow, MD.)

Clinical Summary

Hip dislocations require large amounts of energy, are often associated with fractures of the acetabulum, ipsilateral femur or knee, and can be anterior, posterior, or inferior. Ninety percent of dislocations are posterior, resulting from forces exerted on a flexed hip and knee (eg, a passenger in a motor vehicle accident whose knees hit the dashboard). Anterior hip dislocations occur when there is forced external rotation of the extended hip, which forces the head out of the acetabulum, either by tearing the anterior capsule or fracturing the anterior wall of the acetabulum.

Patients complain of severe hip pain and decreased range of motion. On physical examination, posterior dislocations present with the extremity shortened, internally rotated, adducted, and flexed. With anterior dislocations, the leg is often abducted, externally rotated, and slightly flexed; however, this presentation can vary.

Emergency Department Treatment and Disposition

A neurovascular and radiographic evaluation should occur before and after any attempts at reduction. Treatment for dislocations is early closed reduction, often with conscious sedation, although femoral nerve blocks are an option. Since the muscles around the hip are so strong, the physician should be aware that a general anesthetic with complete paralysis may be required. Posterior dislocations are reduced using in-line traction with the hip and knee flexed to 90 degrees, followed by gentle internal to external rotation. Anterior dislocations are reduced using strong in-line traction with the hip in neutral flexion extension or slight extension, slight adduction and internal rotation, followed by abduction.

Orthopedic consultation should be obtained as early as possible. These patients require admission, with frequent neurovascular evaluation.

Hip replacements have a tendency to dislocate more easily than native hips and usually require less energy for reduction.

Radiographs should be done pre- and postreduction to evaluate for periprosthetic fractures.

Pearls

1. Complications of posterior hip dislocations include sciatic nerve injury and avascular necrosis.
2. Immediate reduction is imperative and should be accomplished within 6 hours. The longer the delay in reduction, the greater the incidence of avascular necrosis.

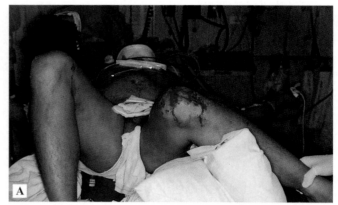

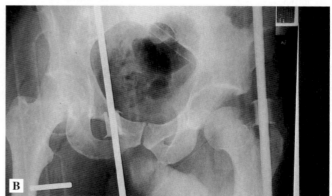

FIGURE 11.60 ■ Hip Dislocation. Typical patient appearance of a left posterior hip dislocation. Note internal rotation of the affected extremity (**A**). Radiograph of patient (**B**). (Photo contributor: Cathleen M. Vossler, MD.)

Clinical Summary

Fractures above the level of the lesser trochanter are termed hip fractures. The femoral head has a tenuous blood supply and hip fractures can compromise blood flow, resulting in avascular necrosis. For classification, hip fractures are generally divided into *intracapsular* (femoral head and neck fractures) and *extracapsular* (trochanteric, intertrochanteric, and subtrochanteric). Accurate classification is important because intracapsular fractures are more likely to be associated with vascular disruption.

Complaints include groin or buttock pain, tenderness, and an inability to bear weight on the affected side. There can be shortening of the affected leg as well as abduction and external rotation.

Radiographic analysis should include an anteroposterior (AP) of the pelvis, so both hips can be compared. Both the Shenton line (the curved line formed by the top of the obturator foramen and the inner side of the neck of the femur) and the neck shaft angle should be evaluated, but can be normal in nondisplaced fractures.

Emergency Department Treatment and Disposition

Fractures of the hip require early orthopedic consultation for admission and, in most cases, surgical reduction and fixation. Femoral head fracture-dislocations are an orthopedic emergency and require immediate reduction. A neurovascular examination should be carefully performed before and after any reduction attempts.

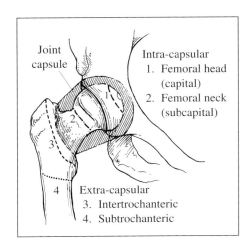

FIGURE 11.61 ■ Hip Fractures. This illustration depicts the different types of proximal femoral fractures.

Pearls

1. Hip pain can be referred in any patient complaining of knee or thigh pain, consider hip fracture.

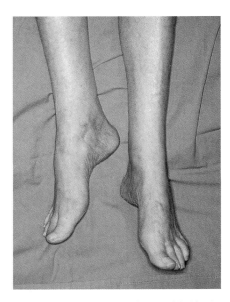

FIGURE 11.62 ■ Hip Fracture. Patients with hip fractures often present with the affected extremity shortened, externally rotated, and abducted. Note the rotation and shortening in this patient with a right intertrochanteric fracture. (Photo contributor: Cathleen M. Vossler, MD.)

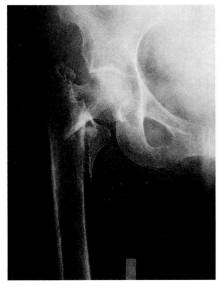

FIGURE 11.63 ■ Hip Fracture. Radiographic examination reveals an intertrochanteric fracture. (Photo contributor: Cathleen M. Vossler, MD.)

2. Fracture-dislocation of the femoral head requires great forces; intraabdominal, and retroperitoneal injuries should be considered.
3. Fractures of the hip may be diagnosed by auscultation of differences in bone conduction between the patient's two extremities. This is performed by placing the stethoscope's diaphragm on the anterosuperior iliac spine and giving the patella soft taps.
4. Any elderly patient with an inability to bear weight has a hip fracture until proven otherwise. Hip fractures can be secondary to osteoporosis so there does not need to be a history of trauma. Since plain films may not be sensitive enough to identify some hip fractures, other imaging such as CT or MRI should be considered.

Clinical Summary

Knee extensor injuries usually occur from three different mechanisms: *quadriceps tendon tear, patellar tendon tear,* and *patellar fracture*. Extension may be limited by any disruption of these three elements. Patients with a history of trauma, other systemic conditions, steroid injections, or fluoroquinolone use are predisposed to rupture.

Quadriceps tendon ruptures are the most common extensor failure and are more often seen in the elderly. Forced flexion during quadriceps contraction (eccentric contraction) may cause rupture; patients may experience sudden buckling and pain. The patella is inferiorly displaced with proximal patellar tenderness, and swelling. A soft tissue defect at the distal aspect of the quadriceps is often apparent.

Patellar tendon rupture occurs in the younger, more active population and results in proximal displacement of the patella with inferior pole tenderness and swelling.

Patellar fractures may be transverse (most common), comminuted, or vertical. They may be caused by direct trauma or as a result of high eccentric tension forces. Tenderness, swelling, and sometimes a palpable defect, are present.

Physical examination will reveal weakness of knee extension against gravity. Patients with complete tears will not be able to extend their knee while those with partial tears will demonstrate weak extension.

Emergency Department Treatment and Disposition

Radiographic evaluation of extensor injuries should include anteroposterior (AP) and lateral views of the knee. Lateral radiographs may help distinguish between the two tendon injuries.

Patients demonstrating either partial or complete tendon ruptures can be discharged with their knee in extension and follow up with orthopedics.

Care must be taken to differentiate between a bipartite patella and a fracture. Nondisplaced and displaced patellar fractures should be treated with splinting in full extension and referred to orthopedics.

Pearls

1. MRI may distinguish partial from complete tears.
2. Patellar fractures may be complicated by future degenerative arthritis.

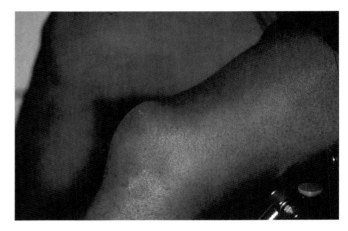

FIGURE 11.64 ■ Quadriceps Tendon Rupture. Inferior displacement of the patella and a distal quadriceps defect suggest quadriceps tendon rupture. (Photo contributor: Robert Trieff, MD.)

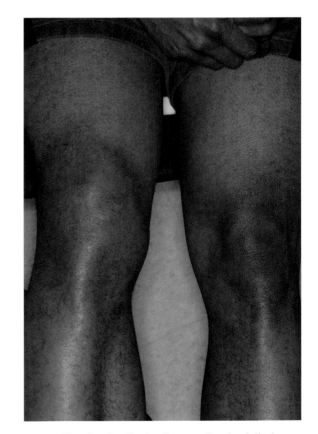

FIGURE 11.65 ■ Patellar Tendon Rupture. Proximal displacement of the patella and inferior pole tenderness in a patient with left patellar tendon rupture. (Photo contributor: Kevin J. Knoop, MD, MS.)

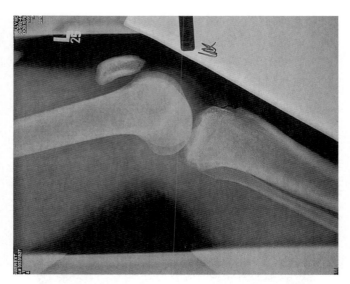

FIGURE 11.66 ■ Patellar Tendon Rupture. A lateral radiograph reveals the proximal patellar displacement seen with complete patellar tendon rupture. (Photo contributor: Kevin J. Knoop, MD, MS.)

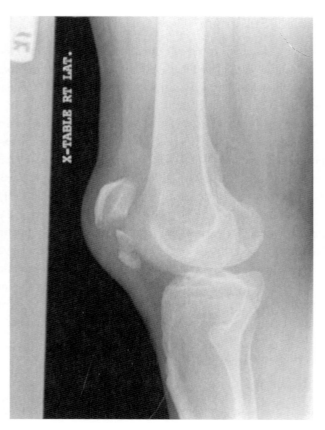

FIGURE 11.67 ■ Patella Fracture. Lateral radiograph of a patient with a fractured patella. The inferior pole of the patella is comminuted and displaced. Internal fixation is indicated if the patient cannot actively extend the knee. (Used with permission from Brunicardi FC, Andersen DK, Billiar TR, et al. *Schwartz's Principles of Surgery.* 8th ed. © 2005 McGraw-Hill, New York, NY.)

Clinical Summary

Patellar dislocations can result from either direct trauma to the patella or powerful quadriceps contraction with knee flexion. Most commonly, the patella dislocates laterally although medial dislocations also occur. Patients who present after a patellar dislocation commonly state that their knee dislocated and this must be ruled out. A hemarthrosis can be present. Common complaints include pain, swelling, and knee deformity. Examination reveals fullness or deformity in the lateral aspect of the knee. The patellar apprehension test is also positive in spontaneously reduced patellar dislocations. This test is done by having the patient extend their knee and gently displacing the patella laterally or medially. The patient will become apprehensive as you attempt to reproduce the dislocation. Radiographic evaluation will confirm the dislocation and will help rule out any associated fracture. Fractures of the patella or lateral femoral condyle occur in 5% of patients.

Emergency Department Treatment and Disposition

Lateral dislocations are reduced by flexing the hip, extending the knee, and gently directing pressure medially on the patella. Reduction is easily accomplished and results in immediate relief of pain. Postreduction films should be taken. After successful reduction, patients require a knee immobilizer in full extension for 4 to 6 weeks. Outpatient referral to a musculoskeletal specialist should be obtained, since these patients require further evaluation.

Pearls

1. A dislocated patella may reduce spontaneously prior to presentation and should be addressed as a possibility in any patient who presents with knee pain. This may be elucidated by inquiring about a knee deformity at the time of injury that is no longer present.

2. Complications of patellar dislocation include degenerative arthritis, recurrent dislocations, and chondral or osteochondral loose bodies.

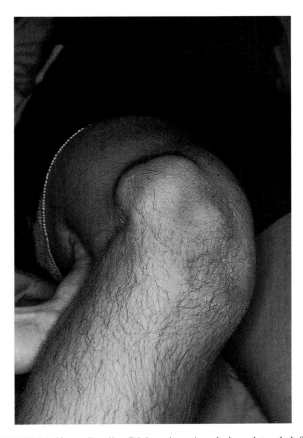

FIGURE 11.68 ■ Patellar Dislocation. An obvious lateral deformity of the right patella in a patient with patellar dislocation. (Photo contributor: Cathleen M. Vossler, MD.)

Clinical Summary

Knee dislocations are classified by the direction of tibial displacement relative to the femur and invariably cause multiple ligamentous injuries. Dislocations can be anterior, posterior, medial, lateral, or rotatory. Knee dislocations are usually the result of motor vehicle crashes, falls, sports, and industrial injuries. Anterior dislocations are more common and usually occur after high-energy hyperextension injuries. Knee dislocations are associated with popliteal artery and common peroneal and tibial nerve injuries. Popliteal artery injury can result from both anterior and posterior dislocations, is more common than nerve injury, and is more devastating. Injury can be present despite normal pulses and, if not identified and repaired within 8 hours, amputation may be necessary. Common peroneal nerve injury can cause decreased sensation on the lateral foot, impaired dorsiflexion and eversion, and impaired sensation over the first dorsal web space. Knee dislocations can spontaneously relocate, so the physician must maintain a high index of suspicion. If a patient presents with a grossly unstable knee after trauma, this is a reduced dislocation and should be evaluated as such.

Patients will complain of pain and ecchymosis will be present; however, an effusion will often be absent since the capsule has been violated. On physical examination, the knee will be grossly unstable since knee dislocations tend to injure most of the ligaments around the knee.

Emergency Department Treatment and Disposition

After a neurovascular examination, radiographic evaluation including an anteroposterior (AP) and lateral of the knee should be done to evaluate for concomitant fractures. Emergent treatment includes early reduction, immobilization, assessment of distal neurovascular function, and emergent orthopedic referral.

Reduction of anterior dislocation is accomplished by flexing the hip 20 degrees and having an assistant apply longitudinal traction on the leg while keeping one hand on the tibia and simultaneously lifting the femur back into position. A posterior splint with the knee in 20 degrees of flexion is used for immobilization and to avoid tension on the popliteal artery. The patient should be admitted for observation and, likely, arteriography.

Pearls

1. Knee dislocations are often associated with a fracture of the tibial plateau.

2. The presence of distal pulses in the foot does not rule out an arterial injury. It has been shown that examination of pulses is not sensitive enough to detect vascular injury after a knee dislocation. You must at least discuss an arteriogram with the orthopaedic or vascular surgeon.

3. Vascular repair after 8 hours of injury carries an amputation rate of greater than 80%.

4. Compartment syndrome is also seen after knee dislocations, usually due to vascular injury and resultant hemorrhage and ischemia.

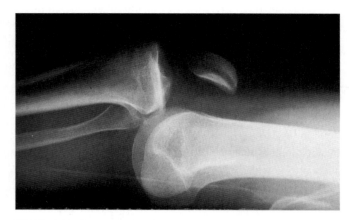

FIGURE 11.69 ■ Anterior Knee Dislocation. A radiograph demonstrating anterior displacement of the tibia in relation to the femur. (Photo contributor: Selim Suner, MD, MS.)

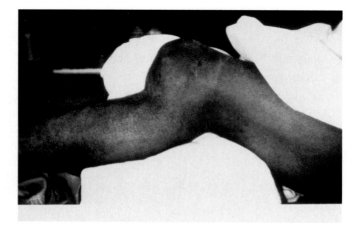

FIGURE 11.70 ■ Posterior Knee Dislocation. Patient demonstrating posterior displacement of the tibia in relation to the femur. (Photo contributor: Paul R. Sierzenski, MD.)

Clinical Summary

While femoral fractures often occur secondary to serious trauma, they can be seen in low-energy injuries such as osteoporosis or stress fractures. The diagnosis is usually evident on visualization of the thigh, and confirmed radiographically. Significant hematoma formation is extremely common. Patients with comminuted femoral shaft fractures are at risk for fat emboli syndrome. For distal fractures, it is important to rule out intraarticular involvement.

Emergency Department Treatment and Disposition

Initial management includes stabilization and evaluation for any life-threatening injuries. It is important to keep in mind that a large amount of blood loss (average 1000 mL) can occur. These patients should have two large-bore intravenous lines and be crossmatched for blood products. Radiographic evaluation of the extremity should be performed and include the hip and knee. The patient may require traction for initial stabilization, and to reduce blood loss and pain. This is accomplished by applying in-line traction, and can be held temporarily in the acute setting with a Hare traction splint.

An open fracture is an orthopedic emergency; these patients require tetanus prophylaxis, antibiotic coverage, and emergent irrigation and debridement in the operating room. Orthopedic consultation should be obtained with any femur fracture since the majority require operative fixation and stabilization.

Pearls

1. Pain can be referred. Any injury between the lumbosacral spine and the knee can be referred to the thigh or knee.

2. Vascular compromise can occur and should be suspected with an expanding hematoma, absent or diminished pulses, or progressive neurologic signs.

3. Femur fractures can mask the clinical findings of a hip dislocation; thus radiographs of the pelvis, hips, and knees should be obtained routinely.

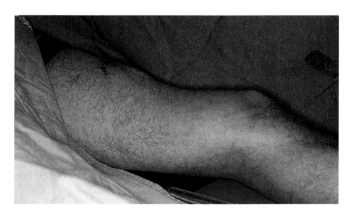

FIGURE 11.71 ■ Midshaft Femur Fracture. A closed midshaft femoral fracture. Note the deformity in the middle of the thigh, consistent with this injury. (Photo contributor: Daniel L. Savitt, MD.)

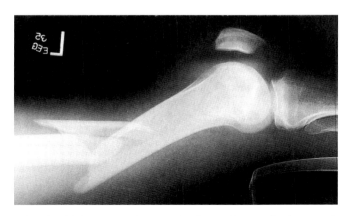

FIGURE 11.72 ■ Femur Fracture. Radiographic examination reveals a comminuted displaced distal femoral fracture. (Photo contributor: Cathleen M. Vossler, MD.)

Clinical Summary

Fibular fractures may be isolated or be associated with injuries of the tibia. Isolated fibular fractures are caused by direct trauma to the lateral leg. Isolated fractures of the fibula are anatomically splinted by an intact tibia. Distal fibular fractures may include a disrupted ankle joint, as evidenced by a widened mortise on the anteroposterior (AP) radiograph. Tibial fractures are classified by their location, amount of displacement, and presence of comminution.

Compartment syndrome can be seen following a tibia fracture and distal neurovascular status should always be documented. Suspect tibial fractures with trauma to the lower extremity, pain, and inability to bear weight.

The Maisonneuve fracture is a combination of an oblique proximal fibular fracture, disruption of the interosseous membrane and tibiofibular ligament distally, and a medial malleolar fracture or tear of the deltoid ligament. This fracture occurs when an external rotational force is applied to the foot, producing a fracture of the proximal third of the fibula. Physical examination findings include tenderness at the medial and anterolateral ankle joint in combination with proximal fibular tenderness.

Emergency Department Treatment and Disposition

Treatment of tibial fractures depends on whether they are open or closed and on the degree of displacement. All open fractures require immediate orthopaedic evaluation. Closed fractures that cannot be reduced may also need open reduction. Patients with isolated nondisplaced tibial fractures may be splinted, started on ice therapy, and referred for outpatient treatment. Displaced tibial fractures should also be evaluated by an orthopaedic surgeon since these are at risk for developing compartment syndrome.

Treatment of fibular fractures is dictated by the degree of pain experienced by the patient and the involvement of the ankle joint. Nondisplaced fractures can be treated with an air cast, while those with displacement should be place in a sugar-tong splint and referred for short-term orthopedic evaluation. Treatment of a Maisonneuve fracture is most commonly operative.

Pearls

1. Early follow up is required for all tibial fractures owing to the risk of compartment syndrome.
2. The peroneal nerve crosses over the head of the fibula and is subject to injury with a Maisonneuve fracture.
3. Some patients with Maisonneuve fracture may complain only of ankle pain. Maisonneuve fracture represents about 1 in 20 ankle fractures, so always examine the proximal fibula in patients complaining of ankle pain.

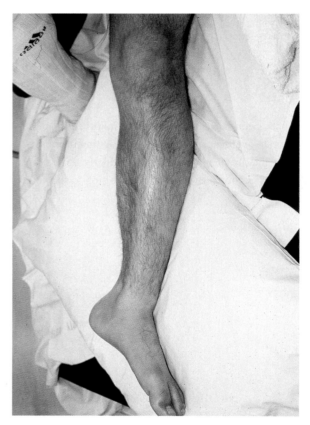

FIGURE 11.73 ■ Tibial-Fibular Fracture. Deformity associated with a midshaft tibial and fibular fracture. (Photo contributor: Kevin J. Knoop, MD, MS.)

Clinical Summary

Fracture blisters are vesicles or bullae that arise secondary to swelling from soft tissue injury. The most commonly affected areas include the tibia, ankle, and elbow. Patients note blister formation within 1 to 2 days after the initial trauma. Patients complain of pain, swelling, ecchymosis, and decreased range of motion. Complications include infection, deep venous thrombosis, and compartment syndrome.

Emergency Department Treatment and Disposition

Blisters are generally left intact, and the underlying fracture is treated.

Pearls

1. Blisters can be seen with other conditions, including barbiturate overdose and burns. In the setting of trauma, however, they frequently indicate an underlying fracture.
2. Blisters are managed in a similar fashion to second-degree burns.

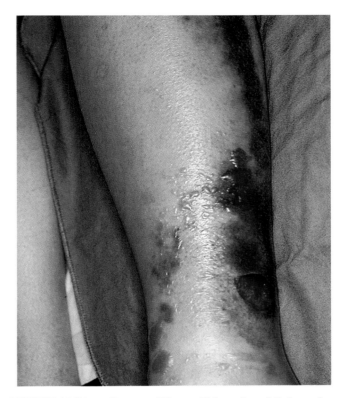

FIGURE 11.74 ■ Fracture Blisters. This patient fell down four steps on the evening prior to presentation. Upon awakening the next morning, he noted ecchymosis, swelling, and blister formation. Radiographs revealed fracture of the fibula. (Photo contributor: Daniel L. Savitt, MD.)

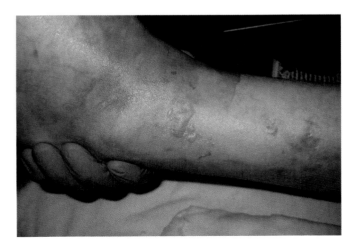

FIGURE 11.75 ■ Fracture Blisters. Blisters associated with an underlying ankle fracture. (Photo contributor: Selim Suner, MD, MS.)

Clinical Summary

Rupture of the Achilles tendon occurs most frequently in middle-aged males involved in athletic activities, but patients with other systemic conditions, steroid injections, or fluoroquinolone use are predisposed. Rupture occurs 2 to 6 cm above the tendon's attachment to the calcaneus. Patients may hear or feel a pop. There is weakness when pushing off of the foot; pain, edema, and ecchymosis may develop. Note that loss of plantarflexion is not necessarily seen as there are other tendons that can compensate. Thompson test can be diagnostic of an Achilles rupture. The patient should be placed in a prone position, the knee and ankle flexed to 90 degrees, and the gastrocnemius muscle should be grasped and squeezed. If the Achilles tendon is even partially intact, then the foot will plantarflex; if completely ruptured, there will be no movement of the foot. Radiographic analysis should include a lateral view of the ankle as the Achilles tendon can sometimes be seen.

Emergency Department Treatment and Disposition

Treatment is either operative or conservative. In either case, the extremity is immobilized in slight plantar flexion and the patient is made non–weight bearing upon emergency department discharge. Acute treatment also involves elevation, analgesia, and ice. These patients can be discharged home with follow-up with orthopedics.

Pearls

1. Approximately 25% of these injuries are initially misdiagnosed as ankle sprains.
2. Palpation of the tendon alone may not detect rupture, as the tendon sheath is often intact.

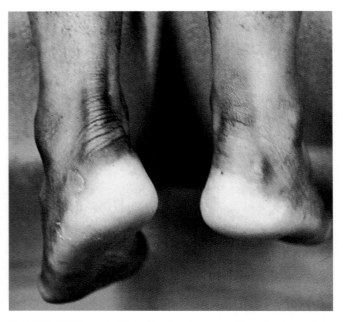

FIGURE 11.76 ■ Achilles Tendon Rupture. Note the loss of the normal resting plantarflexion due to right Achilles tendon rupture. Swelling is also apparent over the injury site. (Photo contributor: Kevin J. Knoop, MD, MS.)

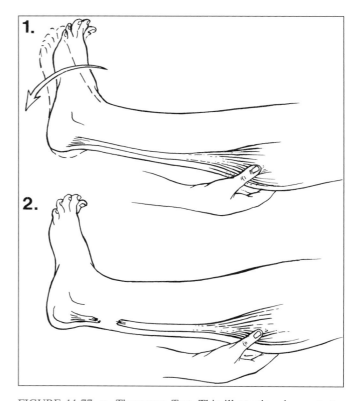

FIGURE 11.77 ■ Thompson Test. This illustration demonstrates the Thompson test, where compression of the gastrocnemius-soleus complex normally produces plantarflexion of the foot (1). If the tendon is completely ruptured, this will not occur (2).

Clinical Summary

The ankle is a hinge joint with the talus sitting in the mortise formed by the distal tibia and distal fibula. Ankle dislocations require forces of great magnitude and usually, the malleoli are also fractured. Posterior and lateral dislocations are the most common, but the ankle can also dislocate medially, superiorly, or anteriorly. A posteriorly dislocated ankle is locked in plantar-flexion with the anterior tibia easily palpable. The foot has a shortened appearance, with the ankle very edematous. Anterior dislocations present with the foot dorsiflexed and elongated. Lateral dislocations present with the entire foot displaced laterally. Ankle dislocations are frequently associated with fractures and are often open.

Emergency Department Treatment and Disposition

A complete neurovascular examination should be performed and if vascular compromise is present, the ankle should be emergently reduced, even if it is open. The skin may also be taut and can be at risk for necrosis. If time permits, radiographic evaluation should include an anteroposterior (AP) and lateral view of the ankle.

To reduce the ankle, gentle traction is applied to the foot with one hand cupping the heel and the other hand on the dorsal aspect of the foot while an assistant applies countertraction. Neurovascular status should be checked before and after any attempts at reduction or immobilization. Reduction usually requires conscious sedation, or general anesthesia. Patients should be placed in a posterior splint with immediate referral to an orthopedic surgeon for hospitalization.

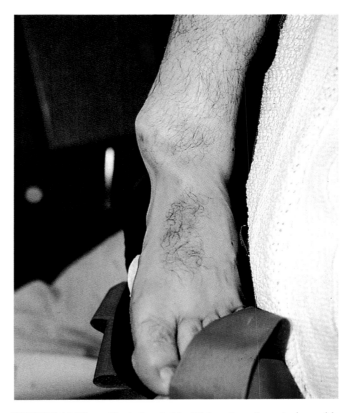

FIGURE 11.78 ■ Posterior Ankle Dislocation. A posterior ankle dislocation is pictured. Radiographs showed an associated fracture. (Photo contributor: Mark Madenwald, MD.)

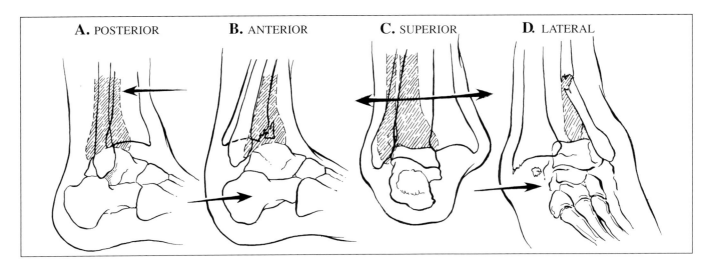

FIGURE 11.79 ■ Ankle Dislocations. This illustration depicts different types of ankle dislocations. Arrows denote direction of the injury force. (Adapted from Simon R. *Emergency Orthopedics: The Extremities.* Norwalk, CT: Appleton & Lange; 1987: p. 402.)

Pearls

1. These injuries are commonly associated with malleolar fractures and often require open reduction and internal fixation.
2. Fifty percent of ankle dislocations are open and require surgical debridement.
3. The subtalar joint may also dislocate and appear clinically similar. The lateral x-ray will show overlap of the talus and calcaneus, while the AP mortise view will show an intact mortise.
4. The worse the ankle appears clinically and radiographically, the easier it is to reduce due to more severe ligamentous disruption.

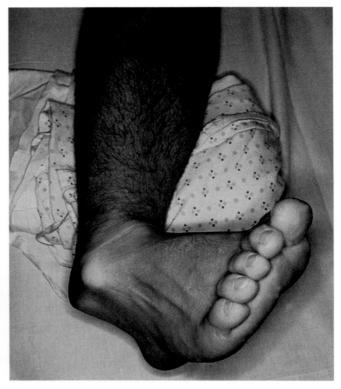

FIGURE 11.81 ■ Subtalar Dislocation. This patient landed on his foot while playing basketball. Neurovascular status was intact, and the ankle, which was promptly reduced after x-ray, showed no associated fracture. (Photo contributor: Kevin J. Knoop, MD, MS.)

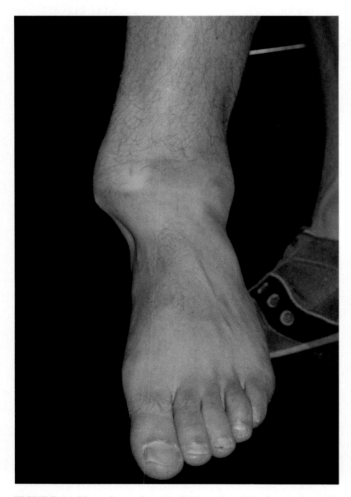

FIGURE 11.80 ■ Lateral Ankle Dislocation. The foot is laterally displaced in this patient with a lateral ankle dislocation. (Photo contributor: Lawrence B. Stack, MD.)

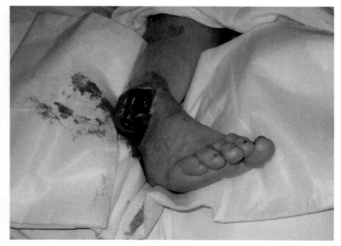

FIGURE 11.82 ■ Open Ankle Fracture-Dislocation. Ankle dislocations are frequently open and have associated fractures. (Photo contributor: Selim Suner, MD, MS.)

Clinical Summary

The calcaneus is the most frequently fractured tarsal bone. Patients present with severe heel pain in association with soft tissue swelling and ecchymosis extending to the arch. Heel contour can be distorted. Radiographs should include antero-posterior (AP) and lateral views of the foot and a Harris axial view. Fractures can involve the tuberosities, the sustentaculum, or the body and are classified as intra- or extraarticular. The Boehler angle should be calculated for all fractures involving the body to rule out a depression, as this will change management. It is normally between 20 and 40 degrees; if approaching or less than 20 degrees a depressed fracture should be suspected.

Emergency Department Treatment and Disposition

CT scans should be obtained to further delineate fracture patterns and rule out involvement of the subtalar joint. Intra-articular fractures require orthopedic consultation; open reduction and internal fixation are usually needed.

Nondisplaced extraarticular fractures generally heal well with bulky compressive dressings, rest, ice, elevation, and non–weight bearing for the first 8 weeks. Orthopaedic referral is necessary since some may require open reduction. Other complications include fracture blisters, nonunion, and chronic pain.

Pearls

1. Calcaneal fracture warrants a diligent search for associated injuries. Twenty percent are associated with spinal fractures, 7% have contralateral calcaneal fractures, and 10% are associated with compartment syndromes. The subtalar joint is disrupted in 50% of cases. A high index of suspicion for thoracic aortic rupture and renal vascular pedicle disruption must be maintained.

2. Minimally displaced fractures of the anterior calcaneous are easily missed and should be suspected in a patient who does not recover appropriately from a lateral ankle sprain.

3. CT scanning is the optimal imaging technique.

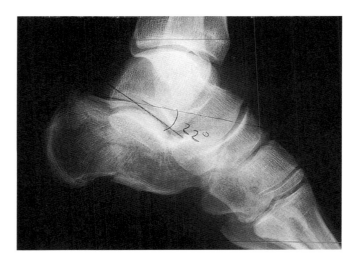

FIGURE 11.84 ■ Calcaneus Fracture. This patient fell from a ladder and struck his heel. A cortical step-off is seen on the inferior aspect of the calcaneus. The Boehler angle has been calculated at approximately 22 degrees. (Photo contributor: Alan B. Storrow, MD.)

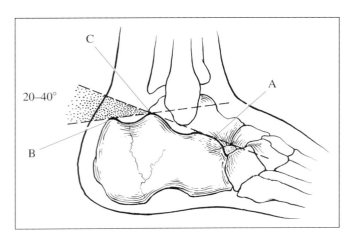

FIGURE 11.83 ■ Calcaneus Fracture: Boehler Angle. The Boehler angle is formed by the intersection of lines drawn tangentially to the anterior (**A**) and posterior (**B**) elements of the superior surface of the calcaneus (**C**). A normal angle is approximately 20 to 40 degrees.

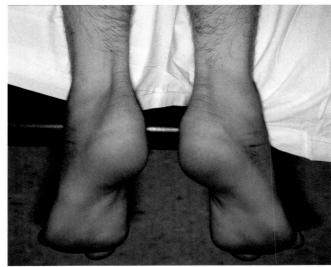

FIGURE 11.85 ■ Bilateral Calcaneal Fracture. A fall from a ladder caused bilateral calcaneal fractures. Note swelling and ecchymosis. (Photo contributor: Lawrence B. Stack, MD.)

Clinical Summary

Classification of these injuries is based on examination; radiographs are often not required to guide management. The most common mechanism is an inversion stress that injures, in order, the anterior talofibular, calcaneofibular, and posterior talofibular ligaments. The medial deltoid is the strongest ligaments; therefore isolated injuries are rare and medial ankle sprains are often associated with lateral malleolar or syndesmotic injuries.

A *Grade 1* sprain is a stretch injury resulting in pain, tenderness, minimal swelling, and maintenance of the ability to bear weight. A *Grade 2* sprain is a partial tear of the ligamentous structures resulting in pain, swelling, local hemorrhage, and moderate degree of functional loss. A *Grade 3* sprain is a complete tear of the ligament or ligaments and presents with positive stress testing, significant swelling, and an inability to bear weight.

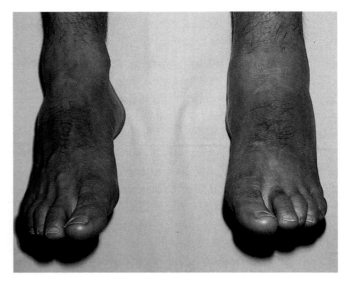

FIGURE 11.86 ■ Ankle Sprain. A Grade 2 left lateral ankle sprain. Note the swelling and asymmetry. (Photo contributor: Kevin J. Knoop, MD, MS.)

Emergency Department Treatment and Disposition

Examination should include an anterior drawer test to assess the integrity of the anterior talofibular ligament. The Ottawa Ankle Rules recommend that radiographs should be performed for the following conditions:

- Tenderness over the lateral or medial malleolus
- Patient is unable to weight bear for four steps both immediately post injury and in the emergency department.

Grade 1 injuries are treated with ice packs, elevation, air cast or splint, and early mobilization. Grade 2 and Grade 3 sprains should receive immobilization in an air cast or posterior splint, ice, elevation and referred to a musculoskeletal specialist.

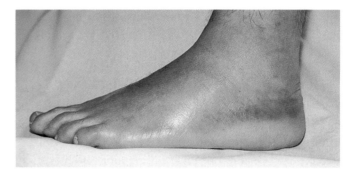

FIGURE 11.87 ■ Ankle Sprain. Note the dependent ecchymosis and swelling in this patient with a Grade 2 left lateral ankle sprain. (Photo contributor: Lawrence B. Stack, MD.)

Pearls

1. Ankle injuries are the most common musculoskeletal problem in emergency medicine.
2. Complications include instability, persistent pain, recurrent sprains, and peroneal tendon dislocation.
3. Both malleoli, the proximal fibula, and the fifth metatarsal should be examined for injury in evaluating a patient with an ankle sprain.

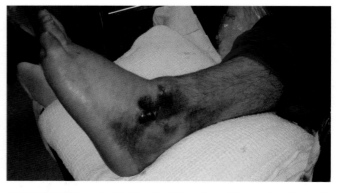

FIGURE 11.88 ■ Ankle Sprain. Marked swelling and ecchymosis in a patient with a probable Grade 3 ankle sprain. (Photo contributor: Selim Suner, MD, MS.)

Clinical Summary

Patients complain of pain, swelling, decreased range of motion, and tenderness over the lateral aspect of the midfoot. Fractures of the fifth metatarsal base have been generically referred to as Jones fractures. However, acute fractures can be divided into two types, depending on their anatomic location. Treatment is determined by this delineation.

The classic Jones fracture is a transverse fracture of the fifth metatarsal at the metadiaphyseal-diaphyseal junction, just distal to the fourth and fifth intermetatarsal joint. It occurs when a force is applied to a plantarflexed and inverted foot.

This is not to be confused with an avulsion fracture of the base of the fifth metatarsal, resulting from a sudden inversion of the foot. The avulsion injury is caused by traction on the lateral cord of the plantar fascia.

Emergency Department Treatment and Disposition

The patient with a Jones fracture should be discharged in a posterior splint and crutches and be non–weight bearing for 6 to 8 weeks. Surgical treatment is sometimes required since there is a risk of nonunion.

The avulsion fracture usually heals rapidly and seldom leads to permanent disability. This patient can be discharged in a hard-soled shoe or walking cast for 2 to 3 weeks and can be weight bearing as tolerated. A significantly displaced fracture may require operative intervention. Both types of patients should be referred to a musculoskeletal specialist as an outpatient.

Pearls

1. The original description of these fractures was by Sir Robert Jones, who personally sustained this injury while dancing. The avulsion fracture is sometimes referred to as a dancer's fracture.
2. The classic Jones fracture has a high incidence of delayed healing and nonunion.

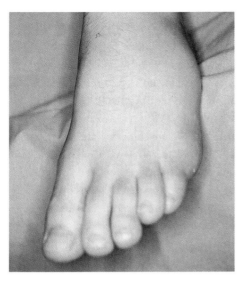

FIGURE 11.89 ■ Jones Fracture. This patient sustained an injury of the fifth metatarsal and presented with pain and swelling over this site. His radiograph revealed a fracture. (Photo contributor: Cathleen M. Vossler, MD.)

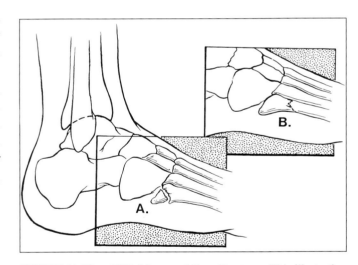

FIGURE 11.90 ■ Fifth Metatarsal Base Fractures. This illustration depicts an avulsion fracture (**A**) and a classic Jones fracture (**B**).

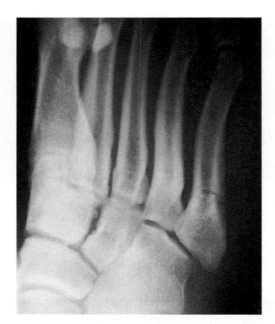

FIGURE 11.91 ■ Jones Fracture. Radiograph with typical appearance for a diaphyseal fracture of the fifth metatarsal base. (Photo contributor: Alan B. Storrow, MD.)

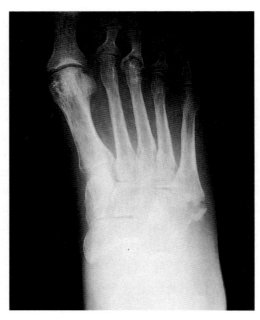

FIGURE 11.92 ■ Fifth Metatarsal Avulsion Fracture. Radiograph illustrating an avulsion-type fracture of the fifth metatarsal base. (Photo contributor: Alan B. Storrow, MD.)

LISFRANC FRACTURE-DISLOCATION

Clinical Summary

The Lisfranc joint (tarsometatarsal joint) connects the midfoot and forefoot. It is defined by the articulation of the bases of the first three metatarsals with the cuneiforms and the fourth and fifth metatarsals with the cuboid. Lisfranc ligament anchors the *second metatarsal base* to the medial cuneiform. Disruption of the Lisfranc joint is typically associated with high-energy mechanisms; however, they may occur with less force. Clinical presentation is variable, but severe midfoot pain and the inability to bear weight are usually present. Radiographs may reveal displacement of the metatarsals in one direction (homolateral) or a split, usually between the first and second metatarsals (divergent).

Emergency Department Treatment and Disposition

Meticulous evaluation of foot radiographs is the key to diagnosis. There are three radiographic findings that suggest a Lisfranc injury. The medial aspect of the second metatarsal should align with the medial borders of the medial cuneiforms on the anteroposterior (AP) foot x-ray. Second, on an AP and an oblique view of the foot, there should not be any widening between the first and second metatarsals. Thirdly, on the oblique view of the foot, the medial aspect of the fourth metatarsal should align with the medial aspect of the cuboid. A disruption of these anatomic relationships is suggestive of a Lisfranc injury. Lisfranc injuries warrant orthopedic evaluation in the emergency department. Closed reduction can be attempted; however, due to significant ligamentous disruption, the injury is often unstable and necessitates operative stabilization. Tenderness over the Lisfranc complex with normal radiographs can reflect a strain of the complex. Weight-bearing radiographs may unmask joint instability, but is often not tolerated in the acute setting. Lisfranc sprains should be placed in a short-leg walking cast.

Pearls

1. Early recognition of Lisfranc fracture-dislocations is facilitated by assessing for the normal bony alignment on x-ray and by searching for frequently associated fractures.
2. Fractures of the second metatarsal base are considered pathognomonic of a Lisfranc injury because these fractures are often associated with disruption of the Lisfranc ligament.

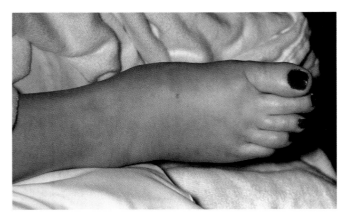

FIGURE 11.93 ■ Lisfranc Fracture-Dislocation. This patient presented with extreme midfoot pain and swelling. (Photo contributor: Lawrence B. Stack, MD.)

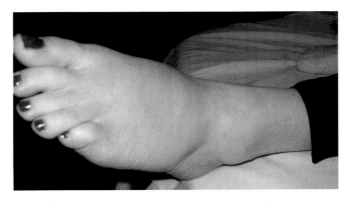

FIGURE 11.94 ■ Lisfranc Fracture-Dislocation. Typical appearance of the swelling associated with this fracture-dislocation. (Photo contributor: Selim Suner, MD, MS.)

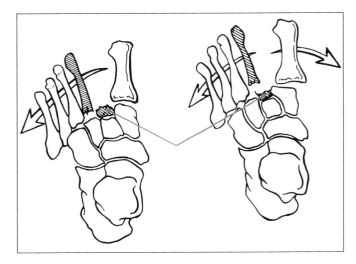

FIGURE 11.95 ■ Lisfranc Fracture-Dislocations. Two different types of Lisfranc fracture-dislocations. Homolateral (*left*) and divergent (*right*).

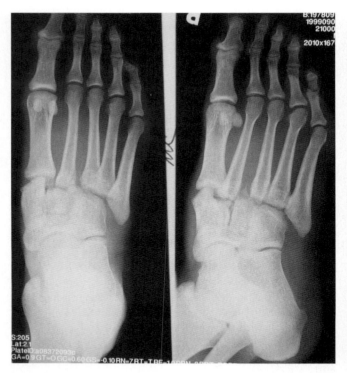

FIGURE 11.96 ■ Lisfranc Injury Radiograph. Note misalignment of the metatarsals, especially the second with the medial cuneiform. (Photo contributor: Selim Suner, MD, MS.)

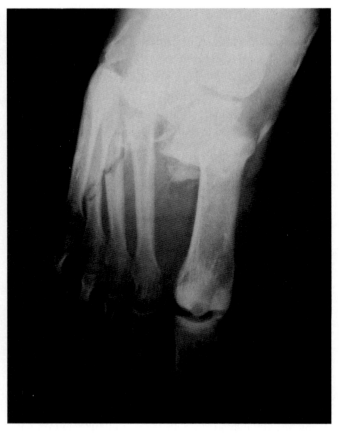

FIGURE 11.97 ■ Lisfranc Fracture-Dislocation. A divergent Lisfranc fracture-dislocation. Note the disruption of the alignment of the second metatarsal and the medial cuneiform. Sometimes these injuries are not as apparent and comparison radiographs are necessary. (Photo contributor: Alan B. Storrow, MD.)

Clinical Summary

Major trauma may result in partial or complete removal of a limb. The high kinetic injury, crush, or avulsion forces required often cause extensive damage and heavy contamination. Other significant injuries to the thorax and abdominal cavities should be considered, and may be life-threatening. Prehospital personnel may be helpful in understanding the mechanism.

Emergency Department Treatment and Disposition

Traumatic limb amputations should be considered life threatening; advanced trauma life support protocols should be rapidly initiated. The injury should be managed as an open fracture with appropriate antibiotics and tetanus prophylaxis. The amputated part should be kept clean, motioned with sterile saline, wrapped in a sterile dressing, placed in a plastic bag, and put on ice. With the possible exception of minor digit amputations, patients should be admitted under trauma and orthopedic consultation for close monitoring of neurologic and vascular status.

While reimplantation is often not possible due to tissue loss and contamination, all patients should receive consideration. Young, healthy individuals with sharp, guillotine injuries without significant avulsion or crushing damage are the best candidates. Radiographs may help delineate the exact spot of injury and reveal associated dislocations or fractures.

Pearls

1. Cooling the amputated part will increase viability from approximately 6 to 8 hours to 12 to 24 hours.
2. Post-reimplantation limb shortening may create significant disability. Proper use of post injury prosthetics may be the better option.

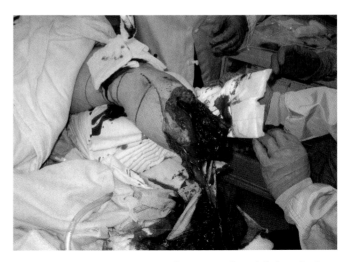

FIGURE 11.98 ■ Lower Extremity Amputation. A below the knee amputation from a motorcycle accident. These injuries are often associated with significant, and potentially life threatening, abdominal or thoracic trauma. (Photo contributor: Selim Suner, MD, MS.)

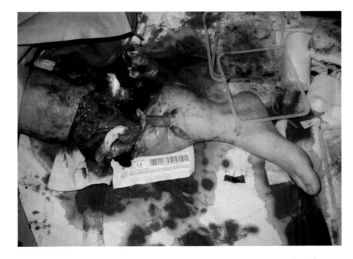

FIGURE 11.99 ■ Lower Extremity Amputation. Amputation from a motor vehicle accident. (Photo contributor: Selim Suner, MD, MS.)

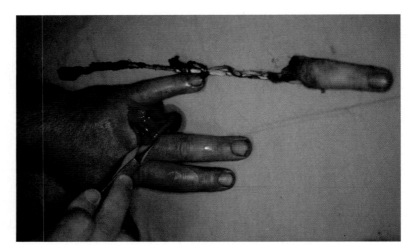

FIGURE 11.100 ▪ Finger Amputation. Digit avulsion and tendon rupture. (Photo contributor: Selim Suner, MD, MS.)

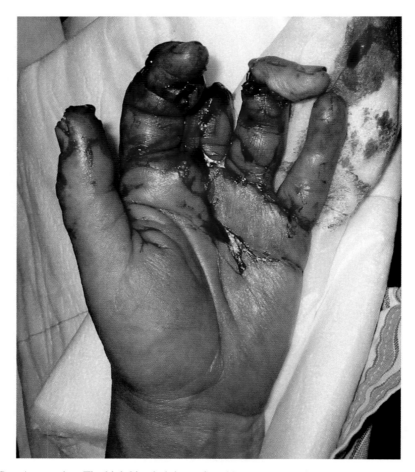

FIGURE 11.101 ▪ Table Saw Amputation. The high kinetic injury of a table saw can produce significant avulsion forces and contamination. (Photo contributor: Selim Suner, MD, MS.)

Chapter 12

EXTREMITY CONDITIONS

Robert J. Tubbs
Daniel L. Savitt
Selim Suner

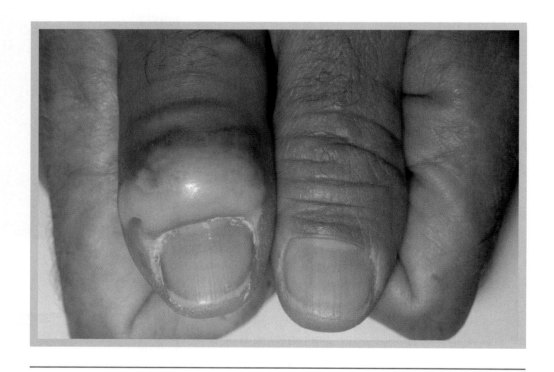

Clinical Summary

Cellulitis, an infection of the skin or subcutaneous tissues, is common. The characteristic findings are: erythema with poorly defined borders, edema, warmth, pain, and limitation of movement. Fever and constitutional symptoms may be present and are commonly associated with bacteremia. Predisposing factors include trauma, lymphatic or venous stasis, immunodeficiency (including diabetes mellitus), and foreign bodies. Common etiologic organisms include group A β-hemolytic *Streptococcus* and *Staphylococcus aureus* in nonintertriginous skin, and gram-negative organisms or mixed flora in intertriginous skin and ulcerations. In immunocompromised hosts, *Escherichia coli, Klebsiella* species, *Enterobacter* species, and *Pseudomonas aeruginosa* are common agents. In recent years, there has been a dramatic increase in the incidence of community-acquired methicillin-resistant *S aureus* (CA-MRSA), particularly in cellulitis associated with a cutaneous abscess. The differential diagnosis includes deep venous thrombosis, venous stasis, erythema nodosum, septic or inflammatory arthritis/bursitis, and allergic reactions.

Emergency Department Treatment and Disposition

Treatment of minor cases commonly consists of immobilization, elevation, analgesia, and oral β-lactam antibiotics with reevaluation in 48 hours. The increase in the incidence of CA-MRSA has prompted some providers, especially in highly endemic areas, to advocate coverage with trimethoprim/sulfamethoxazole in addition to conventional β-lactam antibiotics. Admission and parenteral administration of antibiotics may be necessary for immunocompromised or toxic-appearing patients, or those who do not respond to outpatient therapy.

Pearls

1. Aggressive treatment of cellulitis with broad-spectrum parenteral antibiotics in immunocompromised patients is warranted.
2. Rapidly progressive cellulitis or one that progresses despite treatment with β-lactam antibiotics should raise suspicion for CA-MRSA or deeper infections such as fasciitis.

3. Known risk factors for CA-MRSA include military personnel, prison inmates, and competitive sports players.
4. Routine blood or leading-edge cultures in nontoxic patients are generally low yield.

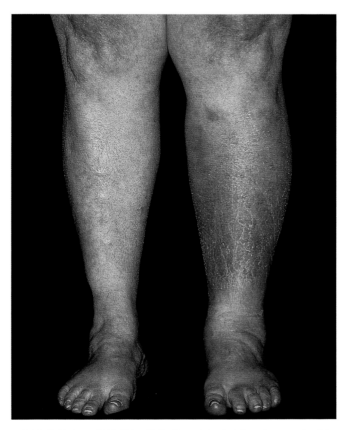

FIGURE 12.1 ■ Cellulitis. Cellulitis of the left leg characterized by erythema and mild swelling. (Photo contributor Frank Birinyi, MD.)

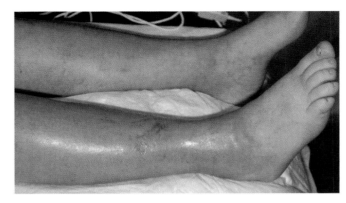

FIGURE 12.2 ■ Cellulitis. Erythema consistent with cellulitis of the right lower extremity. (Photo contributor: Lawrence B. Stack, MD.)

Clinical Summary

A felon is a pyogenic infection of the distal digital pulp space, with pus collecting in the spaces formed by the vertical septa anchoring the pad to the distal phalanx. This condition is characterized by severe pain, exquisite tenderness, and tense swelling of the distal digit with erythema. There may be a visible collection of pus or palpable fluctuance. Complications include deep ischemic necrosis, osteomyelitis, septic arthritis, and septic tenosynovitis. The differential diagnosis includes paronychia, herpetic whitlow, and hematoma following traumatic injury.

Emergency Department Treatment and Disposition

Incision and drainage is generally necessary to treat a felon. To ensure complete drainage of the abscess cavity, all affected compartments should be entered. The packing of the abscess space is made with a small, loose-fitting wick to facilitate drainage. Oral antibiotics directed against gram-positive organisms should be used for 10 days and the packing removed or replaced after 24 to 48 hours.

Pearls

1. Do not extend the incision proximal to the distal flexion crease.
2. Incisions should be made dorsal to the neurovascular bundle; the pincer surfaces (radial aspects of the index and long fingers and ulnar aspect of the thumb and small finger) should be avoided when possible.
3. "Hockey stick" and "fish mouth" incisions are associated with increased occurrence of unnecessary sequelae and are not recommended.
4. If there is radiographic evidence of osteomyelitis, consultation with a hand surgeon is required.

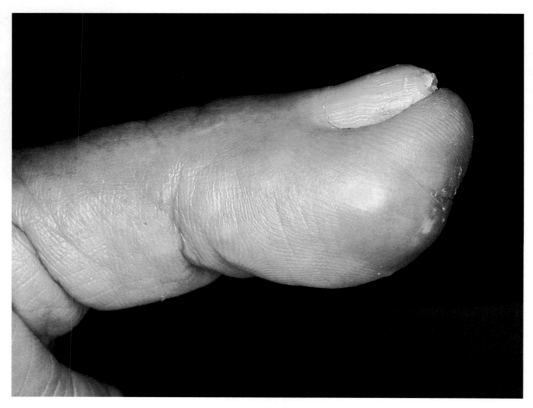

FIGURE 12.3 ■ Felon. Note the area of purulence at the center of the palmar pad in this thumb with a felon. There is also swelling and erythema. (Photo contributor Daniel L. Savitt, MD.)

Clinical Summary

Gangrene denotes tissue that has lost its blood supply and is undergoing necrosis. The term *dry gangrene* is used for tissues undergoing sterile ischemic coagulative necrosis. Patients with atherosclerotic disease and diabetes are at risk for the development of dry gangrene, usually as a result of embolization to the forefoot or toe. *Wet gangrene* is associated with bacterial proteolytic decomposition, and is characterized by its moist appearance, frequently with blistering.

Emergency Department Treatment and Disposition

Hospitalization is usually required. The treatment consists of amputation, debridement, and antibiotic therapy as needed. Wet gangrene requires emergent surgical consultation. Underlying vascular pathology must be evaluated by arteriography and corrected surgically. Patients with systemic toxicity should be resuscitated aggressively.

Pearls

1. Obtain radiographs to help rule out clostridial myonecrosis (gas gangrene, see related item) and osteomyelitis.
2. Aggressive surgical debridement is necessary for cure in most cases of wet gangrene.

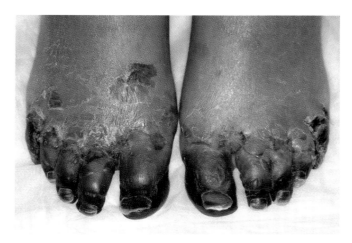

FIGURE 12.4 ■ Dry Gangrene. Dry gangrene of the toes showing the areas of total tissue death, appearing as black, and lighter shades of discoloration of the skin demarcating areas of impending gangrene. (Photo contributor: Lawrence B. Stack, MD.)

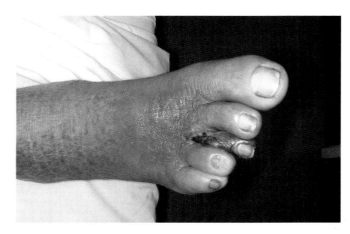

FIGURE 12.5 ■ Wet Gangrene. Note the moist appearance and blistering due to bacterial proteolytic decomposition of gangrenous tissue in this patient with wet gangrene. (Photo contributor: Robert J. Tubbs, MD.)

Clinical Summary

Also referred to as clostridial myonecrosis, this infection causes rapid necrosis and liquefaction of fascia, muscle, and tendon. The vast majority of cases involve *Clostridium perfringens,* which produces several toxins responsible for tissue necrosis, hemolysis, and systemic signs of shock. *Streptococcus pyogenes* accounts for the majority of remaining cases. Myonecrosis is classically associated with trauma (including surgery) and diabetes. There is edematous bronze or purple discoloration, flaccid bullae with watery brown nonpurulent fluid and a foul odor. The classic clinical presentation is pain out of proportion to the appearance of the injury. Low-grade fever and other systemic signs are also typically present, and may develop rapidly.

Crepitance and appearance of gross pockets of air in the tissue may be appreciated but may not be present early in the course. The incubation period for clostridia ranges between 1 and 4 days, but it can be as early as 6 hours. Decreased tissue oxygen tension along with wound contamination are required for the infection to progress. Crepitant cellulitis, synergistic necrotizing cellulitis, acute streptococcal hemolytic gangrene, and streptococcal myositis are some conditions that may be mistaken for clostridial myositis. Often surgical exploration of the fascia and muscle is required to make the correct diagnosis.

Emergency Department Treatment and Disposition

Aggressive resuscitation should be initiated, and consideration given to packed red blood cell transfusion. Broad-spectrum antibiotics, especially clindamycin, in conjunction with penicillin G, in the non—penicillin-allergic patient, are given in the emergency department. Tetanus prophylaxis must not be overlooked. Surgical debridement or amputation, the mainstays of therapy, must be initiated promptly. Hyperbaric oxygen, in conjunction with surgical and antibiotic therapy, may have a synergistic effect in preventing the progression of infection and production of toxin.

Pearls

1. Clostridial infection should be considered in patients presenting with low-grade fever, tachycardia out of proportion to the fever, and pain out of proportion to physical findings.

2. Shock and multiorgan failure may be rapidly progressive. Mortality is 80% to 90% if untreated, 10% to 25% when treated appropriately.
3. Clindamycin may improve survival by inhibiting toxin production.
4. Gram stain yielding gram-positive bacilli with a relative lack of leukocytes can rapidly confirm clinically suspected clostridial myonecrosis.

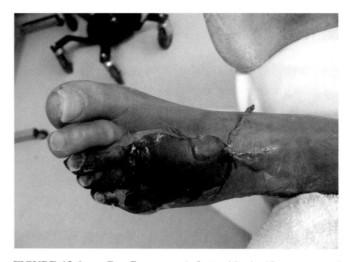

FIGURE 12.6 ■ Gas Gangrene. A foot with significant areas of gangrene and sloughing skin. (Photo contributor: David Kaplan, MD.)

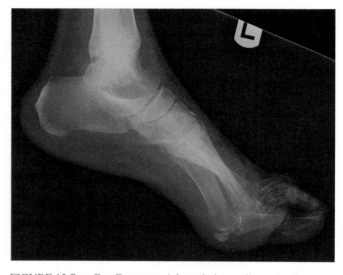

FIGURE 12.7 ■ Gas Gangrene. A lateral view radiograph of the foot in Fig. 12.6 exhibiting pockets of soft tissue gas tracking up the dorsal surface of the foot. (Photo contributor: Douglas Nilson, MD.)

Clinical Summary

This uncommon, severe infection involves the subcutaneous soft tissues, including the superficial and deep fascial layers, with early sparing of the skin and late involvement of the muscle. It is most commonly seen in the lower extremities, abdominal wall, perianal and groin area, and postoperative wounds, but can manifest in any body part. The infection is usually spread from a site of trauma or surgical wound, abscess, decubitus ulcer, or intestinal perforation. Alcoholism, parenteral drug abuse, and diabetes mellitus are predisposing factors. Pain, tenderness, erythema, swelling, warmth, shiny skin, lymphangitis, and lymphadenitis are early clinical findings. Later, there is rapid progression with changes in skin color, formation of bullae with clear pink or purple fluid and cutaneous necrosis within 48 hours. The skin becomes anesthetic and subcutaneous gas may be present. Systemic toxicity may be manifest by fever, dehydration, leukocytosis, and frequently positive blood cultures. Two groups of organisms are implicated in necrotizing fasciitis. Type I includes anaerobic species (*Bacteroides* and *Peptostreptococcus*) and type II group A streptococci alone or with *Staphylococcus aureus*. The differential diagnosis includes cellulitis, osteomyelitis, gas gangrene, streptococcal myonecrosis, infected vascular gangrene, and trauma.

Emergency Department Treatment and Disposition

Prompt diagnosis is critical. If the diagnosis is made within 4 days from symptom onset, the mortality rate is reduced from 50% to 12%. Initial emergency department treatment involves resuscitation with volume expansion, as well as emergent surgical consultation for operative debridement. Prompt initiation of broad-spectrum antibiotics is essential.

Pearls

1. Intravenous calcium replacement may be necessary to reverse hypocalcemia from subcutaneous fat necrosis.
2. Radiographs may be used to detect subcutaneous gas that is not palpable.
3. Hemolysis and disseminated intravascular coagulation (DIC) may be seen in association with necrotizing fasciitis.
4. Antibiotic regimens should include adequate coverage of gram-positive, gram-negative, and anaerobic organisms.
5. Community-acquired MRSA has been implicated in a growing number of cases of necrotizing fasciitis.

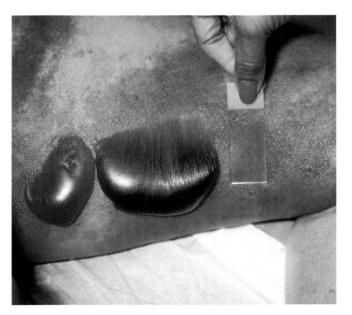

FIGURE 12.8 ■ Necrotizing Fasciitis. Large cutaneous bullae are seen on the leg of this patient with necrotizing fasciitis. Note the dark purple fluid in the bullae. (Photo contributor Lawrence B. Stack, MD.)

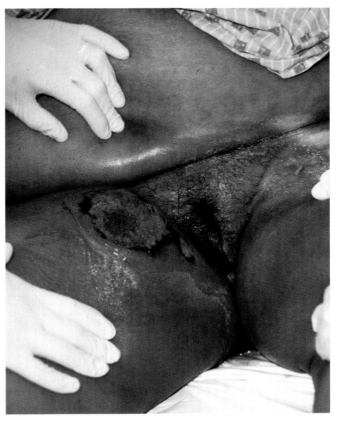

FIGURE 12.9 ■ Necrotizing Fasciitis. Necrotizing fasciitis with cutaneous necrosis can be seen in the inner thigh of this patient. (Photo contributor: Lawrence B. Stack, MD.)

Clinical Summary

Gout is an inflammatory disease characterized by deposition of sodium urate monohydrate crystals in cartilage, subchondral bone, and periarticular structures. An acute attack is characterized by sudden onset of monarticular arthritis, most commonly in the metatarsophalangeal (MTP) joint of the great toe, with swelling, erythema, and tenderness. Gout can also occur in other joints. The deposits of crystals in the tissues about the joint produce a chronic inflammatory response termed a *tophus*.

In pseudogout, calcium pyrophosphate dihydrate (rod- or rhombus-shaped, weakly birefringent) crystals are deposited. Although any joint may be involved, knees and wrists are the most common sites. The acute presenting signs and symptoms are identical with those of gout, but formation of tophi is not seen. Fever, pain, and erythema are common to both entities.

Cellulitis and septic arthritis must be excluded. In the cell count of the synovial fluid from an inflamed joint, 2,000 to 50,000 WBCs with polymorphonuclear neutrophil leukocyte (PMN) predominance is expected. The diagnosis is made by seeing urate or calcium pyrophosphate dihydrate crystals on polarized microscopy coupled with negative Gram stain and cultures.

Emergency Department Treatment and Disposition

Nonsteroidal anti-inflammatory medications are used with excellent results in the acute setting, along with joint immobilization and rest. Colchicine is a reasonable alternative, but it often has side effects such as nausea, vomiting, and diarrhea. It is also associated with serious toxicity, including bone marrow suppression, neuropathy, myopathy, and death (particularly when given intravenously). Intramuscular injection of adrenocorticotropic hormone (ACTH, 40 to 80 units intramuscular or subcutaneous) or steroids may be used in patients with contraindications to colchicine and nonsteroidal anti-inflammatory medications. Allopurinol or probenecid are used in the chronic management of gout and play no role in acute treatment.

Pearls

1. Most (90%) of patients with crystalline-induced synovitis are male and older than 40 years.
2. Serum urate may be *normal* in acute gout.
3. Acute gouty arthritis attacks may be triggered by minor trauma, diuretic or salicylate use, alcohol, or diet.

4. Punched out lesions on subchondral bone may be seen on radiography in chronic tophaceous gout. Chondrocalcinosis may be seen in pseudogout.

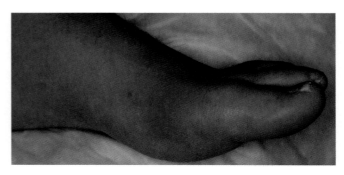

FIGURE 12.10 ■ Podagra. Podagra denotes gouty inflammation of the first MTP joint. Note the swelling and erythema. (Photo contributor: Kevin J. Knoop, MD, MS.)

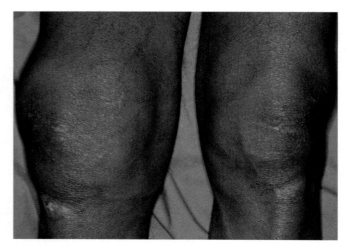

FIGURE 12.11 ■ Gout. Large tophi of gout located in and around the right knee. (Photo contributor: Daniel L. Savitt, MD.)

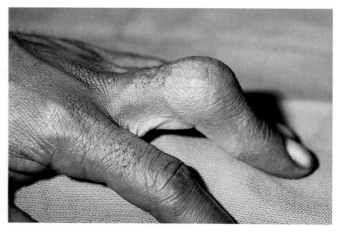

FIGURE 12.12 ■ Gout. The finger is an unusual site for gouty arthritis. (Photo contributor: Alan B. Storrow, MD.)

Clinical Summary

This painful condition is the result of impingement and puncture of the medial or lateral nail fold epithelium by the nail plate, allowing the nail to grow into the dermis. Tenderness and swelling of the nail fold is followed by granulation tissue growth causing sharp pain, erythema, and further swelling. If not promptly treated, the granulation tissue becomes epithelialized, preventing elevation of the nail above the medial or lateral nail groove. Often there is secondary bacterial or fungal infection. Risk factors include cutting the nail too short, tightly-fitting shoes, and trauma. The differential diagnosis includes paronychia, felon, and tumor.

Emergency Department Treatment and Disposition

Early treatment: Elevation of the nail out of nail fold and placement of gauze under nail to prevent contact, in conjunction with warm soaks, is the initial mode of therapy. *Late treatment*: Surgical management involves removal of part of the nail and the inflamed tissue and sometimes destruction of the involved nail matrix. In the emergency department (ED), the lateral portion of the affected nail is removed followed by packing of the paronychial fold with petroleum gauze or other non-adherent dressing. Follow-up by a podiatrist until growth of the nail plate is complete should be considered. The destruction of the nail matrix is required only in patients with recurrent infected ingrown toenails and is not part of routine ED management.

Pearls

1. Ingrown toenail is most common in the great toe, is associated with tight-fitting footwear, and may result from improper nail trimming (ie, cutting the nail too short).
2. Use of antibiotics is not a substitute for surgical excision and will result in only transient improvement of symptoms.

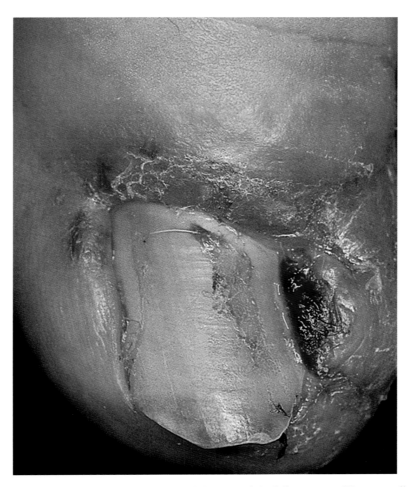

FIGURE 12.13 ■ Ingrown Toenail. An ingrown toenail on the medial aspect of the left great toe. (Photo contributor: Frank Birinyi, MD.)

Clinical Summary

Inflammation of lymphatic channels in the subcutaneous tissues is commonly caused by the spread of local bacterial infection. Group A β-hemolytic streptococcal (GABHS) species are the most frequently implicated agent. Lymphangitis is characterized by red linear streaks extending from the primary site of infection (eg, abscess, cellulitis) to regional lymph nodes (eg, axilla, groin). The lymph nodes are often enlarged and tender. There may be associated peripheral edema of the involved extremity. Lymphangitis may develop within 24 to 48 hours of the initial infection. The differential diagnosis includes cellulitis, trauma, and superficial thrombophlebitis.

Emergency Department Treatment and Disposition

Rest, elevation, and immobilization in addition to antibiotics are the mainstays of treatment. Lymphangitis may be treated with oral antibiotics in afebrile patients who are not immunocompromised. Coverage for *Streptococcus* and *Staphylococcus* is appropriate. Toxic-appearing patients require admission for parenteral antibiotics. Any patient sent home with oral antibiotics should be followed up in 24 to 48 hours. Patients who subsequently do not show improvement require admission for parenteral antibiotic therapy.

Pearls

1. Consider *Pasteurella multocida* with cat and dog bites, *Spirillum minus* with rat bites, and *Mycobacterium marinum* in association with swimming pools and aquaria.
2. Chronic lymphangitis may be associated with mycotic, mycobacterial, and filarial infection.
3. In Africa and Southeast Asia, filariasis (*Wuchereria bancrofti*) is the most common etiologic agent.
4. Aspiration of the leading edge is generally not helpful for acute management.

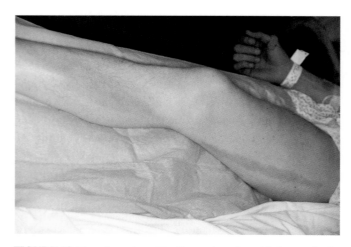

FIGURE 12.14 ■ Lymphangitis. Severe lymphangitis is seen in the lower extremity. The red streak extends from the ankle to the groin and follows lymphatic channels. In this case, the site of infection was the great toe. (Photo contributor: Liudvikas Jagminas, MD.)

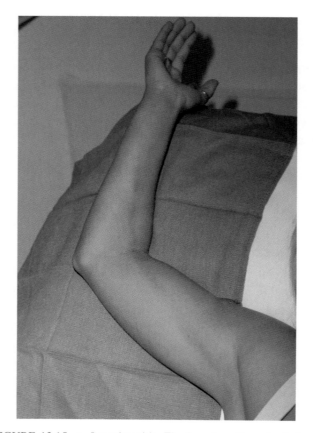

FIGURE 12.15 ■ Lymphangitis. The lymphangitis extends from the wrist to the upper arm. Lymphangitis in the upper extremity commonly arises from nail biting. (Photo contributor: R. Jason Thurman, MD.)

Clinical Summary

Lymphedema occurs from obstruction of lymphatic channels and is associated with malignancy, radiation, trauma, surgery, inflammation, infection, parasitic invasion, paralysis, renal insufficiency, congestive heart failure, cirrhosis, and malnutrition. Lymphedema is characterized by painless pitting edema, fatigue, increase in limb size (particularly during the day), and presence of lymph vesicles. The skin becomes thickened and brown in the late stages. Cellulitis, deep venous thrombosis (DVT), lymphangitis, traumatic hematoma, right heart failure, tuberculosis, and lymphogranuloma venereum should be considered when the diagnosis of lymphedema is made. Imaging techniques of the lymphatic system include radionuclide imaging (lymphoscintigraphy), which is the preferred method, and lymphangiography.

Emergency Department Treatment and Disposition

Control of edema with elevation, pneumatic compression boots and firm elastic stockings, maintenance of healthy skin, and avoidance of cellulitis and lymphangitis are the mainstays of symptomatic treatment. Treatment of the underlying disease may be curative.

Pearls

1. Swelling usually starts distally and progresses proximally.
2. The dorsum of the toes and feet are always involved in lymphedema, unlike other causes of edema.
3. Careful examination for heart failure and screening for renal insufficiency should be completed for all patients with lymphedema.
4. Patients with chronic lymphedema are at risk for development of a rare secondary malignancy, lymphangiosarcoma, characterized by red-blue or purple macular or papular lesions.

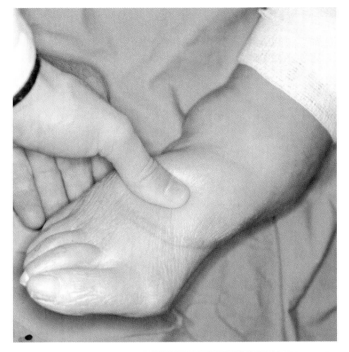

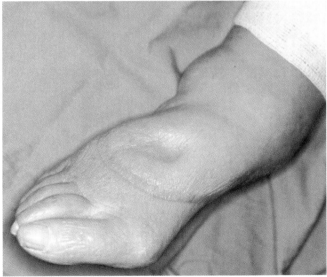

FIGURE 12.16 ■ Pitting Edema. Pitting edema is seen in a woman with lymphedema of the lower extremities. Note how the impression of the thumb remains on the foot. (Photo contributor: Selim Suner, MD, MS.)

Clinical Summary

Bursitis is an inflammatory reaction in a fluid-filled synovial sac, commonly over the subacromial, prepatellar, olecranon, or trochanteric bursa. It is associated with repetitive motion, trauma, or infection. The fluid collection may be bacterial (septic bursitis), gouty, or, most commonly, inflammatory. Bursitis is characterized by pain, tenderness, swelling, warmth, and limited range of motion. It is critical to differentiate septic from benign inflammation.

Since bursitis does not involve the intraarticular space, signs and symptoms should be isolated to the bursal area. Typically, intraarticular arthritis is associated with pain on minor range of motion, while the discomfort of bursitis occurs with stretching of the skin and synovial sac at extreme ranges of joint movement. When this differentiation is difficult by history and examination, fluid aspiration and analysis of the joint fluid for cell count, Gram stain, protein, glucose, and polarized microscopy (see "Crystal-Induced Synovitis," above) may be helpful. Fluid with >50,000 cells per cubic millimeter, polymorphonuclear neutrophil predominance, increased protein, reduced glucose, and a positive Gram stain are associated with bacterial infection.

Emergency Department Treatment and Disposition

Rest, bulky compression dressings, and nonsteroidal anti-inflammatory medications are the initial treatment of choice for inflammatory bursitis. Bursal injection of local anesthetics mixed with corticosteroids can be considered if septic bursitis has been ruled out, usually in patients who have failed treatment with NSAIDs. Reducing the effusion volume by aspiration may provide temporary relief, although the fluid has a propensity to recur. Septic bursitis requires aspiration, gram-positive antibiotic coverage, and consideration of open incision and drainage by orthopedic surgery. Most patients can be treated as outpatients with follow-up.

Pearls

1. Septic joint infections in patients with cancer, who are taking corticosteroids, or who are IV drug users may have lower synovial fluid leukocyte counts (<30,000/mm^3) than usual (>50,000/mm^3).

2. Bursal fluid from a septic bursitis typically has a lower nucleated cell count than septic joint fluid; lower limits of 2000/mm^3 have been proposed.

3. *Staphylococcus aureus* is the most common etiologic agent.

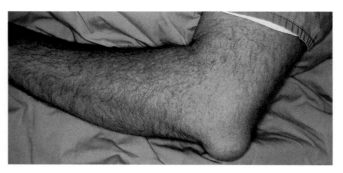

FIGURE 12.17 ■ Olecranon Bursitis. Olecranon bursitis is evident in this flexed elbow. (Photo contributor Selim Suner, MD, MS.)

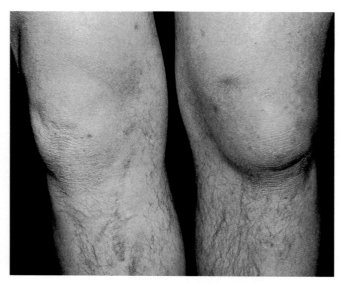

FIGURE 12.18 ■ Prepatellar Bursitis. Local bursal swelling is evident over the left knee. (Photo contributor: Kevin J. Knoop, MD, MS.)

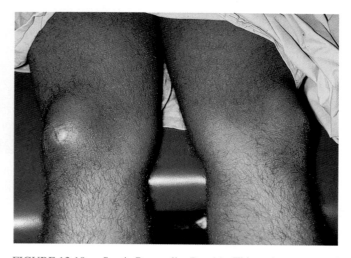

FIGURE 12.19 ■ Septic Prepatellar Bursitis. This patient presented with obvious purulence of his right prepatellar bursal sac. Aspiration confirmed septic bursitis. (Photo contributor Alan B. Storrow, MD.)

Clinical Summary

Palmar space infections occur within the deep fascial spaces of the hand. These infections commonly arise from direct trauma such as puncture wounds to the palm, spread from flexor tenosynovitis of the digits, or hematogenous spread. The palm loses its concavity, and there is dorsal swelling. In addition, tenderness, erythema, warmth, and fluctuance are evident in the palm. A *thenar space* infection is characterized by swelling over the thenar eminence and pain with abduction of the thumb. With a *midpalmar space* infection, motion is limited and painful for the middle and ring fingers. Infection in the web spaces may involve both the palmar and dorsal sides, forming the classic hourglass-shaped abscess (collar button abscess). Cellulitis, local traumatic injury, fractures, and soft tissue mass are included in the differential diagnosis.

Emergency Department Treatment and Disposition

All deep space infections of the hand should be managed by a hand surgeon. Prompt incision and drainage in the operating room is necessary for the best outcome. Parenteral antibiotics against *Staphylococcus aureus* as well as anaerobes should be started in the emergency department.

Pearls

1. Palmar space infections may cause swelling on the dorsal hand due to the dorsal location of hand lymphatics.
2. There may be minimal signs of swelling over the palmar surface.
3. Infections may be associated with compartment syndrome of the hand.

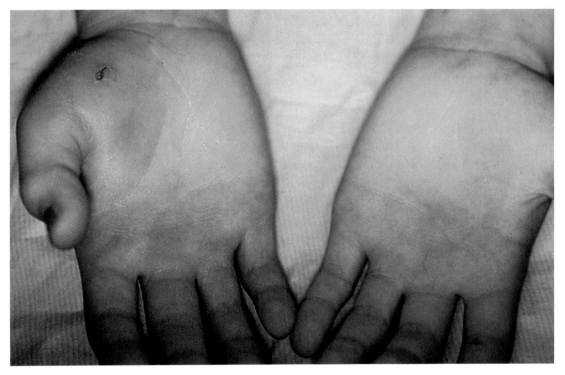

FIGURE 12.20 ■ Palmar Space Infection. Thenar space infection following injury to the thumb. In this palmar view, erythema and swelling in the right thenar area and abduction of the thumb are evident. (Photo contributor: Richard Zienowicz, MD.)

Clinical Summary

Tenosynovitis, an inflammation of the tendon and the surrounding synovial sheath, is characterized by pain and tenderness. Pyogenic flexor tenosynovitis is a very serious infection of the tendon sheath resulting from puncture wounds, local extension, or hematogenous origin. Pyogenic flexor tenosynovitis is characterized by the four cardinal Kanavel signs of: finger held in mild flexion; fusiform swelling of the digit; tenderness along the entire tendon sheath, especially at the palmar surface of the metacarpophalangeal (MCP) joint; and severe pain with passive extension. Tenosynovitis may be complicated by fibrosis and adhesions leading to stiffness, loss of function, and tendon necrosis from destruction of the blood supply.

Inflammatory flexor tenosynovitis is typically due to rheumatoid arthritis, overuse, diabetes mellitus, or connective tissue disorders. The time course is typically more indolent than that of pyogenic flexor tenosynovitis, although the sequelae can be similar. The differential diagnosis includes: cellulitis, traumatic injury, lymphangitis, osteomyelitis, septic arthritis, and allergic reactions.

Emergency Department Treatment and Disposition

It is difficult to distinguish infectious and noninfectious etiologies early in the course of this illness. Early (24 to 48 hours) management of tenosynovitis thought to be noninfectious is accomplished with immobilization and nonsteroidal anti-inflammatory medications. Broad-spectrum parenteral antibiotics, rest, immobilization, elevation, compressive dressing, and emergent consultation with a hand surgeon for incision and drainage are mandated with pyogenic flexor tenosynovitis.

Pearls

1. *Staphylococcus aureus* is the most common organism, but *Streptococcus* as well as gram-negative and anaerobic organisms may also be responsible.
2. The most specific sign of tenosynovitis is pain with passive extension of the digit.
3. Patients with immunocompromised states or recently administered antibiotics may not exhibit the classic tetrad of Kanavel signs.

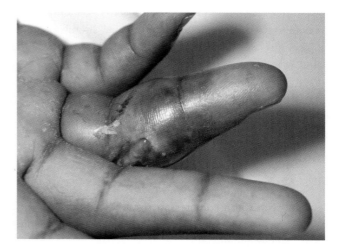

FIGURE 12.22 ■ Flexor Tenosynovitis. Pyogenic flexor tenosynovitis of the fourth finger with fusiform swelling, tenderness along the flexor tendon sheath, and pain on flexion. (Photo contributor: Lawrence B. Stack, MD.)

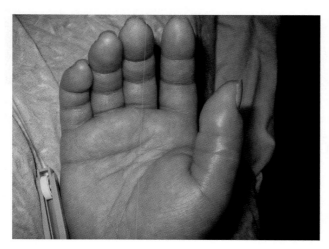

FIGURE 12.21 ■ Tenosynovitis. A suppurative flexor tenosynovitis of the thumb. Note the fusiform swelling and the position of slightly fixed flexion. (Photo contributor: Selim Suner, MD, MS.)

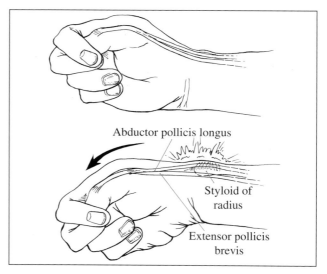

Abductor pollicis longus

Styloid of radius

Extensor pollicis brevis

FIGURE 12.23 ■ Finkelstein Test. Pain over the radial styloid is elicited with ulnar deviation of the wrist as shown.

Clinical Summary

Thrombophlebitis is superficial thrombosis and inflammation of veins or varicosities characterized by redness, tenderness, and potentially palpable, indurated, cordlike venous segments. Common causes of thrombophlebitis are intravenous catheter insertion, irritant solutions through the intravenous line, and trauma. Pregnancy and recent postpartum states have also been associated with increased risk of superficial thrombophlebitis. There is little risk of embolism when this condition is associated with varicose veins or superficial veins distal to the popliteal fossa; however, pulmonary embolism can occur secondary to propagation of the thrombus to more proximal veins of the deep venous system, particularly when the greater saphenous vein is involved. Septic superficial thrombophlebitis, lymphangitis, deep venous thrombosis (DVT), and cellulitis should be included in the differential diagnosis of thrombophlebitis. The patient should be evaluated for the possibility of DVT if no underlying cause of superficial thrombosis is elucidated.

Emergency Department Treatment and Disposition

Elevation with warm compresses, rest, and analgesia is sufficient treatment for uncomplicated superficial thrombophlebitis. Superficial thrombophlebitis with involvement of the saphenofemoral or iliofemoral system requires treatment as a DVT. Admission to the hospital is warranted if there is extensive involvement, septic signs, progression of symptoms despite treatment, or severe inflammatory reactions.

Pearls

1. Thrombophlebitis of the greater saphenous vein may be confused with lymphangitis, since the lymphatic drainage from the leg runs along the vein.
2. The superficial femoral vein, despite its name, is considered a deep vein, and thrombosis involving this requires standard treatment for DVT.
3. Although there are no conclusive studies, anticoagulation should be considered for lower extremity thrombophlebitis involving the greater saphenous vein close to the femoral junction.

4. Thrombophlebitis of the upper extremity is very unlikely to progress to deep venous thrombosis.
5. Suppurative thrombophlebitis should be suspected with high fevers, or signs of extensive erythema or purulent drainage.

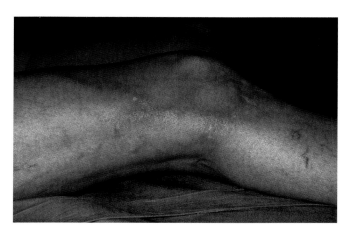

FIGURE 12.24 ■ Thrombophlebitis. This photograph shows thrombophlebitis of the superficial veins in the leg. The thrombosed veins are erythematous, close to the surface, and palpable. (Photo contributor: Lawrence B. Stack, MD.)

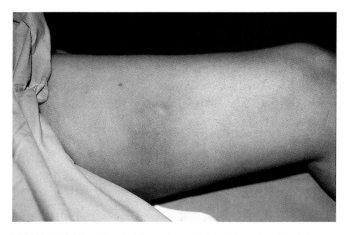

FIGURE 12.25 ■ Septic Thrombophlebitis. Thrombophlebitis may be complicated by bacterial infection. Note the purulence associated with the erythematous thrombosed veins. (Photo contributor: Lawrence B. Stack, MD.)

Clinical Summary

Paronychia is the most common infection seen in the hand and is characterized by inflammation and pus accumulation along a lateral nail fold. Paronychia may spread to involve the eponychium at the base of the nail and the opposite nail fold if untreated. *Staphylococcus aureus* is the most frequently isolated organism, although the infection is generally mixed flora. Felon, dactylitis, herpetic whitlow, hydrofluoric acid burn, and traumatic injury should be considered in the differential diagnosis.

Emergency Department Treatment and Disposition

If paronychia is recognized early, prior to frank abscess formation, warm soaks with or without oral antibiotics may be sufficient. After 2 to 3 days, there may be sufficient accumulation of pus along the eponychial fold to warrant incision and drainage. After digital block, a #11 blade or 18-gauge needle is advanced parallel to the nail and under the eponychium at the site of maximal fluctuance. This should enable easy evacuation of the pus. If pus has collected under the nail (subungual abscess), then a portion of the nail must be removed to provide drainage. Incisions should be packed open with gauze (removed in 24 to 48 hours). Oral antibiotics should be prescribed, and the finger should be reevaluated in 2 to 3 days.

Pearls

1. Paronychia is associated with nail biting, manicure trauma, and small foreign bodies.
2. Superinfection with fungal agents may occur in immuno-compromised patients or chronic, neglected paronychia.
3. Damage to the germinal matrix during excision of the nail plate may result in nail deformity.
4. It is important to distinguish a paronychia from herpetic whitlow, where incision and drainage is contraindicated.
5. Paronychia may occur in the toes as well as the fingers.

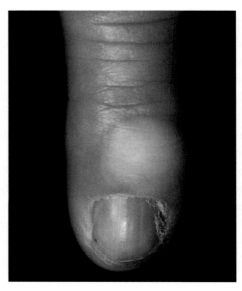

FIGURE 12.26 ■ Paronychia. A paronychia involving one lateral fold and the eponychium. There is swelling, erythema, and tenderness on the dorsum of the distal phalanx. (Photo contributor: Frank Birinyi, MD.)

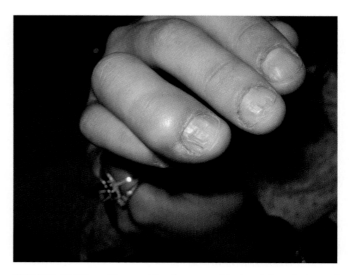

FIGURE 12.27 ■ Paronychia. A paronychia involving the lateral nail fold and eponychium. Note the area of fluctuance along the lateral nail fold and extending along the dorsum of the distal phalanx. (Photo contributor: Selim Suner, MD, MS.)

Clinical Summary

Thrombosis of the subclavian vein (Paget-von Schroetter syndrome) is an uncommon condition, typically occurring in young patients following exercise and compression injury to the subclavian or axillary vein from a narrow thoracic outlet (effort thrombosis). Symptoms of pain, discomfort, and tightness or swelling in the arm are manifest within a day. Pitting edema develops in the fingers, hand, and forearm. There is no arterial insufficiency, and the pulses are palpable. This syndrome is separate from iatrogenic upper extremity thrombosis, generally as a result of vascular access catheters. There is a 15% risk of developing pulmonary embolism from thrombosis of veins in the upper extremity; however, large or fatal emboli from this source are very rare. Ultrasound has become the screening test of choice in most institutions.

Superior vena cava syndrome, trauma to the upper extremity, congestive heart failure, angioedema, and lymphatic obstruction must be considered in the differential diagnosis.

Emergency Department Treatment and Disposition

Treatment consists of elevation, local heat, analgesia, and anticoagulation with heparin for patients presenting with long-term thrombosis. Patients should be admitted to the hospital. In cases of acute thrombosis (within 5 days of symptom onset), thrombolysis with direct catheter infusion of thrombolytic agents may be considered. Surgical thrombectomy has also been employed. Operative correction of anatomic abnormalities should be accomplished to prevent long-term morbidity.

Pearls

1. Swelling of the neck and face may signify thrombosis or compression of the superior vena cava.
2. The superficial veins in the upper extremity are often distended and do not collapse when the arm is elevated.
3. There is a greater incidence of subclavian vein thrombosis in men and in the right arm.
4. Late sequelae related to the thrombus include pain, recurrent swelling, and early fatigue of the upper extremity.
5. Ultrasound may be limited in visualizing nonocclusive mural thrombi, or those located in the proximal subclavian or innominate veins.

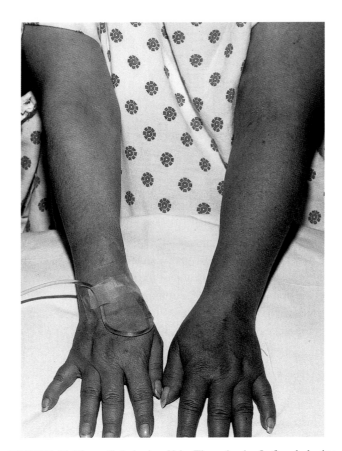

FIGURE 12.28 ■ Subclavian Vein Thrombosis. Left subclavian vein thrombosis manifested by swelling of the upper extremity. (Photo contributor: Frank Birinyi, MD.)

Clinical Summary

Cervical radiculopathy is often caused by compression of a nerve root by a laterally bulging or herniated intervertebral disk. Osteoarthritis and degenerative spondylosis may also cause radiculopathy in the cervical spine. Pain results from injury to the nerve roots and nerves innervating the dura, ligaments, facet joints, and bone. Common clinical features associated with cervical radiculopathy include pain, paresthesia, and root signs (sensory loss, lower motor neuron muscle weakness, impaired reflexes, and trophic changes). The pain is sharp, stabbing, and worse with cough; it often radiates over the shoulder and down the arm. Frequently there is numbness and tingling following a dermatomal distribution. Root signs may be found corresponding to anatomic distribution of nerves. Magnetic resonance imaging (MRI) has become the test of choice to distinguish cervical radiculopathy from disc and bone disease. Electromyelography studies may also be helpful in ruling out other disease processes.

Trauma, myelopathy, plexopathy, neurofibromatosis, metastatic tumor infiltration of nerve roots, neoplasm, shingles, and central cord syndrome should be considered in the differential diagnosis.

Emergency Department Treatment and Disposition

The mainstay of emergency department treatment is pain control and referral to an orthopedic surgeon or neurosurgeon. Although adequate pain control often requires narcotic analgesics, appropriate doses of nonsteroidal anti-inflammatory drugs should also be initiated in patients without contraindications. Since prolonged nerve root compression can lead to permanent neurologic deficits, immediate referral is necessary for progressive neurologic signs. Patients with intractable pain, progressive weakness in the upper extremities, and myelopathy should be admitted to the hospital.

Pearls

1. Most radiculopathies resulting from cervical disk disease is seen in the 30- to 60-year age group and in the C5 to C7 region.

2. Risk factors for cervical radiculopathy include heavy lifting, cigarette smoking, frequent diving from a board, and prior neck trauma.

3. Patients with acute cervical radiculopathy may present with their upper extremity supported by their head to counteract the cervical root distraction caused by the weight of their dependent extremity.

4. CT myelography may be the next most appropriate study in patients with a contraindication to MRI.

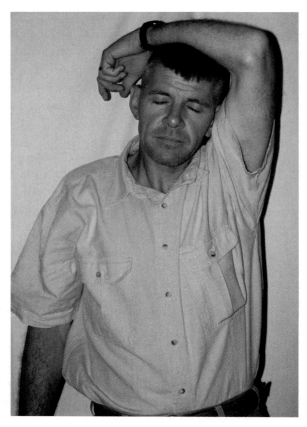

FIGURE 12.29 ■ Cervical Radiculopathy. This is the classic position of relief for cervical radicular pain. This patient presented with severe pain in the neck with radiation to the extremity. The only way the patient was able to get relief was by holding his arm over his head in the position shown. This patient has a C5 to C6 herniated nucleus pulposus. (Photo contributor: Kevin J. Knoop, MD, MS.)

Clinical Summary

Digital clubbing is characterized by bulbous fusiform enlargement of the distal portion of a digit with loss of the angle between the proximal nail fold and the nail plate (Lovibond angle). Associated with the increased tissue mass is enhanced blood flow, excessive curvature of the fingernails, and hyperemic and swollen skin folds around the fingernail. Clubbing may also be seen in the toes. The mechanism underlying clubbing is not known, but it is postulated that the end result is dilatation of the distal digital blood vessels with soft tissue hypertrophy. Clubbing may be hereditary, idiopathic, or acquired and is associated with multiple medical conditions including carcinoma, intrathoracic sepsis, bacterial endocarditis, cyanotic congenital heart disease, esophageal disorders, cirrhosis, inflammatory bowel disease, pulmonary disorders, atrial myxoma, repeated pregnancies, and pachydermoperiostosis. The incidence of clubbing with each of these conditions is variable. Digital clubbing may be reversible in certain disease processes.

Emergency Department Treatment and Disposition

Treatment of the underlying condition is indicated. The disposition depends on the underlying diagnosis and condition of the patient.

Pearls

1. Bone radiographs can be used to diagnose hypertrophic osteoarthropathy. Subperiosteal formation of bone is seen in the distal diaphyses of long bones.
2. Patients rarely recognize clubbing in their own fingers even if the condition is marked.
3. Pseudoclubbing is an overcurvature of the nails in both longitudinal and transverse axes, with preservation of the angle between the proximal nail fold and nail plate.

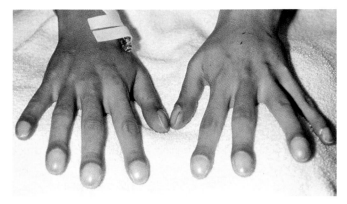

FIGURE 12.30 ■ Clubbing. Marked digital clubbing can be seen in this patient. Note the hyperemia in the skin folds around the nail. (Photo contributor: Alan B. Storrow, MD.)

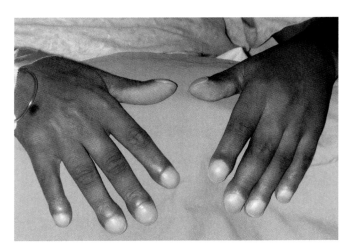

FIGURE 12.31 ■ Clubbing. Note the loss of the angle between the proximal nail fold and the nail plate (Lovibond angle). (Photo contributor: Robert J. Tubbs, MD.)

Clinical Summary

Phlegmasia alba dolens (painful white leg, or milk leg) is caused by massive thrombosis of the iliofemoral veins and characterized by pitting edema of the entire lower extremity, tenderness in the inguinal area, and a pale extremity secondary to arterial occlusion. *Phlegmasia cerulea dolens* (painful blue leg) arises from thrombosis of the veins in the lower extremity including the perforating and collateral veins resulting in venous ischemia with a cool, painful, swollen, tense, and cyanotic-appearing lower extremity. Occasionally there is bullae formation; compartment syndrome and gangrene may follow.

The differential diagnosis includes arterial insufficiency or thrombosis, aortic dissection, abdominal aortic aneurysm, cellulitis, and lymphedema. Doppler ultrasound, impedance plethysmography, and venography (most accurate for determining extent) are used in the diagnosis.

Emergency Department Treatment and Disposition

Systemic anticoagulation with intravenous heparin is indicated for this condition. If there is no improvement in 12 to 24 hours, then iliofemoral venous thrombosis should be suspected. The role of intravenous thrombolytic therapy remains controversial, but can be considered.

Pearls

1. Pregnancy is one risk factor for phlegmasia alba dolens.
2. Forty-four percent of patients with phlegmasia cerulea dolens have an underlying malignancy.
3. Phlegmasia dolens is seen in fewer than 10% of patients with venous thrombosis.
4. Hypotension may result from venous pooling of blood in the lower extremity and diminished venous return.
5. Invasive procedures such as catheter fragmentation and extraction techniques show promise in reducing post-phlebitic syndrome in patients with phlegmasia cerulea dolens.

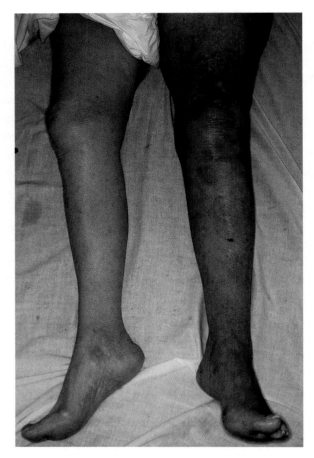

FIGURE 12.32 ■ Phlegmasia Cerulea Dolens. Phlegmasia cerulea dolens of the left lower extremity. Note the bluish discoloration and swelling. (Photo contributor: Daniel L. Savitt, MD.)

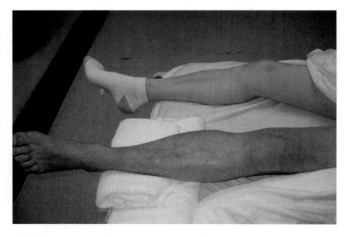

FIGURE 12.33 ■ Phlegmasia Cerulea Dolens. Another example of discoloration and edema secondary to phlegmasia cerulea dolens. (Photo contributor: Selim Suner, MD.)

Clinical Summary

Deep venous thrombosis (DVT) is often encountered in patients with intrinsic coagulopathy or impaired fibrinolysis, or those who have had recent (within 3 months) surgery or trauma. Other associated conditions include immobilization, increased estrogen (pregnancy, oral contraceptives) with smoking, malignancy, prior DVT, inflammatory disease processes, or coronary artery disease. Intravenous catheters are also a major cause of DVT, particularly in the upper extremity. Unilateral swelling and tenderness, classically in the calf and thigh, characterize DVT. Doppler ultrasonography is the screening test of choice in most institutions. In selected low-risk patients a quantitative D-dimer study may be used to rule out DVT.

Fracture, lymphedema, heart failure, compartment syndrome, myositis, arthritis, and superficial phlebitis should also be considered.

Emergency Department Treatment and Disposition

Classic treatment of DVT has been heparin anticoagulation and admission for warfarin loading. However, in recent years low-molecular weight heparin (LMWH) has been shown to be more efficacious for initial treatment. It has also allowed outpatient treatment in a subgroup of patients. Thrombolysis should be reserved for severe cases, where the viability of the extremity is threatened. Although DVT in the calf and superficial veins of the lower extremity do not typically embolize, these thrombi can propagate into the deep venous system and may eventually lead to emboli. Serial diagnostic studies are performed to follow the course of untreated DVT of the distal calf.

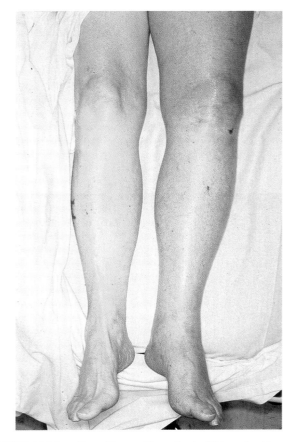

FIGURE 12.34 ■ Deep Venous Thrombosis. This patient has some classic findings of left lower extremity DVT: swelling, erythema, pain, and tenderness. (Photo contributor: Kevin J. Knoop, MD, MS.)

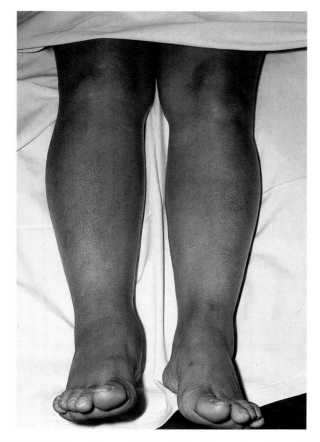

FIGURE 12.35 ■ Ruptured Baker Cyst. Circumferential swelling around the right ankle. MRI revealed a ruptured Baker cyst in the right popliteal fossa. This may mimic acute lower extremity DVT. (Photo contributor: Lawrence B. Stack, MD.)

Pearls

1. A Baker cyst, herniation of the synovial membrane through the posterior knee capsule, may rupture, causing unilateral calf swelling similar to DVT.
2. Patients with unexplained DVT should be screened for occult malignancy.
3. Homan sign (calf pain during passive dorsiflexion) is unreliable in the diagnosis of DVT.
4. Patients with an unclear diagnosis of cellulitis should have an objective study to rule out DVT.
5. It is important to note that the superficial femoral vein is, despite the name, a part of the deep venous system; thrombosis there requires systemic anticoagulation.

Clinical Summary

Dupuytren contracture results from shortening and fibrotic changes of the subcutaneous tissues of the palm and longitudinal bands of the palmar aponeurosis. It may begin as a nodule and then progress to contracture of a finger or fingers. Usually, this is noted at the metacarpophalangeal (MCP) joint, but the proximal interphalangeal (PIP) or distal interphalangeal (DIP) joint, may be involved.

Emergency Department Treatment and Disposition

The only effective treatment is surgery. Patient education and referral to a hand surgeon is recommended. Recurrence and development of a contracture in other areas may occur.

Pearls

1. The flexor tendons are not involved.
2. The ring and small fingers are the most commonly involved.
3. Alcoholic liver disease is associated with an increased risk of development of Dupuytren contracture.

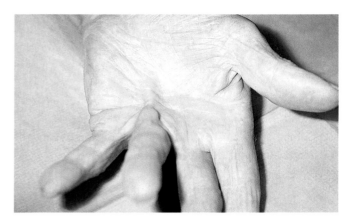

FIGURE 12.36 ■ Dupuytren Contracture. This chronic problem is seen at the most common site: the ring finger. (Photo contributor: Alan B. Storrow, MD.)

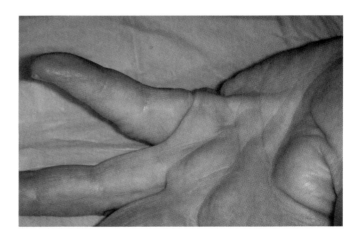

FIGURE 12.37 ■ Dupuytren Contracture. Note the contracture at the metacarpophalangeal joint characteristic of Dupuytren contracture. (Photo contributor: Vineet Mehan, MD.)

Clinical Summary

Achilles tendonitis refers to a spectrum of disease ranging from nonpainful nodules in the actual Achilles tendon to painful swelling of the tendon and paratendon sheath. It most typically develops from overuse, usually after sudden changes in activity or training level. It often occurs in older recreational athletes, who are generally more sedentary and deconditioned, although it may also occur in younger, well-conditioned athletes. Multiple factors generally contribute to the condition, including inappropriate footwear, training on poor surfaces, or prolonged running or jumping. High-risk factors include anatomic abnormalities, such as cavus feet, tibia vara, and heel or forefoot varus deformities. A tight Achilles tendon may develop in women who frequently wear high-heeled shoes, or in patients who wear boots with high heels.

The most common area of pain is typically the area 2 to 6 cm proximal to the insertion site. This is due to a relative paucity of blood vessels in that region, making it more susceptible to inflammation and degeneration from repetitive microtrauma. Patients typically present complaining of pain over the heel. Pain and tenderness increase with dorsiflexion of the foot. In some cases a tendon friction rub may be palpable.

Emergency Department Treatment and Disposition

Careful examination should be performed to distinguish between Achilles tendonitis and tendon rupture. The Thompson test and palpation of the tendon for gaps or discontinuity should be performed on all patients. Any patients with suspicion of partial or complete tendon rupture should be splinted and urgently referred to orthopedic surgery. In cases of tendonitis, gentle progressive stretching and lengthening exercises are helpful. In athletes presenting with tendonitis, a reduction in activity is recommended, especially on hills or climbing. Use of gel heel inserts may be helpful in the short term, by cushioning and raising the heel, thereby decreasing tendon excursion. Use of ice and nonsteroidal anti-inflammatory drugs are generally useful in reducing pain and inflammation. Referral to an orthopedic surgeon for physical therapy is generally indicated in refractory cases.

Pearls

1. Fluoroquinolone use has been reported to increase the risk of Achilles tendonitis and possible tendon rupture. Patients presenting with pain, who are currently taking a fluoroquinolone, should have alternative antibiotic therapy strongly considered.
2. Corticosteroid injection for Achilles tendonitis is very controversial, and should not be performed in the emergency department.
3. Bilateral tendon involvement, especially at the insertion site, suggests a systemic inflammatory condition such as ankylosing spondylitis, reactive arthritis (Reiter syndrome), or psoriatic arthritis.

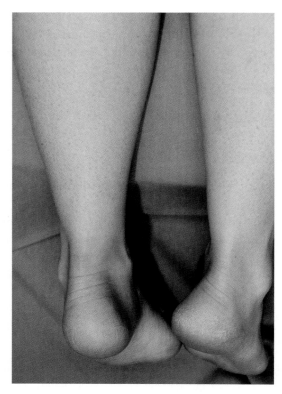

FIGURE 12.38 ■ Achilles Tendonitis. Note the significant erythema and thickening of the Achilles tendon on the patient's left compared to the unaffected right side. (Photo contributor: Kevin J. Knoop, MD, MS.)

GANGLION (SYNOVIAL) CYST

Clinical Summary

Ganglion (synovial) cysts are a cystic swelling overlying a joint or tendon sheath. They are the most common soft-tissue tumors of the hand and wrist, although they can arise over any joint. The etiology is currently debated; the most commonly accepted theory is that the cyst forms secondary to mucoid degeneration of collagen and connective tissues. Other theories postulate a traumatic origin. It is unclear whether repetitive motion leads to causation, although it does appear to provoke symptoms and possibly lead to enlargement of the cyst. They may occur in any age, although the majority arise in patients between the second and fourth decades of life.

Ganglion cysts are composed of collagen fiber walls with clear, highly viscous mucin content within. They may be unilocular or multilocular. The most common presentations include swelling over or in close proximity to a joint, as well as pain, limitation of motion, weakness, and paresthesias. They are rarely greater than 2 cm in diameter. The most common location is dorsally over the scapholunate ligament of the wrist (60%-70%), with the volar wrist the next most common site (20%).

Emergency Department Treatment and Disposition

Ganglion cysts may spontaneously regress; therefore treatment is generally reserved for symptomatic lesions. The treatments include both nonsurgical and surgical options. The most common nonsurgical option is aspiration of the cyst contents, generally using a 16-gauge needle, followed by steroid injection. For recurrent lesions referral to a hand surgeon for excision is generally warranted.

Pearls

1. Transillumination may aid in differentiating a ganglion cyst from a solid tumor; ganglia transilluminate, while solid lesions do not.
2. Patients with chronic dorsal wrist pain of unknown etiology should be screened for occult ganglion cysts.
3. MRI or ultrasound may be useful in detecting occult ganglion cysts.

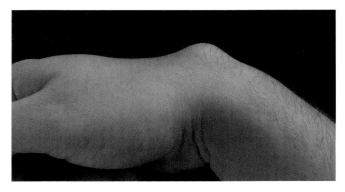

FIGURE 12.39 ■ Ganglion Cyst. This large ganglion cyst is located over the scapholunate ligament, the most common location for this entity. (Photo contributor: Lawrence B. Stack, MD.)

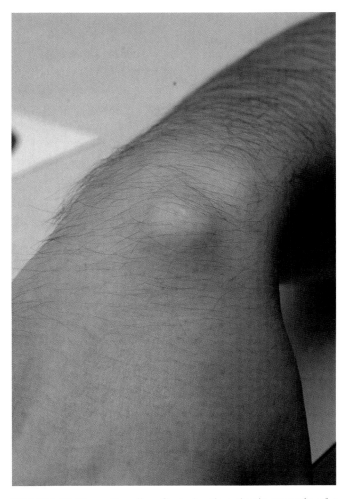

FIGURE 12.40 ■ Ganglion Cyst. Another classic example of a ganglion cyst located over the scapholunate ligament of the wrist. (Photo contributor: Lawrence B. Stack, MD.)

Clinical Summary

Raynaud disease refers to reversible ischemia of peripheral arterioles, usually in response to exposure to cold or emotional stress. The phenomenon is manifested by sharply demarcated color changes of the skin primarily of the digits. In general, it is more prevalent in women and most often affects the hand, although the toes may be involved as well. Cutaneous vasospasm may also affect other areas, including face, ears nose, and nipples.

A typical episode usually starts suddenly with the onset of cold digits associated with sharply demarcated color changes. The skin may be white or blue initially. With rewarming, the skin develops erythema due to a reactive hyperemia. The vasospasm may last for several hours, but usually resolves with removal of the initial stimulus.

The nomenclature for the disease differs somewhat, but in general it is called Raynaud disease, or primary Raynaud phenomenon, if these symptoms occur without evidence of any other associated disease process. In contrast, secondary Raynaud phenomenon occurs when the symptoms occur in association with a related disease process such as systemic lupus erythematosus or scleroderma.

Emergency Department Treatment and Disposition

In an acute episode, the treatment generally involves removal of the inciting stimulus. As many cases are induced by a change in temperature, particularly going from a warm to a cold environment, active rewarming by running the hands under warm water or placing in the axilla are generally effective. Sympathetic stimulation may also trigger an episode, so calming patients who are anxious or removing them from stressful situations may be efficacious.

A thorough history and physical examination should be performed on all patients presenting with an acute episode, with careful attention paid to signs and symptoms of connective tissue disorders. *Acrocyanosis* (Crocq Disease) is a circulatory disorder in which the hands, and less commonly the feet, are persistently cold and blue; some forms are related to Raynaud phenomenon.

Counseling patients about methods for reducing the frequency and duration of attacks is helpful, including avoiding sudden cold exposure, minimizing emotional stress, keeping the digits warm, avoiding cigarette smoking, and avoiding sympathomimetic drugs. Referral for primary care follow-up is recommended for all patients.

Pearls

1. Careful distinction should be made between patients complaining of cold hands or feet and actual Raynaud disease. A history of cool skin and sharply demarcated color changes is essential for the diagnosis.
2. Routine ordering of blood tests, such as ESR or ANA, is not recommended unless other symptoms of connective tissue disorders are present. In these cases close primary care or rheumatology follow-up is recommended.

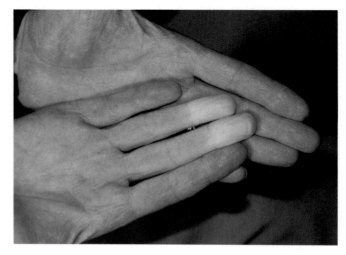

FIGURE 12.41 ■ Raynaud Disease. A patient with sharply demarcated color changes consistent with an acute attack of Raynaud phenomenon due to cold exposure. (Photo contributor: Mary J. Chandler, PA-C.)

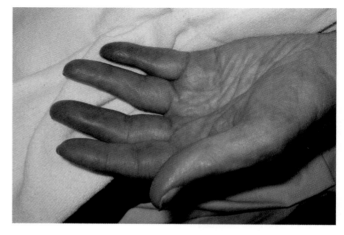

FIGURE 12.42 ■ Acrocyanosis. This patient presented with persistently blue and cold fingers secondary to acrocyanosis. (Photo contributor: Lawrence B. Stack, MD.)

Clinical Summary

An embolus refers to a foreign body in a blood vessel that is carried by the blood to a site distant from its point of origin. Most emboli result from a detached piece of thrombus, generally originating in the heart in the form of left ventricular thrombus following myocardial infarction or from atrial fibrillation. Other sources include atheroemboli from ruptured plaque, tumor, or foreign bodies such as venous or arterial catheters or guidewires.

Acute arterial embolization usually results in distal tissue infarction. Most embolic occlusion occurs at the branch points of arteries, due to the generally abrupt change in diameter at these bifurcation points. The most frequent site of arterial embolism is the bifurcation of the common femoral artery, accounting for 35% to 50% of all cases. Patients generally present with some or all of the "six Ps": pain, pallor, pulselessness, paresthesias, poikilothermia, and paralysis.

The general predictors of degree of ischemic insult include the amount of collateral circulation present, as well as the size of the involved vessel and the size of the obstructing embolus. Generally, patients with long-standing peripheral vascular disease have a greater amount of collateral circulation, and are able to tolerate an acute occlusion better than a patient with normal arteries.

Emergency Department Treatment and Disposition

Acute arterial embolus is a surgical emergency. Immediate initiation of intravenous heparin is indicated to prevent further clot propagation. Consultation with a vascular surgeon is imperative as soon as the diagnosis is suspected, as the rate of limb salvage drastically decreases after 4 to 6 hours. Transfer to a facility with vascular surgery capabilities should be initiated as quickly as possible if the initial facility does not have a vascular surgeon available.

In clear-cut cases of acute arterial embolism the treatment is generally Fogarty catheter embolectomy without prior angiography. In these cases a preoperative angiography only prolongs the limb's ischemic time and decreases the chance of salvage. Ambiguous cases, in which it is difficult to distinguish between acute embolic occlusion and in situ thrombosis, may benefit from preoperative angiography. Emergent surgical intervention may aggravate thrombosis in the case of in situ thrombus formation.

Pearls

1. Acute arterial embolus generally present with sudden onset of severe pain. In contrast, in situ thrombosis tends to have a more subacute presentation.
2. Aortic dissection may mimic acute arterial embolus. Involvement of multiple sites suggests dissection.
3. Intraarterial thrombolytic therapy for acute arterial embolus remains controversial.

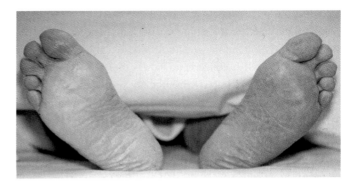

FIGURE 12.43 ■ Arterial Embolus. Note the pallor of this patient's right foot, consistent with an acute arterial embolus, in this case secondary to femoral artery occlusion. (Photo contributor: Lawrence B. Stack, MD.)

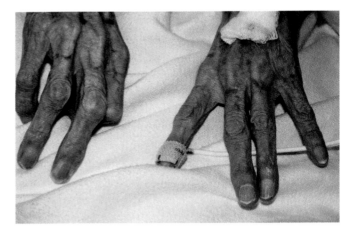

FIGURE 12.44 ■ Arterial Embolus. Pallor in the right hand secondary to arterial embolus, likely from atrial fibrillation. (Photo contributor: Lawrence B. Stack, MD.)

Chapter 13

CUTANEOUS CONDITIONS

J. Matthew Hardin

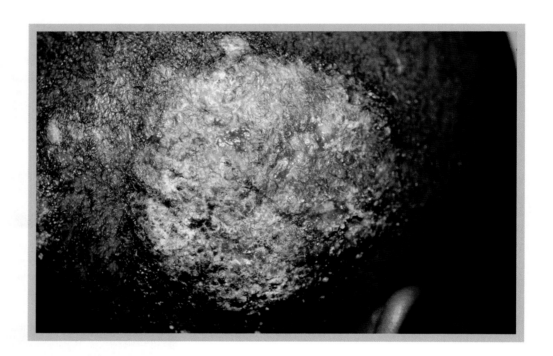

The author acknowledges Christopher R. Sartori, Michael B. Brooks, and Sean P. Collins for portions of this chapter written for the first and second editions.

Clinical Summary

Stevens-Johnson syndrome (SJS) and toxic epidermal necrolysis (TEN) are life-threatening, reactive diseases that represent two ends of a continuum. In general, SJS involves less than 10% BSA epidermal detachment and TEN involves greater than 30% BSA epidermal detachment. Overlap of the two entities occurs in 10% to 30%. Two or more mucosal sites are usually affected. The overall mortality of TEN approaches 30%.

The onset of SJS/TEN begins with fever, systemic toxicity, mucositis, and a generalized, dusky, erythematous rash. Mucositis of the conjunctival, nasal, oral, genital, and rectal mucosa can be the first sign of subsequent skin involvement. Bullae form within the rash and large sheets of epidermis separate from the dermis. The involved skin is exquisitely tender to palpation. The Nikolsky sign is present when lateral pressure on unblistered skin causes the epidermis to slide off. Progression of the involved skin can be rapid, occurring over a single day to slowly evolving over 14 days. In addition to the generalized "skin failure," SJS/TEN is a systemic disease with involvement of the respiratory and gastrointestinal systems. Life-threatening metabolic derangements, sepsis, respiratory failure, and gastrointestinal hemorrhage may occur and are compounded by underlying comorbidities. TEN has a mortality of approximately 50% in elderly patients. With a few exceptions, SJS/TEN results from drug exposure. The main culprits are sulfonamide antibiotics, aromatic anticonvulsants (phenytoin, phenobarbital, and carbamazepine), β-lactam antibiotics, NSAIDs, allopurinol, lamotrigine, tetracyclines, quinolones, abacavir, and nevirapine. Over 200 medications, including over-the-counter medications (pseudoephedrine) and herbal remedies, have been implicated. *Mycoplasma pneumoniae* can cause SJS and vaccinations have been implicated in SJS/TEN.

Emergency Department Treatment and Disposition

Stopping the offending medication is critical. Admission to a burn intensive care unit should be rapidly secured. In the emergency department, attention should be focused on the respiratory status, fluid and electrolyte balance, identification of infectious foci, and ophthalmologic assessment. Supportive care continues to be the foundation. Intravenous immune globulin (IVIG) should be considered with dermatologic and burn consultation.

Pearls

1. The hair-bearing scalp is spared even in severe disease.
2. Neutropenia is associated with a poor prognosis.
3. Cross reactions within the aromatic anticonvulsants are common. The first 8 weeks of treatment have the highest risk of TEN and previous anticonvulsant therapy portends a tenfold increased risk.
4. Patients with previous SJS/TEN to one medication class are not at a higher risk for developing SJS/TEN to other medication classes.

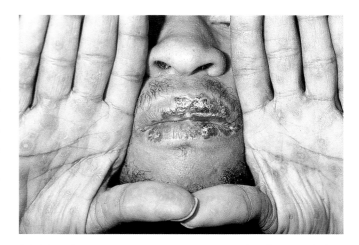

FIGURE 13.1 ■ Stevens-Johnson Syndrome. Note the target lesions on the hands of this patient, as well as the mucosal involvement on the lips. (Photo contributor: Alan B. Storrow, MD.)

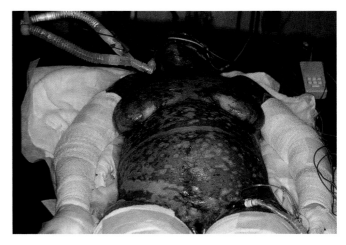

FIGURE 13.2 ■ Toxic Epidermal Necrolysis. Note the widespread erythematous bullae and epidermal exfoliation. (Photo contributor: James J. Nordlund, MD.)

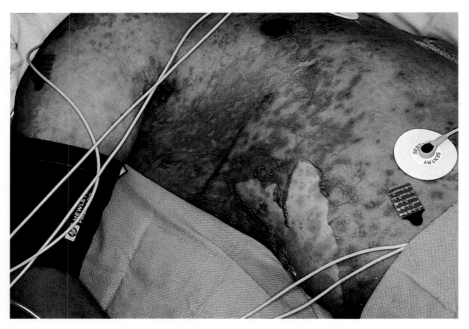

FIGURE 13.3 ▪ Toxic Epidermal Necrolysis. The initial bullae have coalesced, leading to extensive exfoliation of the epidermis. (Photo contributor: Keith Batts, MD.)

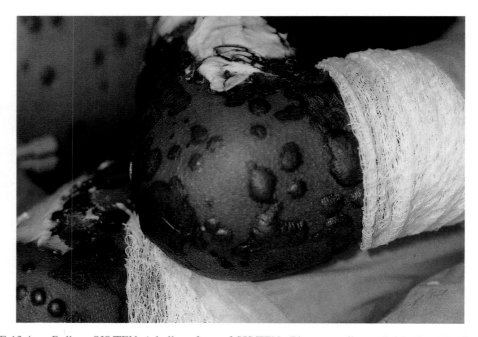

FIGURE 13.4 ▪ Bullous SJS/TEN. A bullous form of SJS/TEN. (Photo contributor: J. Matthew Hardin, MD.)

Clinical Summary

Erythema multiforme (EM) begins with symmetric, erythematous, sharply defined macules on the extremities and trunk. These macules evolve into "targetoid" morphology (a flat, dusky, central purpuric area, surrounded by a raised, edematous ring and peripheral erythema). Bullae may appear in the central dusky area (bullous EM). The mucous membranes, typically the oral mucosa, may become involved. On average, the rash persists for 1 to 4 weeks. The typical targetoid lesions allow for EM to be made clinically (bullae, purpura, and mucosal involvement should prompt a dermatology consultation).

Herpes simplex virus (HSV) is strongly associated with EM; lesions appear approximately 10 days after an outbreak. Since HSV infection (primary or recurrent) may not manifest itself clinically, there may not be a clear association with EM. Other infectious associations include *Mycoplasma pneumoniae*, *Histoplasma capsulatum*, and many other viruses. Medications account for less than 10% of cases; nonsteroidal anti-inflammatory drugs, sulfonamides, anti-epileptics, and antibiotics are responsible for the majority of cases. When associated with bullae, the differential diagnosis includes bullous arthropod reactions, drug-induced EM, and autoimmune bullous diseases (pemphigus vulgaris, paraneoplastic pemphigus, bullous pemphigoid).

Emergency Department Treatment and Disposition

Prevention of HSV recurrences is essential. Use of facial sunblock/sunscreens and lip balms should be encouraged to prevent UVB-induced recurrences. Oral antivirals (acyclovir, valacyclovir, or famciclovir) may be used to prevent both HSV (oral and genital) and EM. Systemic steroids are generally discouraged. With the distinctive clinical findings and no systemic symptoms, patients can be discharged home. Systemic symptoms and atypical presentations require admission and dermatologic consultation.

Pearls

1. The typical "targetoid" lesions are frequently found on the palms and soles.
2. Reassure patients that the lesions will completely resolve.
3. Eye involvement requires ophthalmologic consultation to exclude active HSV infection.

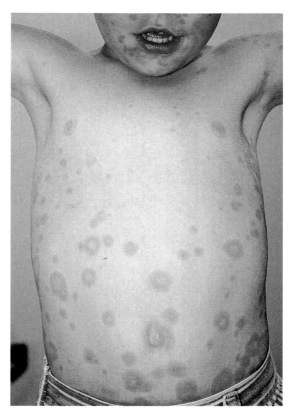

FIGURE 13.5 ■ Erythema Multiforme. Symmetric iris and targetoid patterns with concentric macules and papules. (Photo contributor: Michael Redman, PA-C.)

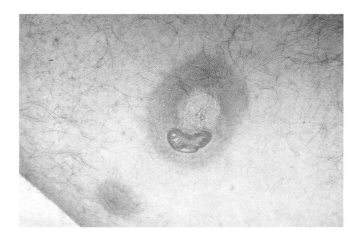

FIGURE 13.6 ■ Bullous Erythema Multiforme. Note the targetoid appearance and vesicle formation. (Photo contributor: J. Matthew Hardin, MD.)

Clinical Summary

Fixed drug eruptions (FDEs) appear 7 to 14 days after first exposure. The lesions can appear anywhere on the body but are most common on the face, lips, hands, feet, and genitalia. Typically, they appear as annular, edematous, well-demarcated plaques. Single or multiple lesions can appear. A central vesicle, bulla, or denuded epidermis may be present. After stopping the offending medication, the lesion(s) fade over several days. Residual hyperpigmentation is common. Reexposure to the offending medication will result in reappearance of the same lesion at the same site. The most common offending medications are sulfonamides, NSAIDs, barbiturates, tetracyclines, and carbamazepine.

Emergency Department Treatment and Disposition

Identify all potential medications (prescription, herbal, and over-the-counter medications) and stop the offending drug. Symptomatic treatment with antihistamines and analgesics is sufficient.

Pearls

1. Pseudoephedrine, a common over-the-counter medication, is a frequent cause of FDEs.
2. Warn patients that hyperpigmentation is expected and may not completely resolve.

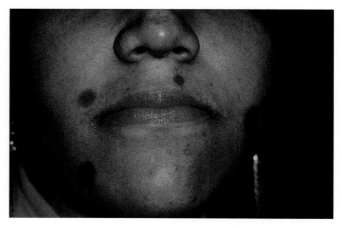

FIGURE 13.8 ■ Fixed Drug Eruption. Recurring reaction to acetaminophen. (Photo contributor: J. Matthew Hardin, MD.)

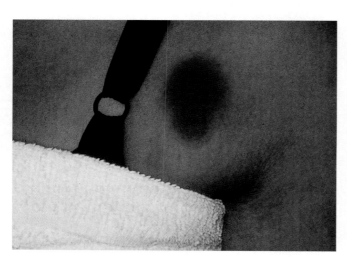

FIGURE 13.7 ■ Fixed Drug Eruption. This red to violaceous, pruritic, sharply demarcated patch is a cutaneous reaction to a drug. Repeated exposure will cause a similar reaction in the same location. (Photo contributor: Department of Dermatology, Wilford Hall USAF Medical Center and Brooke Army Medical Center, San Antonio, TX.)

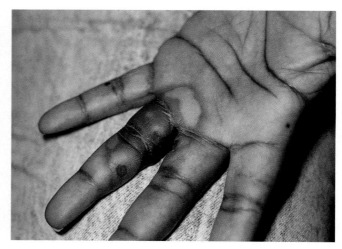

FIGURE 13.9 ■ Fixed Drug Eruption. Recurring reaction to acetaminophen. (Photo contributor: J. Matthew Hardin, MD.)

Clinical Summary

Exanthematous drug eruptions are an adverse hypersensitivity reaction. This symmetric, pruritic, morbilliform, blanching, erythematous eruption is the most frequent of cutaneous drug eruptions. The initially pruritic macules or papules usually become confluent and may progress to an exfoliative dermatitis.

Acute generalized exanthematous pustulosis (AGEP), a type of drug eruption, presents 1 to 5 days after starting a new medication. Typically, a β-lactam or a macrolide antibiotic is implicated. A fever is usually noted with neutrophilia (90% of patients) and eosinophilia (30% of patients). The rash begins with scarlatiniform erythema and quickly becomes generalized, primarily to the head, neck, and trunk. Sterile, nonfollicular pustules develop quickly and are usually less than 5 mm in diameter. Over the next 2 to 4 days, widespread superficial desquamation occurs. (This contrasts with the entire epidermal sloughing of SJS/TEN.) Mucosal sites, especially oral mucosa, can be involved. With the cessation of the offending medication, the rash slowly resolves over 2 weeks. Distinguishing AGEP from cellulitis, erythema multiforme, Stevens-Johnson syndrome, and toxic epidermal necrolysis can be difficult.

Emergency Department Treatment and Disposition

While exanthematous eruptions may resolve despite the drug's continued use, cessation of the causative agent is paramount. It may take as long as 2 weeks for the eruption to fade after discontinuation. Symptomatic management includes antihistamines and topical corticosteroids.

The appearance of AGEP, with pustules, fever, and neutrophilia is difficult to distinguish from an infectious etiology. Treatment is supportive care. The large surface area of desquamation makes secondary infection a major concern, especially in those with comorbidities, the elderly and bedridden patients. A burn ICU may be required if there is significant skin breakdown beyond the superficial desquamation. Differentiation from cellulitis, erythema multiforme, Stevens-Johnson syndrome, and toxic epidermal necrolysis may require a skin biopsy and dermatologic consultation.

Pearls

1. Exanthematous drug eruptions are usually symmetric and pruritic as opposed to viral eruptions, which are usually asymmetric and asymptomatic.

2. Mononucleosis patients taking amoxicillin or AIDS patients taking sulfa drugs frequently experience this reaction.

3. The desquamation seen in AGEP is much more superficial than the full-thickness desquamation seen in Stevens-Johnson syndrome or toxic epidermal necrolysis.

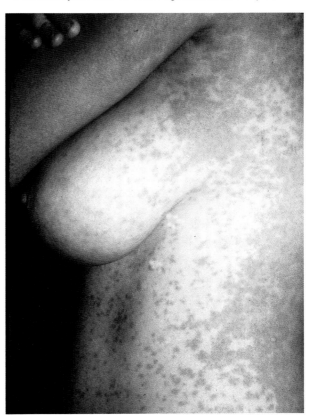

FIGURE 13.10 ■ Exanthematous Drug Eruption. This symmetric, morbilliform, blanching eruption may eventually become confluent, leading to an exfoliative dermatitis. (Photo contributor: GlaxoWellcome Pharmaceuticals.)

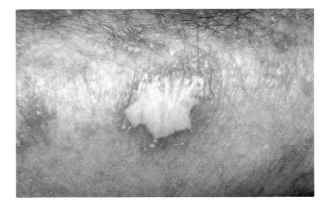

FIGURE 13.11 ■ Acute Generalized Exanthematous Pustulosis. Note the large pustule (sterile) and surrounding smaller pustules. This will eventually slough off and leave a superficial, erythematous erosion. (Photo contributor: J. Matthew Hardin, MD.)

Clinical Summary

Hidradenitis suppurativa (HS) commonly affects overweight, postpubertal females. Males are affected less frequently. This chronic disease involves hair-bearing intertriginous sites such as the axillae, inguinal, perineal, gluteal fold, and inframammary areas. Individual lesions begin with erythematous nodules that become tender and fluctuant. The nodule ruptures with a suppurative discharge and eventual sinus tract formation. This is a primary inflammatory response to the follicle and is not infectious; however, secondary infections are common. Severe hypertrophic scar formation may be dramatic. The differential diagnosis includes granuloma inguinale, mycetoma, tuberculosis, and Crohn disease.

Emergency Department Treatment and Disposition

Hidradenitis suppurativa should be identified and a systemic infection ruled out. Topical and systemic antibiotics help improve lesions, especially if a secondary infection is suspected. Oral doxycycline or minocycline should be tried first with topical clindamycin. In addition, antibacterial soap is helpful to prevent secondary colonization. Incision and drainage should not be performed as this can induce chronic sinus tract formation and scarring. Referral to a dermatologist for long-term management is indicated.

Pearls

1. Many physicians who see HS do not recognize that this disease is not a primary infectious process but rather inflammatory. This often leads to delayed diagnosis and worse skin involvement.
2. One hallmark of hidradenitis is the "double comedones," a blackhead with two or greater surface openings that communicate under the skin.

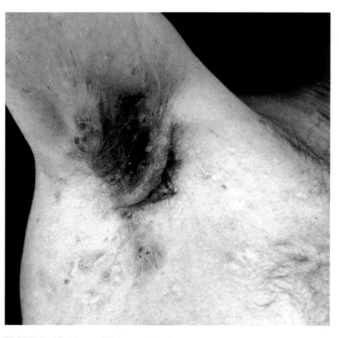

FIGURE 13.13 ■ Hidradenitis Suppurativa. Bulging scar over a fluctuating abscess in the axilla of a 25-year-old man. There are draining sinuses as suggested by the axillary hair matted by dried purulent secretions. There are also multiple depressed scars from previous abscesses. This patient also had acne conglobata. (Used with permission from *Fitzpatrick's Color Atlas & Synopsis of Clinical Dermatology.* 5th ed, Access Medicine, McGraw-Hill.)

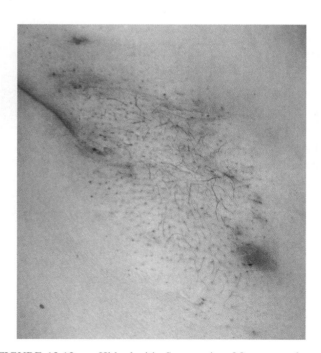

FIGURE 13.12 ■ Hidradenitis Suppurativa. Many comedones, some of which are paired, are a characteristic finding associated with deep, exquisitely painful abscesses and old scars in the axilla. (Used with permission from Wolff K, Johnson RA, Suurmond D. *Fitzpatrick's Color Atlas and Synopsis of Clinical Dermatology.* 5th ed. New York, McGraw-Hill, 2005; p. 15.)

Clinical Summary

Pyogenic granuloma presents as an eruptive, friable papule over weeks. They are frequently located on the extremities, face, or sites of trauma. Children are most commonly affected but they can occur at any age. The lesion will bleed with very little trauma. If the papule is not completely removed, it will recur at the same site. Pregnant women have a higher incidence of pyogenic granulomas (especially on the mouth and gingiva).

Emergency Department Treatment and Disposition

Most emergency department presentations of pyogenic granulomas will be due to prolonged bleeding. Parents are often distraught over the inability to control the brisk bleeding. Silver nitrate applied to the base of the papule is usually effective. Refer patients to a dermatologist for possible biopsy and further treatment.

Pearls

1. An association with isotretinoin, indinavir, and capecitabine has been described.
2. About one-third of these benign lesions follow some form of minor trauma.
3. Biopsy and histology may exclude other vascular tumors.

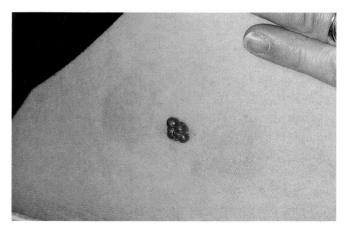

FIGURE 13.15 ■ Pyogenic Granuloma. Note the violaceous color and multilobulated nodule. The hyperpigmented patches on either side are secondary to a bandage. (Photo contributor: J. Matthew Hardin, MD.)

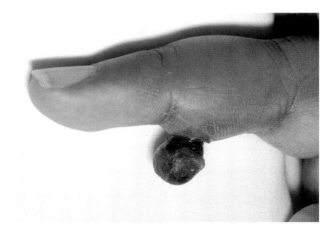

FIGURE 13.16 ■ Pyogenic Granuloma. Friable papule with frequent bleeding. (Photo contributor: Lawrence B. Stack, MD.)

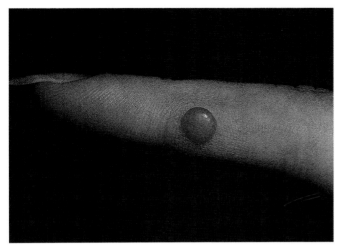

FIGURE 13.14 ■ Pyogenic Granuloma. A solitary, violaceous, pedunculated, vascular nodule formed at the site of an injury. Note that the nodule is well demarcated by a thin rim of epidermis. (Photo contributor: J. Matthew Hardin, MD.)

Clinical Summary

Pyoderma gangrenosum (PG) is an inflammatory condition associated with inflammatory bowel disease (Crohn disease, ulcerative colitis), leukemia, monoclonal gammopathy, polycythemia vera, chronic active hepatitis, HCV, HIV, systemic lupus erythematosis, and pregnancy. Adults (40-60 years old) are commonly affected. The lesion begins on the lower extremities or trunk as a pustule surrounded by erythema. This pustule erodes to form an ulcer. Similar satellite pustules form around the original pustule and erode into ulcers. The lesions eventually coalesce into a large ulcer. The surrounding border is described as "rolled" due to the convex elevation and has a violaceous hue. The ulcers are exquisitely tender to movement and palpation. Another common location for PG is surrounding an ostomy site.

The most concerning diagnosis to exclude is an infectious etiology due to bacterial, mycobacterial, fungal, syphilis, or amebiasis. Spider bites due to *Loxosceles* species can present similarly to PG. Large vessel vasculitis is a consideration as well.

Emergency Department Treatment and Disposition

The diagnosis of PG is based on clinical examination, dermatopathologic evaluation, and exclusion of other causes. This makes PG difficult to diagnose and frequently mistreated. Appropriate cultures and laboratory testing are indicated to exclude an infectious etiology. Broad-spectrum antibiotics are indicated for secondary infections. Dermatology consultation for biopsy and initiation of immunosuppressant therapy may help arrive at a diagnosis sooner.

Pearls

1. Pyoderma gangrenosum is often not thought of until late in the ulcer formation and after multiple skin grafts have failed. Without immunosuppressant therapy, skin grafting is unlikely to succeed.
2. Pyoderma gangrenosum is truly a diagnosis of exclusion as no criteria have defined the illness.

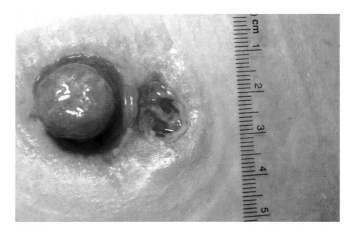

FIGURE 13.17 ■ Pyoderma Gangrenosum. PG starts as a deep-seated nodule surrounded by an erythematous halo with purulence. Note early ulcer formation. An ileostomy site is seen on left of image. PG is commonly associated with inflammatory bowel disease. (Photo contributor: Lawrence B. Stack, MD.)

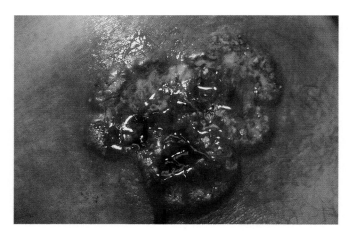

FIGURE 13.18 ■ Pyoderma Gangrenosum. Note the rolled and violaceous borders. This lesion can rapidly enlarge and become secondarily infected. (Photo contributor: J. Matthew Hardin, MD.)

Clinical Summary

Seborrheic dermatitis represents a spectrum of disease ranging from localized to generalized exfoliative erythroderma. All ages are affected. The typical lesions are located on the scalp, external auditory canal, postauricular scalp, eyebrows, eyelids, face (especially the nasolabial folds), axillae, umbilicus, presternal chest, groin, and gluteal fold. The lesions have an erythematous base with yellow, greasy scaling. Infants frequently present with "cradle cap" (yellow greasy scaling lesions on the scalp).

Both infants and adults with seborrheic dermatitis can evolve into a generalized exfoliative erythroderma. This entity is an emergency due to the rapid epidermal turnover, fluid and electrolyte derangements, high-output cardiac failure, sepsis, and respiratory distress syndrome. Other causes of a generalized exfoliative erythroderma include psoriasis, atopic dermatitis, allergic contact dermatitis, drug reactions, Norwegian scabies, and neoplastic causes.

Emergency Department Treatment and Disposition

It is important to emphasize to patients that seborrheic dermatitis is a lifelong disease and has no cure. Treatment is directed at controlling the disease. Localized seborrheic dermatitis is treated with topical 2% ketoconazole applied bid. Scalp seborrheic dermatitis can be treated with selenium sulfide, ketoconazole, or zinc pyrithione shampoos.

Generalized exfoliative erythroderma requires admission dictated by the underlying state of the patient. Emergent consultation with a dermatologist for biopsy and treatment recommendations is indicated.

Pearls

1. New-onset seborrheic dermatitis may herald new HIV infection or immunosuppression.
2. Although there is no cure, reassure patients the rash can be well controlled with topical medications.

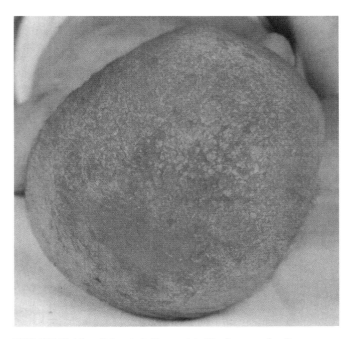

FIGURE 13.19 ■ Seborrheic Dermatitis. Erythema and yellow-orange scales and crust on the scalp of an infant ("cradle cap"). Eczematous lesions are also present on the arms and trunk. (Used with permission from Wolff K, Johnson RA, Suurmond D. *Fitzpatrick's Color Atlas & Synopsis of Clinical Dermatology.* 5th ed. New York, NY: McGraw-Hill; 2005: 51.)

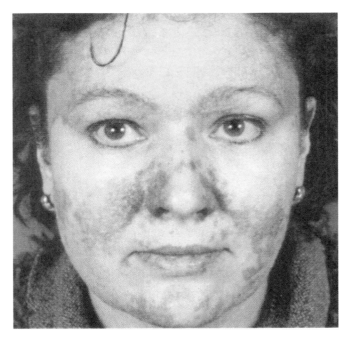

FIGURE 13.20 ■ Erythema and yellow-orange scaling of the forehead, cheeks, nasolabial folds, and chin. Scalp and retroauricular areas were also involved. (Used with permission from Wolff K, Johnson RA, Suurmond D. *Fitzpatrick's Color Atlas & Synopsis of Clinical Dermatology.* 5th ed. New York, McGraw-Hill, 2005; p. 51.)

Clinical Summary

Psoriasis has many forms. The most common is *chronic plaque* psoriasis that presents as stable, symmetric lesions on the trunk and extremities (especially the elbows and knees). The lesions are well-defined, erythematous plaques with a silvery scales. *Inverse* psoriasis represents a form that involves the intertriginous areas. *Guttate* psoriasis presents with an abrupt eruption of 2- to 5-mm erythematous scaly papules on the trunk and extremities. A preceding respiratory infection (usually streptococcal pharyngitis) can precipitate the eruption. This is common in children and young adults. *Pustular* forms of psoriasis can present as localized (nailbed, palms, or soles) or generalized. Pustular psoriasis is characterized by erythema and "lakes of pus." Withdrawal of systemic steroids can precipitate pustular psoriasis (as in patients with COPD and asthma exacerbations treated with systemic steroids).

Emergency Department Treatment and Disposition

Emergency department treatment should ensure no other infectious etiology or systemic symptoms. Pustular forms may need admission to exclude an infectious etiology. Guttate psoriasis responds to amoxicillin, clindamycin, or macrolide antibiotics. Obtain emergent consultation with a dermatologist for patients with generalized presentations and referrals for localized disease.

Pearls

1. Patients withdrawing from steroid treatment may have significant flaring of their psoriasis; make sure to warn any psoriasis patient who is placed on steroids.
2. Medication-induced psoriasis is common with β-blockers.

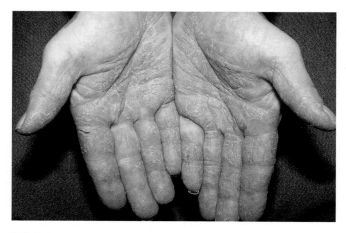

FIGURE 13.21 ■ Psoriasis. Note the erythematous plaques with diffuse fissuring in this case of palmar psoriasis. (Photo contributor: J. Matthew Hardin, MD.)

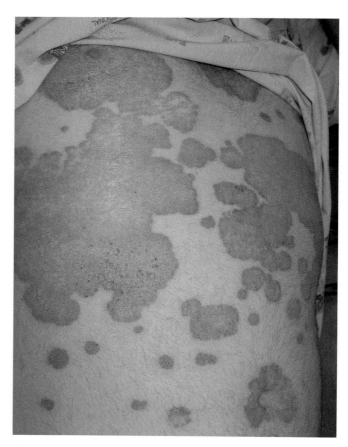

FIGURE 13.22 ■ Psoriasis. Well-defined lesions of chronic plaque psoriasis. (Photo contributor: R. Jason Thurman, MD.)

Clinical Summary

Nummular eczema presents on the extremities and is characterized by an erythematous, edematous, vesicular, and crusted plaque. The lesions enlarge by forming satellite papulovesicles at the periphery that coalesce with the original lesion. Pruritus is the dominant symptom.

Xerotic eczema (also called winter itch, eczema craquele, and asteatotic eczema) presents on the anterior shins, extensor arms, and the flanks. The lesions are erythematous patches with fine, cracked fissures and adherent scaling. The edema and exudate present in nummular eczema is absent. Pruritus can be severe. This is a common finding in the winter and in the elderly.

Emergency Department Treatment and Disposition

Treatment of nummular eczema consists of mid- to high-potency topical steroids under occlusion. Prevention of secondary infection is important as patients cannot resist scratching.

Treatment of xerotic eczema consists of topical emollients (petrolatum) three to four applications per day. Topical steroids may be required for areas with inflammation.

Pearls

1. For nummular eczema, think of the diagnosis when patients present with lesions unresponsive to antibiotics and pruritus is the dominate feature.
2. Both of these entities associated with significant pruritus and secondary infections (especially in the young and the elderly) may occur.

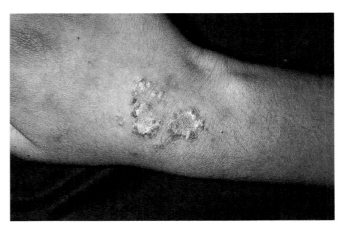

FIGURE 13.23 ■ Eczema. Nummular eczema of the wrist. Note the weepy satellite lesions on the periphery. (Photo contributor: J. Matthew Hardin, MD.)

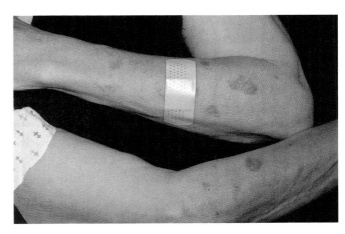

FIGURE 13.24 ■ Eczema. Nummular eczema on the upper extremities. Note the well-defined, erythematous plaques with scaling. This is a common presentation in the elderly. (Photo contributor: J. Matthew Hardin, MD.)

Clinical Summary

Dyshidrotic eczema (also called pompholyx or acute vesiculobullous hand eczema) presents with abrupt appearance of deep-seated, 1- to 2-mm vesicles on the sides of the fingers, palms, and soles. They are extremely pruritic and may coalesce into larger bullae. The lesions may become dry and fissure with healing. The outbreak usually resolves over a few weeks unless secondary infection develops. The differential includes bullous tinea, id reaction, or allergic contact dermatitis (see related items).

Emergency Department Treatment and Disposition

Treatment includes a high-potency topical steroid and prevention of secondary infection. Refer to a dermatologist for long-term treatment.

Pearls

1. These lesions wax and wane with the stress level of the patient.
2. The lesions resemble tapioca pudding.

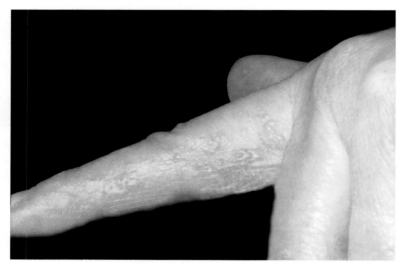

FIGURE 13.25 ■ Dyshidrotic Eczema. In most cases dyshidrotic eczematous dermatitis starts with tapioca-like vesicles on the lateral aspects of the fingers. (Used with permission from *Fitzpatrick's Color Atlas & Synopsis of Clinical Dermatology*. 5th ed, Access Medicine, McGraw-Hill.)

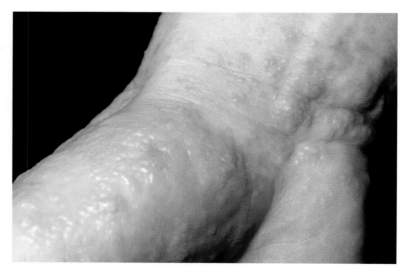

FIGURE 13.26 ■ Dyshidrotic Eczema. The vesicles show confluence and spread to the palm but also to the wrist and dorsal aspect of the hand when the eruption progresses. (Used with permission from *Fitzpatrick's Color Atlas & Synopsis of Clinical Dermatology*. 5th ed, Access Medicine, McGraw-Hill.)

Clinical Summary

Inflammatory tinea capitis and tinea pedis can induce a focal or generalized reaction. These typically result in vesicular or eczematous eruptions, but can be generalized morbilliform eruptions. Characteristically, the secondary id reaction is intensely pruritic. Id reactions are thought to represent a systemic reaction to fungal antigens and can present with systemic symptoms (fever, lymphadenopathy, anorexia, and leukocytosis). The id reaction will not demonstrate fungal elements and will not respond to topical steroids.

Emergency Department Treatment and Disposition

Recognition and treatment of the initial fungal infection (tinea capitis or tinea pedis) is curative. Refer to a dermatologist for follow-up to ensure diagnosis and resolution.

Pearls

1. Repeated evaluation in the emergency department for fungal infection or eczematous rash should prompt further investigation into distant, untreated, and occult fungal infections.
2. Id reactions are intensely pruritic; make sure secondary bacterial infections do not develop from excoriations.

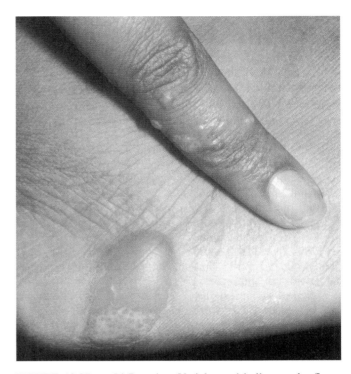

FIGURE 13.27 ■ Id Reaction. Vesicles and bullae on the finger and the lateral foot of a 21-year-old female. Bullous (inflammatory) tinea pedis was present and was associated with dermatophytid reaction. Prednisone was given for 2 weeks; pruritus and vesiculation resolved. (Used with permission from Wolff K, Johnson RA, Suurmond D. *Fitzpatrick's Color Atlas & Synopsis of Clinical Dermatology.* 5th ed. New York, McGraw-Hill, 2005; p. 48.)

Clinical Summary

Atopic dermatitis presents in three overlapping stages: (1) infantile atopic dermatitis, (2) childhood atopic dermatitis, and (3) adult atopic dermatitis. *Infantile* atopic dermatitis begins after 2 months of age and is symmetrically distributed on the cheeks, scalp, neck, forehead, and extensor surfaces of the extremities. The lesions begin as erythema or papules, but, with persistent itching and rubbing, they become thin plaques. If the infant is able to scratch the lesions, they may become exudative and crusted. *Childhood* atopic dermatitis presents with flexural involvement. Other areas frequently involved are the face, neck, and trunk. The scratching induces lichenification of the plaques and the potential for a secondary infection. *Adult* atopic dermatitis is less specific but can present with a childhood-like distribution, papular lesions that coalesce into plaques, and chronic hand dermatitis. Atopic dermatitis can become a generalized exfoliative erythroderma.

The differential diagnoses include seborrheic dermatitis, psoriasis, irritant or allergic contact dermatitis, nummular eczema, and scabies.

Emergency Department Treatment and Disposition

No soaps or detergents with fragrances or masking fragrances should be used. Dryer sheets should not be used for the patient or other family members. Baths should be minimized and only tepid water should be used. After bathing, pat dry the skin and smear a thin film of petrolatum or vegetable shortening over the affected areas. Wearing damp pajamas after application of emollients can help. Dermatologic referral for localized disease is indicated. If a generalized exfoliative erythroderma is present, an emergency department dermatologic consultation is indicated.

Pearls

1. Often called the "itch that rashes" due to the fact that pruritus precedes clinical disease.
2. Using an ice cube over the worst sites can help prevent pruritus.

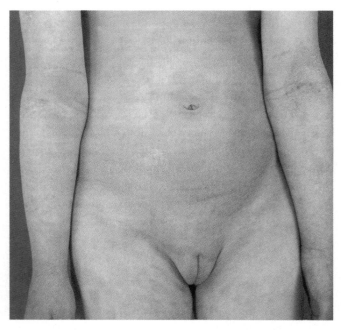

FIGURE 13.28 ■ Atopic Dermatitis. Ill-defined erythema, papules, excoriations, lichenification in the antecubital fossae, with less severe changes on the trunk and thighs. (Used with permission from Wolff K, Johnson RA, Suurmond D. *Fitzpatrick's Color Atlas & Synopsis of Clinical Dermatology*. 5th ed. New York, McGraw-Hill, 2005; p. 40.)

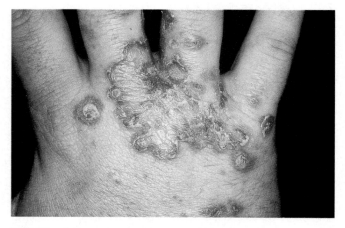

FIGURE 13.29 ■ Atopic Dermatitis. Lichenfied plaques, erosions, and fissures are characteristic of atopic dermatitis. (Photo contributor: James J. Nordlund, MD.)

Clinical Summary

Stasis dermatitis is the direct result of venous insufficiency. It is characteristically distributed on the distal tibia above the medial malleolus. Early in its course, stasis dermatitis presents with erythematous patches. These can progress to scaling and even eczematous and weeping plaques. Patients will often have light brown pigmentation distributed on the lower third of the extremity due to microvasculature extravasation of blood (secondary to increased pressure of the superficial capillaries). Varicose veins are usually present, although may be difficult to visualize in obese patients. Patients with heart failure, cirrhosis, and nephrotic syndrome are at increased risk due to a chronic edematous state.

Emergency Department Treatment and Disposition

Referral to a primary care physician should be initiated to address the underlying etiology (valvular insufficiency, thromboembolic disease, chronic edematous state, etc). In the acute setting, elevation of the extremities and compression hose will temporarily improve venous stasis. Emollients and mid-potency topical steroids are beneficial if there is associated scaling and pruritus.

Pearl

1. Differentiation of stasis dermatitis and cellulitis can be extremely difficult. In the setting of systemic infectious symptoms, cellulitis should be considered.

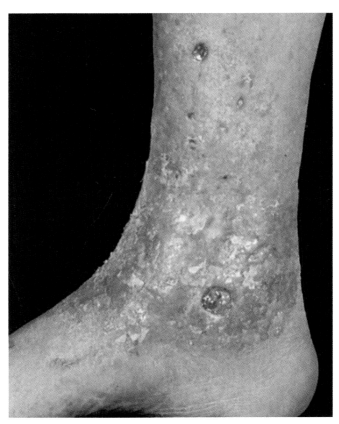

FIGURE 13.31 ■ Stasis Dermatitis. An example of stasis dermatitis showing erythematous, scaly, and oozing patches over the lower leg. Several stasis ulcers are also seen in this patient. (Used with permission from Fauci AS, Braunwald E, Kasper DL, et al. *Harrison's Principles of Internal Medicine*. 17th ed. New York, McGraw-Hill, 2008; p. 315.)

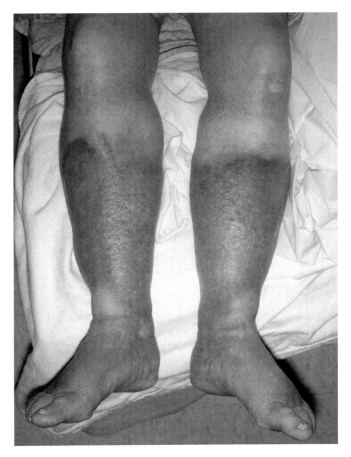

FIGURE 13.30 ■ Stasis Dermatitis. Erythematous patches and mild scaling in a patient with chronic venous insufficiency. (Photo contributor: Lawrence B. Stack, MD.)

Clinical Summary

Acne vulgaris, or common acne, is an inflammation of the pilosebaceous units on the face and trunk. It occurs most commonly in adolescence and produces comedones, pustules, nodules, and cysts. Comedones may be open (blackheads) or closed (whiteheads). Scarring may occur.

Emergency Department Treatment and Disposition

Mild acne is treated with topical clindamycin, erythromycin, or benzoyl peroxide gels. Topical retinoids are another option but require education regarding concentration changes. Oral antibiotics, such as minocycline, may be added if topical treatment is unsatisfactory. Since improvement occurs over a period of months, patients with moderate and severe forms are best referred to a dermatologist.

Pearls

1. Acne vulgaris is typically more severe in males and has a lower incidence in Asians and Blacks.
2. Drugs such as lithium, topical and systemic glucocorticoids, androgens, and oral contraceptives may cause exacerbation.
3. Acne vulgaris is typically worse in fall and winter.

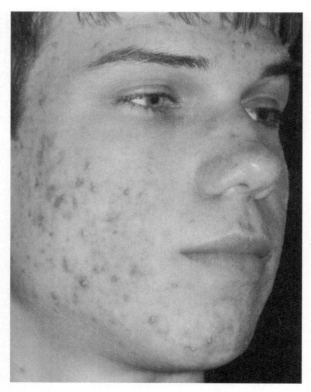

FIGURE 13.32 ■ Acne Vulgaris. A spectrum of lesions is seen on the face of a 17-year-old male: comedones, papules, pustules, and erythematous macules and scars at site of resolving lesions. The patient was successfully treated with a 4-month course of isotretinoin; there was no recurrence over the next 5 years. (Used with permission from Wolff K, Johnson RA, Suurmond D. *Fitzpatrick's Color Atlas & Synopsis of Clinical Dermatology.* 5th ed. New York, McGraw-Hill, 2005; p. 5.)

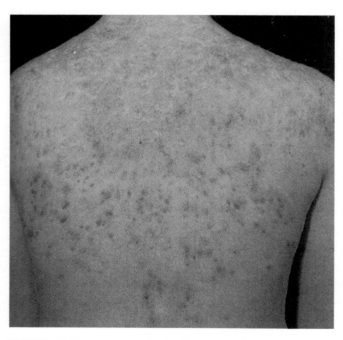

FIGURE 13.33 ■ Acne Vulgaris. Papulopustular acne occurs not only in the face but also on the back, the shoulders and the anterior chest. Lesions are identical to those seen in the face and are coalescing in the midline forming cysts. (Used with permission from Wolff K, Goldsmith LA, Katz SI, et al. *Fitzpatrick's Dermatology in General Medicine.* 7th ed. New York, McGraw-Hill, 2008; p. 695.)

Clinical Summary

Leukocytoclastic vasculitis (LCV) represents the deposition of immune complexes in small blood vessels with subsequent blood vessel destruction and extravasation of blood. Patients present with nonblanching erythematous papules that frequently coalesce into plaques ("palpable purpura"). The lower extremities and dependent areas of the back and the buttocks are most frequently involved. Pruritus can be significant. The face, palms, soles, and mucous membranes are uncommonly involved. Vesicles, ulcers, and necrosis can be seen within the purpuric lesions. The lesions appear over a few days and usually resolve with hyperpigmentation over 4 to 6 weeks or longer. Associated symptoms include fever, arthralgias, myalgias, malaise, and other disease-specific symptoms.

LCV is associated with many chronic diseases (connective tissue diseases, malignancies, viral hepatitis, inflammatory bowel disease, and others), medications (penicillin, sulfonamides, thiazides, allopurinol, phenytoin, NSAIDs, PTU, IV dye, and G-CSF), infections (group A β-hemolytic streptococci, hepatitis A virus, hepatitis B virus, hepatitis C virus, HIV), and idiopathic disorders (Henoch-Schonlein purpura [HSP], acute hemorrhagic edema of childhood, and urticarial vasculitis).

Henoch-Schönlein purpura is a unique form of LCV that presents with palpable purpura of the lower extremities and buttocks. Occasionally, the lesions may be found on the upper extremities, trunk, and face. A recent respiratory infection is commonly elicited. Arthralgias, abdominal pain, and hematuria are also common. Renal vasculitis is common but long-term renal impairment occurs in only 2% of patients. Adults, more pronounced systemic symptoms (fever, arthralgias), and lesions above the waist are associated with more severe renal impairment.

Acute hemorrhagic edema of childhood (AHEC) presents in infants 4 to 24 months of age. A recent bacterial or viral illness is commonly found. Purpuric annular plaques on the face, ears, and extremities appear first and new lesions form proximally. The disease is confined to the skin. The lesions appear worrisome, but the patient is in no distress and nontoxic. Over the course of 2 to 3 weeks, the lesions completely resolve.

Urticarial vasculitis presents with painful urticaria. The lesions are distinguished from common urticaria by their persistence (lasting over 24 hours) and resolution with hyperpigmentation. Urticarial vasculitis can be seen with systemic lupus erythematosus, viral infections (HCV, HBV), medications (including fluoxetine and NSAIDs), and malignancies.

Emergency Department Treatment and Disposition

Recognition that a diverse group of diseases can result in LCV is the first step. Evaluation for systemic symptoms (fever or other signs of infection, hematuria, and GI bleeding) requiring admission should be undertaken. Most cases are self-limited and only require supportive care (rest, elevation, antihistamines, and analgesics). Systemic symptoms require admission and consideration of systemic corticosteroids and other immunosuppressants. Dermatologic referral for mild cases is indicated and, if systemic symptoms present, consultation for biopsy may help rapidly identify the etiology.

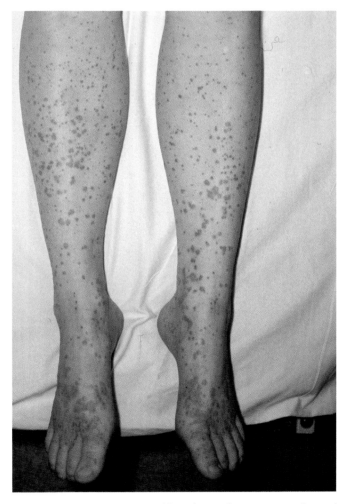

FIGURE 13.34 ■ Vasculitis. Note the erythematous papules and plaques coalescing into larger plaques. If you were to run your finger across these lesions, they would be raised and not blanch. (Photo contributor: Lawrence B. Stack, MD.)

Pearls

1. Failure to recognize systemic symptoms can result in delayed diagnoses and severe morbidity.
2. Vasculitis affects all ages and has equal incidence in males and females. The etiology is often idiopathic.
3. Laboratory examination should include ruling out thrombocytopenic purpura (see related item).

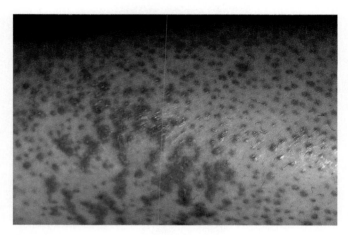

FIGURE 13.35 ■ Vaculitis. Note the erythematous papules coalescing. These would not blanch with pressure. (Photo contributor: J. Matthew Hardin, MD.)

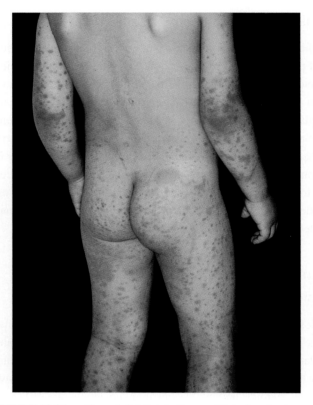

FIGURE 13.37 ■ Henoch-Schönlein Pupura. Note the classic acral distribution of HSP. It is immunoglobulin A (IgA)–mediated and most commonly occurs in children after a streptococcal or viral infection. (Photo contributor: Kevin J. Knoop, MD, MS.)

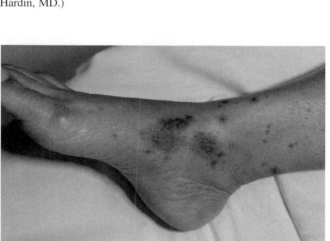

FIGURE 13.36 ■ Vasculitis. These palpable purpura would not blanch with the application of a glass slide, indicating hemorrhage. (Photo contributor: Kevin J. Knoop, MD, MS.)

Clinical Summary

Idiopathic thrombocytopenic purpura (ITP) occurs as a result of platelet injury and destruction. Pinpoint, red, nonblanching petechiae or nonpalpable purpura and ecchymoses are found on the skin and mucous membranes, either spontaneously (platelets < 10,000/mm^3) or at the site of minimal trauma (platelets < 40,000/mm^3). Melena, hematochezia, menorrhagia, and severe intracranial hemorrhages may also occur in conjunction with the purpura. The acute form affects children 1 to 2 weeks after a viral illness; the chronic form occurs most often in adults, with women outnumbering men 3:1. It may present with an associated splenomegaly.

Emergency Department Treatment and Disposition

Hospitalization at the time of diagnosis is recommended because the differential is extensive and the bleeding risks are significant. Platelets are transfused only if there is life-threatening bleeding or the total count is less than 10,000/mm^3. Immunosuppressive drugs, steroids, and intravenous immunoglobulin are of benefit in the acute cases; splenectomy is utilized in chronic cases.

Pearls

1. Petechiae and purpura in a thrombocytopenic patient with splenomegaly make the diagnosis.
2. The acute form of ITP has an excellent prognosis (90% spontaneous remission), whereas the course of chronic ITP is one of varying severity with little hope of remission.

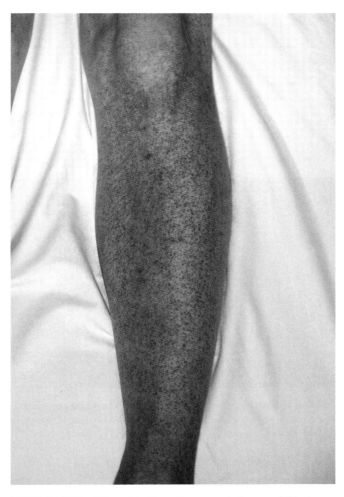

FIGURE 13.38 ■ Idiopathic Thrombocytopenic Purpura. This thrombocytopenic patient with splenomegaly has pinpoint, nonblanching, nonpalpable petechiae. (Photo contributor: R. Jason Thurman, MD.)

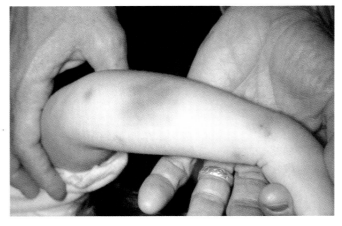

FIGURE 13.39 ■ Idiopathic Thrombocytopenic Purpura. Nonpalpable purpura in ITP. (Photo contributor: Lawrence B. Stack, MD.)

Clinical Summary

The diagnosis of thrombotic thrombocytopenic purpura (TTP) is characterized by the following pentad of symptoms:

1. Microangiopathic hemolytic anemia, with characteristic schistocytes on the peripheral blood smear and a reticulocytosis
2. Thrombocytopenia with platelet counts ranging from 5000 to 100,000/μL
3. Renal abnormalities including renal insufficiency, azotemia, proteinuria, or hematuria
4. Fever
5. Neurologic abnormalities including headache, confusion, cranial nerve palsies, seizures, or coma

The disease affects women more than men and can affect any age group, but it occurs most commonly in ages 10 to 60.

Emergency Department Treatment and Disposition

The cornerstone of therapy is plasma exchange transfusion. Some patients can be treated with plasma infusions alone. It is thought that the transfusions provide a missing substrate and the exchange may remove some unknown toxic substance. Prednisone and antiplatelet therapy with aspirin may be helpful. Patients recalcitrant to standard therapy may be treated with immunosuppressives (vincristine, azathioprine, cyclophosphamide) and even splenectomy. All patients should be admitted.

Pearls

1. Platelet transfusions should be avoided unless there is life-threatening hemorrhage; they can worsen the thrombotic process.
2. Typically TTP is acute and fulminant, but it can become a chronic, relapsing form.
3. Hemoglobin less than 6 g/dL, platelet count less than 20,000, elevated indirect bilirubin and LDH, and a negative Coombs test are typically found.
4. Hemolytic uremic syndrome (HUS), disseminated intravascular coagulation, and the pregnancy-associated HELLP (hemolysis, elevated liver enzymes, low platelet count) syndrome can all present like TTP. HUS and TTP appear to be closely related and may represent variants of a single disease.

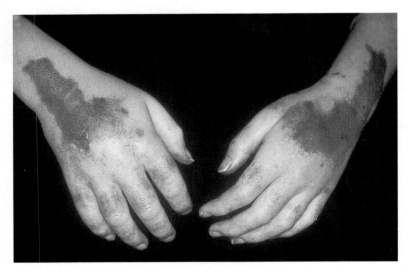

FIGURE 13.40 ■ Thrombotic Thrombocytopenic Purpura. Bleeding at initial presentation is seen in about 30% to 40% of patients with TTP. (Photo contributor: James J. Nordlund, MD.)

Clinical Summary

The first sign of pityriasis rosea (PR) is a well-demarcated, salmon-colored macule that evolves into a larger patch with peripheral scaling (the "herald patch"). Over the following 1 to 2 weeks, generalized, bilateral, and symmetric macules appear along cleavage lines. The macules have a peripheral collarette of fine scaling. This phase gives rise to the "Christmas tree" pattern of lesions on the back. Most patients will have severe itching associated with the generalized eruption. The lesions resolve over the next 6 weeks. Atypical presentations in children include inverse PR (presentation on the face and distal extremities) and papular PR (scaling papules rather than macules). An association with *Human Herpes Virus 7* has been postulated but definitive causality has not been established.

Emergency Department Treatment and Disposition

Reassure the patient that this disease is both benign and self-limited. Pruritus can be treated with oral antihistamines, low-to-mid topical steroids and oatmeal baths. Antibiotics do not shorten the disease course; however, in a small study, high-dose acyclovir was shown to clear the eruption.

Pearls

1. In patients with risk factors for syphilis and HIV, appropriate screening tests should be performed.
2. Patients should be warned of the extended course of PR and given appropriate antihistamines and follow-up.
3. Atypical presentations are seen in dark-skinned individuals.

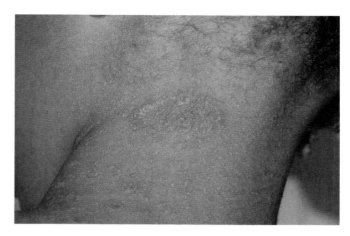

FIGURE 13.41 ■ Pityriasis Rosea Herald Patch. The herald patch of PR, a well-demarcated salmon-colored macule with scales, frequently precedes the generalized phase by 1 to 2 weeks. (Photo contributor: Lawrence B. Stack, MD.)

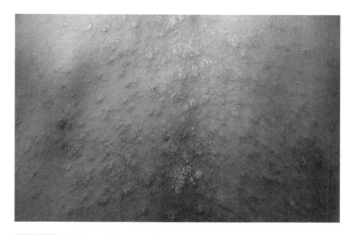

FIGURE 13.42 ■ Pityriasis Rosea. An exanthematous, papulosquamous eruption, with the long axis of the oval papules following the lines of cleavage in a Christmas tree-like eruption. (Photo contributor: David Effron, MD.)

Clinical Summary

Livedo reticularis presents as a macular, reticulated (lace-like) patch of nonpalpable cutaneous vasodilatation in response to a variety of vascular occlusive processes. This pattern predominates in the peripheral or acral areas and may or may not be associated with purpura. In time, the overlying epidermis and dermis may infarct and form ulcerations or develop palpable dermal papules or nodules. Livedo reticularis is usually representative of a severe underlying systemic disease. Inflammatory vascular diseases (livedo vasculitis, polyarteritis nodosa, lupus erythematosus), septic emboli (meningococcemia), tumors (pheochromocytoma), and systemic illnesses associated with mechanical vessel blockage (anticardiolipin antibody syndrome, polycythemia vera, sickle cell anemia, cholesterol embolus) are a few diseases associated with or responsible for livedo reticularis. It can also occur independent of any disease association.

Emergency Department Treatment and Disposition

The treatment of livedo reticularis is management of the underlying disorder and avoiding exposure to cold.

Pearls

1. Livedo reticularis is an inflammatory vascular disease usually found symmetrically on the ankles and dorsum of the feet. It consists of painful stellate-shaped ulcerations surrounded by an erythematous livedo pattern.
2. Cholesterol emboli usually occur after an intraarterial procedure. Pain often precedes the livedo pattern of purpura on the distal extremities.
3. Patients with anticardiolipin antibody syndrome have extensive livedo reticularis and recurrent arterial and venous thromboses involving multiple organ systems.

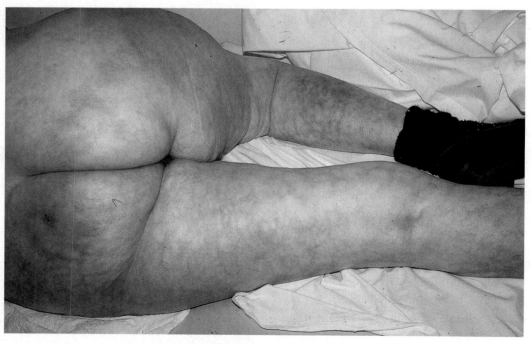

FIGURE 13.43 ■ Livedo Reticularis. Note the reticulated (lacelike) blanching erythema symmetrically distributed over the lower extremities. (Photo contributor: James J. Nordlund, MD.)

Clinical Summary

Acute urticaria develops over days to weeks and presents with transient wheals. Generally, acute urticaria resolves within 6 weeks, whereas chronic urticaria lasts longer than 6 weeks. Common triggers include medications (penicillin, aspirin), foods (chocolate, shellfish, nuts, eggs, milk, and others) and infections (streptococcal, hepatitis B and C, mononucleosis, and helminths), and physical factors (exercise, pressure, cold, vibratory and solar-induced urticaria).

Dermatographism is the production of linear wheals and surrounding erythema after stroking the skin. It is considered an exaggerated physiologic response to friction and can be found in up to 5% of the population. Persistent dermatographism can be seen with scratching and tight clothing. This is seen primarily in children and young adults and generally improves over 5 to 10 years.

Angioedema develops acutely with subcutaneous edema, but no overlying epidermal changes. Life-threatening laryngeal edema can rapidly occur. Angiotensin-converting enzyme (ACE) inhibitors frequently cause angioedema of the face, lips, and tongue. Urticaria is not present with ACE inhibitor associated angioedema. NSAID-induced angioedema occurs within minutes of ingestion and is associated with urticaria. Other triggers for angioedema include medications (penicillin, sulfonamides), foods (as with urticaria), insect envenomations, radiocontrast media, cold urticaria, solar urticaria, vibratory urticaria, and idiopathic urticaria. Hereditary and acquired C1 esterase inhibitor deficiencies also cause angioedema.

Emergency Department Treatment and Disposition

Triggers of urticaria and angioedema should be investigated and, if present, stopped. ACE inhibitor and NSAID are class specific; therefore, patients should never use these medication classes again. H1 and H2 blockers usually help with urticaria. Systemic steroids and epinephrine are used in severe reactions. Hereditary C1 esterase inhibitor deficiency can be treated with fresh frozen plasma or C1 inhibitor concentrate. Prevention with androgens (danazol, stanazol) may be used prior to surgical procedures. Acquired C1 esterase inhibitor requires treatment of the underlying malignancy.

Pearls

1. More than 50% of chronic urticaria is idiopathic.
2. Wheals in the same location lasting more than 24 hours are concerning for urticarial vasculitis and require a confirmatory skin biopsy.
3. Fifty percent of ACE inhibitor–associated angioedema occurs within the first week of treatment. The other 50% can occur at any time.

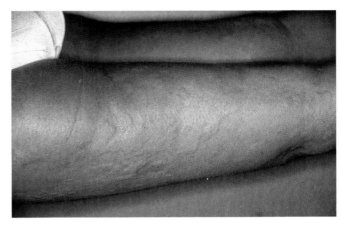

FIGURE 13.44 ■ Urticaria. Note the classic raised plaques on the lower extremity of this patient with urticaria. (Photo contributor: James J. Nordlund, MD.)

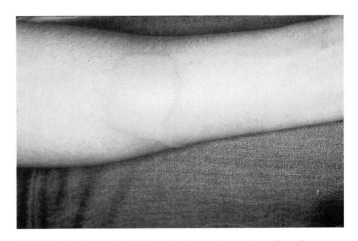

FIGURE 13.45 ■ Cold Urticaria. Plaque formation after placement of an ice cube on the skin confirms cold urticaria. (Photo contributor: James J. Nordlund, MD.)

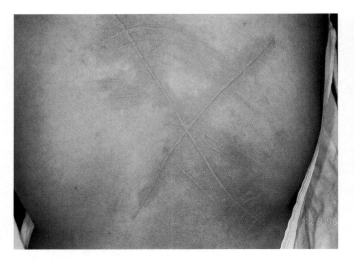

FIGURE 13.46 ■ Dermatographism. Note the linear wheal with surrounding erythematous flare after scratching and stroking. (Photo contributor: J. Matthew Hardin, MD.)

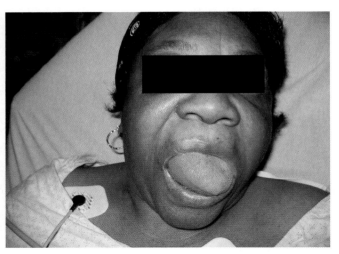

FIGURE 13.48 ■ Angioedema. ACE inhibitor-induced angioedema of the tongue can produce airway difficulties. (Photo contributor: Selim Suner, MD, MS.)

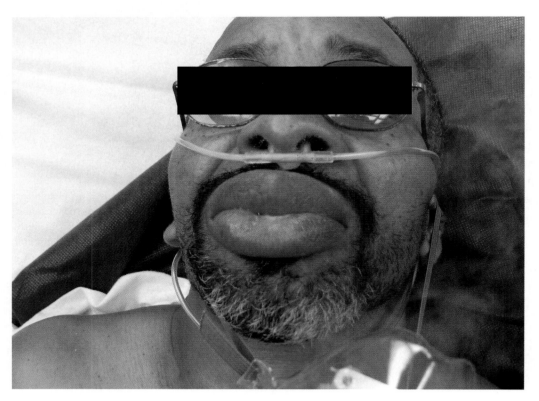

FIGURE 13.47 ■ Angioedema. ACE inhibitor-induced angioedema of the lips. (Photo contributor: R. Jason Thurman, MD.)

Clinical Summary

Allergic contact dermatitis occurs after previously sensitized skin is rechallenged with the same allergen. It represents a delayed type hypersensitivity reaction. Papules and vesicles first develop that can become a generalized morbilliform eruption. Pruritus is a dominant feature. The most common causes of allergic contact dermatitis are nickel, toxicodendrons (poison ivy, poison oak, and poison sumac), neomycin, fragrances, balsam of Peru, formaldehyde, bacitracin, and rubber compounds.

Emergency Department Treatment and Disposition

Identification of the causative agent and prevention of further contact is critical. Supportive care is given with antihistamines and topical steroids. Systemic steroids may be needed for generalized eruptions.

Pearls

1. Toxicodendron allergic contact dermatitis requires a minimum 3 week taper of oral prednisone. Otherwise, a worse rebound effect often occurs.
2. Patients can develop a second allergic contact dermatitis to topical treatments (containing fragrances, preservatives, and antibiotics).
3. Neomycin causes an allergic contact dermatitis in up to 15% of the general population.

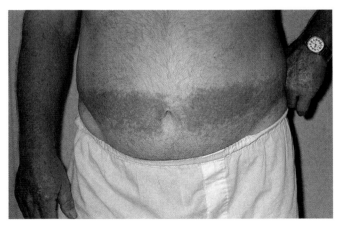

FIGURE 13.49 ■ Contact Dermatitis. Erythematous eruption in a waist band distribution. (Photo contributor: J. Matthew Hardin, MD.)

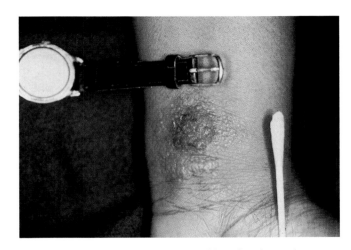

FIGURE 13.50 ■ Contact Dermatitis. Note that the erythematous, edematous base of the eruption corresponds to the posterior surface of the watch. Superimposed on the erythematous base are multiple vesicles with exudate and crust. (Photo contributor: the Department of Dermatology, Wilford Hall USAF Medical Center and Brooke Army Medical Center, San Antonio, TX.)

Clinical Summary

Phytophotodermatitis and phototoxic drug reactions result from exposure of a substance (photosensitizer) that, upon absorption of UV radiation, becomes activated. As the photosensitizer returns to the inactive state, the release of energy induces a local reaction. The photosensitizer can access the skin topically (phytophotodermatitis) or internally (phototoxic drug reaction). The most common phytophotodermatitis photosensitizers are furocoumarins (found in celery, parsley, and limes). Phototoxic drug reactions are most commonly caused by NSAIDs, sulfonamides, thiazide diuretics, and tetracyclines.

These reactions occur in only sun-exposed sites and can appear hours to days after initial exposure. The clinical presentation is that of sunburn. Hyperpigmentation may last for months after initial reaction.

Emergency Department Treatment and Disposition

Identification of possible causes is the first step. Avoidance of these agents is essential.

Pearls

1. Remember that only sun-exposed sites are involved (verses allergic contact dermatitis).
2. Topical exposures to plants cause streaming and linear lesions, whereas ingestion of photosensitizers cause more diffuse reactions.

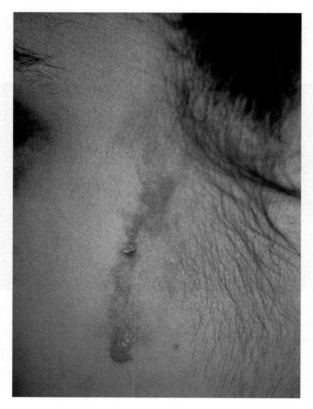

FIGURE 13.51 ■ Phytophotodermatitis. This linear, photo-distributed, eczematous plaque resulted from contact with a plant-derived photosensitizer (lime juice). This frequently resolves with hyperpigmentation. (Photo contributor: the Department of Dermatology, Wilford Hall USAF Medical Center and Brooke Army Medical Center, San Antonio, TX.)

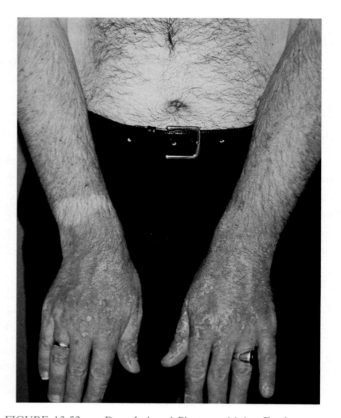

FIGURE 13.52 ■ Drug-Induced Photosensitivity. Erythematous reaction to ultraviolet radiation associated with carbamazepine use. (Photo contributor: the Department of Dermatology, Naval Medical Center, Portsmouth, VA.)

Clinical Summary

Erythema nodosum (EN) can present at any age but is most common in young, adult females. The most typical presentation is bilateral, erythematous, subcutaneous, tender nodules on the pretibial and lateral lower extremities (usually spares the posterior calves). Rarely, the nodules can be found on the thighs, upper extremities, and face. Concomitant symptoms often include lower extremity edema and arthralgias. Systemic symptoms can occur and include fever, headache, and gastrointestinal complaints. Generally, the nodules resolve over days to weeks with flattening and a change in color to a blue-green (like a deep bruise). There is no ulceration and the skin slowly returns to normal.

Multiple etiologies can present with EN. Infectious causes include streptococcal, tuberculosis, *Yersinia*, *Salmonella*, *Shigella*, coccidioidomycosis, histoplasmosis, sporotrichosis, blastomycosis, and toxoplasmosis. EN has also been associated with sarcoidosis and inflammatory bowel disease. Oral contraceptives, sulfonamides, bromides, and iodides are known to be common causative agents, among many others.

Emergency Department Treatment and Disposition

With the many etiologies of EN, it is critical to exclude and treat an infectious, systemic, or medication cause. Supportive care with elevation of the extremity, rest, and NSAIDs is prudent. Recurrences do occur and should prompt a further workup for occult infection or medication. Referral to a dermatologist for a biopsy may help confirm the diagnosis.

Pearls

1. The patient's history is very helpful in determining possible etiologies. A complete medication, travel, and past medical history must be performed.

2. Systemic glucocorticoids can be considered, but only when the etiology is clearly known and infectious agents are excluded.

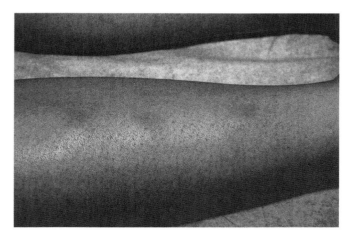

FIGURE 13.53 ■ Erythema Nodosum, Acute. Erythema nodosum, acute phase. Note the pretibial, erythematous and subcutaneous nodules. (Photo contributor: J. Matthew Hardin, MD.)

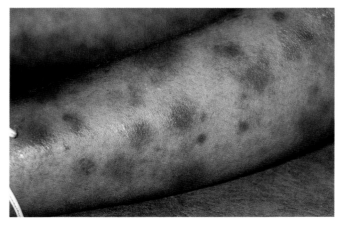

FIGURE 13.54 ■ Erythema Nodosum, Resolving. Note the bruise-like appearance of the resolving phase. (Photo contributor: J. Matthew Hardin, MD.)

Clinical Summary

Borrelia burgdorferi is the tick-borne spirochete responsible for Lyme borreliosis, and erythema chronicum migrans (ECM) is the pathognomonic rash of Lyme disease occurring early in the infection. The initial prodromal symptoms of fever, myalgias, arthralgias, and headache are followed by a macule or papule progressing to a plaque at the site of the bite. This plaque expands its red, raised border as it clears centrally, leading to an annular appearance. The plaque may burn and is rarely pruritic. On average, there are 9 days between the time of the bite and the appearance of the rash.

Emergency Department Treatment and Disposition

The duration of antibiotic treatment (10 to 30 days) depends on the severity of the symptoms. Doxycycline is the drug of choice. Pregnant or lactating females and children younger than 8 years of age should be treated with amoxicillin, penicillin, or cefuroxime. Erythromycin is a suitable alternative. Patients with minimal symptoms may be treated on an outpatient basis. Those patients with significant toxicity and complications require admission, supportive care, and IV antibiotics.

Pearls

1. An annular plaque arising at the site of a tick bite in a patient with systemic symptoms should be treated as Lyme disease until proved otherwise.
2. Stage I of Lyme disease consists of constitutional symptoms and the characteristic rash of ECM.
3. Stage II of Lyme disease consists of neurologic (aseptic meningitis, encephalitis, bilateral Bell palsy) and cardiac (myocarditis, conduction blocks) manifestations.
4. Stage III of Lyme disease consists of asymmetric, episodic, oligoarticular arthritis.
5. The annular plaque may resemble a fixed drug eruption, tinea corporis, urticaria, or the herald patch of pityriasis rosea.

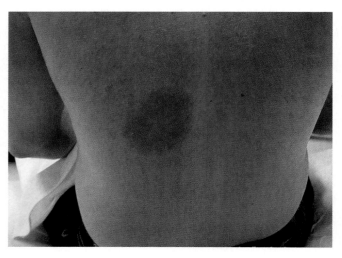

FIGURE 13.55 ■ Erythema Chronicum Migrans. The eruption of Lyme disease forms at the site of the tick bite. The initial papule forms into a slowly enlarging oval area of erythema with central clearing. (Reprinted with permission of *Annals of Emergency Medicine* 2005;46:224. Photo contributor: Shannon B. Snyder, MD.)

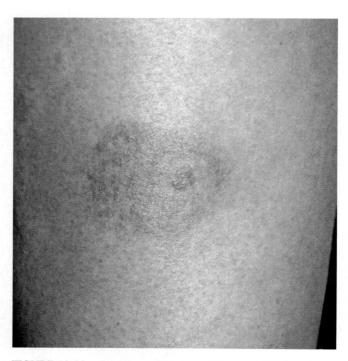

FIGURE 13.56 ■ Erythema Chronicum Migrans. ECM from Lyme disease. (Photo contributor: David Effron, MD.)

Clinical Summary

Rickettsia rickettsii is transmitted by the bite of an infected tick. Fever, rigors, headache, myalgias, and weakness occur 7 to 10 days after inoculation. The initially blanching macular eruption begins at approximately 4 days on the distal extremities and somewhat later on the palms and soles. It soon becomes petechial as it spreads centrally to involve the trunk and abdomen. However, it can present without obvious cutaneous manifestations.

Emergency Department Treatment and Disposition

Doxycycline or chloramphenicol is required for this potentially fatal illness. Doxycycline is the drug of choice, yet it should be avoided in pregnant or lactating women and children younger than 8 years of age. Mildly ill patients may be treated with oral antibiotics on an outpatient basis as long as close follow-up can be arranged. More severely ill patients should be admitted because their care can be complicated by circulatory collapse and coma. Approximately 20% of untreated patients will die; overall mortality is 3% to 7%.

Pearls

1. Palmar and plantar petechiae in a severely ill patient should be treated as Rocky Mountain spotted fever until proven otherwise. Treatment should not be delayed until laboratory confirmation is obtained.
2. Most cases occur between April and October, with the highest US incidence occurring in the Southeast and South-Central states.
3. Doxycycline therapy also treats Lyme disease, ehrlichiosis, and relapsing fever, all of which can be confused with RMSF.

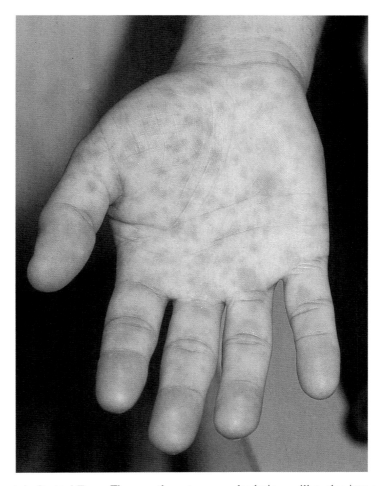

FIGURE 13.57 ■ Rocky Mountain Spotted Fever. These erythematous macular lesions will evolve into a petechial rash that will spread centrally. (Photo contributor: Daniel Noltkamper, MD.)

Clinical Summary

Disseminated gonococcus (GC) is a systemic infection, with septic vasculitis following the hematogenous dissemination of the organism *Neisseria gonorrhea*. The spectrum of disease varies from skin lesions alone to skin lesions with tenosynovitis or septic arthritis. The initial lesion is an erythematous macule that evolves into a necrotic, purpuric vesicopustule. These purpura are few in number, asymmetric, and predominantly distal in location.

Emergency Department Treatment and Disposition

Therapy consists of intravenous or intramuscular ceftriaxone or cefotaxime until symptoms either improve or resolve, followed by an additional 7 days of orally administered cefixime. If susceptible, ciprofloxacin, ofloxacin, or levofloxacin can be used. Hospitalization is recommended for noncompliant patients or cases noted to have an associated septic arthritis.

Pearls

1. The most common symptom of disseminated GC is arthralgia of one or more joints, primarily involving the hands or knees.
2. Skin lesions develop in up to 70% of cases and will resolve within 4 days regardless of antibiotics.
3. Less than one-third of patients will have urethritis.
4. The purpura of septic vasculitis (of whatever bacterial etiology) tend to be fewer in number, asymmetric, and distal in location.
5. Infectious arthritis or tenosynovitis must be considered when the patient presents with joint complaints.

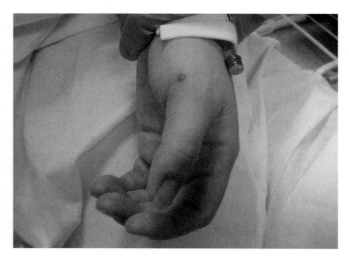

FIGURE 13.58 ■ Disseminated Gonococcus. Vesiculopustule on the hand of a patient with disseminated gonococcus. (Photo contributor: Stephan E. Russ, MD.)

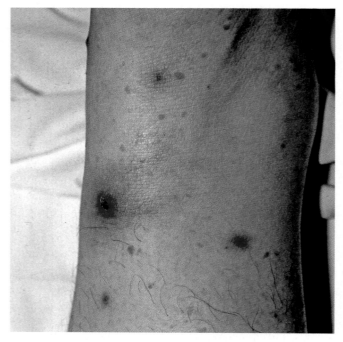

FIGURE 13.59 ■ Disseminated Gonococcus. Erythematous macules of disseminated gonococcus. (Photo contributor: David Effron, MD.)

Clinical Summary

Infective endocarditis is an illness characterized by fever, valve destruction, and peripheral embolization manifested by rare, usually distal purpura. *Streptococcus viridans* is the most common causative organism. Janeway lesions occur in 5% of cases and consist of nontender, small, erythematous macules on the palms or soles. Osler nodes occur in 10% of cases and consist of transient, tender, purplish nodules on the pulp of the fingers and toes. Splinter hemorrhages are black, linear discolorations beneath the nail plate. They are present in 20% of cases and are more suggestive of subacute bacterial endocarditis (SBE) if present at the proximal or middle nail plate. Murmurs, retinal hemorrhages, septic arthritis, and significant embolic episodes such as pulmonary embolism or stroke may also be present.

Emergency Department Treatment and Disposition

Antibiotics must be appropriate for the infectious agent; however, therapy is often required before the diagnosis is confirmed or the infecting organism is known. All toxic patients require admission, as do all febrile patients who have prosthetic valves or who are intravenous drug abusers. Vancomycin and gentamicin, or nafcillin and gentamicin should be considered empirically pending the blood culture results. Patients with rheumatic or congenital valve abnormalities may receive streptomycin with penicillin or vancomycin.

Pearls

1. Janeway lesions, Osler nodes, and splinter hemorrhages in a febrile patient with a murmur are virtually diagnostic of infective endocarditis.
2. Rheumatic heart disease is the most common predisposing factor; the mitral valve is the most common site of damage.
3. Congenital heart disease, intravenous drug abuse, and prosthetic heart valves are additional predisposing factors for the development of infective endocarditis.

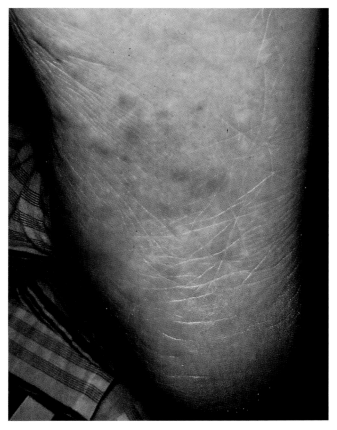

FIGURE 13.60 ■ Janeway Lesions. Peripheral embolization to the sole, resulting in a cluster of erythematous macules known as Janeway lesions. (Photo contributor: the Department of Dermatology, Wilford Hall USAF Medical Center and Brooke Army Medical Center, San Antonio, TX.)

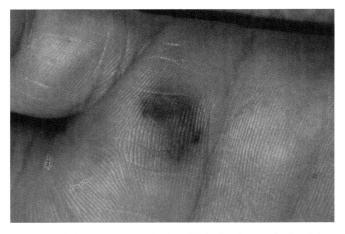

FIGURE 13.61 ■ Janeway Lesion. Embolization to the hand in a patient with infectious endocarditis. (Photo contributor: Alan B. Storrow, MD.)

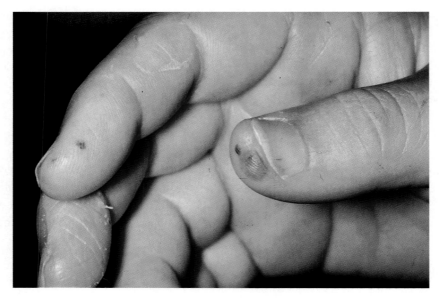

FIGURE 13.62 ▪ Osler Nodes. Subcutaneous, purplish, tender nodules in the pulp of the fingers known as Osler nodes. (Photo contributor: the Armed Forces Institute of Pathology, Bethesda, MD.)

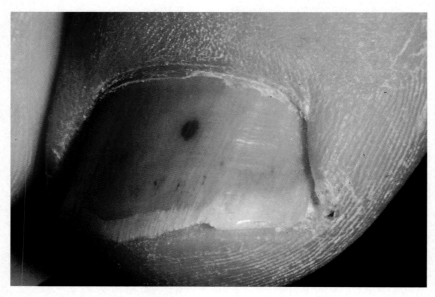

FIGURE 13.63 ▪ Splinter Hemorrhages. Note the splinter hemorrhages along the distal aspect of the nail plate, due to emboli from subacute bacterial endocarditis. (Photo contributor: the Armed Forces Institute of Pathology, Bethesda, MD.)

Clinical Summary

Erysipelas is a group A streptococcal cellulitis involving the skin to the level of the dermis. The plaque is typically erythematous, edematous, and painful, with an elevated, well-demarcated border. The associated edema tends to make the plaque appear shiny. Erysipelas frequently occurs on the face and lower extremities.

Emergency Department Treatment and Disposition

All infections require rest, elevation, heat, and antibiotics. Mild presentations may be treated on an outpatient basis with oral dicloxacillin, penicillin, or erythromycin. More severe illness or toxicity requires hospitalization and intravenous antibiotics (nafcillin, oxacillin, cefazolin, or penicillin).

Pearls

1. The well-demarcated, tender, shiny, erythematous plaque is diagnostic of erysipelas.
2. This same shiny, erythematous plaque on the face of a febrile child may be caused by *Haemophilus influenzae*, necessitating intravenous chloramphenicol or a cephalosporin.
3. Lymphatic streaking is more common in erysipelas than cellulitis.

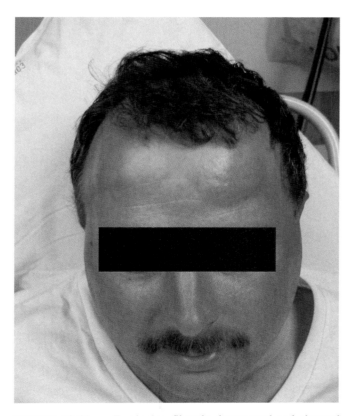

FIGURE 13.64 ■ Erysipelas. Sharply demarcated and elevated erythema of erysipelas. (Photo contributor: R. Jason Thurman, MD.)

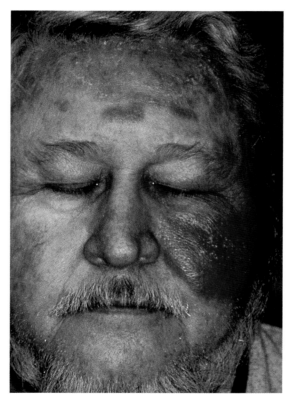

FIGURE 13.65 ■ Erysipelas. Note the well-demarcated, edematous, erythematous, shiny plaque. (Photo contributor: the Department of Dermatology, Wilford Hall USAF Medical Center and Brooke Army Medical Center, San Antonio, TX.)

Clinical Summary

Hot-tub folliculitis is a pruritic, follicular, pustular eruption confined to the hair follicle and is secondary to a cutaneous infection with *Pseudomonas aeruginosa*. Headache, sore throat, earache, and fever may accompany the pustules, which usually localize to the trunk and proximal extremities.

Emergency Department Treatment and Disposition

The folliculitis usually involutes in 7 to 10 days without treatment, although ciprofloxacin may be used. Acetic acid compresses and local wound cleansing may speed recovery. In addition, the hot tub or source of exposure must be decontaminated to avoid reexposure.

Pearls

1. Pruritic pustules confined to the hair follicles of the trunk and proximal extremities are diagnostic of folliculitis.
2. Other forms of folliculitis should be treated with cleaning, topical antibiotics, and, if refractory, oral antibiotics such as cephalexin.
3. This may also result from contact with chemicals (exfoliative beauty aids) or repetitive physical trauma (friction from tight clothing).

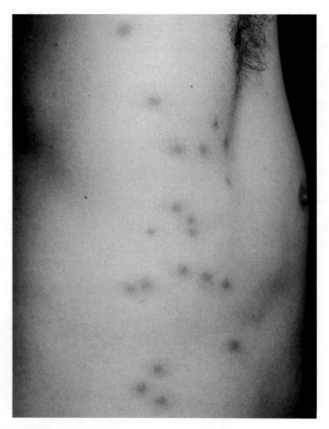

FIGURE 13.66 ■ Hot Tub Folliculitis. Note the pustules localized to the hair follicles of the trunk and proximal extremity. (Photo contributor: Jeffrey S. Gibson, MD.)

Clinical Summary

Ecthyma gangrenosum is a *Pseudomonas aeruginosa* infection that usually occurs in the septic, immunocompromised, or neutropenic patient. The initially erythematous macules develop bullae or pustules surrounded by violaceous halos. The pustules become hemorrhagic and rupture, forming painless ulcers with necrotic, black centers.

Emergency Department Treatment and Disposition

These patients are usually septic and immunocompromised. Admission is usually required for the patient to receive antipseudomonal antibiotics and general supportive care.

Pearls

1. Consider ecthyma gangrenosum when examining a septic patient who presents with bullae or pustules that rupture and form painless, necrotic ulcers.
2. It is important to consider underlying immunodeficiency when making this diagnosis.
3. Necrotizing vasculitis, fixed drug eruptions, pyoderma gangrenosum, and brown recluse spider bites must all be considered in the differential diagnosis.

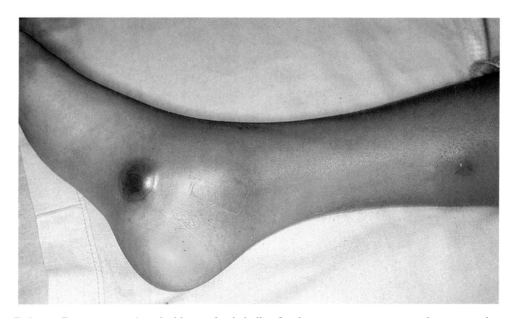

FIGURE 13.67 ■ Ecthyma Gangrenosum. A typical hemorrhagic bulla of ecthyma gangrenosum secondary to pseudomonal sepsis. (Photo contributor: James Mensching, MD.)

Clinical Summary

Initial papules of secondary syphilis are usually asymptomatic, though they may be painful or pruritic. They appear 2 to 10 weeks after the primary chancre. Headache, sore throat, fever, arthralgias, myalgias, and generalized lymphadenopathy may also present. Exanthematous papules are symmetric and nondestructive, usually forming a pityriasis rosea–like pattern on trunk, palms, and soles. Later lesions are firm, pigmented papules with a coppery tint and adherent scales. Macerated papules may form on mucous membranes; "motheaten" alopecia on scalp; and condylomata lata in the intertriginous areas.

Emergency Department Treatment and Disposition

Penicillin is the agent of choice. Tetracycline, doxycycline, erythromycin, or multidose ceftriaxone are used in cases of penicillin allergy. Jarisch-Herxheimer reaction may occur several hours after treatment, correlating with the spirochete clearance from the blood. This lasts approximately 24 hours; it may be more threatening than the disease. Increasing fever, rigors, myalgias, headache, tachycardia, hypotension, and a drop in the leukocyte and platelet count may occur. Fluid resuscitation to maintain blood pressure and supportive care may be needed.

Pearls

1. Scaly palmar and plantar papules are strongly suggestive of secondary syphilis, the incidence of which is rising.
2. These scaling red-brown papules appear 2 to 10 weeks after the spontaneous resolution of the initial painless chancre.

3. Tertiary syphilis occurs in untreated or poorly treated patients and may manifest itself as general paresis, tabes dorsalis, optic atrophy, and aortitis with aneurysms.
4. Syphilis is "the great imitator." It may resemble psoriasis, drug eruptions, pityriasis rosea, viral exanthems, tinea corporis, tinea versicolor, and condyloma acuminata. A positive serologic test for syphilis makes the diagnosis.

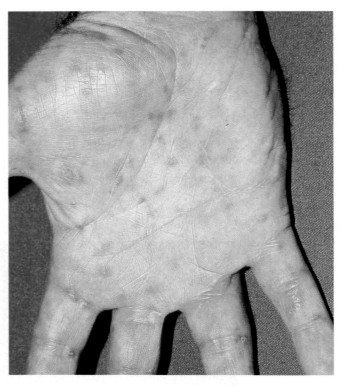

FIGURE 13.69 ■ Secondary Syphilis. These firm, pigmented, erythematous papules are characteristic of secondary syphilis. (Photo contributor: Lynn Utecht, MD.)

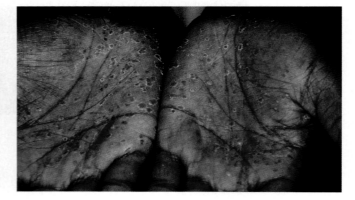

FIGURE 13.68 ■ Secondary Syphilis. Eruptive, scaly, copper-colored papules on foot may be the initial presentation. They are usually symmetric, asymptomatic, and nondestructive. (Photo contributor: the Department of Dermatology, Wilford Hall USAF Medical Center and Brooke Army Medical Center, San Antonio, TX.)

FIGURE 13.70 ■ Secondary Syphilis. These firm, pigmented papules with a coppery tint and adherent scale are characteristic. (Photo contributor: the Department of Dermatology, Wilford Hall USAF Medical Center and Brooke Army Medical Center, San Antonio, TX.)

Clinical Summary

Dissecting cellulitis of the scalp occurs predominately in young black males. This condition, along with acne conglobata (acne fulminans without systemic symptoms), hidradenitis suppurativa, and pilonidal cysts is known as the "follicular occlusion tetrad." Clinically, patients present with multiple, fluctuant abscesses on the vertex and occiput of the scalp. Sinus tracts form between the abscesses. Over time, scarring alopecia can result. Most patients are young and the psychological impact can be significant.

Emergency Department Treatment and Disposition

Exclusion of an acute secondary infection is essential. Incision and drainage of new, rapidly forming abscesses may be indicated. Antibiotics help prevent further abscesses and tetracyclines help decrease the inflammatory component. This is an inflammatory condition and antibiotics alone are not adequate. Refer patient to a dermatologist for biopsy and possible isotretinoin treatment.

Pearls

1. Recurrent scalp abscesses and draining sinus tracts that are unresponsive to antibiotics should prompt consideration for this diagnosis.
2. Early diagnosis can prevent further scarring and alopecia.

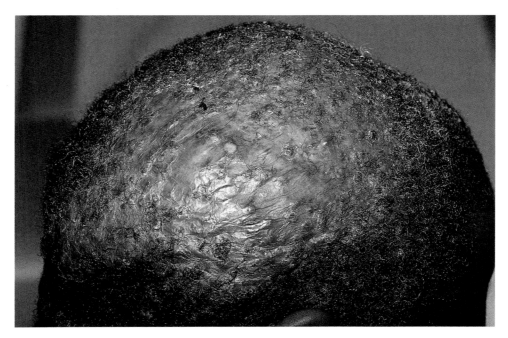

FIGURE 13.71 ■ Dissecting Cellulitis of the Scalp. This is resolving with scarring alopecia. (Photo contributor: J. Matthew Hardin, MD.)

Clinical Summary

Squamous cell carcinoma (SCC) is the second most common skin cancer. It is associated with a higher incidence in males, increased age, chronic sun exposure, immunosuppressive treatment, and chronic burns or scars. Initially, SCC presents with erythematous macules that develop into firm papules and plaques. Most are located on the sun-exposed sites of the head, neck, and upper extremities.

Emergency Department Treatment and Disposition

After ensuring a secondary infection is not present, prompt outpatient dermatologic referral is indicated.

Pearls

1. There is a higher risk of metastasis with SCC versus basal cell carcinoma (although still very low).
2. Any persistent nodule, plaque, or ulcer should be examined for SCC.

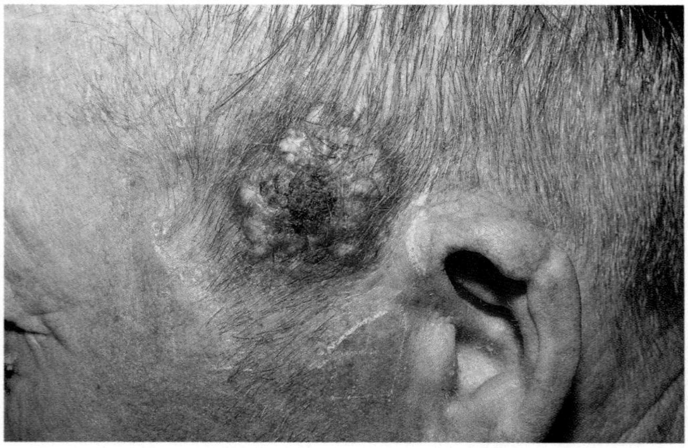

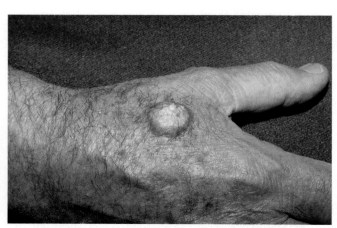

FIGURE 13.73 ■ Squamous Cell Carcinoma. This nodule with central ulceration slowly developed over 1 year. (Photo contributor: J. Matthew Hardin, MD.)

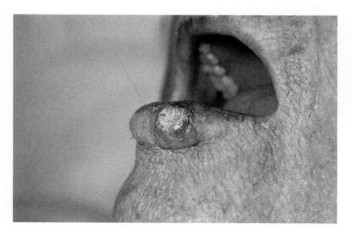

FIGURE 13.72 ■ Squamous Cell Carcinoma. The lower lip is exposed to more sunlight and is therefore involved more frequently. (Photo contributor: J. Matthew Hardin, MD.)

FIGURE 13.74 ■ Squamous Cell Carcinoma. This nodule has a central keratogenous core. (Photo contributor: J. Matthew Hardin, MD.)

Clinical Summary

Basal cell carcinoma (BCC) is the most common nonmelanoma skin cancer. BCC can present anywhere on the body but is most common on the sun-exposed areas. The typical lesion begins as a pearly papule with telangiectasias (nodular BCC). The lesion may ulcerate and bleed. Other forms of BCC include superficial BCC (pink, scaly plaque with pearly border), pigmented BCC (appears as a nodular or superficial BCC with dark brown to black center), and morpheaform BCC (appears as a rapidly expanding scar).

Emergency Department Treatment and Disposition

After ensuring a secondary infection is not present, prompt outpatient dermatologic referral is indicated. Surgical excision and topical chemotherapy are therapeutic options.

Pearls

1. The metastatic potential of BCC is very low (0.1%).
2. BCC is rare in brown and black-skinned persons.

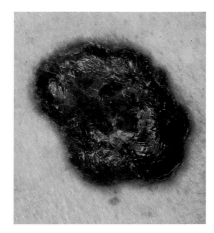

FIGURE 13.76 ■ Pigmented Basal Cell Carcinoma. This pigmented basal cell carcinoma consists of a firm, translucent, brownish-black ulcerated nodule with an irregular surface and asymmetry of its border. (Photo contributor: the Department of Dermatology, Wilford Hall USAF Medical Center and Brooke Army Medical Center, San Antonio, TX.)

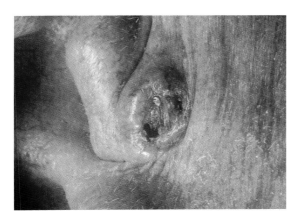

FIGURE 13.75 ■ Basal Cell Carcinoma. Nodular basal cell carcinoma consists of a firm, centrally ulcerated (rodent ulcer) nodule with a raised, rolled, pearly, telangiectatic border. (Photo contributor: the Department of Dermatology, Wilford Hall USAF Medical Center and Brooke Army Medical Center, San Antonio, TX.)

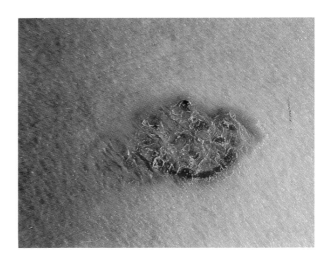

FIGURE 13.77 ■ Basal Cell Carcinoma. A superficial multicentric basal cell carcinoma is frequently psoriasiform in nature. Note the flat, erythematous, scaly plaque with its elevated, irregular border. (Photo contributor: the Department of Dermatology, Wilford Hall USAF Medical Center and Brooke Army Medical Center, San Antonio, TX.)

Clinical Summary

Melanoma is a potentially fatal cutaneous tumor derived from epidermal melanocytes. Any age can be affected but the peak incidence is 20- to 45-year old patients (much younger than basal cell or squamous cell carcinomas). The most significant risk factor is a primary relative with melanoma. Evaluation of any pigmented lesion should include the ABCDE rule (A for asymmetry, B for irregular borders, C for color variegation, D for diameter greater than 6 mm, and E for elevation or thickening). Any lesion with these characteristics is considered suspicious for melanoma.

Emergency Department Treatment and Disposition

Prompt outpatient dermatologic referral is indicated.

Pearls

1. The palms, soles, and subungual sites are most common with dark-skinned individuals.
2. Melanoma can occur in sites not exposed to the sun (genitalia/buttocks).

3. Any growing pigmented or nonpigmented lesion should be referred to dermatology.
4. Most patients will not have new moles after 35 years old. A new mole in this setting should be evaluated by dermatology.

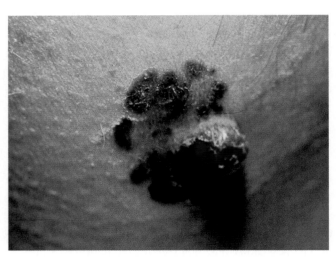

FIGURE 13.79 ■ Nodular Melanoma. This melanoma has progressed to an exophytic tumor, which was deeply invasive histopathologically. (Photo contributor: the Department of Dermatology, Wilford Hall USAF Medical Center and Brooke Army Medical Center, San Antonio, TX.)

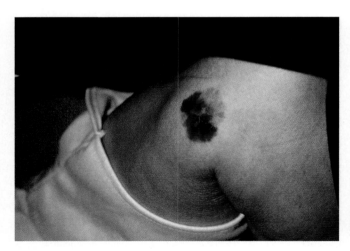

FIGURE 13.78 ■ Melanoma. This lesion demonstrates asymmetry, color variegation, and a diameter greater than 6 mm. (Photo contributor: J. Matthew Hardin, MD.)

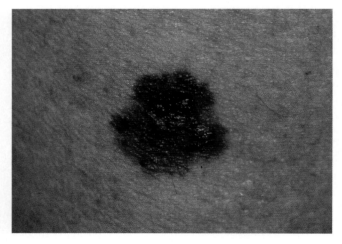

FIGURE 13.80 ■ Melanoma. Note the asymmetry, irregular border, and focal hyperpigmentation in this melanoma. (Photo contributor: the Department of Dermatology, Wilford Hall USAF Medical Center and Brooke Army Medical Center, San Antonio, TX.)

Clinical Summary

Herpes zoster is a dermatomal, unilateral reactivation of the varicella zoster virus. Pain, tenderness, and dysesthesias may present 4 to 5 days prior to an eruption composed of umbilicated, grouped vesicles on an erythematous, edematous base. The vesicles may become purulent or hemorrhagic. Nerve involvement may actually occur without cutaneous involvement. Ophthalmic zoster involves the nasociliary branch of the fifth cranial nerve and presents with vesicles on the nose and cornea (Hutchinson sign). Ramsay Hunt syndrome is a herpes zoster infection of the geniculate ganglion that presents with decreased hearing, facial palsy, and vesicles on the tympanic membrane, pinna, and ear canal.

The most likely differential diagnosis is herpes simplex infection, which is usually recurrent. The prodromal pain must be differentiated from potential pleural, cardiac, or abdominal origin. Tzanck smear of the floor of a vesicle demonstrating multinucleated giant cells makes the diagnosis of a herpes-family infection (see related item).

Emergency Department Treatment and Disposition

Uncomplicated cases of herpes zoster can be managed with supportive care, especially pain control. Admission to the hospital for intravenous acyclovir is usually reserved for complicated cases involving multiple dermatomal distributions or the ophthalmic branch of the trigeminal nerve, disseminated disease, or immunocompromised patients. Acyclovir, famciclovir, or valacyclovir hasten the healing and decreases the pain if started within 72 hours of vesicle appearance. These agents have also been shown to reduce the duration of postherpetic neuralgia. Prednisone may also prove useful. Herpes zoster keratitis requires immediate ophthalmologic consultation to avoid any potential vision loss.

Pearls

1. Dermatomally grouped, umbilicated vesicles on an erythematous base are diagnostic of herpes zoster.
2. The thorax is the most common area involved, followed by the face (trigeminal nerve).
3. The nonimmune or immunocompromised should avoid lesional contact from prodrome until reepithelialization, since the crusts can contain the varicella zoster virus.
4. Typically, an infected patient may transmit chickenpox to a nonimmune individual.
5. Zoster during pregnancy seems to have no deleterious effects on the mother or baby.

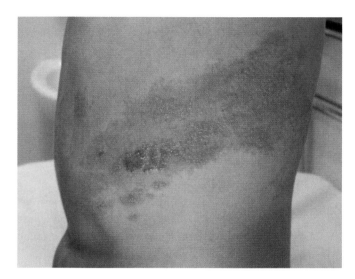

FIGURE 13.81 ■ Herpes Zoster. Umbilicated, grouped, dermatomal vesicles on an erythematous base in a patient with herpes zoster. (Photo contributor: Selim Suner, MD, MS.)

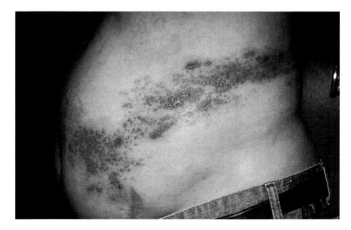

FIGURE 13.82 ■ Herpes Zoster. This eruption consists of a dermatomal distribution of umbilicated vesicles on an erythematous base. Note the occasional cluster of hemorrhagic vesicles. Tzanck smear was positive. (Photo contributor: the Department of Dermatology, Wilford Hall USAF Medical Center and Brooke Army Medical Center, San Antonio, TX.)

Clinical Summary

Primary or recurrent herpes simplex virus (HSV) infection commonly presents as grouped vesicles on an erythematous base. Plaques and erosions also occur.

Herpetic whitlow is a painful HSV infection of the distal finger characterized by edema, erythema, vesicles, and pustules an erythematous base. Fever, lymphangitis, and regional adenopathy are often present.

Herpes gladiatorum spreads via direct skin-to-skin contact in sports such as rugby and wrestling. The condition may become latent, and tends to recur at the site of the primary lesion. Cutaneous lesions of the primary infection may occur alone or with fever, lymphadenopathy, myalgia, pharyngitis, malaise, blepharitis, or keratoconjunctivitis.

Incubation may take 2 to 14 days. Stinging, burning, and pruritus at the inoculation site typically precede the eruptions. Diagnosis is made on identification of the characteristic lesions most easily during the vesicular phase. Later, crusted and dried vesicular fluid may be confused with impetigo. Viral cultures taken from scraping the base of an unroofed vesicle may confirm the diagnosis. A Tzanck smear may provide more immediate confirmation.

Emergency Department Treatment and Disposition

Oral antivirals in addition to analgesics and antipyretics are useful. To be most effective, antivirals must be started within 72 hours of the eruption and should be initiated if prodromal symptoms (burning, stinging) occur. Topical antibiotic ointments help prevent secondary infection and speed healing.

Pearls

1. Wear protective gloves; herpetic infections are an occupational hazard in the medical and dental professions.
2. Wrestlers with vesicles and ulcers may not participate.

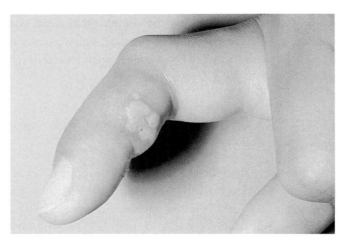

FIGURE 13.84 ■ Herpetic Whitlow. Note the cluster of vesicles on an erythematous base. (Photo contributor: Lawrence B. Stack, MD.)

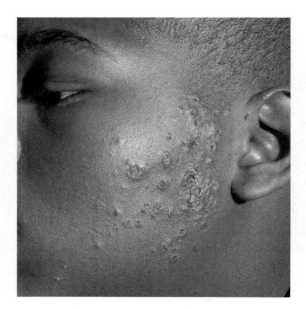

FIGURE 13.85 ■ Herpes Gladiatorum. Primary herpes gladiatorum in a wrestler. Note the varied stages of lesions, from vesicular to dried crusts. (Photo contributor: Lawrence B. Stack, MD.)

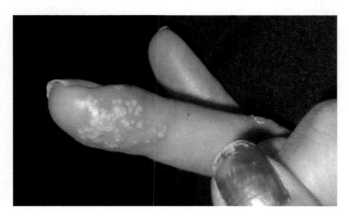

FIGURE 13.83 ■ Herpetic Whitlow. Painful, grouped, confluent vesicles on an erythematous base on the distal finger. (Photo contributor: Selim Suner, MD, MS.)

Clinical Summary

Autoimmune bullous diseases are uncommon but have dramatic presentations. *Bullous pemphigoid* (BP) results from autoantibodies to the epidermal basement membrane that results in tense bullae. The elderly are primarily affected and the bullae are frequently located on the proximal extremities. In *Pemphigus vulgaris* (PV) the autoantibodies are directed against the epidermal keratinocytes. This results in flaccid bullae (more superficial bullae). PV bullae and subsequent erosions commonly present in the oral pharynx, scalp, and trunk. *Paraneoplastic pemphigus* presents with severe oral ulcerations (similar to SJS/TEN, see related item) and resolves with treatment of the associated malignancy.

Emergency Department Treatment and Disposition

Considering an autoimmune bullous disease in the differential is the first step. Admission with early dermatologic consultation for histologic and immunofluorescent studies should be considered. Systemic steroids and immunosuppressant therapy are required for control. Patients with significant body surface area involvement should be treated in a burn unit.

Pearls

1. Oral ulcerations should always raise the suspicion of autoimmune bullous diseases.
2. The high morbidity and mortality of this disease is now significantly lower due to modern steroid-sparing immunosuppressants and wound care.

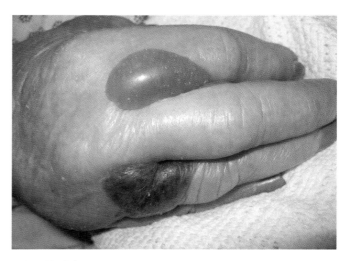

FIGURE 13.87 ■ Bullous Pemphigoid Tense bullae on in the distal extremities are a common presentation of BP. (Photo contributor: Selim Suner, MD, MS.)

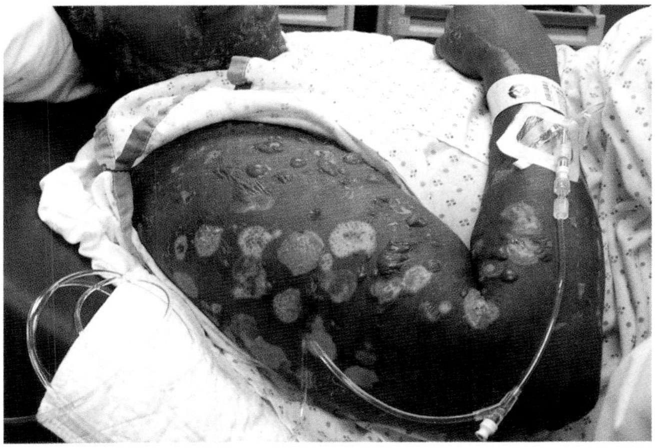

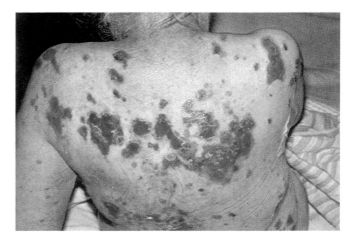

FIGURE 13.86 ■ Bullous Pemphigoid. Tense blister formation among confluent erosions and plaques. (Photo contributor: Lawrence B. Stack, MD.)

FIGURE 13.88 ■ Pemphigus Vulgaris. Multiple flaccid bullae now de-roofed and at risk for secondary infection. (Photo contributor: J. Matthew Hardin, MD.)

Clinical Summary

Sweet syndrome, also known as acute febrile neutrophilic dermatosis, is characterized by fever, peripheral neutrophilia, and a nonvasculitic neutrophilic cutaneous eruption. The lesions are tender, well-demarcated violaceous to erythematous plaques that may have a central yellowish discoloration and can occur anywhere on the body, but most frequently on the upper extremities, neck, and face. The plaques generally cause a burning pain and are nonpruritic. While the cause of Sweet syndrome is unknown, it is thought to represent an abnormal immunological response. It seems to respond to anti-inflammatory and immunomodulatory treatment. Twenty percent of patients with Sweet syndrome have an associated malignancy. Other associated illness include bacterial and viral infections, inflammatory bowel disease, autoimmune disorders, and collagen vascular disease.

Emergency Department Treatment and Disposition

Diagnostic criteria for Sweet syndrome include abrupt onset of the characteristic lesions and histopathology consistent with Sweet syndrome, along with 2 of 4 minor criteria: leukocytosis, good response to glucocorticoids (but not to antibiotics), antecedent fever or infection, accompanying fever, arthralgia, or underlying malignancy. Management includes prednisone 40 mg/day tapered over 4 to 6 weeks, dermatology referral for diagnosis confirmation, and outpatient evaluation for malignancy.

Pearls

1. Sweet syndrome is four times more common in females.
2. Malignancies associated with Sweet syndrome include acute myeloid leukemia, and solid tumors of the breast, genitourinary and gastrointestinal tracts.

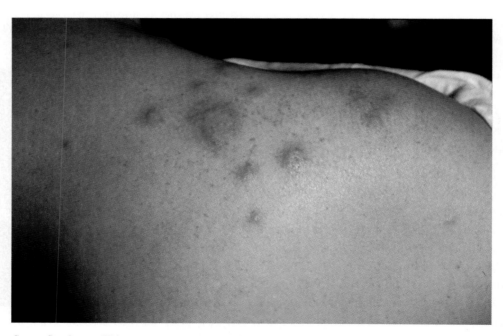

FIGURE 13.89 ■ Sweet Syndrome. This young woman complained of sudden onset of fever and painful skin lesions. Her WBC was 22,000 with neutrophilia. This constellation of symptoms suggests Sweet syndrome, and was confirmed by histology. (Photo contributor: Lawrence B. Stack, MD.)

Clinical Summary

Tinea corporis includes all dermatophyte infections excluding the scalp, face, hands, feet, and groin. The dermatophytosis is pruritic and consists of a well-circumscribed scaly plaque with a slightly elevated border and central clearing. This annular configuration is most commonly found on the trunk and neck. Skin scrapings viewed with KOH preparation exhibit septate hyphae.

Tinea faciale is a dermatophyte infection of the facial skin. It commonly appears as a well-circumscribed erythematous patch. *Tinea manus* is a dermatophyte infection of the hands.

Tinea cruris, or "jock itch," is a pruritic dermatophytosis of the intertriginous areas, usually excluding the penis and scrotum. The scaly, erythematous plaque spreads peripherally, with central clearing. The borders of the plaque are usually well defined.

Tinea pedis, or "athlete's foot," consists of erythema and scaling of the sole, maceration, occasional vesiculation, and fissure formation between and under the toes. These pruritic, painful fissures may become secondarily infected. Frequently the toenails are also affected.

Tinea capitis is scalp ringworm, or a dermatophytosis of the scalp. It presents as a pruritic, erythematous, scaly plaque with broken or missing hairs frequently referred to as "gray patch" or "black dot" ringworm. This may develop into a *kerion*. A kerion is a delayed-type hypersensitivity reaction to the fungus, where the initial erythematous, scaly plaque becomes boggy with inflamed, purulent nodules and plaques. The hair follicle is frequently destroyed by the inflammatory process in a kerion, leading to a scarring alopecia.

Emergency Department Treatment and Disposition

Initial treatment consists of topical antifungal medications. Griseofulvin or ketoconazole are reserved for resistant cases. It is important to treat for 1 to 2 weeks beyond the point of clinical cure to ensure successful eradication of the fungus. Decreasing the amount of perspiration by using topical powders may help prevent recurrences.

Systemic antifungals are required for several weeks to treat *tinea capitis* successfully. Systemic antibiotics and corticosteroids are usually added when treating a *kerion*. Selenium sulfide lotion used as a shampoo may actually decrease the duration of the infection. Ketoconazole is reserved for resistant cases.

Pearls

1. The scale is usually located at the leading edge of erythema and provides the best yield for scraping as part of the KOH examination.
2. The recurrence rate is high, especially for tinea manus.
3. Warmth and moisture are predisposing factors.
4. Macerated areas may become secondarily infected by bacteria.
5. Tinea capitis is a disease of childhood; it is rare in immunocompetent adults.

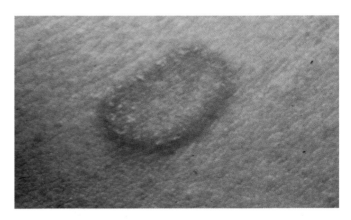

FIGURE 13.90 ■ Tinea Corporis, Ringworm. This dermatophytosis is ringworm, a well-defined, pruritic, scaly plaque with a raised border and central clearing (annular). KOH preparation is positive. (Photo contributor: the Department of Dermatology, Wilford Hall USAF Medical Center and Brooke Army Medical Center, San Antonio, TX.)

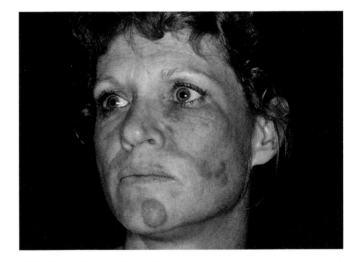

FIGURE 13.91 ■ Tinea Faciale. Note the sharply marginated, polycyclic, scaly plaque with central clearing localized to the face. KOH preparation is positive. (Photo contributor: the Department of Dermatology, Wilford Hall USAF Medical Center and Brooke Army Medical Center, San Antonio, TX.)

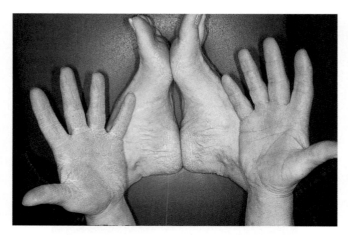

FIGURE 13.92 ■ Tinea Manus. This dermatophytosis is usually unilateral when it involves the hands. Note the diffuse hyperkeratosis of the left hand as well as involvement of both feet (tinea pedis). (Photo contributor: James J. Nordlund, MD.)

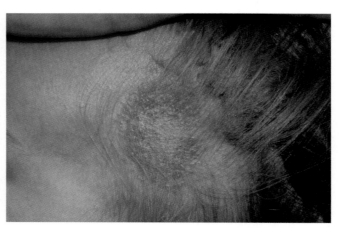

FIGURE 13.95 ■ Tinea Capitis. The appearance of a "ringworm" like infection of the scalp dictates treatment for tinea capitis. (Photo contributor: Kevin J. Knoop, MD, MS.)

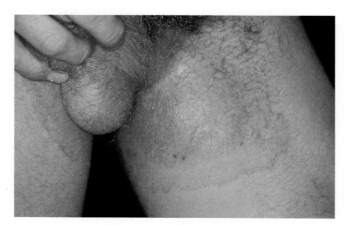

FIGURE 13.93 ■ Tinea Cruris. This dermatophytosis is commonly called "jock itch." Note the erythematous, scaly plaque with its well-defined border. It characteristically does not involve the scrotum or penis. KOH preparation is positive. (Photo contributor: James J. Nordlund, MD.)

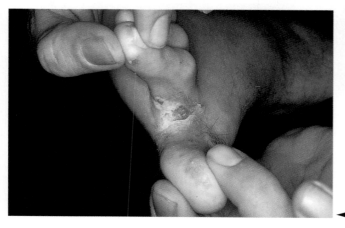

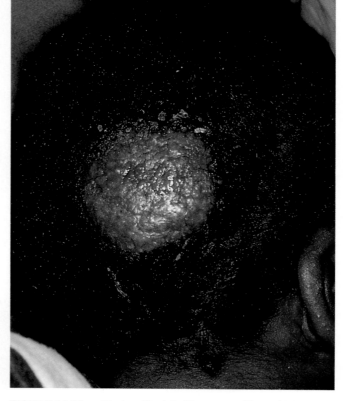

FIGURE 13.96 ■ Kerion. Occipital boggy swelling with hair loss consistent with kerion. (Photo contributor: Anne W. Lucky, MD.)

FIGURE 13.94 ■ Tinea Pedis. A pruritic, scaling hyperkeratotic rash involving the soles of the feet and extending to the interdigital spaces is pathognomonic for tinea pedis. (Photo contributor: James J. Nordlund, MD.)

Clinical Summary

Tinea versicolor, or pityriasis versicolor, is a chronic, superficial fungal infection that involves the trunk and extremities with little or no facial involvement. The fungus is part of normal skin flora. Finely scaling brown macules are present in fair-skinned patients, whereas scaly hypopigmented macules are often noted in dark-skinned patients. These sharply demarcated macules are intermittently pruritic.

Emergency Department Treatment and Disposition

Treatment consists of short applications of selenium sulfide lotion, topical antifungal creams, or topical ketoconazole. Resistant cases require referral and consideration of oral ketoconazole. Ultraviolet exposure is required to regain any lost pigment.

Pearls

1. Tinea versicolor is more common in adolescents and young adults.
2. Clinically active areas or areas colonized with the fungus may be identified by orange fluorescence noted on the Wood lamp examination.
3. Application of cocoa butter or greasy emollients predisposes children to this condition.

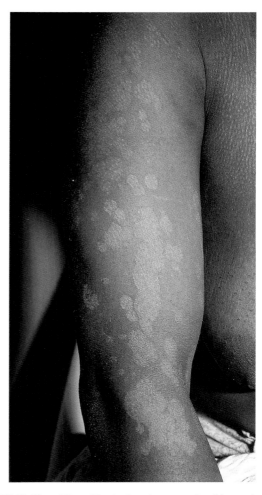

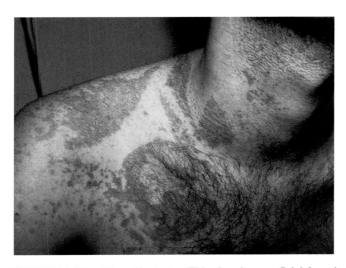

FIGURE 13.97 ■ Tinea Versicolor. This chronic superficial fungal infection leads to the formation of multiple well-defined, scaly brown macules on the trunk and extremities. (Photo contributor: the Department of Dermatology, Wilford Hall USAF Medical Center and Brooke Army Medical Center, San Antonio, TX.)

FIGURE 13.98 ■ Tinea Versicolor. An example of hypopigmented areas on dark skin. (Photo contributor: James J. Nordlund, MD.)

Clinical Summary

Onychomycosis is an invasion of the nails by any fungus. Four clinical subtypes are noted. *Distal subungual* presents as discolorations of the free edge of the nail with hyperkeratosis leading to a subungual accumulation of friable keratinaceous debris. *White superficial* consists of sharply outlined white areas on the nail plate which leave the surface friable. *Proximal subungual* presents as discolorations which start proximally at the nail fold. *Candidal onychomycosis* encompasses the entire nail plate, leaving the surface rough and friable.

Emergency Department Treatment and Disposition

The most common treatment consists of oral griseofulvin, fluconazole, luconazole, or terbinafine. Candidal infections require oral ketoconazole. Toenail onychomycosis is very difficult to eradicate.

Pearls

1. All that causes the nail plate to separate from the nail bed is not necessarily fungus. Psoriasis and various other nail dystrophies, such as distal onycholysis caused by excessive water exposure or drugs, must be differentiated from this fungal infection.
2. Distal subungual is the most common type of onychomycosis.

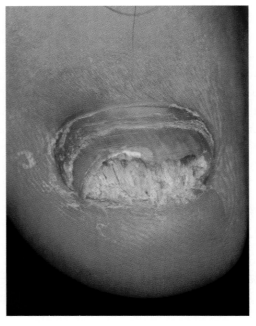

FIGURE 13.99 ■ Onychomycosis. Invasion of the nail bed by fungus. (Photo contributor: Lawrence B. Stack, MD.)

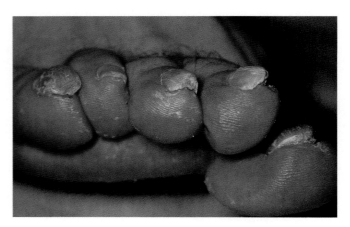

FIGURE 13.100 ■ Onychomycosis. Note that multiple nail beds have been invaded by the fungus, leading to chronic hyperkeratosis and subungual accumulation of friable keratinaceous debris. (Photo contributor: the Department of Dermatology, Wilford Hall USAF Medical Center and Brooke Army Medical Center, San Antonio, TX.)

Clinical Summary

Vitiligo is an acquired loss of pigmentation that commonly involves the backs of the hands, face, and body folds. There is a positive family history in 30% of the cases. Initially the disease is limited, but it then slowly progresses over years. Vitiligo is secondary to absence of epidermal melanocytes, which may be due to an autoimmune phenomenon against melanocytes. Approximately half of these cases begin in patients less than 20 years of age.

Emergency Department Treatment and Disposition

Vitiligo requires referral to a dermatologist for PUVA (psoralen plus ultraviolet A), topical therapy, or skin grafting. The best results from therapy occur on the face and neck.

Pearls

1. Vitiligo occurs at sites of trauma (Koebner phenomenon).
2. Wood lamp examination helps identify hypopigmented areas in patients with light complexions.
3. Tinea versicolor, in contrast, has a scale and positive KOH preparation.

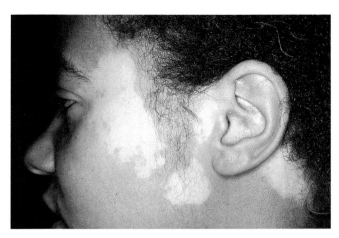

FIGURE 13.101 ■ Vitiligo. Note the hypopigmented areas characteristic of vitiligo. (Photo contributor: James J. Nordlund, MD.)

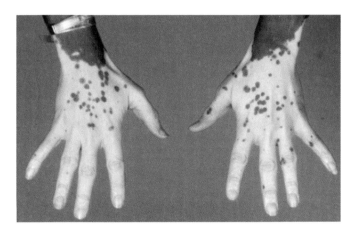

FIGURE 13.102 ■ Vitiligo. Characteristic lesions display an acral distribution and striking depigmentation as a result of loss of melanocytes. (Used with permission from Fauci AS, Braunwald E, Kasper DL, et al. *Harrison's Principles of Internal Medicine.* 17th ed. New York, McGraw-Hill, 2008; p. 312.)

Clinical Summary

Transmission of scabies occurs after direct skin contact with an infected individual and possibly from clothing and bedding infested with the mite. The female mite burrows into the individual's skin and deposits two to three eggs daily. Fecal pellets (scybala) are also deposited in the burrow and may be responsible for the localized pruritus. Nocturnal pruritus is characteristic of scabies. The pink-white, slightly elevated burrows are typically found in the web spaces of the hands and feet, penis, buttocks, scrotum, and extensor surfaces of the elbows and knees. Norwegian scabies tends to cause asymptomatic crusting, rather than the typical inflammatory papules and vesicles, as well as nail dystrophy and keratosis.

Emergency Department Treatment and Disposition

Topical permethrin or lindane is commonly used to treat scabies. Each of these products should be applied thoroughly and then, after 8 to 12 hours, washed from the skin. Lindane should be avoided during infancy and pregnancy because of reports of infant neurotoxicity following systemic absorption through the skin.

Pearls

1. Ivermectin given as a single 200-μg/kg dose or a 5% sulfur ointment can also be used for treatment.

2. Oral antipruritic therapy and analgesics will help alleviate discomfort.

3. Intimate contacts and all family members in the same household should be treated.

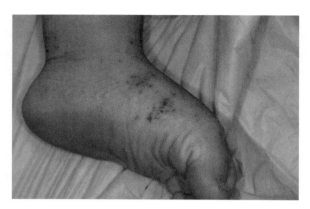

FIGURE 13.104 ■ Scabies. Burrows and erosions from itching on the foot of a patient with scabies. (Photo contributor: David Effron, MD.)

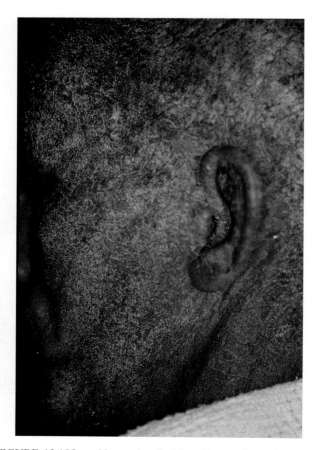

FIGURE 13.105 ■ Norwegian Scabies. Gray scales and crusting consistent with Norwegian scabies. In these patients, many thousands (versus a few dozen) mites are present. (Photo contributor: Lynn Utecht, MD.)

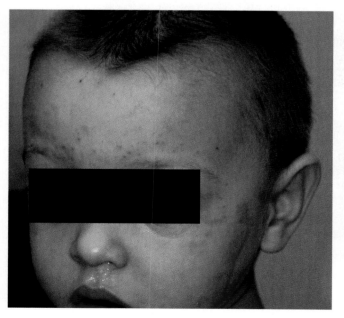

FIGURE 13.103 ■ Scabies. Burrows on the forehead of a young patient with scabies. (Photo contributor: David Effron, MD.)

Clinical Summary

Uremic frost is a classic manifestation of chronic renal failure; it is rarely seen today. It develops as a result of accumulation of urea in sweat. In advanced uremia, the accumulation of urea in sweat may reach such a critical level that, upon its evaporation, a fine white powder is left on the skin surface. Associated hyperkalemia may also be present owing to renal failure.

Emergency Department Treatment and Disposition

Treatment of the underlying condition that resulted in the patient's uremia may prevent further accumulation of uremic frost. Typically, urgent dialysis is indicated.

Pearls

1. Although rare today, this condition may be seen in patients without adequate air conditioning who are poorly controlled on dialysis.
2. For patients presenting with altered mental status, attention to the airway, oxygenation, and rapid assessment and treatment of associated metabolic disorders, such as hyperkalemia, are indicated.

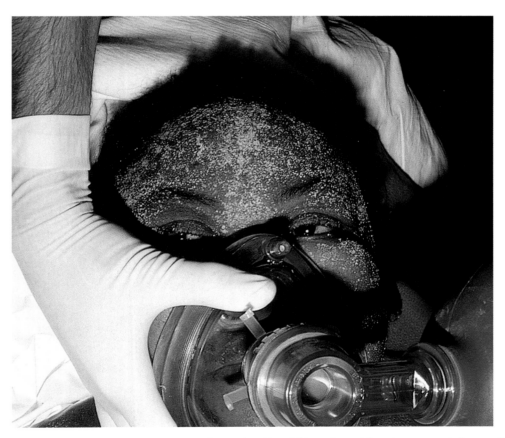

FIGURE 13.106 ■ Uremic Frost. Note the fine white powder on the skin of this patient with end-stage renal disease. (Photo contributor: Richard C. Levy, MD.)

Clinical Summary

Anthrax is usually a disease of herbivores; humans are infected when they come into contact with infected animals or contaminated animal products. Recently, anthrax has received increased international attention as a potential biological warfare agent. There are three distinct clinical manifestations of anthrax.

Cutaneous anthrax accounts for about 95% of human cases. After direct contact on exposed skin, the infection begins as a pruritic papule. It enlarges into an ulcer surrounded by vesicles in 1 to 2 days and then eventually becomes a characteristic black, necrotic central eschar surrounded by nonpitting edema. Systemic manifestations (fever, hypotension, tachycardia) may accompany cutaneous involvement.

Respiratory anthrax (woolsorters disease) occurs after exposure to anthrax spores and presents as an upper respiratory infection. Within 1 to 4 days, the disease progresses to severe respiratory distress, hypoxia, and hypotension. Death uniformly occurs within 24 hours after the onset of the fulminant phases of the infection.

Gastrointestinal anthrax is rare and occurs 3 to 7 days after exposure to contaminated animal meat. Initially it presents as a nonspecific gastroenteritis with fever, vomiting, diarrhea, and malaise. The disease then progresses to hematemesis, bloody diarrhea, sepsis, and shock. Death usually occurs 2 to 5 days after symptom onset.

Emergency Department Treatment and Disposition

Admission is indicated for patients with anthrax. Intravenous penicillin is the primary treatment for all forms. Ciprofloxacin or doxycycline are alternatives. Oral ciprofloxacin is recommended for postexposure prophylaxis.

Pearls

1. Gastrointestinal and inhalation anthrax are almost uniformly fatal, even with antibiotic therapy.
2. Human-killed vaccine is available and recommended for mill workers and veterinarians at high risk for exposure.
3. A classic pathologic finding for inhalation anthrax is hemorrhagic mediastinitis; this may be manifested on chest radiography as a widened mediastinum.
4. Decontamination of suspected anthrax spore exposure consists of removal of exposed clothing (place in a sealed plastic bag) and washing of the exposed area with soap and water.
5. Cutaneous anthrax resembles staphylococcal infection, tularemia, and plague.

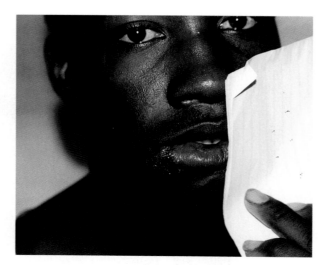

FIGURE 13.107 ■ Anthrax. Note the early ulcer of cutaneous anthrax on the right lower lip. (Photo contributor: Thea James, MD.)

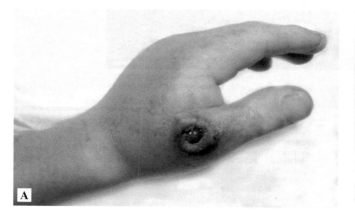

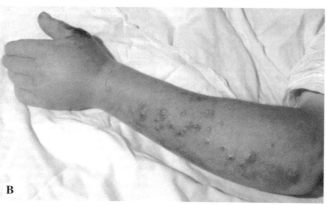

FIGURE 13.108 ■ Anthrax. (**A**) A black eschar with a central hemorrhagic ulceration on the thumb associated with massive edema of the hand. (**B**) A nodular lymphangitis extending proximally from the primary lesion on the thumb. (Used with permission from Wolff K, Johnson RA, Suurmond D. *Fitzpatrick's Color Atlas & Synopsis of Clinical Dermatology.* 5th ed. New York, McGraw-Hill, 2005; p. 631.)

Clinical Summary

Intertrigo is a dermatitis occurring on apposed surfaces of skin, such as the creases of the neck, folds of the groin and armpit, or a panniculus. It is characterized by a tender, red plaque with a moist, macerated surface. A candidal infection may result and often becomes secondarily infected with skin flora. Erythema, fissures, burning, itching, exudates, and fever may also accompany intertrigo.

Emergency Department Treatment and Disposition

Local care, empiric topical antifungal treatment, and good personal hygiene are recommended. Intravenous antibiotics initiated in the emergency department directed against skin flora are recommended if there is secondary infection.

Pearls

1. Necrotizing fasciitis of the abdominal wall should be considered in the differential.
2. Topical corticosteroids should be avoided because of atrophy risk.

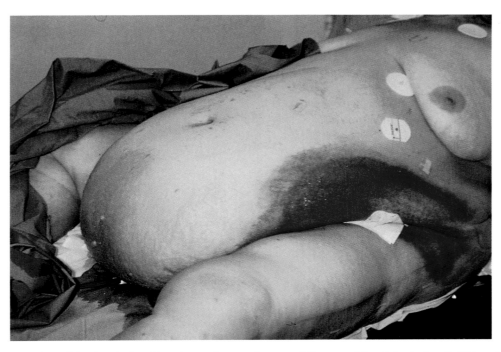

FIGURE 13.109 ■ Intertrigo of the Panniculus. Note the exudate, erythema, and fissures of the abdominal wall. This patient also had fever, suggesting secondary infection. (Photo contributor: Lawrence B. Stack, MD.)

Clinical Summary

Abdominal striae are linear, depressed, pink or bluish scar-like lesions that may later become silver or white. They are caused by weakening of the elastic cutaneous tissues from chronic stretching. They most commonly occur on the abdomen but are also seen on the buttocks, breasts, and thighs. Striae are commonly seen in obesity, pregnancy, Cushing syndrome, and chronic topical corticosteroid treatment. In Cushing syndrome, a state of adrenal hypercorticism, the skin becomes fragile and easily breaks from normal stretching.

Emergency Department Treatment and Disposition

This finding seldom presents as a condition requiring acute treatment; thus, attention is directed to determining and treating the underlying cause.

Pearls

1. Recent striae (pink or blue) with moon facies, hypertension, renal calculi, osteoporosis, and psychiatric disorders are suggestive of Cushing syndrome.

2. The striae caused by pregnancy typically fade with time, unlike those associated with Cushing syndrome.

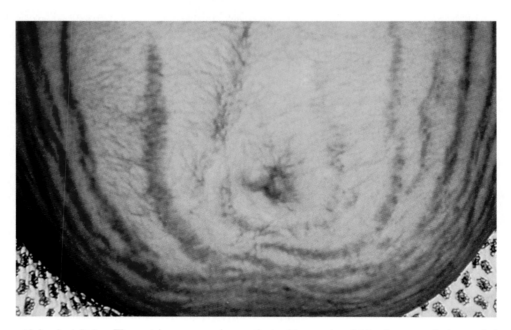

FIGURE 13.110 ■ Abdominal Striae. These striae are seen in a patient with recent weight gain, moon facies, and altered mental status. The patient was diagnosed with Cushing syndrome. (Photo contributor: Geisinger Medical Center, Department of Emergency Medicine, Danville, PA.)

Clinical Summary

Melasma is commonly seen on the face of young adult females. It consists of symmetric, light to dark brown patches. The most common sites are on the malar cheek, lateral forehead, upper cutaneous lip and mandible. Factors associated with accentuation of melasma include sunlight exposure, pregnancy (often called "the mask of pregnancy"), and oral contraceptives.

Emergency Department Treatment and Disposition

Most patients will be concerned about accentuation of their previously imperceptible melasma. Ruling out pregnancy or confirming exogenous estrogens in any patient presenting with melasma should be performed first. Essential to any treatment of melasma is strict sun avoidance. Referral to a dermatologist can be made on a nonurgent basis.

Pearls

1. Sun exposure on other parts of the body can cause accentuation of facial melasma.
2. The pigmentation usually resolves over weeks.
3. Melasma may or may not return with subsequent pregnancy.

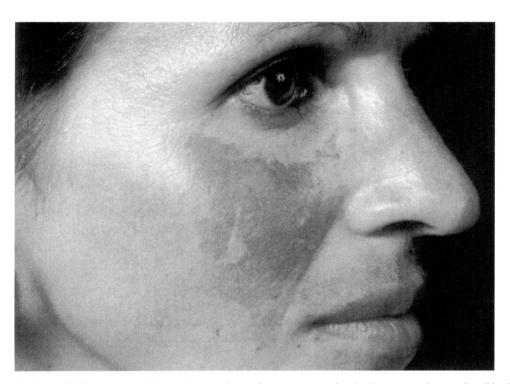

FIGURE 13.111 ■ Melasma. Well-demarcated, hyperpigmented macules are seen on the cheek, nose, and upper lip. (Used with permission from Wolff K, Johnson RA, Suurmond D. *Fitzpatrick's Color Atlas & Synopsis of Clinical Dermatology.* 5th ed. New York, McGraw-Hill, 2005; p. 349.)

Clinical Summary

Jaundice presents as light yellowing of the skin, mucous membranes, and sclera; it is generally detectable when bilirubin levels are about 3.0 mg/dL. Many patients may not be aware of the faint yellowing of their skin and present with seemingly unrelated symptoms. Be aware that up to 50% of patients with jaundice will have pruritus. The most important diagnoses to rule out are: hemolytic anemias, viral hepatitis, chronic alcohol abuse, autoimmune hepatitis, medications, primary biliary cirrhosis, primary sclerosing cholangitis, cholelithiasis, surgical strictures, and obstructive malignancies. Acetaminophen, penicillins, and oral contraceptives are some of the more common medications associated with jaundice.

Emergency Department Treatment and Disposition

As the etiology of jaundice is broad, a thorough history focusing on associated symptoms (fever, pruritus, vomiting, hematochezia, melena, and abdominal pain), previous surgical procedures, and medication history (including over-the-counter medications) is essential. Physical findings of fever, abdominal tenderness, and hepatomegaly should be sought. Work-up of jaundiced patients should include white blood cell count and differential, liver function tests including bilirubin levels, hepatitis viral screening, and imaging studies.

Pearls

1. Patients who consume large amounts of β-carotene (found in squash and carrots) may have mild yellowing of their skin but will lack scleral icterus or elevations in bilirubin.
2. Women starting oral contraceptives may experience cholestasis in the first few months that may cause jaundice.

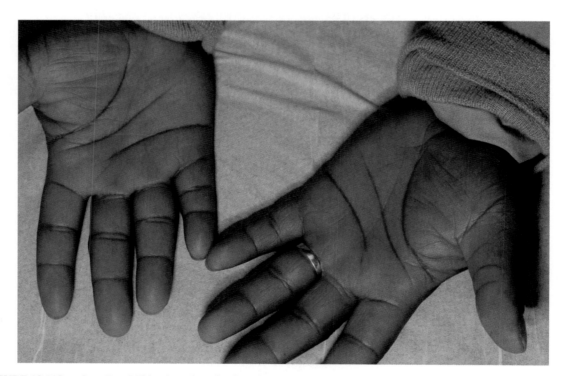

FIGURE 13.112 ■ Jaundice. Mild palmar jaundice in a dark-skinned patient. (Photo contributor: Kevin J. Knoop, MD, MS.)

Clinical Summary

Alopecia is defined by loss of hair. It can be classified into *scarring* (absence of follicles) and *nonscarring* (presence of follicles) alopecia. Scarring alopecia is commonly caused by discoid lupus erythematosus (erythematous mottled pigmentation and atrophic scalp scarring) and folliculitis decalvans (multiple crops of pustules on the scalp). Occasionally, prolonged bacterial and inflammatory fungal infections (kerion) can induce scarring on the scalp. Nonscarring alopecia results from alopecia areata (annular areas of alopecia on the scalp or beard area), telogen effluvium (diffuse scalp shedding of hair 2 to 3 months after a stressful event, illness, or new medication), anagen effluvium (diffuse scalp shedding after chemotherapy), trichotillomania (constant pulling of the hair), traction alopecia (chronic tension of braided hair causing alopecia), and tinea capitis. Syphilis can cause a patchy, "moth-eaten" alopecia.

Emergency Department Treatment and Disposition

Evaluation of alopecia in the emergency department should focus on the history and infectious etiologies. Treatment for tinea capitis and kerions requires systemic antifungals, long-term treatment, and periodic laboratory monitoring. Referral to a dermatologist or primary care physician is recommended. In an at-risk patient, screening for syphilis should be considered. Bacterial infections should be treated with antibiotics after bacterial cultures are obtained. Other forms of alopecia can be referred to a dermatologist.

Pearls

1. Thallium and arsenic poisoning can cause alopecia.
2. Any scaling patch of alopecia should be scraped and examined for fungal organisms.
3. Patchy alopecia in sexually active patients should prompt screening for syphilis.

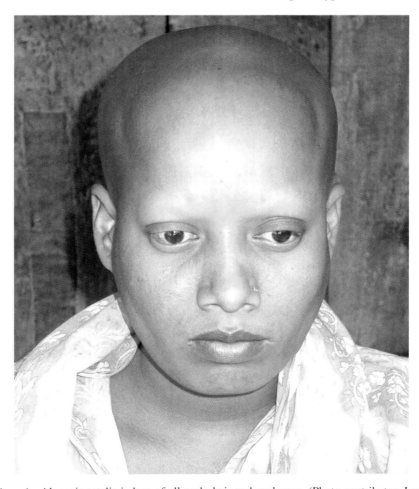

FIGURE 13.113 ■ Alopecia. Alopecia totalis is loss of all scalp hair and eyebrows. (Photo contributor: Lawrence B. Stack, MD.)

Clinical Summary

Systemic lupus erythematosus (SLE) has four cutaneous manifestations: malar rash, discoid rash, photosensitivity, and oral ulcers. Eighty percent of patients have skin findings at some point of the disease. The malar "butterfly" rash presents with erythema and mild edema over the bridge of the nose and malar cheeks. Similar erythematous patches may be seen on the ears, neck, and chest. Discoid lesions can appear at any site but are usually found above the neck, including the scalp. They are characterized as annular, erythematous macules, or plaques that eventually become atrophic and scarred.

Emergency Department Treatment and Disposition

Urgent referral to a dermatologist or rheumatologist is essential for early diagnosis and prevention of other systemic manifestations.

Pearls

1. Consider any suspicious rash on the face a manifestation of SLE and refer to a dermatologist early.
2. The malar rash resolves without scarring, whereas discoid lesions result in permanent scarring.

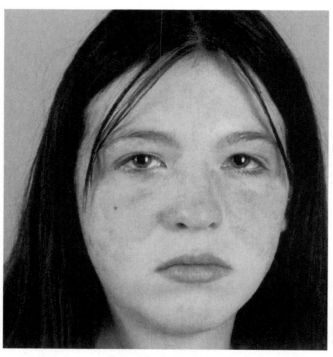

FIGURE 13.114 ■ Butterfly Rash of SLE. Bright red, sharply defined erythema with slight edema and minimal scaling in a "butterfly pattern" on the face. This is the typical "malar rash." Note also that the patient is female and young. (Used with permission from Wolff K, Johnson RA, Suurmond D. *Fitzpatrick's Color Atlas & Synopsis of Clinical Dermatology.* 5th ed. New York, McGraw-Hill, 2005; p. 385.)

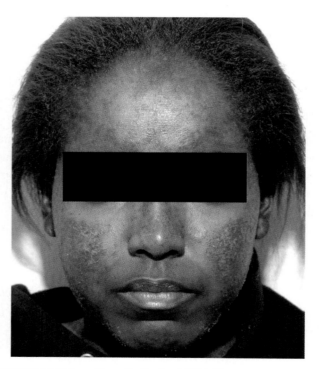

FIGURE 13.115 ■ Butterfly Rash of SLE. The appearance of the malar "butterfly" rash in a dark-skinned individual. (Photo contributor: Lawrence B. Stack, MD.)

Clinical Summary

Porphyrias are associated with enzymatic defects in heme biosynthesis. Porphyria cutanea tarda (PCT) presents as a condition of fragile skin and vesicles found on the dorsum of the hands, especially after trauma. The classic symptoms are easily traumatized skin, leading to blisters in sun-exposed areas, erosions, milia, and hypertrichosis. It may be induced by ethanol, estrogens, oral contraceptives, iron overload, and certain environmental exposures. The typical bullae and erosions may also occur in other areas, especially the feet and nose. In contrast to other porphyrias, PCT is not associated with life-threatening respiratory failure, abdominal pain, or peripheral autonomic neuropathies. Confirmation of the diagnosis requires 24-hour urine testing for various porphyrins. Other forms of porphyria, other bullous diseases, systemic lupus erythematosus (SLE), sarcoidosis, and Sjögren syndrome must be considered in the differential.

Emergency Department Treatment and Disposition

Laboratory examination may begin in the emergency department with blood chemistries, porphyrin studies, and consideration of appropriate biopsies. Treatment includes discontinuation of any drugs that might initiate PCT. Phlebotomy and the use of chloroquine can be considered.

Pearls

1. PCT is the most common type of porphyria.
2. Examination of the urine may reveal orange-red fluorescence with a Wood lamp.
3. This condition is sometimes termed *fragile skin*.

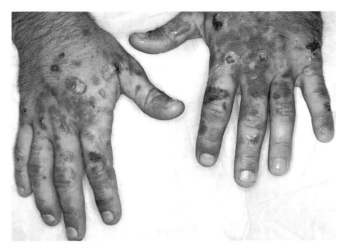

FIGURE 13.116 ■ Porphyria Cutanea Tarda. Blisters and erosions of PCT. (Photo contributor: Selim Suner, MD, MS.)

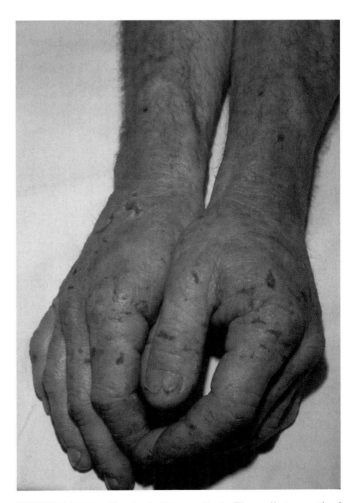

FIGURE 13.117 ■ Porphyria Cutanea Tarda. The easily traumatized skin and erosions of PCT. (Photo contributor: Alan B. Storrow, MD.)

Specialty Areas

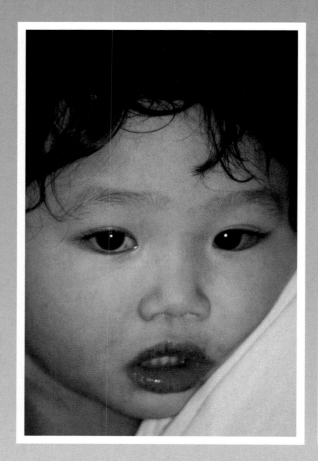

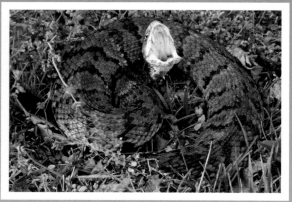

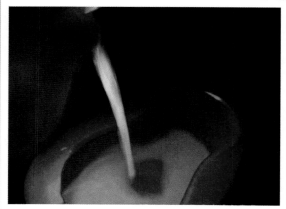

Chapter 14

PEDIATRIC CONDITIONS

Matthew R. Mittiga
Javier A. Gonzalez del Rey
Richard M. Ruddy

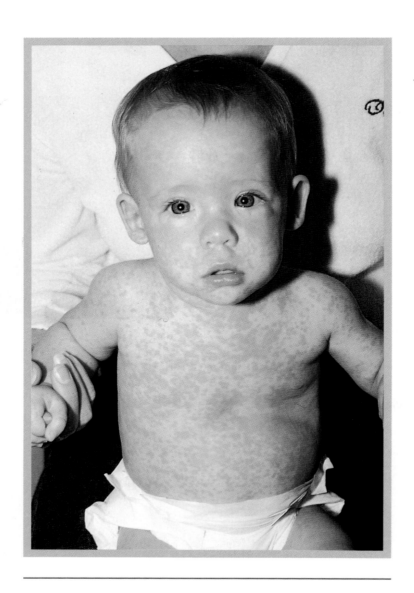

Clinical Summary

Erythema toxicum neonatorum is a benign, self-limited eruption of unknown etiology that occurs in up to 70% of term newborns characterized by discrete, small, erythematous macules or patches up to 2 to 3 cm in diameter with 1- to 3-mm firm pale yellow or white papules or pustules in the center. The trunk is predominantly involved. This rash usually presents within the first 24 to 72 hours of life. The distinctive feature of erythema toxicum is its evanescence or disappearance with each individual lesion usually disappearing within 2 or 3 days. New lesions may occur during the first 2 weeks of life. The neonate should appear well and lack any systemic signs of illness other than occasional peripheral eosinophilia. Wright-stained slide preparations of the scraping from the center of the lesion demonstrate numerous eosinophils. The differential diagnosis includes transient neonatal pustular melanosis, newborn milia, miliaria, neonatal herpes simplex, bacterial folliculitis, candidiasis, and impetigo of the newborn.

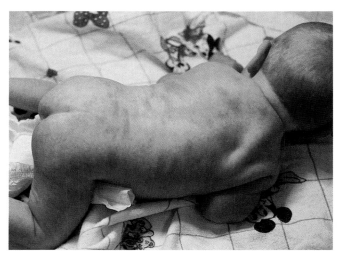

FIGURE 14.1 ■ Erythema Toxicum. Newborn infant with diffuse macular rash of erythema toxicum. (Photo contributor: Kevin J. Knoop, MD, MS.)

Emergency Department Treatment and Disposition

As this condition is self-limiting, no therapy is indicated in the setting of a well-appearing newborn with normal activity and appetite. Parents can be educated and reassured about the evanescence of the rash. In cases where impetigo, *Candida,* or herpes infections are suspected, a smear from the center of the lesion and bacterial and viral cultures may be necessary to make a final diagnosis.

Pearls

1. Erythema toxicum is the most common rash of the newborn.
2. The lesions may present anywhere on the body but tend to spare the palms and soles.
3. Laboratory evaluation is usually unnecessary.

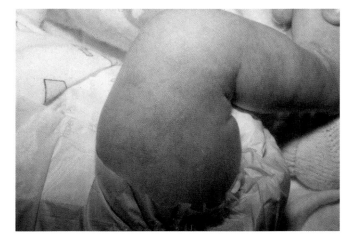

FIGURE 14.2 ■ Erythema Toxicum. Close up of lower extremity of a neonate with erythema toxicum. (Photo contributor: Robert W. Hickey, MD.)

Clinical Summary

Nevus simplex (salmon patch) is the most common vascular lesion in infancy, present in about 40% of newborns. It appears as a slightly pink to deep scarlet macule or patch on the nape of the neck, the glabella, mid-forehead, or upper eyelids. Lesions generally fade over the first 2 years of life but may become more prominent with crying or straining.

Emergency Department Treatment and Disposition

Parental education and reassurance can be helpful, but no treatment is indicated. Pulsed dye laser may be considered for persistent lesions that are cosmetically undesirable.

Pearls

1. Salmon patches are composed of ectatic dermal capillaries.
2. Salmon patches appear symmetrically and cross the midline in contrast to the unilateral distribution of a port-wine stain.
3. When seen on the nape of the neck, this lesion is referred to as a *stork bite* or as an *angel's kiss* when appearing on the forehead.
4. About 5% appearing at the nape of the neck will remain permanently or recur.

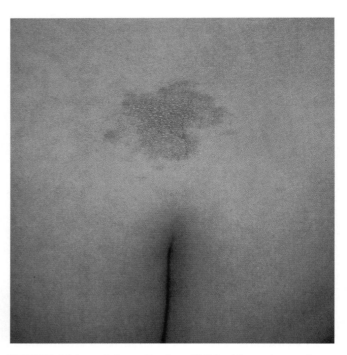

FIGURE 14.4 ■ Salmon Patches. Child with patch over lower back consistent with salmon patches. (Photo contributor: Anne W. Lucky, MD.)

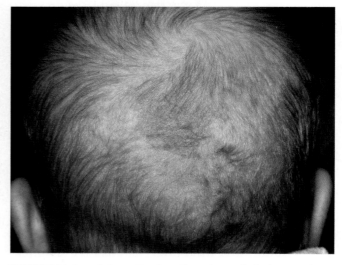

FIGURE 14.5 ■ Salmon Patches. Posterior scalp lesion consistent with a salmon patch. (Photo contributor Andrew H. Urbach, MD.)

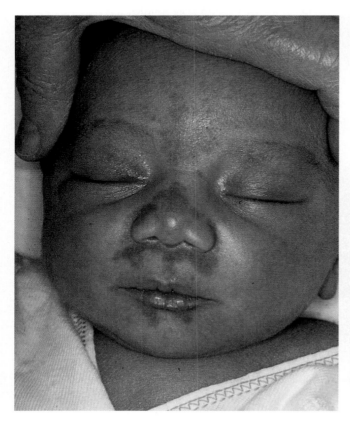

FIGURE 14.3 ■ Salmon Patches. Newborn with characteristic salmon patches over his face. (Photo contributor: Anne W. Lucky, MD.)

Clinical Summary

Neonatal jaundice occurs when total serum bilirubin is sufficiently elevated to cause yellowing of the skin, sclerae, and/or mucous membranes. This correlates with a total bilirubin concentration in excess of 5 mg/dL and progresses in a head-to-toe fashion as bilirubin levels increase. Most cases of physiologic (<12 mg/dL) jaundice are self-limited, without sequelae, appear on the second or third day of life, and peak between the third and fifth day (preterm infants peak later). Causal factors include an increase of bilirubin production following breakdown of fetal red blood cells, a temporary decrease in conjugation of these by-products by the immature newborn liver, and increased enterohepatic circulation (present in all newborns). Risk factors for unconjugated hyperbilirubinemia include maternal diabetes, prematurity, drugs, polycythemia, traumatic delivery with cutaneous bruising or hematoma, and breastfeeding. Most infants with jaundice have no "disease," but a careful history and organized approach is necessary to identify potentially pathologic causes. Kernicterus results from extreme unconjugated hyperbilirubinemia causing neuronal death and pigment deposition in the basal ganglia and cerebellum, associated with bilirubin encephalopathy which manifests in a multitude of irreversible neurologic abnormalities.

Emergency Department Treatment and Disposition

Initial laboratory workup should include blood type, Coombs test, complete blood count with smear for red cell morphology, reticulocyte count, and indirect and direct bilirubin levels. Initial management should ensure adequate hydration and treatment of the underlying condition. The level of serum bilirubin at which to start phototherapy is dependent upon the infant's postnatal age in hours, gestational age, and an assessment of risk factors. Guidelines exist to initiate phototherapy to maintain the bilirubin level below 20 mg/dL. Exchange transfusion is considered if the serum level remains elevated (22-25 mg/dL) despite appropriate phototherapy.

Pearls

1. Onset of clinical jaundice in the first 24 hours of life strongly suggests the presence of a pathologic process.
2. Conjugated (direct) serum bilirubin concentration exceeding 10% of total serum bilirubin or 2 mg/dL suggests hepatobiliary disease or metabolic disorder.
3. Bilirubin levels at which to initiate phototherapy or exchange transfusion should be modified for prematurity, sepsis, low birth weight, and other risk factors.

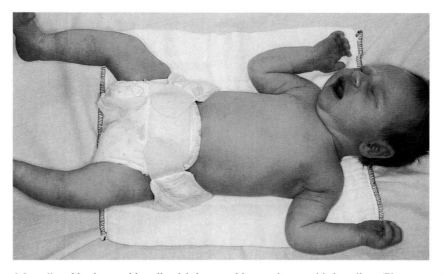

FIGURE 14.6 ■ Neonatal Jaundice. Newborn with yellowish hue to skin consistent with jaundice. (Photo contributor: Kevin J. Knoop, MD, MS.)

Clinical Summary

Neonatal galactorrhea occurs in up to 6% of term newborns and is usually secondary to transplacental transfer of maternal estrogen. These hormonal effects (maternal estrogens and possibly endogenous prolactin) lead to palpable breast buds in approximately one-third of all term newborns. Males and females are equally affected. In most cases, the breast enlargement and galactorrhea begin to subside after the second week of life and have almost always resolved by 2 months of age. In an occasional female infant, the hypertrophy and galactorrhea may persist up to 6 months. These infants are occasionally predisposed to infections (mastitis or abscess) possibly incited by repetitive manipulation of the enlarged breast bud. The differential diagnosis includes early mastitis with purulent discharge that may resemble normal neonatal milk production.

Emergency Department Treatment and Disposition

Treatment is not necessary; reassurance for parents with the routine scheduled office visits to follow up to resolution is very important.

Pearls

1. Newborns with hypertrophied mammary tissue and evidence of clear colostrum-like secretion in the absence of erythema, tenderness, and/or fluctuance usually do not present with neonatal mastitis.
2. Persistence of enlarged breast buds beyond 6 months of age should prompt endocrinologic follow up.
3. In an older child, galactorrhea may be the presenting sign of hypothyroidism or elevated prolactin levels.

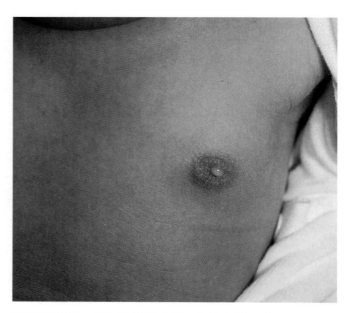

FIGURE 14.7 ■ Witch's Milk. Milky fluid draining from the nipple in a newborn. (Photo contributor: Michael J. Nowicki, MD.)

Clinical Summary

Neonatal mastitis is an infection of the breast tissue that occurs in full-term neonates with a peak incidence in the third week of life. Females are affected more often than males in a 2:1 distribution. Clinically it manifests as swelling, induration, erythema, warmth, and tenderness of the affected breast. In some cases purulent discharge may be expressed from the nipple. Fever may be present in 25% to 40% of affected patients. Bacteremia is rare. *Staphylococcus aureus* is the most common pathogen causing 75% to 85% of cases. Rarely, Gram-negative organisms, group B, or group D *Streptococcus* are the cause. If treatment is delayed, mastitis may progress rapidly with involvement of subcutaneous tissues and subsequent toxicity and systemic findings. In the initial stages, neonatal mastitis may mimic mammary tissue hypertrophy owing to maternal passive hormonal stimulation. Minor trauma, cutaneous infections, and duct blockage may precede this infection.

Emergency Department Treatment and Disposition

Institution of treatment is important to avoid cellulitic spread and breast tissue damage. In cases of mild cellulitis with no associated fluctuance in an otherwise well-appearing, afebrile neonate, culture of nipple discharge and antibiotic coverage (anti-staphylococcal penicillin or first-generation cephalosporin) and close follow up complete the treatment. Adjustment of coverage can be made once results of cultures or Gram stain are available, especially in the presence of Gram-negative bacilli. In cases involving systemic signs of infection, rapid subcutaneous spreading or toxicity, a complete sepsis workup should be performed, and hospitalization is indicated. If no organism is seen initially on Gram stain, parenteral anti-staphylococcal penicillin and an aminoglycoside or cefotaxime alone should be used. In cases of palpable fluctuance, prompt surgical consultation should be obtained to assess the need for needle aspiration or incision and drainage. Conservative treatment with intravenous antibiotics often results in resolution of the fluctuance without surgical intervention. Recovery is usually within 5 to 7 days.

Pearls

1. Antibiotic choice should include coverage for *S aureus*.
2. Maintain a low threshold for initiating a sepsis workup and intravenous antibiotics.
3. Delays in the diagnosis and treatment may lead to distortion of the nipple, impairment of the secretory capacity of the breast, and reduction in the size of the adult breast.

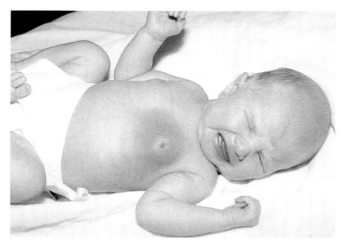

FIGURE 14.8 ■ Neonatal Mastitis. Neonate with left-sided breast swelling, erythema, and purulent discharge. (Photo contributor: Raymond C. Baker, MD.)

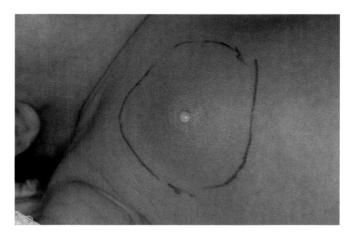

FIGURE 14.9 ■ Neonatal Mastitis. Neonate with marked swelling, erythema, and purulent discharge. (Photo contributor: Emergency Medicine Department, Naval Medical Center, Portsmouth, VA.)

Clinical Summary

An umbilical granuloma is granulation tissue with incomplete epithelialization that persists following cord separation. Usually parents describe a persistent discharge from the umbilicus after the cord has dried and separated. The granuloma is soft, pink, wet, and friable. An umbilical polyp is a rare anomaly resulting from the persistence of the omphalomesenteric duct or the urachus and may have a similar appearance. This polyp is usually firm and resistant, with a mucoid secretion. Omphalitis, an infection of the umbilicus and surrounding structures, should be considered.

Emergency Department Treatment and Disposition

Cleaning and drying of the umbilical cord base with alcohol several times a day may prevent granuloma formation. Cauterization of the granuloma by application of a silver nitrate stick is the treatment of choice. It is important to protect the surrounding skin (apply Vaseline) and remove excess silver nitrate to avoid chemical burns. The cauterization may need to be repeated at 3-day intervals if drainage persists.

Pearls

1. An umbilical granuloma is the most common umbilical abnormality in neonates.
2. Commonly, the only sign of granuloma formation is the presence of nonpurulent discharge noted in the diaper area that is in contact with the umbilicus.
3. Omphalitis presents with redness of the periumbilical area typically tracking upward in the midline and often with a purulent discharge from the umbilicus. Omphalitis can progress to abdominal wall cellulitis or peritonitis and requires a full sepsis work up and hospital admission for treatment with broad spectrum parenteral antibiotics.

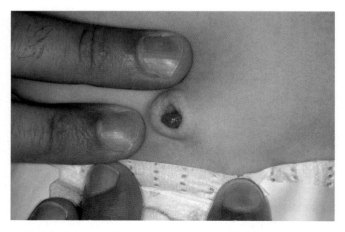

FIGURE 14.10 ■ Umbilical Granuloma. Newborn infant with umbilical granuloma visible in umbilicus. (Photo contributor: Anne W. Lucky, MD.)

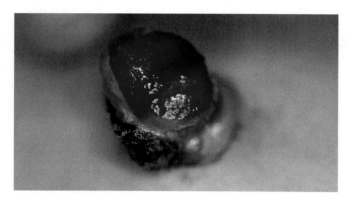

FIGURE 14.11 ■ Omphalomesenteric Duct. This red mass resembling a granuloma was found to be an omphalomesenteric duct. (Photo contributor Kevin J. Knoop, MD, MS.)

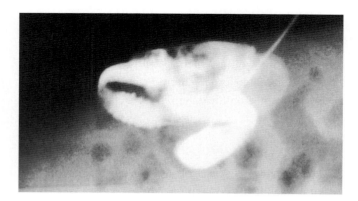

FIGURE 14.12 ■ Fistulogram. A fistulogram confirms the diagnosis of persistent omphalomesenteric duct. (Photo contributor: Kevin J. Knoop, MD, MS.)

Clinical Summary

Hypertrophic pyloric stenosis (HPS) is characterized by progressive postprandial, nonbilious vomiting that steadily increases in frequency and amount due to hypertrophy of the pyloric musculature and edema of the pyloric canal, producing gastric outlet obstruction. It is usually diagnosed in infants from birth to 5 months, most commonly at 2 to 8 weeks of life. The vomiting may become forceful and is then described as projectile (although this pattern is not always present). There is a familial tendency, and white males are more frequently affected. During the physical examination, peristaltic waves may be observed traveling from the left upper to right upper quadrants. The hypertrophy of the antral and pyloric musculature produces the "olive" to palpation (best palpated in the epigastrium or right upper quadrant after emptying the stomach with a nasogastric tube). As a result of persistent vomiting, hypochloremic, hypokalemic metabolic alkalosis with varying degrees of dehydration and failure to thrive may occur when the diagnosis is not made early in the course. The finding of a pyloric olive is pathognomonic. Ultrasound is a useful diagnostic tool to confirm the diagnosis when the olive is not evident on examination or early in the course. The differential diagnosis includes intestinal obstruction or atresia, malrotation with volvulus, hiatal hernia, gastroenteritis, adrenogenital syndrome, increased intracranial pressure, esophagitis, sepsis, gastroesophageal reflux, and poor feeding technique.

Emergency Department Treatment and Disposition

Treatment includes correction of electrolyte imbalances and dehydration, as well as emergent surgical consultation for curative Ramstedt pyloromyotomy. Patients may benefit from a nasogastric tube on low intermittent suction.

Pearls

1. Hypertrophic pyloric stenosis is the most common cause of metabolic alkalosis in infancy.
2. Clinical suspicion can be heightened with serial examinations and observation of the child after oral fluid challenges for persistent projectile vomiting.
3. Clinical manifestations of pyloric stenosis begin at a mean age of 3 weeks after birth.

4. Pyloric ultrasonography is the diagnostic study of choice.
5. Projectile vomiting can also be a result of increased intracranial pressure.

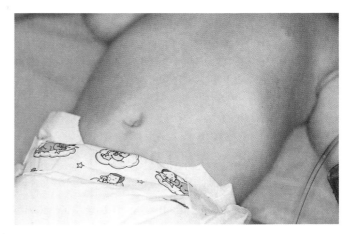

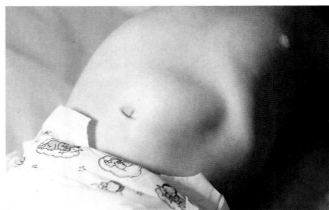

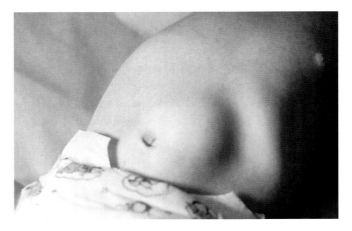

FIGURE 14.13 ■ Gastric Wave of Hypertrophic Pyloric Stenosis. A gastric wave can be seen traversing the abdomen in this series of photographs of a patient with HPS. (Photo contributor: Kevin J. Knoop, MD, MS.)

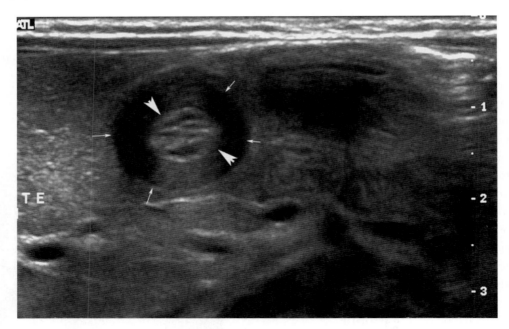

FIGURE 14.14 ■ Ultrasound Target Sign in HPS. This transverse ultrasound shows redundant, infolded mucosa (arrowheads) between muscular components (arrows), referred to as the "target sign." (Photo contributor: Lawrence B. Stack, MD.)

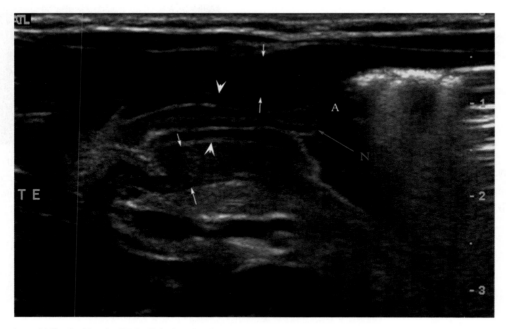

FIGURE 14.15 ■ Antral Nipple Sign in HPS. This longitudinal sonogram shows two-layered, thickened mucosa (arrowheads) surrounded by muscular components (arrows). Redundant pyloric mucosa protrudes into the fluid in the gastric antrum (A), forming the "antral nipple sign" (N) in HPS. (Photo contributor: Lawrence B. Stack, MD.)

Clinical Summary

Erythema infectiosum is a viral infection caused by parvovirus B19 presenting most commonly between 4 and 10 years of age. It is characterized initially by bright red macular erythema of the cheeks with sparing of the nasal ridge and perioral areas followed by an erythematous maculopapular eruption on the extensor surfaces of extremities that evolves with central clearing into a reticulated, lacy pattern. It may present with low-grade fever, malaise, sore throat, arthritis, or arthralgias. The differential diagnosis includes morbilliform eruptions caused by viruses such as measles, rubella, roseola, and infectious mononucleosis. Bacterial infections (eg, scarlet fever), drug reactions, and other skin conditions such as guttate psoriasis, papular urticaria, atopic dermatitis, and erythema multiforme are also included in the differential.

Emergency Department Treatment and Disposition

Treatment is aimed at symptomatic relief. Parents can be reassured that this exanthem is benign and self-limited. Once the rash appears, the patient is no longer contagious. It is important to educate the patient and family about the possible risk of parvovirus B19 as a cause of hydrops fetalis or fetal deaths early in pregnancy and the issue of an aplastic crisis in patients with hematologic problems such as sickle cell disease, hereditary spherocytosis, other hemolytic anemias, or immunocompromise.

Pearls

1. Recrudescence of the lacy, reticular rash may occur with exercise, overheating, emotional upset, or sun exposure as a result of cutaneous vasodilatation.

2. Parvovirus B19 is the most common cause of hydrops fetalis.

3. In young adults, parvovirus B19 causes papular purpuric gloves and socks syndrome.

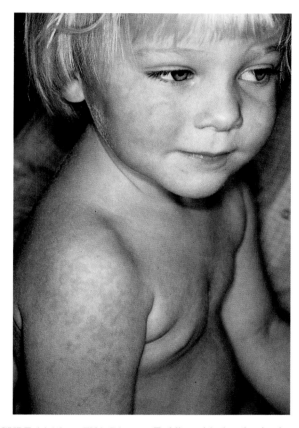

FIGURE 14.16 ■ Fifth Disease. Toddler with the classic slapped-cheek appearance of fifth disease caused by parvovirus B19. Note the lacy reticular macular rash on the shoulder and upper extremity. (Photo contributor: Anne W. Lucky, MD.)

Clinical Summary

The typical presentation of roseola infantum involves a prodrome characterized by a 3- to 5-day history of high fever in a child 6 months to 3 years of age. Fussiness may be present, but the child is often otherwise well-appearing. This is followed by defervescence and the appearance of the typical exanthem which is composed of erythematous macules and papules on the trunk, neck, proximal extremities, and occasionally the face. The rash fades in a few days. The causative agent in most cases is human herpesvirus 6 (HHV-6). The differential diagnosis includes common viruses such as measles, rubella, parvovirus B19, or infectious mononucleosis. Bacterial infections (eg, scarlet fever), drug reactions, and other skin conditions such as guttate psoriasis, papular urticaria, and erythema multiforme are also included in the differential.

Emergency Department Treatment and Disposition

As with most viral infections, only supportive therapy is necessary. Special attention should be paid in maintaining fluid intake, fever control for the patient's comfort, and parental education about the benign, self-limiting characteristics of this illness.

Pearls

1. Rashes *during* the febrile course of an illness are not roseola.

2. With defervescence and appearance of the rash, the patient is no longer contagious.

3. The most frequent complication of roseola is febrile seizures.

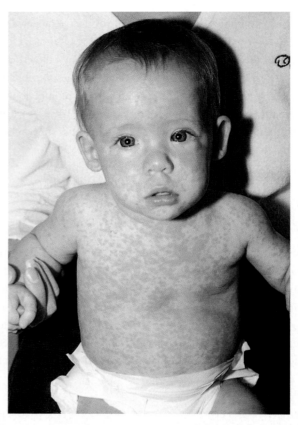

FIGURE 14.17 ■ Roseola Infantum (Exanthem Subitum). Toddler with maculopapular eruption of roseola. (Photo contributor: Raymond C. Baker, MD.)

Clinical Summary

Impetigo is a focal bacterial infection of the superficial skin that is caused by *Streptococcus pyogenes* (group A β-hemolytic *Streptococcus*) and *Staphylococcus aureus*. It most commonly affects children 2 to 5 years of age and usually involves the face and extremities. It begins as small vesicles or pustules with very thin roofs that rupture easily with the release of a cloudy fluid and the subsequent formation of a honey-colored crust. The lesions may spread rapidly by autoinoculation secondary to scratching and coalesce to form larger areas of infection. The differential diagnosis includes second-degree burns, varicella, herpes simplex infections, nummular dermatitis, superinfected eczema, and scabies.

Emergency Department Treatment and Disposition

These lesions are highly contagious and spread by direct contact. Good hand washing and personal hygiene should be emphasized to the patient and family. Application of topical antibacterials, such as mupirocin ointment, has proved to be as effective as oral antibiotics. If lesions are multiple and extensive, oral antibiotic coverage is indicated and should be directed against the organisms mentioned above. Effective oral agents include first-generation cephalosporins, dicloxacillin, amoxicillin with clavulanic acid, or clindamycin.

Pearls

1. Inflicted cigarette burns may resemble the lesions of impetigo.
2. Poststreptococcal glomerulonephritis can be a complication of impetigo caused by group A β-hemolytic *Streptococcus*.

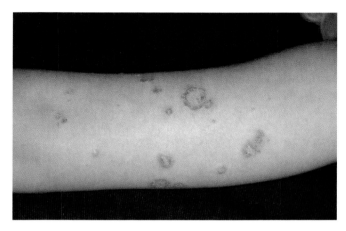

FIGURE 14.19 ■ Impetigo. The crusting lesions of impetigo on an extremity. (Photo contributor: Anne W. Lucky, MD.)

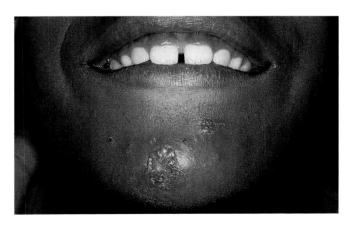

FIGURE 14.18 ■ Impetigo. Young girl with crusting impetiginous lesions on her chin. (Photo contributor Michael J. Nowicki, MD.)

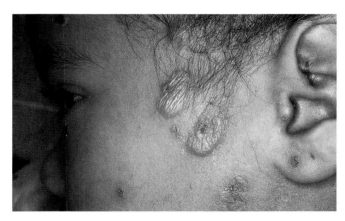

FIGURE 14.20 ■ Bullous Impetigo. A child with impetiginous lesions on the face. Note the formation of bullae. (Photo contributor Anne W. Lucky, MD.)

Clinical Summary

Measles presents as an acute febrile illness with a 3- to 4-day prodromal period characterized by dry cough, coryza, and conjunctivitis associated with fever (38.38°C-40°C [101°F-104°F]), chills, and malaise. Kopliks spots, the pathognomonic sign of measles, appear as 1- to 3-mm red papules with gray-white centers on the buccal mucosa. They usually present 1 to 2 days before the development of the characteristic erythematous maculopapular rash. This rash appears during the third or fourth day of the illness. It usually begins as dark red to purple macules and papules on the forehead, around the hairline, behind the earlobes, and spreads with a cephalocaudad progression. Individual lesions often progress to confluence. It tends to fade in the same order that it appeared. Most cases recover without complications; others may develop otitis media, croup, pneumonia, encephalitis, myocarditis, and rarely subacute sclerosing panencephalitis (SSPE), a very late complication. The differential diagnosis of the characteristic rash is vast and includes exanthem subitum, rubella, infections caused by echovirus, coxsackie and adenoviruses, toxoplasmosis, infectious mononucleosis, scarlet fever, Kawasaki disease, drug reactions, Rocky Mountain spotted fever, and meningococcemia.

Emergency Department Treatment and Disposition

Supportive therapy includes bed rest, antipyretics, and adequate fluid balance. Complications should be treated according to the presentation. Currently available antivirals are not effective. Postexposure prophylaxis includes administration of the measles-mumps-rubella (MMR) vaccine within 72 hours of exposure to a patient with active measles. Passive immunization with IVIG is effective for prevention and attenuation of measles if given within 6 days of the initial exposure. During outbreaks, MMR vaccine can be given to infants younger than 12 months. However, such infants require an additional two doses of MMR at the recommended ages after their first birthday. The use of gamma globulins and steroids in SSPE is limited.

Pearls

1. Measles is now rare in the United States but remains endemic in other parts of the world.
2. MMR vaccine is preferable to IVIG in postexposure prophylaxis.
3. Morbilliform means measles-like.

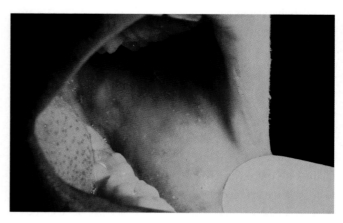

FIGURE 14.21 ■ Kopliks Spots. Tiny white dots (Kopliks spots) are seen on the buccal mucosa. (Photo contributor Lawrence B. Stack, MD.)

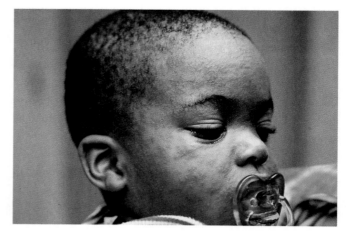

FIGURE 14.22 ■ Measles. School-age child with a morbilliform rash on his face consistent with measles. (Photo contributor: Javier A. Gonzalez del Rey, MD.)

Clinical Summary

Chickenpox results from primary infection with varicella zoster virus and is characterized by a generalized pruritic vesicular rash, fever, and mild systemic symptoms. The skin lesions have an abrupt onset, develop in crops, start on the trunk and spread outward, and evolve from erythematous, pruritic macules to papules and vesicles (rarely bullae) that finally crust over within 48 hours. The classic lesions are teardrop vesicles surrounded by an erythematous ring ("dewdrop on a rose petal"). The most common complication of varicella is occasional secondary bacterial infection, usually with *Streptococcus pyogenes* or *Staphylococcus aureus*. Other complications from varicella include encephalitis, glomerulonephritis, hepatitis, pneumonia, arthritis, and meningitis. Cerebellitis (manifested clinically as ataxia) may develop and is usually self-limited. Although several illnesses can present with vesiculobullous lesions, the typical case of varicella is seldom confused with other problems. Common viral infections that manifest with vesicular rashes include herpes simplex, zoster, coxsackie, influenza, echovirus infections, and vaccinia. On occasion varicella can be confused with papular urticaria.

Emergency Department Treatment and Disposition

Suspected varicella infection should lead to strict isolation early in the emergency department or office encounter. Most patients do not develop any complications. Treatment should be supportive and directed to pruritus and fever control (avoid salicylates because of their association with Reye syndrome). Oral acyclovir initiated within 24 hours of the onset of the rash may result in a modest decrease in the duration of symptoms and in the number and duration of skin lesions. Acyclovir is not recommended routinely for treatment of uncomplicated varicella in an otherwise healthy child less than 12 years of age. In the immunocompromised host, VZIG (varicella zoster immunoglobulin) and intravenous acyclovir are indicated.

Pearls

1. Skin lesions in varicella present in successive crops so that macules, papules, vesicles, and crusted lesions may all be present at the same time.
2. Healthy children are no longer contagious when all lesions have crusted over (usually 4-5 days from the development of the initial lesions).

3. Consider oral acyclovir for those at risk for more severe infection, including anyone older than 12 years, persons with chronic diseases, and persons taking chronic aspirin or corticosteroid therapy. Postexposure prophylaxis for susceptible individuals includes varicella zoster immune globulin (VZIG) within 96 hours of exposure in high-risk patients (immunocompromised patients or pregnant women) or immunization with varicella vaccine within 72 hours of exposure in non–high-risk patients.
4. Vaccination has greatly reduced frequency and added to atypical presentation.

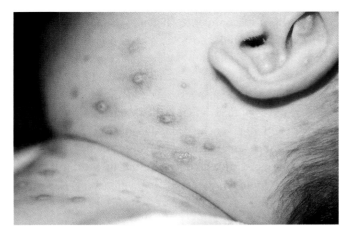

FIGURE 14.23 ■ Varicella (Chickenpox). Multiple umbilicated cloudy vesicles of varicella. (Photo contributor: Lawrence B. Stack, MD.)

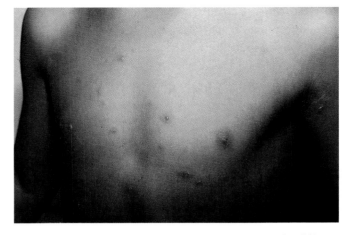

FIGURE 14.24 ■ Varicella (Chickenpox). Vesicles in different stages of maturation. Note the clear vesicle on an erythematous base ("dewdrop on a rose petal") in the center of the chest. (Photo contributor: Judith C. Bausher, MD.)

Clinical Summary

Zoster (shingles) represents a reactivation of latent varicella zoster virus (VZV) and has been noted as early as the first week of life in infants born to mothers who contracted varicella during pregnancy. These lesions present as clustered vesicles in a dermatomal distribution. Pain is intense and in certain cases can persist beyond 1 month after the lesions have disappeared (known as postherpetic neuralgia). The diagnosis is usually made clinically; however, tissue cultures, direct fluorescent antibodies, and Tzanck smears (see Fig. 25.28) can be done from vesicle scrapings for confirmation. Impetigo and cutaneous burns (cigarette) may mimic the appearance of herpetic vesicles. Varicella (chickenpox) is more diffusely spread, although a small crop of lesions may mimic zoster. Zoster also may be confused with herpes simplex virus (HSV) infection; although a close examination should reveal a dermatomal distribution in zoster.

Emergency Department Treatment and Disposition

Currently, acyclovir (800 mg orally five times per day for 7 to 10 days initiated within 48 hours of the onset of the rash in children ≥12 years) is the treatment of choice for zoster infections in both immunocompromised and immunocompetent children. Pain relief and prevention of secondary infection are also important. Intravenous antiviral therapy is recommended for immunocompromised patients. There is no pediatric formulation of famciclovir or valacyclovir, and there is insufficient data on their use in children.

Pearls

1. Zoster can occur in children of all ages.
2. A vesicular rash with a dermatomal distribution is diagnostic of zoster.
3. The most common sites for the development of zoster lesions are those supplied by the trigeminal nerve and the thoracic ganglia.
4. A patient with zoster can transmit chickenpox (varicella) to a nonimmune child or adult.

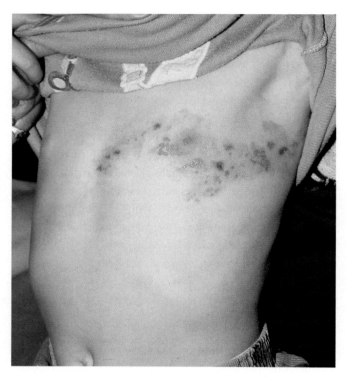

FIGURE 14.25 ■ Herpes Zoster. Vesicles in a classic thoracic dermatomal distribution are seen in this child. (Photo contributor: Frank Birinyi, MD.)

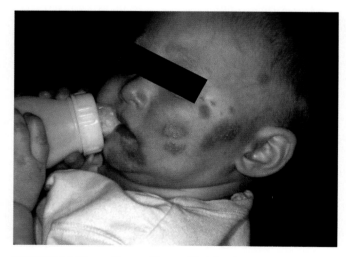

FIGURE 14.26 ■ Herpes Zoster. Vesicles in a trigeminal nerve distribution. (Photo contributor: Anne W. Lucky, MD.)

Clinical Summary

Hand, foot, and mouth disease is a seasonal (summer–fall) viral infection caused by coxsackievirus A16. Toddlers and school-age children are affected most commonly. It is characterized by a prodrome of fever, malaise, sore throat, and anorexia over 1 to 2 days, followed by the appearance of the characteristic enanthem in the posterior oropharynx and on the tonsillar pillars consisting of small, red macules evolving into small vesicles 1 to 3 mm in diameter that rapidly ulcerate. The oral manifestations are followed by a vesicular eruption characterized by 3- to 7-mm erythematous macules with a central gray vesicle on the hands and feet involving the palmar and plantar surfaces as well as the interdigital surfaces. Nonvesicular lesions may also be present on the buttocks, face, and legs.

Emergency Department Treatment and Disposition

Supportive therapy (fluid maintenance with fever and pain control) is the mainstay of treatment. The duration and characteristics of the illness should be discussed with the parents. In most cases, the course is self-limited resolving in 7 to 10 days, and the prognosis excellent. Rare secondary complications such as myocarditis, pneumonia, and meningoencephalitis may occur.

Pearls

1. The child is contagious until all vesicles have resolved.
2. The oral lesions tend to involve the posterior oropharynx as contrasted to those of herpetic gingivostomatitis that involve the anterior structures of the mouth.
3. Varicella vesicles are located more centrally, are more extensive, and usually spare the palms and soles.

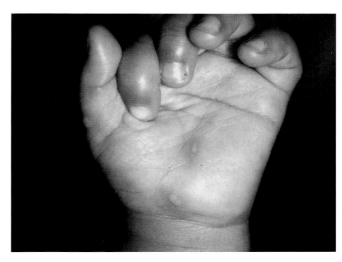

FIGURE 14.28 ■ Hand, Foot, and Mouth Disease. Erythematous vesicular rash scattered on the palms consistent with coxsackievirus. (Photo contributor: Lawrence B. Stack, MD.)

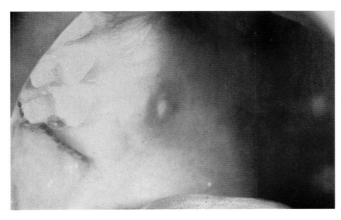

FIGURE 14.27 ■ Hand, Foot, and Mouth Disease. Discrete vesicular erosions on the posterior oropharynx and soft palate secondary to coxsackievirus. (Photo contributor: James F. Steiner, DDS.)

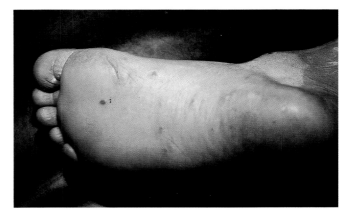

FIGURE 14.29 ■ Hand, Foot, and Mouth Disease. Vesicular rash of the feet consistent with coxsackievirus. (Photo contributor: Raymond C. Baker, MD.)

Clinical Summary

Cold panniculitis represents acute cold injury to the subcutaneous fat. It manifests as erythematous, indurated plaques on exposed skin, especially the perioral areas and cheeks. Lesions appear 24 to 72 hours after exposure to cold and gradually soften and return to normal over 1 to 2 weeks usually without permanent sequelae. This phenomenon is caused by subcutaneous fat solidification and necrosis when exposed to low temperature. It is much more common in infants. It is believed to occur because of the inherent properties of infants' fat containing higher concentrations of saturated fatty acids. The differential diagnosis includes facial cellulitis, frostbite, trauma, pressure erythema, giant urticaria, and contact dermatitis.

Emergency Department Treatment and Disposition

Treatment is supportive. Parental education and reassurance is very important.

Pearls

1. Because these lesions may also be painful, the differentiation of cold panniculitis from cellulitis may be difficult. The absence of systemic symptoms, especially fever, and the history of cold exposure are very suggestive of cold panniculitis.
2. The lesions may resolve with resulting hyperpigmentation of the affected area.

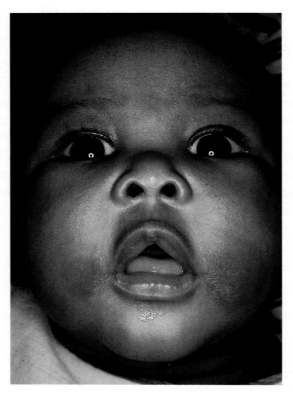

FIGURE 14.30 ■ Cold Panniculitis. Infant with cheek erythema, swelling, and discoloration consistent with popsicle panniculitis or cold injury. (Photo contributor: Anne W. Lucky, MD.)

Clinical Summary

Herpetic gingivostomatitis is a viral infection commonly seen in infants and children caused by herpes simplex virus (HSV). Patients usually present with fever, malaise, decreased oral intake, cervical adenopathy, and pain in the mouth and throat. Vesicular and ulcerative lesions appear throughout the oral cavity. The gingiva becomes very friable and inflamed, especially around the alveolar rim. Increased salivation with foul breath may be present. Although fever resolves in 3 to 5 days, children may have difficulty eating for 7 to 14 days. Sometimes, autoinoculation produces vesicular lesions on the fingers (herpetic whitlow).

Emergency Department Treatment and Disposition

Treatment includes pain control, hydration, and consideration of oral acyclovir therapy. The pain may be significant and often requires oral narcotic pain medications. Control of the pain will allow the patient to consume fluids and remain well hydrated. Acyclovir has been shown to reduce the duration of pain, gingival swelling, oral lesions, fever, and viral shedding if initiated within the first 72 hours of illness. Avoidance of citrus juices or spicy food is recommended. Cold clear fluids, popsicles, and ice cream may be useful in small children. Not infrequently, admission for intravenous hydration is necessary. Adequate fever control is also necessary for patient comfort and to avoid an increase in fluid losses. Topical pain control may be achieved by using mixtures of antihistamine (diphenhydramine elixir) and antacid (1:1) applied to lesions with a Q-tip. In small children, local application of viscous lidocaine should be avoided, since patients may develop toxic serum levels due to altered absorption from inflamed oral mucosa leading to seizures.

Pearls

1. Most of these lesions are in the anterior two-thirds of the oral cavity. Posterior lesions sparing the gingiva are most commonly seen in coxsackievirus infections.
2. Primary herpes simplex virus infection in childhood is usually asymptomatic.
3. After primary oral infection, HSV remains latent in the trigeminal ganglion until reactivated as herpes labialis.

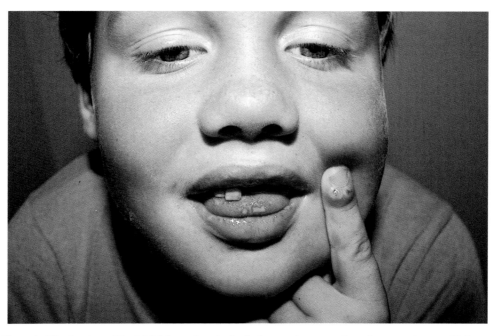

FIGURE 14.31 ■ Herpetic Gingivostomatitis. Multiple oral vesicular lesions and tongue ulcerations consistent with herpes gingivostomatitis. Vesicular lesions from autoinoculation are present on the finger (herpetic whitlow). (Photo contributor: Michael J. Nowicki, MD.)

Clinical Summary

Meningococcemia is an acute febrile illness with generally rapid onset of marked toxicity and petechial rash involving the skin and mucous membranes. The petechiae progress to become palpable purpura and may coalesce to become purpura fulminans. It progresses rapidly to hypotension with multisystem failure. In cases of fulminant disease, this shock stage is accompanied by disseminated intravascular coagulation and massive mucosal hemorrhages. Prodrome symptoms may include upper respiratory infection and malaise. Children less than 5 years of age are at greatest risk.

Emergency Department Treatment and Disposition

In stable patients in whom the diagnosis of meningococcemia is entertained, cultures of blood, spinal fluid, nasopharynx, complete blood count, platelet count, and coagulation studies should be obtained. Consider bedside screening studies, liver function tests, and other studies as indicated. These patients should be admitted for close monitoring to institutions capable of delivering critical care services. Broad-spectrum parenteral antibiotics should be used for initial coverage until the organism is identified and sensitivities are available due to the overlap of this clinical syndrome with that of other organisms causing sepsis. In the unstable septic patient, adequate ventilation and cardiac function must be ensured. Hemodynamic monitoring and support (fluids and vasoactive drugs) are of paramount importance. Peripheral and central venous catheters and urinary and arterial catheters are usually necessary for optimal care of these patients.

Pearls

1. Skin scrapings of the purpuric lesion can be microscopically examined for the presence of Gram-negative diplococci and may be cultured for organisms.
2. A child with a fever and an evolving petechial rash must be presumed to have meningococcemia.

3. A quadrivalent meningococcal conjugate vaccine is now available and recommended for all children older than 11 years of age.
4. Prophylaxis for all close contacts is recommended with rifampin for 48 hours, or a single dose of ceftriaxone or ciprofloxacin.

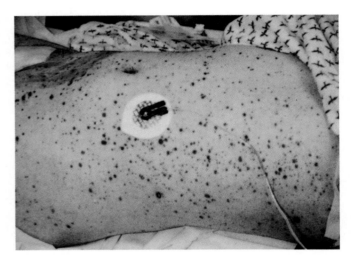

FIGURE 14.32 ■ Meningococcemia. Diffuse petechiae in a patient with meningococcemia. (Photo contributor: Richard Strait, MD.)

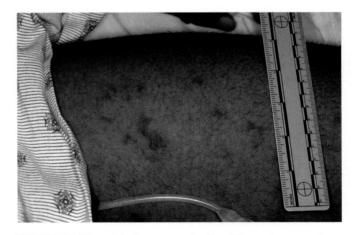

FIGURE 14.33 ■ Meningococcemia. Petechiae and purpura in an adolescent patient with meningococcemia. (Photo contributor: Kevin J. Knoop, MD, MS.)

Clinical Summary

Acute urticaria (defined as <6 weeks duration) is a common condition of childhood caused by histamine release associated with an infection, an insect sting or bite, or ingestion of certain foods or medications. It is characterized by the sudden onset of pruritic, transient, erythematous, well-circumscribed wheals scattered over the body. The lesions blanch with pressure and may vary from pinpoint size to several centimeters in diameter. They can have a central clearing or associated tense edema. Individual lesions usually resolve in 1 to 3 hours, and most urticarial reactions last 24 to 48 hours. On rare occasions, they may take weeks to resolve. Infrequently, there may be systemic reactions such as wheezing, stridor, or angioedema. The differential diagnosis includes erythema multiforme, Henoch-Schönlein purpura (HSP), arthropod bites, contact dermatitis, reactive erythemas, allergic vasculitis, juvenile rheumatoid arthritis, mastocytosis, and pityriasis rosea.

Emergency Department Treatment and Disposition

Treatment is symptomatic. If the offending agent can be identified, avoidance is recommended. Oral antihistamines are useful in the control of pruritus. If a systemic reaction is also part of the initial presentation, steroids and subcutaneous epinephrine should be considered. In many instances it is very difficult to identify the etiologic agent. Unless there is evidence of acute angioedema, most cases can be discharged home on oral antihistamines to follow up with a primary care physician.

Pearls

1. By definition, a lesion of urticaria must change or resolve within 24 hours of its appearance.
2. The most common causes of urticaria in children are viral illnesses and certain foods. In young children egg, milk, soy, peanut, and wheat are the most common allergens. In older children fish, seafood, nuts, and peanuts are more common causes.
3. The addition of an H2 antagonist may be helpful when H1 agents alone are ineffective.
4. Upon discharge, any patient who demonstrated signs of a systemic reaction should be provided with an epinephrine autoinjection device.

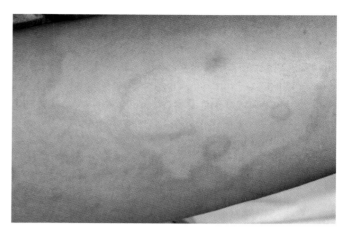

FIGURE 14.34 ■ Urticaria. Well-circumscribed, raised, pruritic extremity lesions consistent with urticaria. (Photo contributor: Anita P. Sheth, MD.)

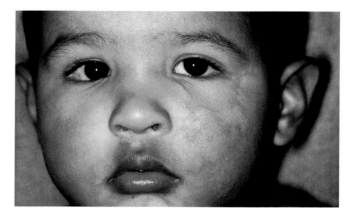

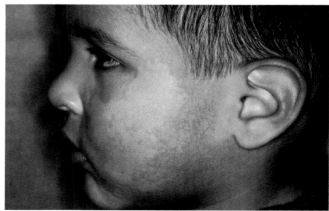

FIGURE 14.35 ■ Urticaria. Preschool child with annular, raised pruritic lesions with the central clearing and tense edema of polycyclic urticaria. The lesions had completely disappeared after about 5 minutes. (Photo contributor: Kevin J. Knoop, MD, MS.)

Clinical Summary

Staphylococcal scalded skin syndrome most commonly affects infants and children less than 5 years of age and is caused by an exfoliative exotoxin-producing strain of *Staphylococcus aureus*. Initial presentation includes fever, malaise, and irritability following an upper respiratory infection with pharyngitis or conjunctivitis. Patients develop a diffuse faint erythematous rash that becomes tender to touch. Crusting around the mouth, eyes, and neck is not uncommon. Within 2 to 3 days, the upper layers of epidermis may be easily removed; finally flaccid bullae develop with subsequent exfoliation of the skin. In young patients, this exfoliation may involve a large surface area with significant fluid and electrolyte losses. The differential diagnosis includes toxic epidermal necrolysis, exfoliative erythroderma, bullous erythema multiforme, bullous pemphigoid, bullous impetigo, sunburn, acute mercury poisoning, toxic shock syndrome, and epidermolysis bullosa.

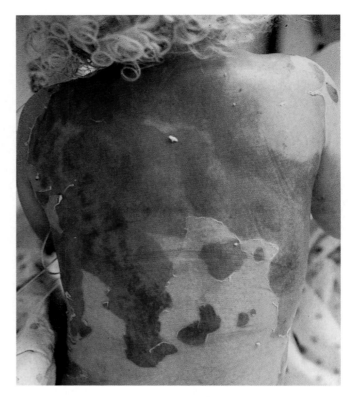

Emergency Department Treatment and Disposition

Treatment is directed at the eradication of *S aureus*, thus terminating the production of toxin. Semisynthetic penicillinase-resistant penicillins or clindamycin should be used intravenously. Admission is usually necessary, especially in young infants. This age group requires careful attention to fluid and electrolyte losses and the prevention of secondary infection of the denuded skin. Management of pain associated with the rash may require narcotic analgesics.

Pearls

1. The wrinkling or peeling of the upper layer of the epidermis (pressure applied with a Q-tip or gloved finger) that occurs within 2 or 3 days of the onset of this illness is known as Nikolsky sign.
2. The fluid in the bullae of staphylococcal scalded skin syndrome is sterile. The toxin is produced at a remote site and delivered to the skin via the bloodstream.
3. Infants with involvement of large areas of the body surface are at increased risk for hypothermia.
4. Corticosteroids are contraindicated in the treatment of staphylococcal scalded skin syndrome.

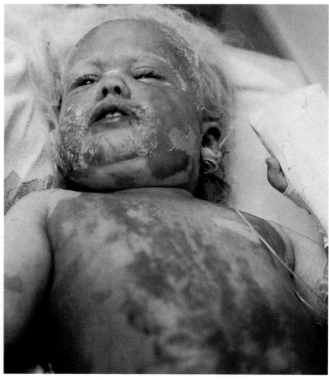

FIGURE 14.36 ■ Staphylococcal Scalded Skin Syndrome. Toddler with diffuse macular peeling eruption consistent with scalded skin syndrome from *S aureus*. (Photo contributor: Judith C. Bausher, MD.)

Clinical Summary

Scarlet fever manifests as erythematous macules and papules that result from an erythrogenic toxin produced by group A β-hemolytic *Streptococcus*. The most common site for invasion by this organism is the pharynx and occasionally skin or perianal areas. The disease usually occurs in children (2-10 years of age) and less commonly in adults. The typical presentation of scarlet fever includes fever, headache, sore throat, nausea, vomiting, and malaise followed by the scarlatiniform rash. The rash is typically erythematous; it blanches (in severe cases may include petechiae), and owing to the grouping of the fine papules gives the skin a rough, sandpaper-like texture. It initially occurs centrally on the face, often with perioral sparing, neck, and upper trunk but quickly becomes generalized and typically desquamates after 5 to 7 days. On the tongue, a thick, white coat and swollen papillae give the appearance of a strawberry ("strawberry tongue"). Palatal petechiae and tender anterior cervical lymphadenopathy may be present. A similar syndrome is caused by staphylococci producing an exfoliative exotoxin, which can be differentiated from the streptococcal infection because of the absence of pharyngitis, strawberry tongue, and negative throat cultures. The differential diagnosis also includes enteroviral infections, viral hepatitis, infectious mononucleosis, toxic shock syndrome, drug eruptions, rubella, mercury intoxication, and Kawasaki disease.

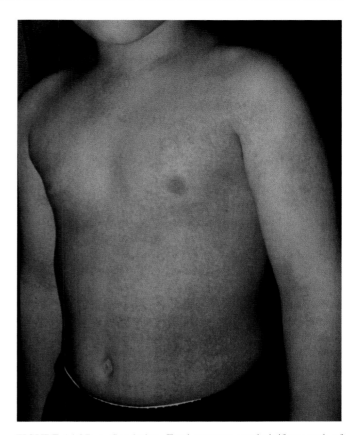

FIGURE 14.37 ■ Scarlatina. Erythematous scarlatiniform rash of scarlet fever. (Photo contributor: Lawrence B. Stack, MD.)

Emergency Department Treatment and Disposition

Penicillin, either a single intramuscular (IM) dose of benzathine penicillin G or oral penicillin V for 10 days, is the treatment of choice. Alternatives include erythromycin or clindamycin in penicillin-allergic patients.

Pearls

1. Petechiae (commonly found as part of the scarlatiniform eruption) in a linear pattern seen along the major skin folds in the axillae and antecubital fossae are known as "Pastia lines."

2. In darker skin colors, the rash may be difficult to differentiate and may consist only of punctate papular elevations called "goose flesh."

3. There has never been an isolate of group A *Streptococcus* that is resistant to penicillin.

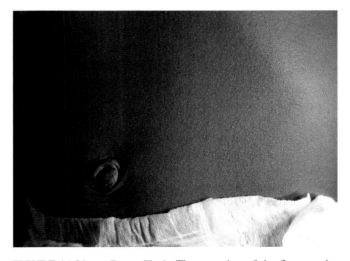

FIGURE 14.38 ■ Goose Flesh. The grouping of the fine papules gives the skin a "goose flesh" texture in darker skin colors. (Photo contributor: Kevin J. Knoop, MD, MS.)

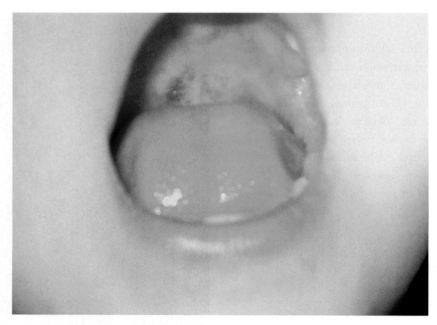

FIGURE 14.39 ■ Palatal Petechiae. Petechiae present on the posterior soft palate of a child with group A streptococcal infection. (Photo contributor: Hannah F. Smitherman, MD.)

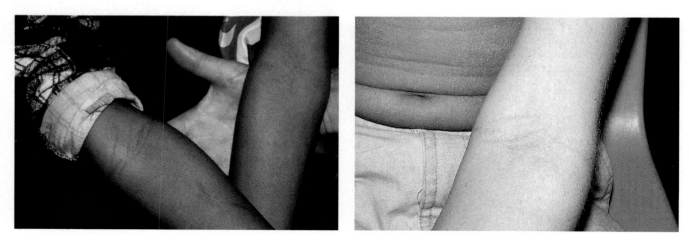

FIGURE 14.40 ■ Pastia Lines. Confluent petechiae in a linear pattern in the antecubital fossa consistent with Pastia lines are seen in these patients with scarlet fever. Left: The forearm on the right belongs to the patient's sister and does not show Pastia lines. Right: Pastia lines in a Caucasian patient. A classic sandpaper rash is also evident on the arm and trunk. (Photo contributor: Stephen W. Corbett, MD.)

Clinical Summary

Blistering distal dactylitis is a cellulitis of the fingertip caused by Group A β-hemolytic streptococci or *Staphylococcus aureus* infection in children from infancy to teenage years. The typical lesion is a fluid-filled, painful, tense blister with surrounding erythema located over the volar fat pad on the distal portion of a finger or toe. Polymorphonuclear leukocytes and gram-positive cocci can be found in the Gram stain of the purulent exudate from the lesion. The differential diagnosis includes bullous impetigo, burns, friction blisters, and herpetic whitlow.

Emergency Department Treatment and Disposition

There is usually a rapid response to incision and drainage of the blister and a 10-day course of antibiotic therapy (dicloxacillin, cephalexin, or erythromycin).

Pearl

1. Nonpurulent fluid and vesicular lesions becoming confluent multilocular bullae are characteristic of herpetic whitlow and help distinguish it from blistering distal dactylitis.

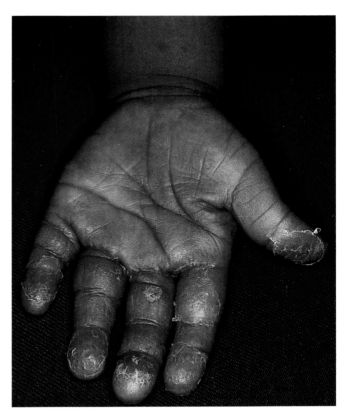

FIGURE 14.41 ■ Blistering Distal Dactylitis. Blistering rash of the distal fingers with surrounding erythema typically caused by *Streptococcus*. Note the location of the rash over the volar finger pads. (Photo contributor: Anne W. Lucky, MD.)

Clinical Summary

Also known as "anaphylactoid purpura," Henoch-Schönlein purpura (HSP) is a systemic vasculitis of small vessels characterized by 2- to 10-mm erythematous hemorrhagic papules in a symmetric, acral distribution usually involving the buttocks and extremities (see Fig. 15.23). It is a disease of children (commonly aged 3-12 years) and young adults. The classic exanthem consists of urticarial wheals, erythematous maculopapules, and larger palpable ecchymotic-looking areas. There is often associated abdominal pain (caused by edema and hemorrhage of the intestinal wall) and arthritis. Mucosal involvement is rare; however, edema of the scalp, hands, scrotum, and periorbital tissue is not uncommon. Gastrointestinal symptoms (abdominal pain, occult and gross bleeding, and intussusception) may precede the rash. Renal involvement is the most frequent and serious complication and usually occurs during the first month. It commonly manifests as microscopic hematuria and may progress to glomerulonephritis. Hypertension is uncommon. The diagnosis is made by history and clinical examination. Laboratory tests are usually normal (platelets, complement level, and antinuclear antibodies) except for the urinalysis, which may be positive for blood or protein in 50% of the patients. The prognosis is excellent, with full recovery in most instances. The course of HSP is marked by relapses and remissions in 50% of patients (rash seems to recur within the first 6 weeks). Prognosis is dictated by the renal involvement. Overall, approximately 1% of patients progress to end-stage renal disease. During the initial phases of the disease, the diagnosis may be difficult. The rash may be confused with drug reactions, erythema multiforme, urticaria, and even physical abuse. Other causes of purpura, such as bleeding disorders or infection (meningococcemia), should be included in the differential diagnosis.

Emergency Department Treatment and Disposition

Treatment is supportive. Corticosteroids (1-2 mg/kg/day for 5-7 days) may be used to treat severe abdominal pain. They are not recommended routinely for rash or joint pains. In cases where intussusception is suspected, prompt surgical consultation and diagnostic ultrasonography or air-contrast enema are indicated. Ultrasound is the preferred imaging modality in HSP because it identifies intussusception throughout the bowel and not just in the ileocolic area. Patients with HSP limited to the skin and joints with minimal urinary findings can be managed as outpatients. Severe abdominal pain, gastrointestinal hemorrhage, intussusception, and severe renal involvement are indications for admission.

Pearls

1. All children presenting to the emergency department with suspected HSP should have a stool occult blood test performed if they have abdominal pain and a urinalysis to monitor for nephritis. Stools show gross or occult blood in more than half of cases.

2. Intussusception associated with HSP is seen in 2% of patients, most commonly in boys, particularly those about 6 years of age. The intussusception is often ileo-ileal.

3. The typical rash occurs in 100% of cases and is the presenting feature in 50% of cases. Joint symptoms may precede the rash as the presenting complaint in 25% of patients. Ankles and knees are the most commonly affected joints.

4. Monthly urinalysis should be performed for 3 months following diagnosis to screen for delayed renal involvement.

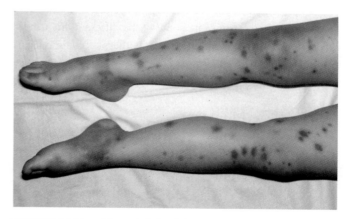

FIGURE 14.42 ■ Henoch-Schönlein Purpura. These erythematous, hemorrhagic papules and petechiae in a symmetric acral distribution are classic findings in HSP. This child presented with no other symptoms. (Photo contributor: Lawrence B. Stack, MD.)

Clinical Summary

Hemangiomas are benign vascular tumors characterized by a rapid proliferative phase followed by a spontaneous involutional phase. They are the most common soft tissue tumors of infancy. The appearance of hemangiomas is determined by the lesion's depth, location, and stage of evolution. A strawberry hemangioma lies in the upper dermis and often originates as an erythematous macular patch, a pale macule, or a localized telangiectasia with a pale halo. The lesion grows and becomes vascularized during the first 2 months of life. The classic presentation is a bright red, slightly elevated, noncompressible plaque. It commonly regresses by 2 to 3 years of age. Localized hemangiomas can affect the airway, eyes, or other areas where they occur. The differential diagnosis includes vascular malformations, malignant vascular neoplasms, pyogenic granulomas, and giant melanocytic birthmarks.

Emergency Department Treatment and Disposition

Most cases require no therapy because strawberry hemangiomas usually regress without residua. Treatment of hemangiomas in general is indicated when there is an obstruction of a vital orifice (ie, airway, mouth, or nares) or vision (eyelids) or if hematologic or cardiovascular complications are present. Education and parental reassurance are important because there is great pressure to treat for cosmetic reasons. Oral corticosteroids, intralesional corticosteroids, pulsed dye laser, and recombinant interferon-α are some of the different therapeutic modalities available. In complex cases, dermatologic consultation is recommended.

Pearls

1. Kasabach-Merritt syndrome (hemolytic anemia, thrombocytopenia, and coagulopathy) is associated with Kaposiform hemangioendothelioma or tufted angiomas and not with common hemangiomas as was previously thought.

2. As many as 20% of affected infants have multiple lesions.

3. In contrast to hemangiomas, vascular malformations, such as port-wine stains, do not proliferate or involute. They persist throughout life and grow in proportion with the child.

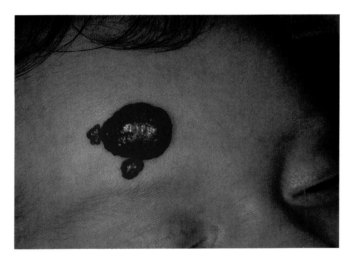

FIGURE 14.43 ■ Strawberry Hemangioma. Raised umbilicated vascular lesion on the right forehead consistent with strawberry hemangioma. (Photo contributor: Anne W. Lucky, MD.)

Clinical Summary

Orbital (postseptal) cellulitis is a serious bacterial infection characterized by fever, painful purple-red eyelid swelling, restriction of eye movement, proptosis, and variable decreased visual acuity. It may begin with eye pain and low-grade temperature. In general, it is caused by *Streptococcus pneumoniae, Haemophilus influenzae, Moraxella catarrhalis, and Staphylococcus aureus*. It usually arises as a complication of ethmoid or maxillary sinusitis. If not treated promptly, it can lead to blindness, cavernous sinus thrombosis, meningitis, subdural empyema, or brain abscess. Periorbital (preseptal) cellulitis usually presents with edema and typically circumferential erythema of the eyelids and periorbital skin, minimal pain, and fever. Proptosis and ophthalmoplegia are not characteristic. Preseptal cellulitis usually results from trauma, contiguous infection, or in rare instances, from primary bacteremia among young infants. Common organisms are *S aureus* and group A *Streptococcus*.

Emergency Department Treatment and Disposition

A broad-spectrum parenteral antibiotic with staphylococcal coverage, ophthalmologic consultation, and admission are indicated in cases of orbital cellulitis. Orbital CT with contrast is needed to assess for abscess requiring surgical drainage. In febrile or ill-appearing patients with periorbital cellulitis, admission with broad-spectrum antibiotic therapy is indicated. Mild cases (especially those with history of trauma, eg, abrasion, insect sting) can be treated as outpatients with close follow-up.

Pearls

1. Conjunctiva is typically unaffected in periorbital cellulitis.
2. Proptosis and limitation of ocular motility are seen more frequently in older children with orbital cellulitis.

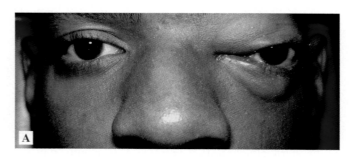

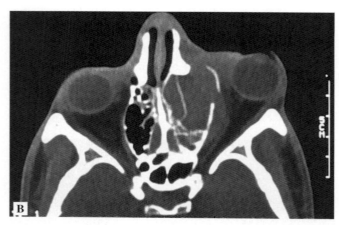

FIGURE 14.45 ■ Orbital Cellulitis. Left ethmoid sinusitis with extension into the orbital space, periosteal abscess formation and proptosis is seen in this patient (**A**) and on CT (**B**). (Photo contributor: Lawrence B. Stack, MD.)

FIGURE 14.44 ■ Orbital Cellulitis. Left orbital cellulitis with decreased range of motion secondary to edema. Note the injected conjunctiva. (Photo contributor: Javier A. Gonzalez del Rey, MD.)

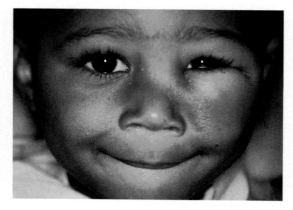

FIGURE 14.46 ■ Periorbital Cellulitis. Left periorbital cellulitis with edema and erythema of the eyelids. Note that the conjunctiva is clear and not injected. (Photo contributor: Kevin J. Knoop, MD, MS.)

Clinical Summary

A branchial (aka pharyngeal) cleft cyst arises from the incomplete obliteration of one the branchial clefts during embryogenesis. There are four paired branchial arches that form on the external surface of the embryo. The spaces in between these arches are the branchial clefts. The branchial arches ultimately develop into structures of the head and neck. As the obliteration of the clefts occurs, a portion of a cleft may remain forming a cystic space. The anatomic location of a branchial cleft cyst depends upon the specific arch/cleft involved. Involvement of the first branchial cleft may result in a cyst in the region of the parotid gland, the pre or postauricular area, or inferior to the angle of the mandible. A second cleft anomaly may be found along the anterior border of the sternocleidomastoid muscle or deep into it in the vicinity of the carotid arteries. Third and fourth arch/cleft anomalies are very unusual. The cysts usually present clinically when they become infected and enlarge acutely usually in association with an upper respiratory infection.

Emergency Department Treatment and Disposition

The diagnosis of these lesions is suggested by history and physical examination. Treatment includes antibiotics to decrease the inflammation if there is an associated infection. Ensure that there is no evidence of airway compromise. Complete excision of these lesions is necessary in order to prevent recurrence. Consultation with an otolaryngologist is appropriate.

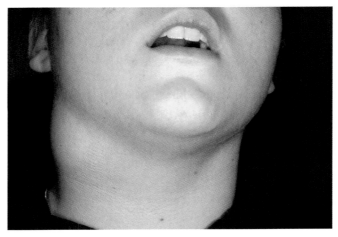

FIGURE 14.48 ■ Second Branchial Cleft Cyst. **Right neck mass seen** in second branchial cleft cyst. (Photo contributor: Scott Manning, MD.)

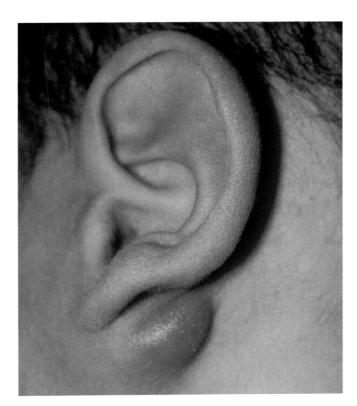

FIGURE 14.47 ■ First Branchial Cleft Cyst. Periauricular mass from a first branchial cleft cyst. (Photo contributor: Lawrence B. Stack, MD.)

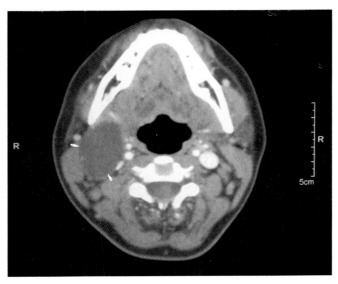

FIGURE 14.49 ■ Second Branchial Cleft Cyst. Neck computed tomography showing second branchial cleft cyst. (Photo contributor: Scott Manning, MD.)

Pearls

1. Branchial cleft anomalies are second only to thyroglossal duct cysts in frequency of congenital head and neck lesions in children.

2. Malformations of the second branchial cleft represent approximately 95% of branchial cleft anomalies and give rise to cysts in the region of the sternocleidomastoid muscle.

3. These lesions may be intimately involved with major vessels and nerves. Excision by a specialist familiar with the underlying anatomy is recommended.

Clinical Summary

A thyroglossal duct cyst arises from the incomplete obliteration of the thyroglossal duct during fetal development. It usually presents as a painless, midline, anterior neck mass that moves with swallowing and protrusion of the tongue. It may occur anywhere from the base of the tongue to the sternal notch and may rapidly enlarge if infected. Infection of the cyst often occurs in association with upper respiratory symptoms.

Emergency Department Treatment and Disposition

The diagnosis of this lesion is suggested by history and physical examination. Antibiotics are indicated if the lesion has rapidly enlarged due to infection. Common pathogens include *Haemophilus influenzae*, *Staphylococcus aureus*, and *Staphylococcus epidermidis*. Treatment involves excision of the entire tract following resolution of any associated infection. Referral to an otolaryngologist is appropriate.

Pearls

1. A thyroglossal duct cyst is the most frequent congenital head and neck lesion in children.
2. In approximately 1% of patients with this lesion, the only functional thyroid tissue is located within the cyst. Therefore, patients should be screened by history for symptoms of hypothyroidism. If symptoms are present, a serum TSH should be sent, and ultrasound of the midline neck should be considered prior to surgical removal.
3. The cyst typically moves cranially with protrusion of the tongue or with swallowing due to its relationship with the hyoid bone.

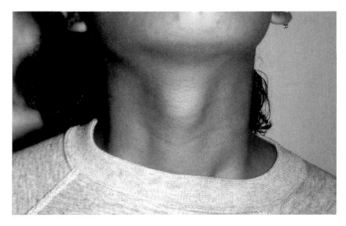

FIGURE 14.50 ■ Thyroglossal Duct Cyst. A midline mass is seen in thyroglossal duct cyst. (Photo contributor: Lawrence B. Stack, MD.)

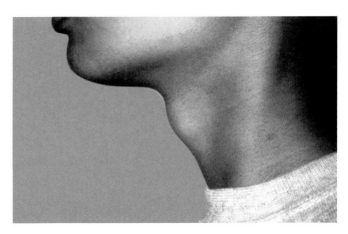

FIGURE 14.51 ■ Thyroglossal Duct Cyst. Lateral view of thyroglossal duct cyst. (Photo contributor: Lawrence B. Stack, MD.)

Clinical Summary

Cystic hygromas are lymphatic malformations found most commonly in the neck in infants and children less than 2 years of age. They present as nontender, compressible, unilocular, or multilocular masses with thin, transparent walls and are filled with straw-colored fluid. Unlike hemangiomas, these lesions rarely undergo spontaneous regression. The vast majority tend to grow and infiltrate adjacent structures. In cases where the tongue is involved, they may produce tracheal compression and respiratory difficulty. The differential diagnosis includes branchial arch remnants, thyroglossal cysts, cystic teratomas, cervical lymphadenopathy, and other primary neoplastic diseases.

Emergency Department Treatment and Disposition

Elective surgical removal is the treatment of choice in the vast majority of cases, since these lesions do not regress and may affect local tissues. Extent of the lesion should be evaluated prior to its removal (x-rays and computed tomography). The earlier these lesions can be removed, the better the cosmetic result. Aspiration of the lesion, with or without injection of a sclerosing agent, is another therapeutic option.

Pearls

1. Rapid enlargement of a cystic hygroma is most likely due to bleeding or infection. This can result in airway compromise.
2. Chromosomal aberrations are found in a significant number of infants with cystic hygromas. These lesions are frequently associated with Noonan, Turner, and Down syndromes.

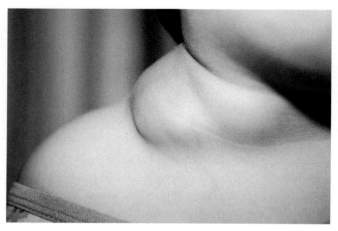

FIGURE 14.52 ■ Cystic Hygroma. A bright, supraclavicular, soft, boggy, compressible mass consistent with cystic hygroma. (Photo contributor: Richard M. Ruddy, MD.)

Clinical Summary

Catscratch disease is a benign, self-limited condition caused primarily by *Bartonella henselae* that manifests with regional lymphadenopathy (Fig. 14.54), which usually follows (1-3 weeks) red-brown, nontender papules at the presumed site of bacterial inoculation. A history of contact with or scratch from a cat is usually present. Lymphadenopathy may persist for months and in rare cases patients may develop complications such as encephalitis, osteolytic lesions, hepatosplenic lesions, weight loss, prolonged fever, and fatigue. The differential diagnosis includes lymphogranuloma venereum, bacterial adenitis, sarcoidosis, infectious mononucleosis, tumors (benign or malignant), tuberculosis, tularemia, brucellosis, and histoplasmosis.

Emergency Department Treatment and Disposition

The disease is usually self-limited and management is primarily symptomatic. Parents and patients should be reassured that the nodes are benign and frequently resolve within 2 to 4 months. In cases of painful, fluctuant nodes, needle aspiration may be necessary for relief of symptoms. Antibiotic therapy should be considered for acutely or severely ill patients or for prolonged adenopathy. If the diagnosis is in doubt, IgM and IgG antibody titers to *Bartonella* species can be sent. Several anecdotal reports have suggested that oral antibiotics such as azithromycin, rifampin, trimethoprim-sulfamethoxazole, and ciprofloxacin or intravenous gentamicin may be effective. Surgical excision of the affected nodes is generally unnecessary.

Pearls

1. Catscratch disease is the most common cause of regional adenopathy and should be considered in all children or adolescents with persistent lymphadenopathy.
2. Parinaud oculoglandular syndrome is characterized by a unilateral conjunctivitis and preauricular lymphadenopathy caused by *B henselae*.

3. Even in the presence of severe and multiple hepatic lesions, liver transaminase levels are normal and hepatomegaly is rare.

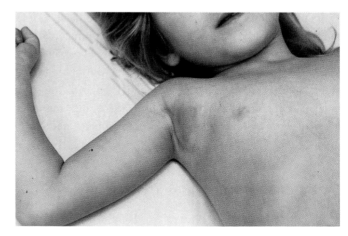

FIGURE 14.53 ■ Catscratch Disease. An erythematous, tender, suppurative node is seen in a young febrile patient with a history of cat scratch on the extremity. The node required drainage 2 days later. (Photo contributor: Kevin J. Knoop, MD, MS.)

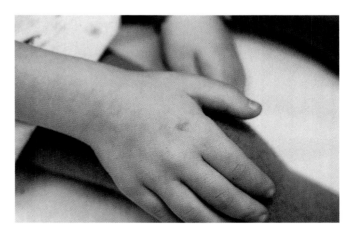

FIGURE 14.54 ■ Catscratch Disease. The precipitating wound that caused the suppurative node in Fig. 14.53. (Photo contributor: Kevin J. Knoop, MD, MS.)

Clinical Summary

Epiglottitis is a life-threatening condition characterized by sudden onset of fever, irritability, sore throat, moderate to severe respiratory distress with stridor, and variable degrees of drooling. The patient generally appears toxic and prefers a sitting position, leaning forward with neck extension in a sniffing position with an open mouth. Since the release of the Hib vaccine there has been a dramatic decrease in the incidence as well as a shift in the bacterial etiology. Most cases are now caused by streptococci, staphylococci, nontypeable *H influenzae*, and *Candida albicans*. Adults typically have a more indolent course characterized by "severe" sore throat and odynophagia. Direct thermal injury has been reported as a noninfectious cause. On soft tissue lateral neck x-ray, the epiglottis is seen as rounded and blurred (thumbprint sign). Epiglottitis may progress to complete obstruction if not treated. Differential diagnosis includes acute infectious laryngitis, acute laryngotracheo-bronchitis (croup), acute spasmodic laryngitis, membranous (bacterial) tracheitis, anaphylactic reaction, foreign body aspiration, retropharyngeal abscess, and extrinsic or intrinsic compression of the airway (tumors, trauma, cysts).

Emergency Department Treatment and Disposition

Immediate intervention is required. If epiglottitis is suspected, child should be allowed to remain in a position of comfort, and manipulation kept to a minimum if the patient is maintaining an adequate airway. If impending respiratory failure is present, an airway must be established. If possible, this should be done in the operating room or designated area where advanced airway management with sedation is available. An experienced anesthesiologist and surgeon should be available in case a surgical airway is needed. Once the airway has been controlled, the patient should be sedated to avoid accidental extubation and appropriate antibiotic therapy should be instituted (ceftriaxone or ampicillin-sulbactam) and adjusted once culture results are available.

Pearls

1. Definitive diagnosis of epiglottitis requires direct visualization of a red, swollen epiglottis, preferably in an operating room with advanced airway measures readily available.
2. Allow the child to remain undisturbed in a position of comfort while preparing for airway management. An agitated child is at increased risk for suddenly losing the airway.

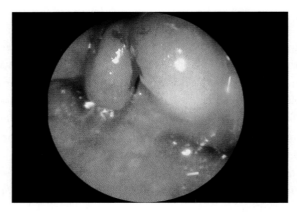

FIGURE 14.55 ■ Epiglottitis. Endoscopic view of almost complete airway obstruction secondary to epiglottitis. Note the slit-like opening of the airway. (Photo contributor: Department of Otolaryngology, Children's Hospital Medical Center, Cincinnati, OH.)

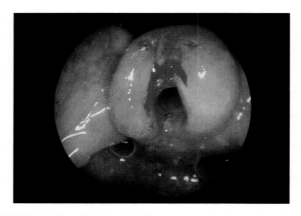

FIGURE 14.56 ■ Epiglottitis. The same patient immediately after extubation. Although erythema and some edema persist, the airway is widely patent. (Photo contributor: Department of Otolaryngology, Cincinnati Children's Hospital Medical Center, Cincinnati, OH.)

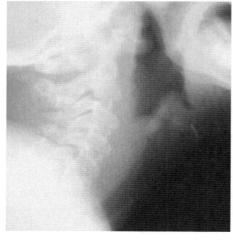

FIGURE 14.57 ■ Epiglottitis. Lateral soft-tissue x-ray of the neck demonstrating thickening of aryepiglottic folds and thumbprint sign of epiglottis. (Photo contributor: Richard M. Ruddy, MD.)

Clinical Summary

Retropharyngeal abscess (RPA) usually presents with fever, difficulty in swallowing, excessive drooling, sore throat, changes in voice, or neck stiffness. Limitation in neck movement on examination, especially with hyperextension, or torticollis may be an important finding. The resultant edema represents cellulitis and suppurative adenitis of the lymph nodes located in the prevertebral fascia and is seen on a soft tissue lateral x-ray of the neck as prevertebral soft tissue thickening. The RPA may be preceded by an upper respiratory infection, pharyngitis, otitis media, or a wound infection following a penetrating injury into the posterior pharynx. It is helpful for the examiner to be familiar with the normal laryngeal structures. The differential diagnosis includes pharyngitis, acute laryngotracheobronchitis, epiglottitis, membranous (bacterial) tracheitis, cervical adenitis, infectious mononucleosis, peritonsillar abscess, foreign body aspiration, and diphtheria. These patients may present with stiff neck mimicking meningitis.

Emergency Department Treatment and Disposition

This illness requires immediate intervention to prevent respiratory compromise and airway obstruction. The first step is to evaluate the airway and establish an artificial one if necessary. Antibiotic coverage should be initiated immediately (clindamycin $\pm$ third-generation cephalosporin or a β-lactamase-resistant penicillin). Analgesia should be administered as needed. Radiologic evaluation includes soft tissue lateral neck x-ray and neck CT with contrast to define the extent of infection. In the absence of obstruction, medical treatment with IV antibiotics for 24 to 48 hours is first-line therapy. If impending obstruction is present or the infection is unresponsive to IV antibiotic therapy, needle aspiration or incision and drainage should be performed in the operating room. These patients require hospitalization and immediate otolaryngologic or surgical consultation.

Pearls

1. On lateral soft tissue x-ray of the neck, the prevertebral soft tissue can measure up to 7 mm in width at the level of C2. At C6, it can measure up to 14 mm in width. This represents approximately one-half the width of the corresponding vertebral body.

2. The prevertebral soft tissue may appear falsely enlarged during neck flexion or crying.

3. The peak incidence occurs in 3- to 5-year olds. It is rare beyond 6 years of age because the retropharyngeal lymph nodes involute after this age.

4. Retropharyngeal abscesses in older patients most commonly arise as a complication of trauma or an immunocompromised state.

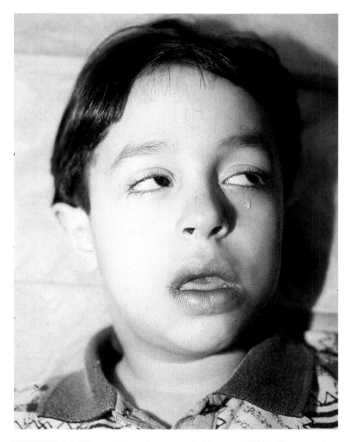

FIGURE 14.58 ■ Retropharyngeal Abscess. This ill-appearing 6-year-old child presented with a several-day history of fever, neck pain, sore throat, cough, and headache. Soft tissue lateral radiography of the neck showed thickened prevertebral tissues opposite C2 to C4. Computed tomography (CT) showed the airway narrowed to a width of 5 mm within the oropharynx. (Photo contributor: Mark Ralston, MD.)

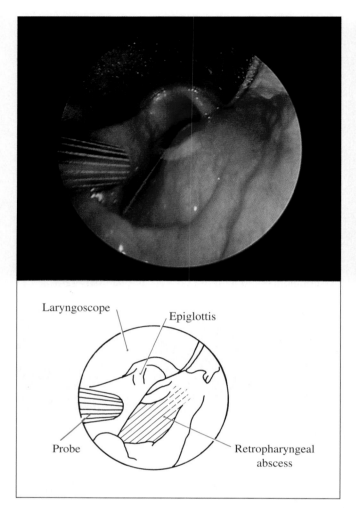

FIGURE 14.59 ■ Retropharyngeal Abscess. Endoscopic view of a retropharyngeal abscess. Note the massive swelling posteriorly. (Photo contributor: Department of Otolaryngology, Cincinnati Children's Hospital Medical Center, Cincinnati, OH.)

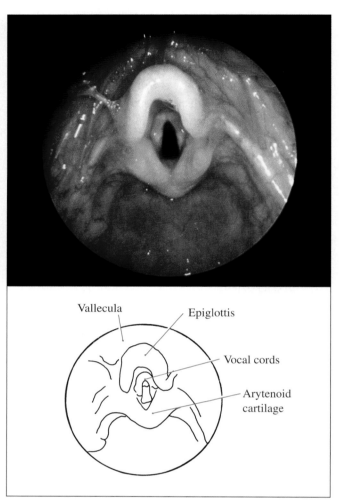

FIGURE 14.61 ■ Normal Laryngeal Structures. Endoscopic view of a normal epiglottis and surrounding structures. (Photo contributor: Department of Otolaryngology, Cincinnati Children's Hospital Medical Center, Cincinnati, OH.)

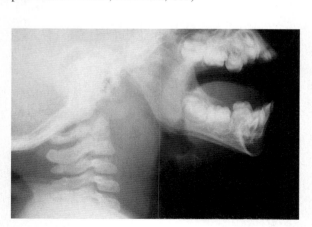

FIGURE 14.60 ■ Retropharyngeal Abscess. Lateral soft tissue neck x-ray demonstrating prevertebral soft tissue density consistent with retropharyngeal abscess. (Photo contributor: Richard M. Ruddy, MD.)

Clinical Summary

The majority of button battery ingestions occur in children less than 5 years of age. The most important factors in determining both symptoms at presentation, as well as management, are location within the gastrointestinal tract and duration of contact with the mucosal surface. Batteries that are lodged in the esophagus may be asymptomatic initially or may present with pain, drooling, dysphagia, poor intake, cough, vomiting, or fever. Mechanisms of injury associated with button battery ingestion include electrical-current-induced soft tissue injury and liquefaction necrosis resulting from alkali exposure due to battery leakage or the de novo synthesis of alkali at the surface of the battery.

Emergency Department Treatment and Disposition

Plain radiographs should be obtained to locate the battery within the gastrointestinal (GI) tract. Button batteries can be distinguished from coins on plain x-ray by demonstration of a double contour. Button batteries that are lodged in the esophagus can lead to potentially fatal complications and require immediate removal in consultation with a gastroenterologist or surgeon. This is best accomplished with direct visualization by endoscopy and with a definitive airway in place to prevent aspiration of the battery upon removal from the esophagus. Batteries that have passed into the stomach are likely to traverse the GI tract without complication. X-rays can be repeated at weekly intervals until passage is documented. Instructions detailing concerning symptoms (abdominal pain, abdominal distention, hematemesis, or blood in the stools) should be provided to the parents at the time of discharge.

Pearls

1. Button batteries with a diameter of 20 mm or greater that remain in the stomach beyond 48 hours should be considered for removal.
2. Button batteries lodged in the nasal cavity or external auditory canal also require emergent removal to prevent complications such as perforation or stenosis.
3. Heavy metal poisoning due to absorption of button battery components though the GI tract is extremely rare.

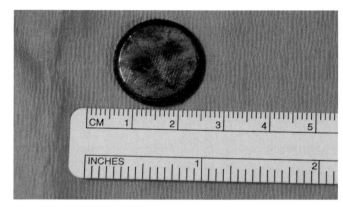

FIGURE 14.63 ■ Disk Battery. This battery was retrieved after ingestion. (Photo contributor: Lawrence B. Stack, MD.)

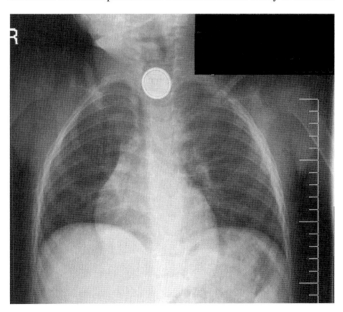

FIGURE 14.62 ■ Disk Battery Ingestion. Chest x-ray showing circular "coin-like" appearance with a second concentric ring from the plastic insulating grommet. This identifies the foreign body as a disk battery. (Photo contributor: Scott Manning, MD.)

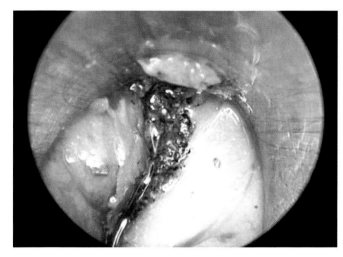

FIGURE 14.64 ■ Disk Battery Ingestion. This endoscopic view shows esophageal necrosis after disk battery lodged in the esophagous. (Photo contributor: Scott Manning, MD.)

Clinical Summary

Membranous tracheitis is an acute bacterial infection (*Staphylococcus aureus, Haemophilus influenzae,* streptococci, and pneumococci) of the upper airway capable of causing life-threatening airway obstruction. It may present as a primary infection or occur as a bacterial complication of a viral infection of the upper respiratory tract. The infection produces marked swelling and thick, purulent secretions of the tracheal mucosa below the vocal cords. The secretions can form a thick plug that may ultimately lead to an acute tracheal obstruction. Patients appear toxic, with high fever and a croup-like syndrome that can progress rapidly. The usual treatment for croup is ineffective in these patients. The characteristic "membranes" may be seen on x-rays of the airway as edema with an irregular border of the subglottic tracheal mucosa. On direct laryngoscopy, copious purulent secretions can be found in the presence of a normal epiglottis. The differential diagnosis includes acute laryngotracheobronchitis, retropharyngeal abscess, peritonsillar abscess, foreign-body aspiration, and acute diphtheric laryngitis.

Emergency Department Treatment and Disposition

Otolaryngologic consultation should be obtained as soon as the diagnosis is considered. Direct visualization of the trachea is more important than a possible radiologic diagnosis. Aggressive airway management, including endotracheal intubation, may be needed to protect the airway and allow for repeated suctioning to prevent acute airway obstruction. The patient should be admitted to the intensive care unit for close monitoring and sedation needs. Appropriate antibiotic coverage against suspected organisms should be instituted immediately.

Pearls

1. Bacterial tracheitis often presents with acute, severe airway obstruction after a short prodrome. It should be suspected in all patients with an atypical croup-like presentation: unusual age group, toxicity, not improving with routine croup therapy, and unusual roentgenographic changes of the trachea.

2. Up to 50% of soft tissue films may delineate a subglottic membrane.

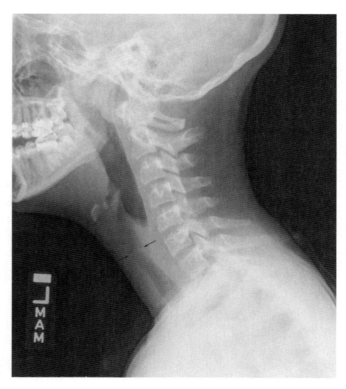

FIGURE 14.65 ■ Membranous Tracheitis. Lateral soft tissue x-ray of the neck in a 13-year-old girl with the acute onset of stridor after 3 days of sore throat. Membranes (arrows) are visible in the subglottic region. (Photo contributor: Matthew R. Mittiga, MD.)

Clinical Summary

There are several fracture patterns that are unique to children. Physeal fractures, torus (buckle) fractures, greenstick fractures, and bowing fractures or deformities all occur secondary to the physiologic differences between immature and mature bone. Physis (growth plate) fractures are common because of the relative weakness of the growth plate compared to the cortical lamellar bone. This weakness is related to the relatively large ratio of cells to matrix in the physis. The Salter-Harris (SH) classification was designed to describe each type of physeal fracture, its prognosis, and its treatment.

SH type I: Fracture that extends only through the growth plate. It is a very difficult radiologic diagnosis since the fracture line is not visible unless the fracture is displaced. It is usually a clinical diagnosis, but occasionally a physeal widening is observed on the x-ray.

SH type II: Fracture along the growth plate with an oblique extension through a piece of the metaphysis. This is the most common growth plate fracture.

SH type III: Fracture through the growth plate that extends into the epiphysis and articular cartilage into the joint space.

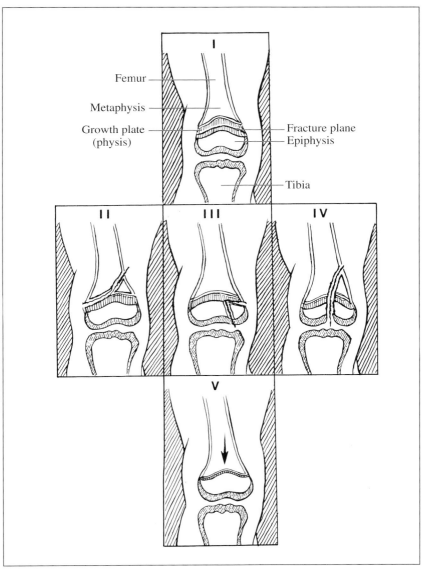

FIGURE 14.66 ■ Salter-Harris Fracture Classification. Salter-Harris classification for physeal (growth plate) fractures.

SH type IV: Fracture through the growth plate that extends into both the metaphysis and the epiphysis and into the joint space.

SH type V: Crushing injury resulting in compression of the growth plate.

Emergency Department Treatment and Disposition

Immobilization by splinting is the treatment of choice in types I and II (minimum of 3 weeks). In these cases, reduction is easy to achieve and maintain. Growth is generally unimpaired. Types III and IV may require open reduction to avoid later traumatic arthritis and, in some cases, growth arrest. Type V fractures are rare and require very close follow-up because of arrest of growth caused by the death of the germinal cells. Types III, IV, and V require immediate orthopedic consultation.

Pearls

1. After initial assessment and evaluation, always suspect SH type I if there is evidence of tenderness and swelling around the growth plate area despite negative x-rays.
2. Comparison views of the unaffected side may be useful in diagnosing SH types I and V.
3. Types I and II generally possess a substantial potential for remodeling and have a very good prognosis. Types III and IV threaten growth potential and articular integrity and require anatomic (often surgical) reduction. Type V is very high risk for growth arrest.

Clinical Summary

This painful condition is commonly the first clinical manifestation of sickle cell disease. It usually presents in children younger than 5 years of age. The pain and abnormalities are the result of infarction of the small bones of the hands or feet. These children present acutely ill, with fever, refusal to bear weight, and swollen hands and feet. They may have a marked leukocytosis, and the initial x-rays may be normal. It is not until 1 to 2 weeks later that subperiosteal new bone, cortical thickening, and even complete bone destruction can be seen. The differential diagnosis includes osteomyelitis, trauma, cold injuries, acute rheumatic fever, juvenile rheumatoid arthritis, and leukemia.

Emergency Department Treatment and Disposition

The most important aspects in the treatment of vaso-occlusive crisis in sickle cell disease include an adequate fluid balance, oxygenation, and analgesia. Therapy should be individualized. Codeine, hydromorphone, morphine, and ketorolac are analgesic agents commonly used in the treatment of children with painful sickle crisis. If fever is present, bacterial infection should be assumed until proven otherwise. Complete blood count (CBC), reticulocyte count, and blood cultures should be obtained from all febrile sickle cell patients. Empiric broad-spectrum antibiotic coverage should be instituted immediately (a third-generation cephalosporin, such as ceftriaxone, is a good choice). In cases of dactylitis, very close follow-up is necessary not only for the management of sickle cell disease but to reevaluate the radiologic changes in the small bones of the hands and feet. In most instances, the previously described changes disappear; however, in rare cases, shortening of the fingers and toes has been described as the result of severe bone infarcts.

Pearls

1. Most clinical manifestations of sickle cell disease occur after the first 5 to 6 months of life. The hemolytic anemia gradually develops over the first 2 to 4 months (changes that follow the replacement of fetal hemoglobin by hemoglobin S) and leads to the clinical syndromes associated with an increased percentage of SS hemoglobin.

2. Sickle cell patients are at high risk for infection from encapsulated organisms due to their functional asplenia. The most common organisms causing osteomyelitis in sickle cell patients are *Salmonella* sp, *Staphylococcus aureus*, and *Streptococcus pneumoniae*.

3. Dactylitis can often be differentiated from osteomyelitis based on the symmetrical involvement of multiple bones and a negative blood culture.

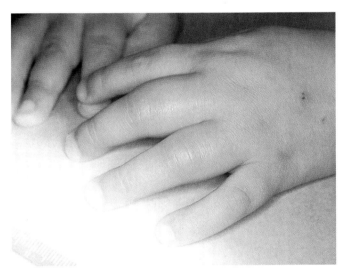

FIGURE 14.67 ■ Acute Sickle Dactylitis. Bilateral cylindrical swelling of soft tissue of the hands in sickle cell disease consistent with vaso-occlusive crisis or dactylitis. (Photo contributor: Donald L. Rucknagel, MD, PhD.)

Clinical Summary

A single strand of hair or thread may encircle a finger, a toe, or the penis, leading to circumferential strangulation of the appendage. Children in their first year of life are particularly at risk from inadvertent attachment of a parent's hair or loose thread. The affected digit appears edematous, erythematous, and painful. If not corrected, vascular compromise or infection can ensue. The differential diagnosis includes insect bites, trauma, cellulitis of the digit, osteomyelitis, or ainhum (dactylosis spontanea).

Emergency Department Treatment and Disposition

Visualization of the constricting material may be difficult. Edema, erythema, and periarticular skin folds may hide the hair or thread. It is imperative to carefully retract the skin around the proximal aspect of the edema. A magnifying lens may be helpful in identifying the band. Since the removal can be painful, consider a digital block prior to removal. A topical anesthetic may also be applied to assist in reducing local pain. Using a small hemostat, grasp a portion of the material, cut it with a surgical blade, and unwind it. Occasionally, hair-removing agents have been used to remove hair fibers. This is not advisable on deeply cut skin and will be ineffective for synthetic fibers. Elevation of the involved digit after removal of the constricting agent provides resolution of the edema and erythema within 2 to 3 days. In some cases the digit's blood supply may have been irreversibly compromised. Subspecialty consultation should be considered whenever neurovascular integrity is in question or if the constricting band cannot be visualized and removed.

Pearls

1. In the vast majority of cases, a clear line of demarcation can be identified between the normal tissue and the affected area (Fig. 14.68).
2. Irritability may be the only presenting symptom. Examination for hair tourniquets should be included in the evaluation of any inconsolable infant.
3. There may be an insidious onset with re-epithelialization over the hair tourniquet leaving it difficult to visualize.

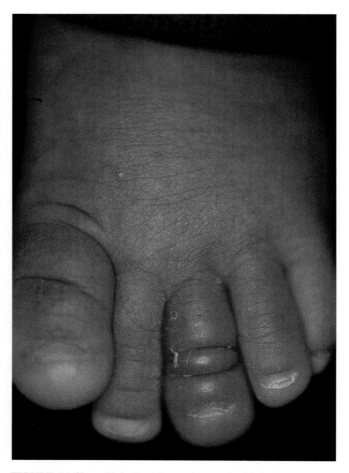

FIGURE 14.68 ■ Hair Tourniquet. A strand of hair has encircled the middle toe in two places, causing erythema and swelling. (Photo contributor: Kevin J. Knoop, MD, MS.)

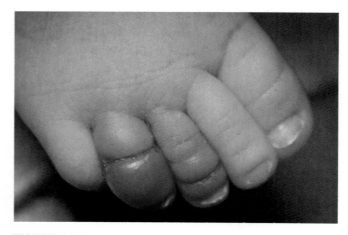

FIGURE 14.69 ■ Hair Tourniquet. Erythema distal to the hair tourniquet of the affected toes due to strangulation by the tourniquet. (Photo contributor: Robert W. Hickey, MD.)

Clinical Summary

Failure to thrive (FTT) is the inability to maintain a normal growth pattern in weight, stature, and occasionally in head growth. Definitions are varied and include a fall in weight below the third percentile relative to age or growth deceleration that crosses two major percentiles on a standardized growth chart. It is most common in infancy, and the condition is nonorganic (50%), organic (25%), or mixed (25%) in etiology. The diagnosis is made after complete history and physical examination with comparison of the measurements of length (supine in children <3 years of age), weight, and head circumference (maximal occipital-frontal circumference) to standard measurements. In cases of deficient caloric intake or malabsorption, the patient's head circumference is normal and the weight is reduced out of proportion to height. The differential diagnosis of failure to thrive is lengthy. Nonorganic disorders include poor feeding technique, disturbed maternal-child interaction, emotional deprivation, inadequate caloric intake, and child neglect. Organic causes are numerous.

Emergency Department Treatment and Disposition

Depending on history, physical findings, and the social situation, most cases can be managed as outpatients. The primary care provider can assist in determining whether outpatient management is indicated. If the diagnosis of failure to thrive is made in the emergency department, admission is suggested to complete the evaluation. This could be the only indication of a poor social environment or inadequate access to medical care. Initial laboratory investigations should include a complete blood count, electrolytes, BUN, creatinine, glucose, urinalysis, and stool examination if the stool pattern is abnormal. More specific testing should be directed by findings in the history and physical examination. Early involvement of social services may facilitate the evaluation and follow-up. Treatment will vary according to the underlying disorder and often involves a team approach, employing the assistance of nutritionists, psychologists, and home health workers.

Pearls

1. Failure to thrive in neglected children is accompanied by signs of developmental delays, emotional deprivation, apathy, poor hygiene, withdrawn behavior, and poor eye contact.

2. The major contributor to failure to thrive is caloric inadequacy. Dietary history should include details of formula preparation, volume consumed, and, in toddlers, the volume of juice consumed.

3. Standardized growth charts can be downloaded for free at www.cdc.gov/growthcharts.

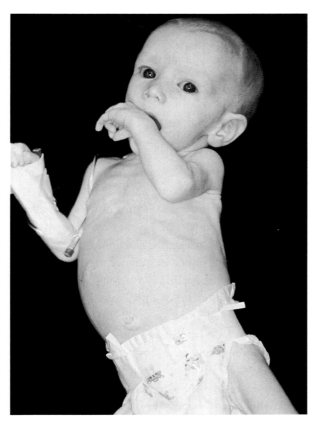

FIGURE 14.70 ■ Failure to Thrive. This infant has not been able to maintain a normal growth pattern and appears cachectic. (Photo contributor: Kevin J. Knoop, MD, MS.)

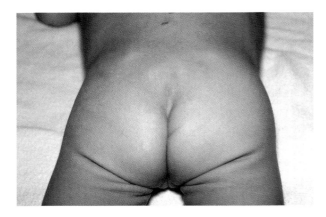

FIGURE 14.71 ■ Failure to Thrive. Accentuation of the gluteal folds secondary to loss of subcutaneous fat in an infant with FTT. (Photo contributor: Andrew H. Urbach, MD.)

Clinical Summary

The etiology of dental caries is multifactorial with an interplay between microflora (plaque colonized with *Streptococcus mutans*), substrate (fermentable carbohydrates from breast milk, formula, or juice), and host (saliva and teeth). Nursing or milk bottle caries results from prolonged and frequent night time breastfeeding or sleeping with a bottle containing milk or sugar-containing juices. The sugars are fermented by the bacteria in plaque, lowering the pH in the mouth and resulting in demineralization of the tooth enamel. The condition generally occurs before 18 months of age and is more prevalent in medically underserved children. Upper central incisors are most commonly involved. Dental referral is indicated.

Emergency Department Treatment and Disposition

Parental education and immediate referral to a dentist is necessary to prevent complications. If untreated, the caries may destroy the teeth and spread to contiguous tissues. These patients have a high risk for microbial invasion of the pulp and alveolar bone with the subsequent development of a dental abscess and facial cellulitis. In these cases, aggressive treatment with antibiotics (penicillin) and pain control, with prompt dental referral for definitive care, is necessary.

Pearls

1. The role of the emergency department physician is to recognize this pattern of dental decay (upper incisors most commonly) and initiate dental referral and parental education.

2. Nursing or bottle caries tends to spare the lower front teeth because of the shielding of the lip and tongue and the increased exposure to saliva from the sublingual glands that washes away cariogenic substrates.

3. The newborn mouth is generally devoid of micro-organisms. Newborns and infants are colonized with *S mutans* from parents and family members. Education on avoidance of sharing utensils and cups may help delay colonization of infants.

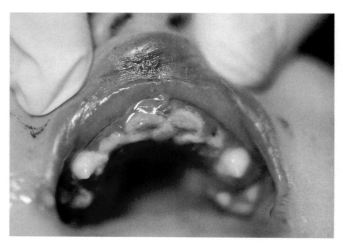

FIGURE 14.72 ■ Nursing Bottle Caries. Extensive tooth decay from sleeping with bottle containing milk or sugar-containing juices. (Photo contributor: Lawrence B. Stack, MD.)

Clinical Summary

Nursemaid's elbow is a condition that occurs commonly in children younger than 6 years of age who are usually picked up or pulled by the arm while the arm is extended at the elbow with the forearm pronated. The peak incidence is 2 to 3 years of age. The children present unwilling to supinate or pronate the hand on the affected side. Generally they hold the affected arm close to their side in a passive pronation with partial flexion at the elbow. Radiographic studies should be considered only in patients with an unusual mechanism of injury or those who do not become rapidly asymptomatic after the reduction maneuver. The differential diagnosis includes radial head fracture or complete dislocation, posterior elbow dislocation, condylar and supracondylar fractures of the distal humerus, or buckle fracture of radius or ulna.

Emergency Department Treatment and Disposition

Carefully palpate for tenderness at all points of the affected arm. There should be minimal to no tenderness to palpation. Orthopedic consultation is generally not indicated unless an underlying fracture is diagnosed. Reduction is usually achieved by one of two maneuvers: (1) while supinating the forearm, pressure is applied over the radial head and the elbow is flexed, or (2) while holding the elbow in extension, hyperpronation of the forearm is maintained until reduction is achieved. A palpable click over the radial head is evident upon successful reduction. The patient usually begins using the arm normally within minutes. When the injury has been present for several hours, reduction may be difficult, and it may take several hours to recover full function of the elbow.

Pearls

1. Radiographs of radial head subluxation typically appear normal.
2. Immobilization after reduction is not necessary.
3. If the patient remains symptomatic after reduction attempts, obtain x-rays to assess for fractures.

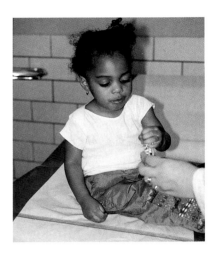

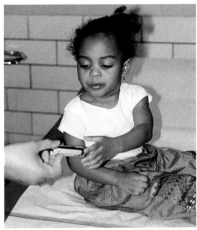

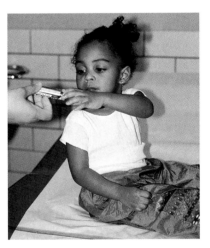

FIGURE 14.73 ■ Nursemaid's Elbow. This child presents with pseudoparalysis of the right arm after a pulling injury. Note how she avoids use of the affected arm and preferentially uses the other arm. (Photo contributor: Kevin J. Knoop, MD, MS.)

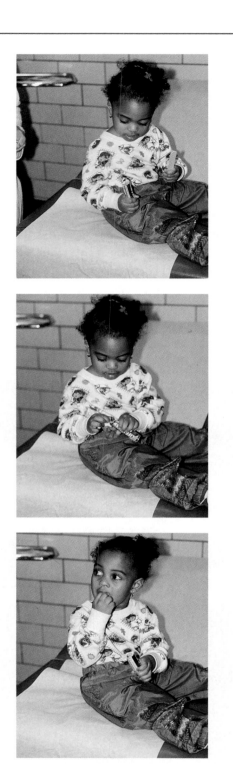

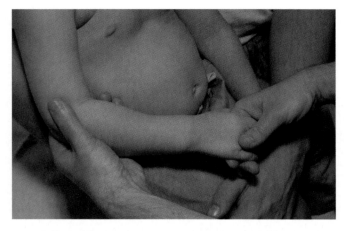

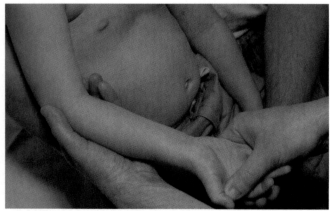

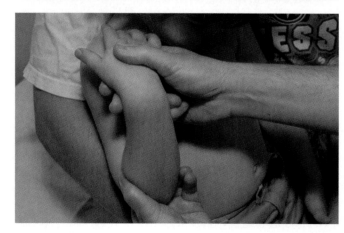

FIGURE 14.75 ■ Nursemaid's Elbow Reduction. Simultaneous suponation with elbow flexion technique for reduction of Nursemaid's elbow. (Photo contributor: R. Jason Thurman, MD.)

FIGURE 14.74 ■ Nursemaid's Elbow—Reduced. After reduction, there is initial reluctance to use the injured arm. With distraction and encouragement, the patient demonstrates successful use of the extremity. (Photo contributor: Kevin J. Knoop, MD, MS.)

Clinical Summary

Inguinal hernias are common in childhood with an incidence as high as 4%. Premature infants have an even higher incidence, and boys are approximately 10 times more likely than girls to develop an inguinal hernia. There are two types of inguinal hernias: indirect (common) and direct (rare). Indirect inguinal hernias result from failure of the processus vaginalis to obliterate toward the end of fetal development. With the presence of a patent processus vaginalis, the possibility for protrusion of intra-abdominal viscera through the internal inguinal ring exists producing the hernia. Indirect inguinal hernias are more common on the right and present as a bulge in the groin by parental history or on physical examination. Maneuvers that increase intra-abdominal pressure, such as crying in an infant or blowing bubbles in an older child, may make the hernia easier to visualize. Associated symptoms such as vomiting, abdominal distention, lack of bowel movements, blood in the stool, lethargy, or irritability suggest incarceration or strangulation of the hernia. Incarceration is most common in the first year of life.

Emergency Department Treatment and Disposition

The differential diagnosis includes hydrocele, lymphadenopathy, and an undescended or retractile testicle. With the history of a bulge but a normal physical examination in the emergency department, outpatient referral to a pediatric surgeon for timely evaluation and repair is appropriate. If a hernia is palpable, it is imperative to ensure that it can be easily manually reduced. Reduction of an incarcerated inguinal hernia may be facilitated by adequate pain control and sedation. The reduction technique

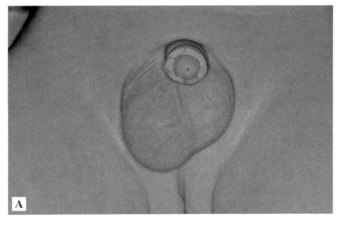

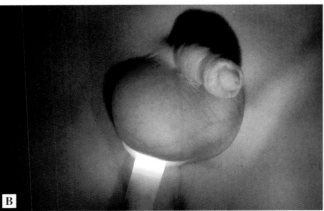

FIGURE 14.76 ■ Hydrocele. Painless scrotal swelling (**A**) which transilluminates (**B**). This patient had an inguinal hernia which was repaired electively. (Photo contributor Kevin J. Knoop, MD, MS.)

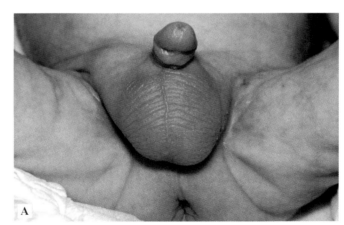

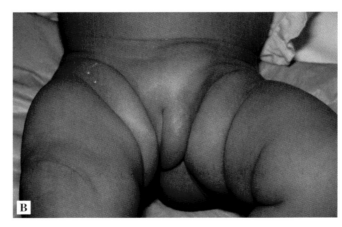

FIGURE 14.77 ■ Inguinal Hernia. Right inguinal hernia in a male infant (**A**). Left inguinal hernia in a female infant (**B**). (Photo contributor: Lawrence B. Stack, MD.)

consists of gentle traction inferiorly on the hernia sac with some pressure from above to straighten the inguinal canal. The contents of the sac can be completely reduced approximately 80% of the time. There is a high rate of early recurrence of incarceration. Admission to the hospital with repair in 24 to 48 hours after the associated edema has subsided is advisable. Immediate operative repair is indicated for any incarcerated hernia that can not be manually reduced.

Pearls

1. Transillumination of the scrotum using an otoscope or pen light may aid in differentiation of hernia and hydrocele. Hydroceles will transilluminate whereas hernias will not.
2. The Trendelenburg position may aid in hernia reduction.
3. Palpate both testicles in the scrotum prior to diagnosing an inguinal hernia.

Clinical Summary

Enterobius vermicularis is a threadlike white worm that infects the colon and causes intense pruritus of the perianal region, where the gravid adult female migrates to deposit eggs at night. Female worms measure 8 to 13 mm in length and can be observed moving about the perianal area at night. On rare occasions this nematode can lead to vulvovaginitis. The diagnosis can be made by direct visualization of the nematode by the parents or by using a piece of transparent adhesive tape and touching it to the perianal area upon awakening in the morning. This tape is then applied to a glass slide for microscopic examination under low power to look for eggs. The differential diagnosis includes perianal irritation, cellulitis, fissures, hemorrhoids, and contact dermatitis.

Emergency Department Treatment and Disposition

The treatment of choice is mebendazole (100 mg regardless of weight) or pyrantel pamoate (11 mg/kg to a maximum of 1 g).

Either of these drugs is given as a single dose and repeated in 2 weeks to treat secondary hatchings of the organism. Because of the high frequency of reinfection, families should be treated as a group.

Pearls

1. Reinfection from other infected individuals (daycare cohorts) or autoinfection is necessary to maintain enterobiasis in the individual, since these nematodes usually die after depositing their eggs in the perianal region. Frequent hand washing may reduce chances of infection as transmission occurs by the fecal-oral route.

2. Enterobius vermicularis is the most common intestinal nematode in the United States, affecting 5% to 15% of the population. Many infections are asymptomatic.

3. Suspect pinworm infection in children who present with nocturnal restlessness. These patients are often evaluated for urinary tract infection because the scratching of the perineal area is misinterpreted by the parents and treating clinicians as painful urination.

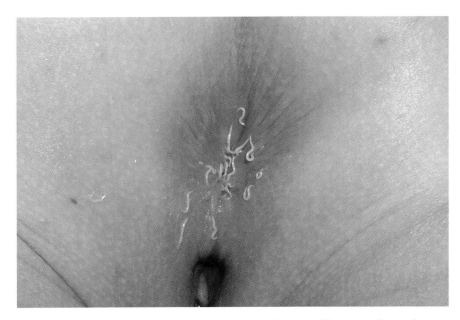

FIGURE 14.78 ■ Pinworms. Multiple tiny pearly-white worms are seen at the anus. (Photo contributor: Lawrence E. Heiskell, MD.)

Clinical Summary

Oculogyric crisis (OGC) is the most common of the ocular dystonic reactions. It includes blepharospasm, periorbital twitches, and protracted staring episodes. Usually it occurs as a side effect of neuroleptic drug treatment. OGC represents approximately 5% of the dystonic reactions. The onset of a crisis may be paroxysmal or stuttering over several hours. Initial symptoms include restlessness, agitation, malaise, or a fixed stare followed by the more characteristically described maximal upward deviation of the eyes bilaterally in a sustained fashion. The eyes may also converge, deviate upward and laterally, or deviate downward. The most frequently reported associated findings are backward and lateral flexion of the neck, widely opened mouth, tongue protrusion, and ocular pain. A wave of exhaustion follows some episodes. Other features noted during attacks include eye blinking, lacrimation, pupil dilation, drooling, facial flushing, vertigo, anxiety, and agitation. Several medications have been associated with the occurrence of OGC: cetirizine, neuroleptics, amantadine, benzodiazepines, carbamazepine, chloroquine, levodopa, lithium, metoclopramide, and nifedipine. Careful history and physical examination should exclude the possibility of focal seizures, meningitis, encephalitis, head injury, conversion reaction, and other types of movement disorders.

Emergency Department Treatment and Disposition

Treatment in the acute phase in children involves reassurance, discontinuation of the causative agent, and diphenhydramine at a dosage of 1.25 mg/kg initially; this may be repeated if there is no effect. For moderate to severe cases, give the initial dose parenterally. Occasionally, doses up to 5 mg/kg are required. The treatment with diphenhydramine should be continued every 6 hours for 1 to 2 days. Benztropine can also be used; however, benztropine is not approved for children below 3 years of age, and this agent has been noted to cause dystonic reactions. Close monitoring of patients with these drug side effects is important during treatment and for a few hours thereafter, because dystonic reactions are occasionally accompanied by fluctuations in blood pressure and disturbances of cardiac rhythm.

Pearls

1. The abrupt termination of the symptoms at the conclusion of the crisis, after the use of diphenhydramine, is diagnostic and most striking.
2. In infants presenting with "seizures," unusual behavior, eye deviation, and a history of reflux treated with metoclopramide, the possibility of OGC should be considered. Although the overall incidence of extrapyramidal effects associated with metoclopramide is 0.2%, pediatric and geriatric patients are affected more commonly, with an incidence as high as 10%. These side effects usually occur within a few days of initiation of the medication and are more common at higher doses.

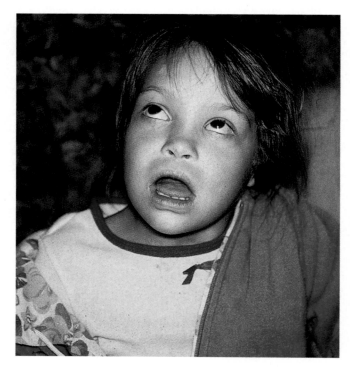

FIGURE 14.79 ■ Oculogyric Crisis. This 6-year-old boy developed extrapyramidal symptoms, including opisthotonos and oculogyric crisis, after his dosage of risperidone was increased. Benadryl 12.5 mg PO given at home resolved the opisthotonos. Persistent oculogyric crisis (upward gaze deviation) and hypertonia resolved completely after Benadryl 25 mg IM. (Photo contributor: Mark Ralston, MD.)

KAWASAKI DISEASE

Clinical Summary

Kawasaki disease (KD), also known as mucocutaneous lymph node syndrome, is an acute self-limited vasculitis of unknown etiology occurring most commonly in young children with a peak incidence between 1 and 2 years of age. The classic diagnosis is made clinically and is based on the presence of greater than or equal to 5 days of fever and greater than or equal to four of the five principal clinical features (fever, generalized erythematous maculopapular rash, bilateral nonexudative conjunctivitis, erythema of the lips and oral mucosa, changes in the distal extremities, and cervical lymphadenopathy). The fever is typically spiking and remittent with peak temperatures often greater than 40°C (104°F). Changes in the extremities are distinctive. Erythema and induration of the palms and soles occurs acutely followed in 2 to 3 weeks by desquamation of the fingers and toes beginning in the periungual region. One to two months after the onset of the fever, deep transverse grooves across the nails (Beau lines) may appear. The rash usually appears within 5 days of the onset of fever and most commonly is a nonspecific, diffuse maculopapular eruption. Early desquamation may occur in the perineal region, especially in infants. Conjunctival injection involves the bulbar conjunctivae, spares the limbus, and is not associated with an exudate. Changes of the lips and oral cavity include dry, red, cracked lips, strawberry tongue, and diffuse erythema of the oropharyngeal mucosa. Cervical lymphadenopathy is usually unilateral, confined to the anterior cervical triangle, and is greater than or equal to 1.5 cm in diameter. Incomplete KD (ie, does not meet all of the classic criteria) may be diagnosed based on fever for greater than or equal to 5 days, two or three clinical criteria, associated elevation of ESR ($\geq$40 mm/h) or CRP ($\geq$3 mg/dL), and greater than or equal to three supplemental laboratory criteria (albumin $\leq$3 g/dL, anemia for age, elevation of alanine aminotransferase, platelet count after 7 days $\geq$450,000/mm^3, white blood cell count $\geq$15,000/mm^3, and urine $\geq$10 white blood cells/high-power field). Incomplete KD is more common in infants. Coronary artery aneurysms or ectasia develop in 15% to 25% of untreated children with KD and may lead to ischemic heart disease, myocardial infarction, or sudden death. KD is a generalized vasculitis and may cause aseptic meningitis, urethritis, myocarditis, arthritis, liver dysfunction, abdominal pain, and gallbladder hydrops.

The differential diagnosis of KD includes scarlet fever, staphylococcal scalded skin syndrome, toxic shock syndrome, viral infections (measles, adenovirus, enterovirus, Epstein-Barr virus), bacterial cervical lymphadenitis, drug hypersensitivity reaction, Stevens-Johnson syndrome, and acrodynia.

Emergency Department Treatment and Disposition

If suspected, consultation with a cardiologist or other specialist in Kawasaki disease is highly recommended for confirmation of diagnosis as well as treatment alternatives. A baseline echocardiogram should be obtained to document the status of the coronary arteries. Treatment includes hospitalization, administration of IVIG 2 g/kg infused over 8 to 10 hours, and initiation of high-dose aspirin 80 to 100 mg/kg/day in four divided doses. Approximately 90% of patients will defervesce with this regimen. Failure to respond is usually defined as persistent or recurrent fever greater than or equal to 36 hours after completion of the initial IVIG infusion. Retreatment with IVIG 2 g/kg is recommended. With IVIG treatment in the acute phase of the disease, the risk of coronary artery abnormalities is decreased to less than 5%.

Pearls

1. Children with Kawasaki disease are commonly irritable and difficult to console.
2. Kawasaki disease is the leading cause of acquired heart disease in children in the United States. Echocardiography should be considered in any infant less than 6 months of age with fever of greater than or equal to 7 days duration, laboratory evidence of inflammation, and no other explanation for the febrile illness.
3. Even when treated with high-dose IVIG regimens within the first 10 days of illness, approximately 5% of children with Kawasaki disease develop at least transient coronary artery dilation.
4. Annual vaccination against influenza should be provided to all patients receiving aspirin therapy to avoid Reye syndrome.

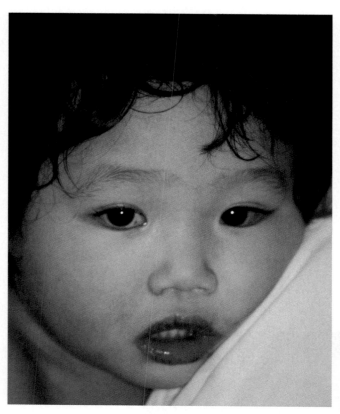

FIGURE 14.80 ■ Kawasaki Disease. Irritability in an infant with Kawasaki disease. Note also the conjunctivitis, and red, cracked lips. (Courtesy of Tomisaku Kawasaki, MD.)

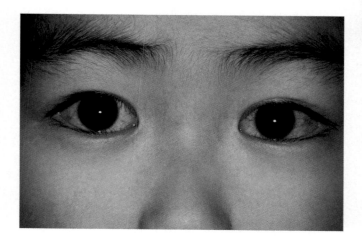

FIGURE 14.81 ■ Conjunctivitis. Note the intense redness of the bulbar conjunctiva seen in this patient with Kawasaki disease. (Courtesy of Tomisaku Kawasaki, MD.)

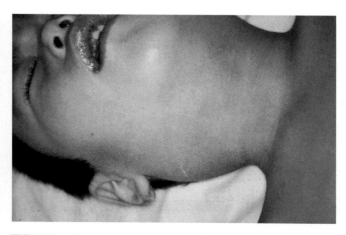

FIGURE 14.82 ■ Lymphadenopathy. Visible cervical lymphadenopathy is seen in this child with Kawasaki disease. (Courtesy of Tomisaku Kawasaki, MD.)

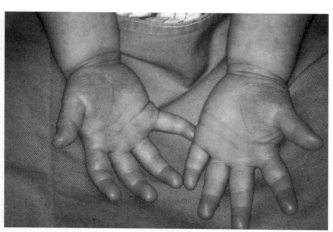

FIGURE 14.83 ■ Extremity Findings. Red swollen hands are present in this patient with Kawasaki disease. (Courtesy of Tomisaku Kawasaki, MD.)

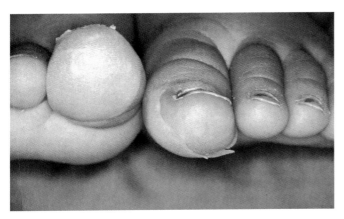

FIGURE 14.84 ■ Periungual Desquamation. This finding typically begins 2 to 3 weeks after the onset of Kawasaki disease, in contrast to perineal desquamation that occurs during the early course of the disease in infants. (Courtesy of Tomisaku Kawasaki, MD.)

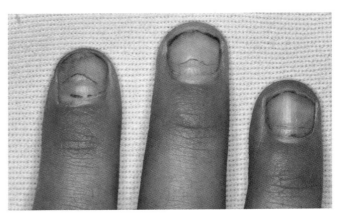

FIGURE 14.85 ■ Beau Lines. Deep transverse grooves across the nails may appear 1 to 2 months after the onset of fever. (Courtesy of Tomisaku Kawasaki, MD.)

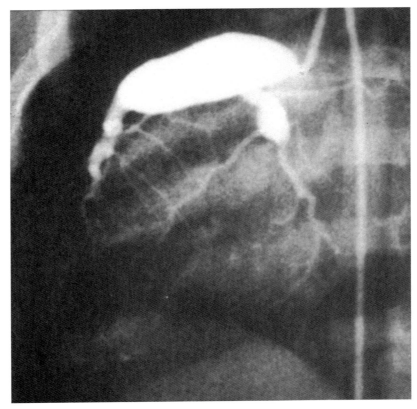

FIGURE 14.86 ■ Coronary Artery Aneurysms. A large coronary artery aneurysm is seen in this patient with Kawasaki disease. (Courtesy of Tomisaku Kawasaki, MD.)

Chapter 15

CHILD ABUSE

Robert A. Shapiro
Charles J. Schubert
Kathi L. Makoroff
Megan L. McGraw

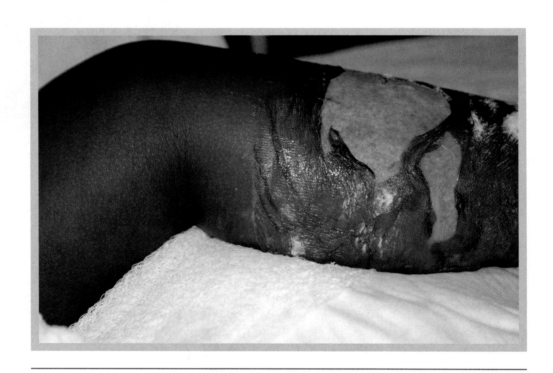

Clinical Summary

Burns in children are frequently the result of child abuse. The most common types of pediatric burns from abuse are immersion burns and contact burns. Certain clues may assist the physician in differentiating accidental burns from inflicted burns, but often considerable doubt remains even after a careful evaluation.

In an *immersion burn*, a child is held firmly and deliberately immersed and will have burn margins that are sharp and distinct. If the child has little opportunity to struggle, few or no burns from splashing liquid will occur. In contrast, a child who accidentally comes into contact with a hot liquid will move about in an attempt to escape further injury. This movement causes the burn margins to be less distinct and may result in additional small burns as hot liquid splashes onto the skin. Children who are "dipped" into a bath of hot water often show sparing of their feet and/or buttocks because they are held firmly against the tub's relatively cooler porcelain bottom. A child who has had a hand dipped into hot water and held there may reflexively close the fingers, sparing the palm and fingertips.

Contact burns usually have a distinct and recognizable shape. Contact burn patterns most commonly associated with abuse include burns from curling irons, hair dryers, heater elements, and cigarettes. A child who has multiple contact burns or burns to areas that are unlikely to come in contact with the hot object accidentally should be evaluated for abuse.

Emergency Department Treatment and Disposition

Document thoroughly all burns that may be due to abuse. Draw sketches and take photographs of the injuries. Obtain a skeletal survey in children under the age of 2 years. Report any suspected abuse immediately to local child protective agency before discharge from the emergency department. Provide standard burn therapy.

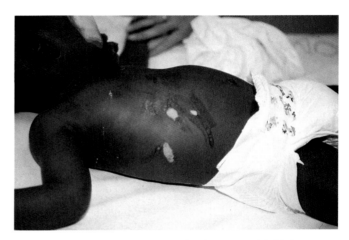

FIGURE 15.2 ■ Contact Burn (Curling Iron). Multiple contact burns on the chest and abdomen from a curling iron. Accidental curling iron burns occur, but because this infant has so many burns, the injury is suspicious for abuse and should be reported. (Photo contributor: Robert A. Shapiro, MD.)

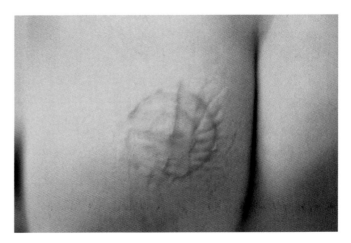

FIGURE 15.3 ■ Contact Burn (Hair Dryer). The heated grid from the end of a hair dryer caused this child's burns. The burn size and pattern marks of the burn matched exactly the hair dryer grid that was found in the child's home. (Photo contributor: Robert A. Shapiro, MD.)

FIGURE 15.1 ■ Immersion Burns. Immersion burns are often associated with toilet-training accidents. This girl was plunged into hot water after soiling herself. She shows sparing of the buttocks, which contacted the surface of the bathtub and avoided being burned. (Courtesy of *The Visual Diagnosis of Child Physical Abuse.* American Academy of Pediatrics, 1994.)

Pearls

1. If the history or developmental abilities of the child do not correlate with or explain the examination, suspect physical abuse.
2. Maintain a high index of suspicion whenever caring for a pediatric burn patient. Look carefully for other signs of abuse, such as bruising or fractures.

3. Cigarette burns may resemble impetigo from insect bites and accidental burns from a cigarette are usually single, superficial, and not completely round. Common sites of accidental cigarette burns are the face, trunk, and hands.
4. Bullous impetigo can resemble second-degree burns. Contact dermatitis and cellulitis may resemble first-degree burns.
5. Injuries due to suspected child abuse may be photographed without parental consent in most states.

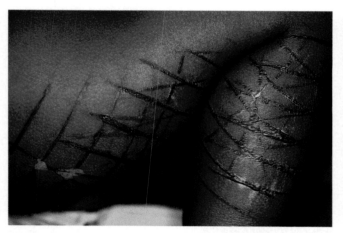

FIGURE 15.4 ■ Contact Burn (Heater Grate). This child was held against a heater grate. The pattern became more obvious with the child's knee flexed—the position of the leg at the time of the injury. (Photo contributor: David W. Munter, MD.)

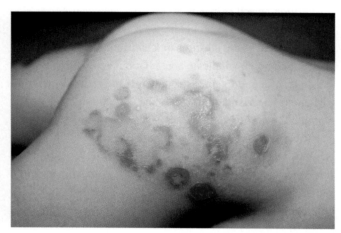

FIGURE 15.6 ■ Impetigo. These circular lesions of impetigo resemble healing cigarette burns. (Photo contributor: Michael J. Nowicki, MD.)

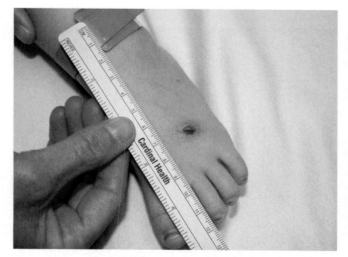

FIGURE 15.5 ■ Contact Burn (Cigarette). Cigarette burns are circular injuries with a diameter of about 8 mm. Children who accidentally run into a lit cigarette often have burns to the face or distal extremities. Accidental burns may be less distinct or deep compared with inflicted burns. (Photo contributor: Kathi L. Makoroff, MD.)

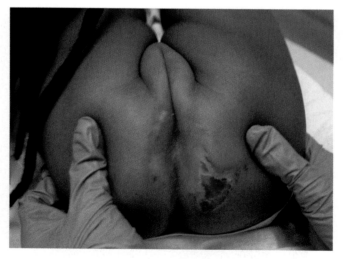

FIGURE 15.7 ■ Buttock Burn from Diarrhea. This patient was given a pediatric laxative and has a diarrheal stool following. The affected skin does not involve the area around the anus or the gluteal clefts. (Photo contributor: Cincinnati Children's Hospital Medical Center.)

Clinical Summary

Bruises are the most common manifestation of physical child abuse. Child abuse should be suspected whenever bruises are (1) over soft body areas, such as the thighs, buttocks, cheeks, abdomen, and genitalia; (2) more numerous than usual; (3) of different ages (suggests repeated episodes of abuse); (4) the shape of objects such as belts, cords, or hands (demonstrates the injuries were inflicted); or (5) noted in young, nonambulating children.

The time period over which a bruise heals can be variable and color of the bruise should not be used for dating purposes. Bite marks have special forensic characteristics. Recognition of an adult bite may indicate abuse. Compared with an adult's, the shape of a child's bite is rounder. If the impressions from the canines are visible in the bite, the perpetrator's age can be estimated. (Most children under 8 years have <3 cm between their canines.) Dried saliva within the bite can also be used to identify the perpetrator. The bites of animals are usually smaller and the shape of the arch mark is narrower than a human's. Sharp animal canines often cause tearing of the skin instead of the crushing seen in human bites.

Emergency Department Treatment and Disposition

Completely undress the child and look for additional signs of abuse. Obtain a complete history of all injuries. Sketch and photograph the injuries. Obtain a complete blood count and bleeding studies (prothrombin time and partial thromboplastin time [PT and PTT]) to rule out a bleeding diathesis as the cause of the findings. For children less than 2 or 3 years of age who have extensive injuries, obtain a skeletal survey, alanine transferase (ALT), aspartate aminotransferase (AST), amylase, and urinalysis.

If human bites are found or suspected, consider consultation with a forensic dentist. All suspected human bites should be photo documented. If indicated, collect swabs for DNA forensic analysis from the unwashed, fresh bites, which may contain saliva from the perpetrator. Run a moistened swab

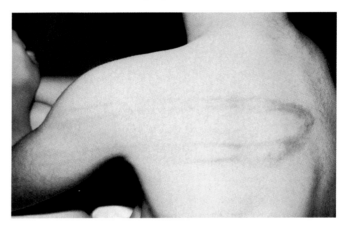

FIGURE 15.9 ■ Looped Pattern Markings. Loop marks are clearly seen within the bruising on this child's back. The loop marks indicate that an extension cord, belt, or some similar object was used to punish him. (Photo contributor: Robert A. Shapiro, MD.)

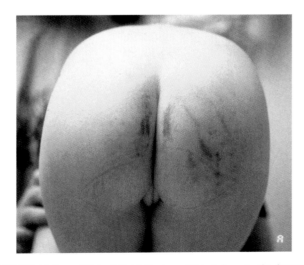

FIGURE 15.8 ■ Gluteal Fold Bruises. This injury to the buttocks demonstrates linear, parallel bruises near the gluteal folds. Forceful spanking causes gluteal fold bruises. They do not indicate a separate trauma in addition to the spanking. (Photo contributor: Charles Schubert & Robert A. Shapiro, MD.)

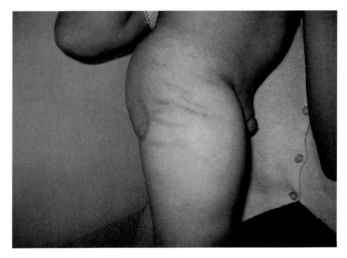

FIGURE 15.10 ■ Looped Pattern Markings. Subtle loop and linear marks are seen on the thigh and buttock of this child. (Photo contributor: Cincinnati Children's Hospital Medical Center.)

followed by a dry swab over the bite and clearly document the chain of evidence.

Report suspected abuse to the legally mandated child protection agency before the child is discharged from the emergency department.

Pearls

1. Determination of the age of a bruise is imprecise. Bruises that are "fresh" (<48 hours) are usually recognizable because they are tender, red, and swollen. Occasionally, bruises may not be visible for up to 48 hours after an injury.
2. Children may deny abuse when questioned because of threats made to them. The child in Fig. 15.20 initially denied that he had been gagged. He told the examining physician that he had spilled some cleaning fluid onto his lips.
3. When a parent or caretaker inflicts an injury while disciplining a child, the incident must be reported to the local child protection agency. Even if corporal punishment is lawful in a given state, the infliction of an injury is never lawful.

4. Place a millimeter ruler or coin next to a pattern injury before taking photographs so that measurements can be made.
5. Consent is not required in most states to photograph injuries suspicious for child abuse.
6. Bleeding disorders—such as idiopathic thrombocytopenic purpura (ITP), Henoch-Schönlein purpura, and leukemia can mimic child abuse.
7. Folk remedies, such as cupping and coining, may result in soft tissue findings that are not reportable as abuse.
8. Bruises on the pinna of the ear are highly concerning for physical abuse.

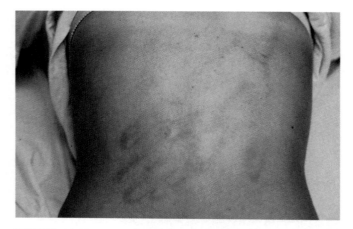

FIGURE 15.12 ■ Hand-Print Bruise. Bruise from a slap showing the outline of her father's hand is clearly seen on the back of this adolescent. (Photo contributor: Robert A. Shapiro, MD.)

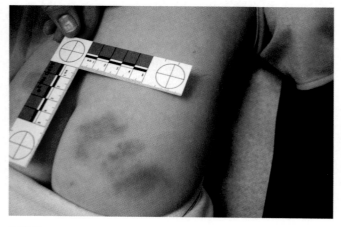

FIGURE 15.13 ■ Linear Bruises. These linear, parallel bruises on the buttocks with unaffected skin between them are indicative of an injury caused by an object. Common objects that cause injuries like these include belts, fingers, cords, and rulers. (Photo contributor: Kathi L. Makoroff, MD.)

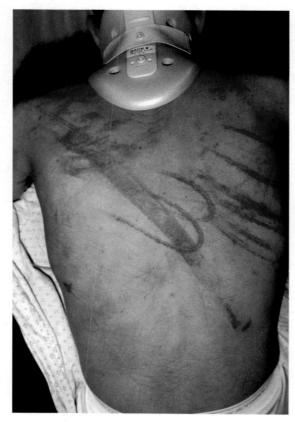

FIGURE 15.11 ■ Looped Pattern Markings. Loop and linear marks are seen on the back of this child. (Photo contributor: Alan B. Storrow, MD.)

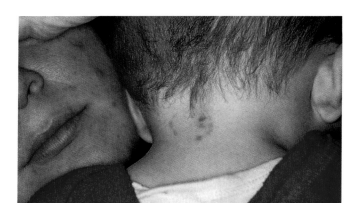

FIGURE 15.14 ■ Bite Mark (Child). Distinct impressions of teeth are seen in this injury with the outlines of the upper and lower oral arches. Note the size of the mother's mouth in relation to the size of the bite on the neck, making an adult an unlikely source. (Photo contributor: Kevin J. Knoop, MD, MS.)

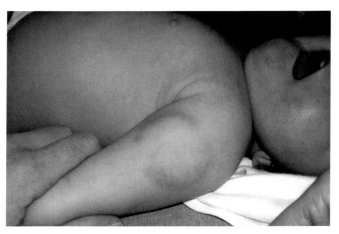

FIGURE 15.16 ■ Bite Mark (Adult). This bite mark on this child's arm is more consistent with an adult bite. (Photo contributor: Megan McGraw, MD.)

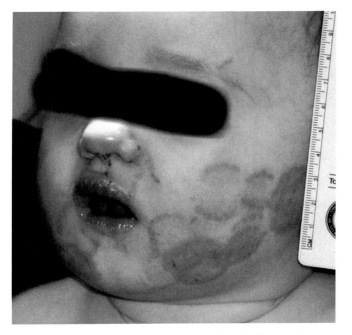

FIGURE 15.15 ■ Bite Mark (Child). Multiple bite marks were inflicted on this child's face by another child. (Photo contributor: Cincinnati Children's Hospital Medical Center.)

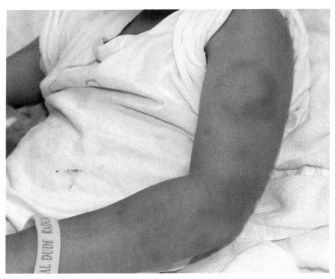

FIGURE 15.17 ■ Bruises. Bruises cover this child's left arm. The circular bruise on the upper arm is a human bite. Saliva from the perpetrator may be present within the bite and sampled for DNA analysis. (Photo contributor: Robert A. Shapiro, MD.)

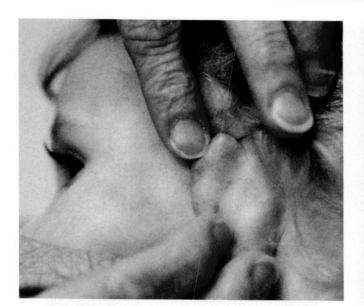

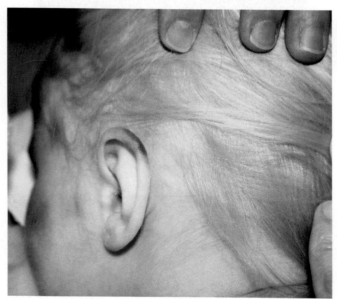

FIGURE 15.18 ■ Pinch Marks on Pinna. Children may be pulled up or along by their ears, causing this injury. A child's ears should be inspected for this injury whenever abuse is suspected. (Photo contributors: Robert A. Shapiro, MD and Kathi L. Makoroff, MD.)

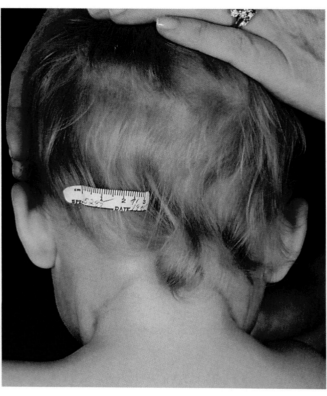

FIGURE 15.19 ■ Strangulation Bruise. This child was beaten while at the sitter's and suffered circumferential linear neck abrasions consistent with attempted strangulation. There is also occipital ecchymosis from the abuse. (Photo contributor: Barbara R. Craig, MD.)

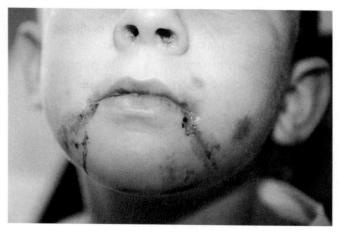

FIGURE 15.20 ■ Gagging Bruise. This child had a sock stuffed into his mouth and tied around his head. The bruises in the corners of the child's mouth are indicative of gagging. Additionally, there are circular bruises on his left and right cheeks caused from the perpetrator's fingers while holding the child still to insert the sock. Pattern markings within the bruises match the fabric pattern of the sock. (Photo contributor: Robert A. Shapiro, MD.)

Clinical Summary

Whenever bruising is excessive, is not associated with a compatible history, or occurs in an unusual distribution, seek a specific etiology. It may be appropriate to suspect and report child abuse when these conditions exist but also consider other diagnoses. It is important to consider other diagnoses when considering injuries potentially caused from abuse.

Common Childhood Bruising

Accidental trauma in ambulatory children is most likely to occur on the forehead and the extensor surfaces of the tibia, elbow, and knee.

Mongolian Spots

Mongolian spots or congenital dermal melanocytosis are bluish sacral or truncal lesions, most often seen in non-Caucasian infants and young children. Mongolian spots may be limited to only a few lesions, or may extend up the back and shoulders.

Cupping, Coining, and Moxibustion

Families sometimes practice traditional folk remedies with their children, such as cupping, coining, and moxibustion. Each of these practices leaves markings on the child's skin, which may be interpreted as child abuse. In cupping, a flammable object is ignited and placed into a cup. After the flames have extinguished, the cup is inverted and placed onto the child's skin. As the warm air within the cup cools, a vacuum is produced. This remedy leaves circular suction markings. Coining is done by rubbing a coin up and down the child's back, just lateral to the spine. This results in petechiae and chronic skin changes on the back. Coining and cupping should not be painful to the child and neither should be reported as child abuse. In moxibustion, a flammable object, such as a thread, is ignited on or near the child's skin. Moxibustion may cause superficial burns. Whether moxibustion is reported as child abuse would depend on the physical findings and the judgment of the physician.

Henoch-Schönlein Purpura

Henoch-Schönlein purpura (HSP) is a vasculitis of the small blood vessels. The skin lesions are usually small, symmetric, palpable purpuras. They may appear in a linear pattern and are often confined to the lower extremities. Associated symptoms may include joint and abdominal pain.

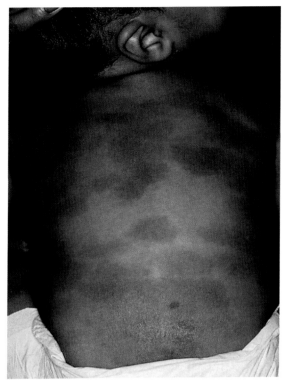

FIGURE 15.21 ■ Mongolian Spots. Numerous congenital dermal melanocytosis or mongolian spots on this youngster extend up the back and shoulders. (Photo contributor: Douglas R. Landry, MD.)

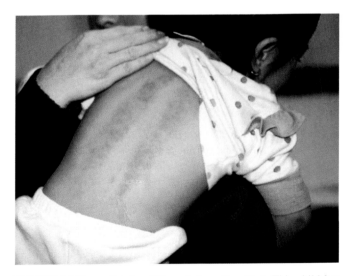

FIGURE 15.22 ■ Coining (Cheut Sah or Cao Gio). This child has petechiae and bruising along her spine. Her parents were practicing the Southeast Asian practice of coining, a healing remedy, in which a coin is rubbed along the spine to heal an illness. (Photo contributor: Charles Schubert, MD.)

Idiopathic Thrombocytopenic Purpura

Idiopathic thrombocytopenic purpura (ITP) is an acquired platelet disorder that results in abnormal bleeding. It is most common in 1- to 4-year-old children. The presenting complaint is most often abnormal bruising. The bruises can appear anywhere on the body and are numerous, mimicking child abuse. The child may also have epistaxis, hematuria, or other bleeding.

Hemophilia

Hemophilia is usually diagnosed soon after birth because of abnormal bleeding. Ecchymoses and soft-tissue swelling are greater than would be expected, given the history of trauma.

Emergency Department Treatment and Disposition

A hematologist should be consulted for children with platelet disorders and coagulopathies. HSP requires supportive care and close follow-up. The most serious complication of HSP is bowel obstruction from intussusception.

Pearls

1. Mongolian spots can exist anywhere on the body and occasionally appear in Caucasian children. They are noted first in the newborn period.
2. Consider HSP in school-age children with purpura of the lower extremities.
3. Consider ITP in preschool children who have multiple ecchymosis and petechiae without other signs or indications of abuse.
4. Vitamin K deficiency is a cause of bleeding in infancy.
5. Trauma to the forehead may cause bilateral eye ecchymosis within a few days and can be mistaken for eye trauma.

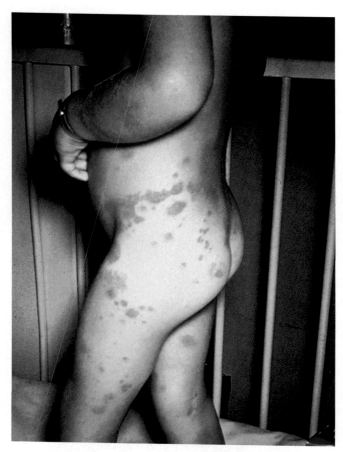

FIGURE 15.23 ▪ Henoch-Schönlein Purpura (HSP). This child has palpable purpura on the extensor surfaces of the legs. HSP should be considered whenever there is symmetric ecchymosis along the extensor surfaces of the extremities and buttocks. Migratory arthritis and abdominal pain may be present. (Photo contributor: Ralph A. Gruppo, MD.)

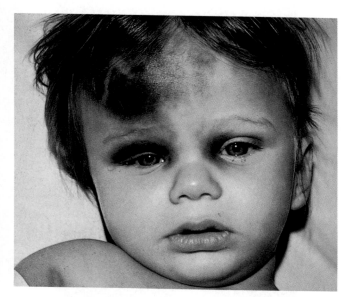

FIGURE 15.24 ▪ Hemophiliac with Bruising. This child's bruising is due to factor VIII deficiency. The degree of bleeding within the ecchymosis is more extensive than that seen in children without coagulopathies. (Photo contributor: Ralph A. Gruppo, MD.)

Clinical Summary

Certain fractures should always raise a suspicion of child abuse: metaphyseal corner fractures, posterior rib fractures, scapular fractures, fractures in a nonambulating child, and untreated healing fractures. Fractures incompatible with the history and those for which no explanation is available are also suspicious of child abuse.

Normal pediatric radiographic variants, periosteal changes caused by conditions other than healing fractures, and illnesses that cause fragile bones may all be mistaken for fractures due to child abuse. A pediatric radiologist should be consulted if any doubt exists about the radiographic interpretation. Specific disorders that can be mistaken for child abuse include osteogenesis imperfecta, copper deficiency, osteopetrosis, rickets, scurvy, hypervitaminosis A, osteomyelitis, severe prematurity, tumors, leukemia, prostaglandin E overdose, and infantile cortical hyperostosis (also known as Caffey disease).

Conditions that cause bone fragility must be considered when unexpected fractures are discovered, even though such cases are rare. The most frequently discussed bone fragility disorder is osteogenesis imperfecta (OI), a rare inherited connective-tissue disorder. Associated features seen in some children with OI include blue sclerae, wormian bones (seen on the skull x-ray), and osteopenia. A family history of bone fragility, hearing loss, and short stature is often present. In rare instances, children with OI lack these associated features.

Emergency Department Treatment and Disposition

If abuse is suspected in a child under 2 or 3 years of age, obtain a skeletal survey. The skeletal survey should include a minimum of 19 films, including frontal views of the appendicular skeleton and frontal and lateral views of the axial skeleton.

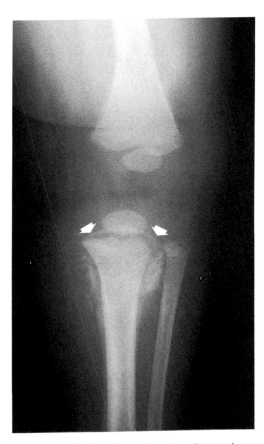

FIGURE 15.25 ■ Healing Corner Fracture. Impressive periosteal elevation, causing the bucket-handle appearance in this metaphyseal fracture. This fracture is most often seen as the result of shaking or pulling. (Photo contributor: Alan E. Oestreich, MD.)

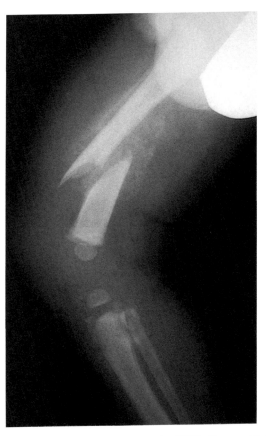

FIGURE 15.26 ■ Spiral Femur and Proximal Tibia Fracture. Note displaced spiral femur fracture with faint callus formation and more solid (older) periosteal reaction of the proximal tibia. Child abuse is likely because there are two injuries which occurred at different times and no treatment was obtained. (Photo contributor: Alan E. Oestreich, MD.)

Coned down views over a joint may be needed for best visualization of metaphyseal injuries. Oblique views are useful for hand, rib, and nondisplaced lone bone-shaft fractures. All images obtained (including those of the chest) should use bone technique. Ideally, all studies should be read by a radiologist while the patient is still in the emergency department. Consider computed tomography or magnetic resonance imaging of the head in infants with skull fractures when abuse is suspected. Suspected abuse must be reported immediately to the appropriate child protection agency. Fractures should be managed appropriately.

Pearls

1. Suspect abuse when a child has multiple fractures, fractures of different ages, unsuspected (occult) fractures, or fractures without a consistent trauma history.
2. Accidental trauma that includes rotational forces can result in a spiral fracture (eg, spiral femur fractures in young ambulatory children).
3. Obtain a skeletal survey in any child under 2 years of age who has any injuries suspicious of abuse.
4. Radiographic signs of healing are typically first seen 10 days after a fracture.
5. Fractures that are not immobilized have a larger callus than immobilized fractures.

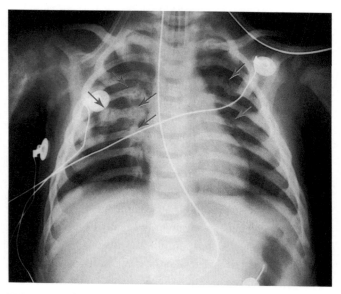

FIGURE 15.28 ■ Multiple Healing Rib Fractures. There are healing rib fractures of the right posterior fifth, sixth, and seventh ribs, the right lateral sixth rib, and the left posterior fourth rib. The surrounding callus indicates the fractures are older than 10 days. An acute fracture is seen on the left posterior sixth rib. (Photo contributor: Alan E. Oestreich, MD.)

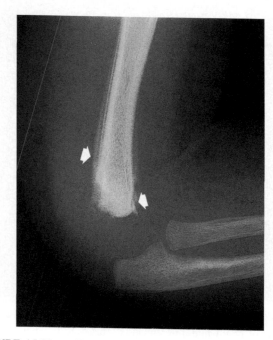

FIGURE 15.27 ■ Healing Fracture of the Distal Humerus. The periosteal reaction along the distal humerus dates this fracture older than 10 days. No treatment was obtained for the acute injury. (Photo contributor: Alan E. Oestreich, MD.)

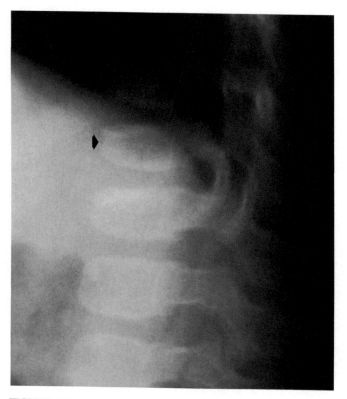

FIGURE 15.29 ■ Compression Fracture. The wedging of T-12 (*arrow*) and probably L-1 indicates vertebral compression fractures. These fractures are the result of significant forces applied to the spinal column and are often indicative of child abuse. (Photo contributor: Alan E. Oestreich, MD.)

Clinical Summary

Infants and children who are violently shaken may suffer inflicted head injury, commonly referred to as "shaken baby syndrome." Typically, the infant is held by the chest and violently shaken back and forth. This shaking results in intracranial hemorrhages, most commonly subdural and subarachnoid hemorrhages. Cerebral edema and cerebral contusions can also be seen. There are often no external signs of trauma, although infants and children who are shaken may also have fractures, abdominal trauma, bruises, and other injuries. Neurologic symptoms such as vomiting, apnea, seizures, irritability, or altered mental status are commonly seen but may be absent. Retinal hemorrhages are seen in 80% of shaken babies. The hemorrhages may be unilateral or bilateral. Inflicted head injury should be strongly considered when retinal hemorrhages are found in any child less than 2 years of age.

Emergency Department Treatment and Disposition

CT or MRI of the head should be obtained and the patient treated in the usual fashion. A report of suspected child abuse must be made to the child protective agency. A skeletal survey should also be obtained and other injuries noted. An ophthalmologist should document and follow the patient's retinal injuries.

Pearls

1. Child abuse should be suspected in any nonambulatory infant with facial bruising.
2. Infants and children with inflicted head injury may have no external signs of trauma and minimal neurologic deficits.
3. Retinal hemorrhages from CPR and mechanisms other than major trauma (birth, severe hypertension, coagulopathies, sepsis, simple falls) are typically less extensive than those seen with inflicted head injury.
4. A history indicating that a short fall caused the intracranial injury should be highly suspected.

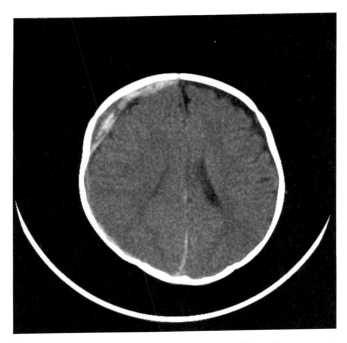

FIGURE 15.30 ■ Acute Subdural Hematoma. There is a crescent-shaped, hyperdense collection, indicating an acute subdural hematoma over the right cerebral hemisphere. In addition, the right side of the brain demonstrates mass effect. (Photo contributor: Cincinnati Children's Hospital Medical Center.)

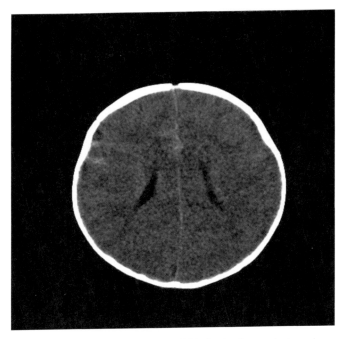

FIGURE 15.31 ■ Brain Edema. This brain demonstrates edema and loss of gray-white differentiation. These are findings that can be seen in children with inflicted head injury. (Photo contributor: Cincinnati Children's Hospital Medical Center.)

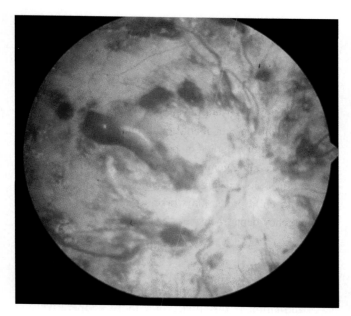

FIGURE 15.32 ■ Retinal Hemorrhages. Multiple retinal hemorrhages are present. (Photo contributor: Rees W. Shepherd, MD.)

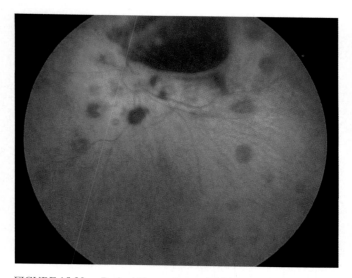

FIGURE 15.33 ■ Retinal Hemorrhages. Multiple discreet subhyaloid hemorrhages are seen. (Photo contributor: John D. Baker, MD and Massie Research Laboratories, Inc.)

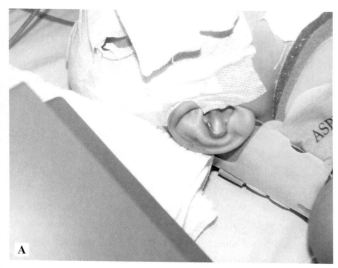

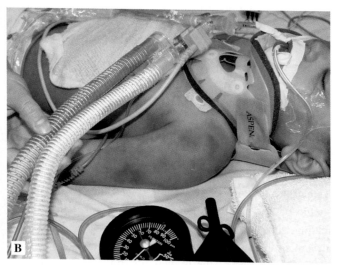

FIGURE 15.34 ■ Inflicted Head Injury. This child was a victim of inflicted head injury. Unlike most victims of inflicted head injury, he also has signs of cutaneous injury. Bruises on his right pinna (**A**) and left upper arm (**B**) were noted on examination. (Photo contributor: Robert A. Shapiro, MD.)

Clinical Summary

Child sexual abuse is a not uncommon presenting complaint to the emergency department. The child's interview is best left to abuse professionals. The emergency department physician must recognize and document injuries from abuse and treat medical sequela.

The genital examination of prepubertal girls is usually limited to inspection of the external genitalia and hymen for injury and infection. An internal inspection is rarely required. Children should first be examined in the "frog-leg" position. The child can lie on the examination table or sit on a parent's lap, whichever makes her most comfortable. Position the patient in a supine position with her knees flexed and out. The soles of her feet should be opposed. Alternatively, the child can be placed in a knee-chest position. The knee-chest position is particularly useful to visualize vaginal foreign bodies as well as the posterior hymeneal rim.

First, examine the perineum for trauma, condylomata, herpetic lesions, or discharge. Next examine the hymen. To visualize the hymen, hold the labia majora between the thumb and index fingers of each hand. Apply lateral and posterior traction to the labia while pulling them outward. When done properly, this procedure is not painful and provides excellent visualization of the hymen. If the hymen cannot be visualized in the supine frog-leg position, the knee-chest position should be attempted. Examine the hymen for indications of trauma, such as swelling, ecchymoses, or tears. In pubertal girls, a cotton swab or Foley catheter can help the examiner inspect the edges of the hymen for injury. The redundant hymeneal edges can often be spread with a cotton swab providing the necessary visualization. If needed, a deflated Foley catheter can be inserted into the vagina and inflated with 10 mL of air. Gentle traction can then be placed on the catheter by pulling until the balloon spreads the hymeneal edges. By moving the inflated balloon from side to side, different sections of the hymen can be exposed.

Emergency Department Treatment and Disposition

If sexual abuse is suspected, a report of alleged sexual abuse must be made to the child protective agency and police. Concerning or abnormal examination findings should be photo documented and the child referred for a definitive examination by a child abuse expert. Forensic evidence must be collected if semen, blood, saliva, hair, or skin of the alleged perpetrator may be on the child's clothing or body. This is usually reserved for sexual assault within the past 72 hours but local practice may differ. Screening tests for sexually transmitted infections should be considered but presumptive STD treatment should be withheld in the prepubertal child unless medically necessary. Confirmatory studies of positive screening tests will be indicated, ascending genital infection is rare and the incidence of infection is low in prepubertal girls. Confirm the child's safety with child protection workers prior to discharge from the emergency department.

Pearls

1. Allow the child to sit on her mother's lap during the examination if this makes her more cooperative and less fearful.

2. Speculum examinations are rarely indicated in prepubertal girls and are reserved for removal of an intravaginal foreign body or evaluation of intravaginal trauma. General anesthesia is usually indicated before inserting a speculum into a prepubertal child.

3. Apply caudal traction to the labia during examination to prevent a superficial tear of the posterior fourchette.

4. If a portion of the hymen cannot be visualized because it is adherent to the adjacent labia or to itself, gently touch the adherent tissue with the contralateral labia to pull it free. A drop of saline placed onto the posterior hymen may also separate adherent tissues without causing discomfort to the child. The prepubertal hymen is very sensitive to touch—do not use a cotton swabs or attempt manual manipulation.

5. The inner hymeneal ring is usually smooth and uninterrupted. Notches at 3 and 9 o'clock are normal. Minor irregularities are likely to be insignificant.

6. The shape and appearance of the prepubertal hymen is variable. Annular and crescentic configurations are the most common. Hymens may also be septate, imperforate, or cribriform (multiple small openings).

7. A normal examination does not exclude sexual abuse. The majority of abused prepubertal girls have normal genital examinations. Examination findings specific for sexual abuse are found in approximately 2% to 6% of girls who report abuse.

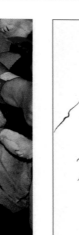

FIGURE 15.35 ■ Child Sitting in Mother's Lap for Genital Examination. This young girl is being examined while she sits on her mother's lap. Many children are most comfortable when examined while held by a parent. Her legs are in the "frog-leg" position as labial traction is applied. (Photo contributor: Cincinnati Children's Hospital Medical Center.)

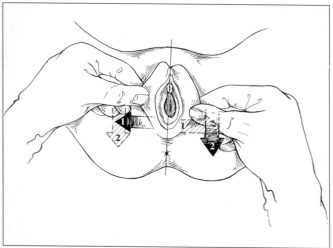

FIGURE 15.36 ■ Labial Traction Examination Technique. Position the child in a supine position with her knees out and soles together. Hymenal inspection in prepubertal girls is best accomplished when lateral (1) and posterior (2) traction to the labia is applied as shown here. (Adapted from Giandino AP, et al. *A Practical Guide to the Evaluation of Sexual Abuse in the Prepubertal Child*. Sage Publications; 1992.)

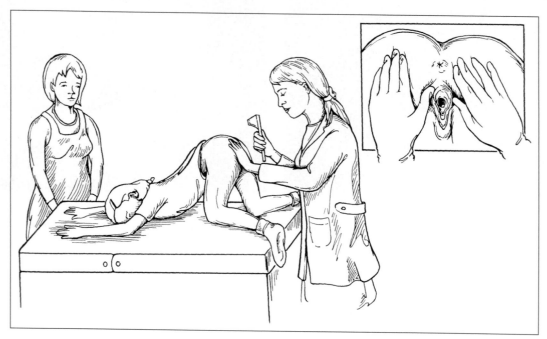

FIGURE 15.37 ■ Knee-Chest Examination Technique. This position is used to exam the posterior hymenal rim and vaginal vault. Children may feel exposed and vulnerable in this position. Position the child on her hands and knees, knees spread wider than her shoulders and chest on the examination table with a swayed backbone. (Reproduced with permission from Pearlman MD, Tintinalli JE, Dyne PL. *Obstetric & Gynecologic Emergencies: Diagnosis and Management*. New York: McGraw-Hill; 2004.)

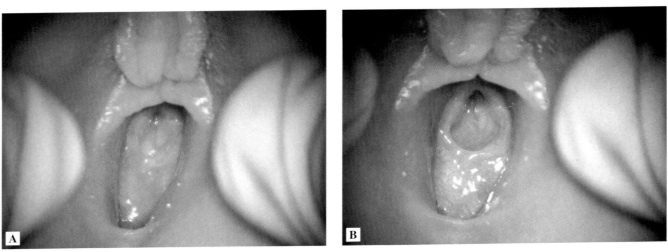

FIGURE 15.38 ■ Proper Labial Traction Allows Visualization of the Prepubertal Hymen. **(A)** Lateral labial traction only. The hymenal margins cannot be visualized. **(B)** Lateral, posterior, and caudal labial traction provides complete visualization of the hymenal rim. (Photo contributor: Cincinnati Children's Hospital Medical Center.)

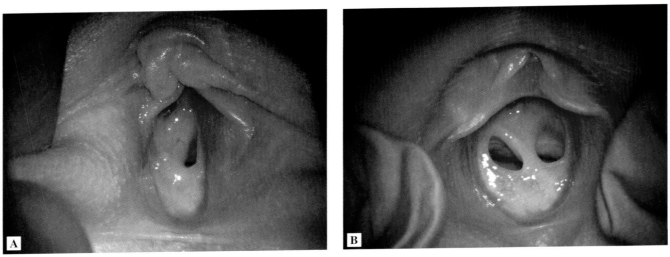

FIGURE 15.39 ■ Proper Labial Traction Allows Visualization of the Prepubertal Hymen. **(A)** The hymen is partially visible with lateral traction only. **(B)** With optimal traction, a hymenal septum is found which creates the appearance of two vaginal openings. A septum is a normal hymenal variant. See Fig 15.44—vaginal duplication. (Photo contributor: Cincinnati Children's Hospital Medical Center.)

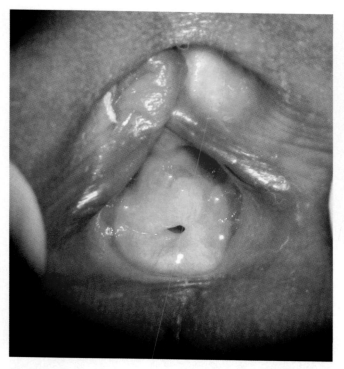

FIGURE 15.40 ■ Normal Estrogenized Newborn Hymen. Infants often have thickened annular hymens. Maternal estrogens cause this effect. Do not confuse with traumatic swelling. (Photo contributor: Cincinnati Children's Hospital Medical Center.)

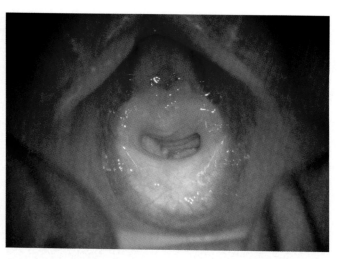

FIGURE 15.42 ■ Normal Crescentic Hymen. The hymen is crescent shaped without any defects. Hymenal tissue may be absent near the urethra between 10 and 2 o'clock. Using a "clock face" analogy, the superior portion of the hymen near the urethra is the 12 o'clock position. (Photo contributor: Cincinnati Children's Hospital Medical Center.)

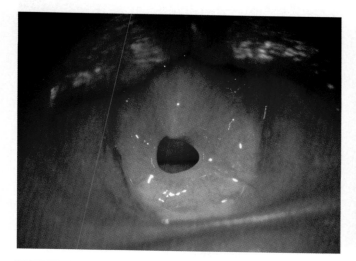

FIGURE 15.41 ■ Normal Annular Hymen. The hymen is doughnut shaped without any defects. (Photo contributor: Cincinnati Children's Hospital Medical Center.)

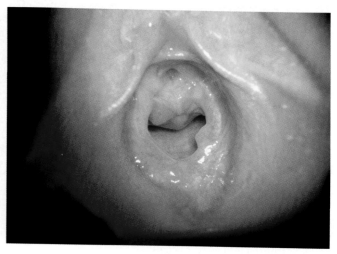

FIGURE 15.43 ■ Normal Hymenal Mound—Crescentic Hymen. The hymen is crescent shaped, tissue is absent near the urethra between 11 and 1 o'clock. A nonspecific mound of hymenal tissue is noted at 3 o'clock. (Photo contributor: Cincinnati Children's Hospital Medical Center.)

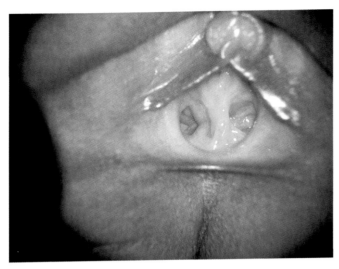

FIGURE 15.44 ■ Vaginal Duplication. The hymenal septum noted in this photograph extends into the vagina. Consider a pelvic ultrasound and referral to pediatric gynecology in patients with a thick septated hymen or septated vagina. Imaging studies in this patient demonstrated a bicornuate uterus as well. (Photo contributor: Cincinnati Children's Hospital Medical Center.)

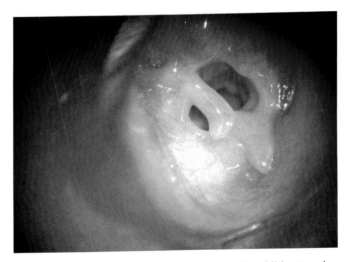

FIGURE 15.45 ■ Hymenal Tag and Septum. In addition to a hymenal septum, this examination demonstrates a redundant hymenal tag. This is not a traumatic finding. Tags and septa often resolve spontaneously during puberty. (Photo contributor: Cincinnati Children's Hospital Medical Center.)

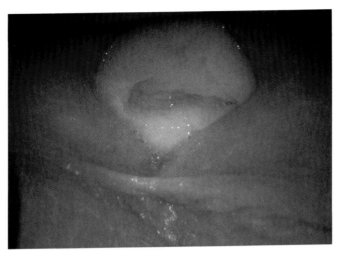

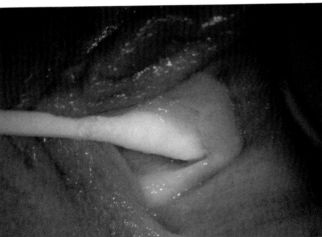

FIGURE 15.46 ■ Cotton Swab Technique to Better Visualize the Adolescent Hymen. The adolescent hymen is usually thick and redundant. A cotton swab can be used to expand redundant tissue for better visualization of possible disruptions and trauma. (Photo contributor: Cincinnati Children's Hospital Medical Center.)

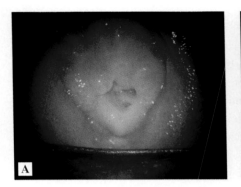
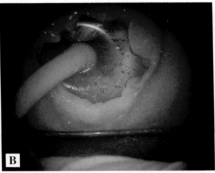
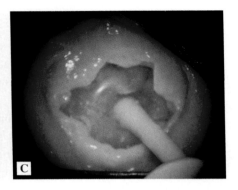

FIGURE 15.47 ■ Foley Catheter Technique to Better Visualize the Adolescent Hymen. In addition to using a cotton swab to examine a redundant hymen (**A**), a Foley catheter can be inserted into the adolescent vagina, filled with 10 cc of air and gently retracted (**B**). Side-to-side displacement of the catheter exposes different hymenal sections for inspection (**C**). (Photo contributor: Cincinnati Children's Hospital Medical Center.)

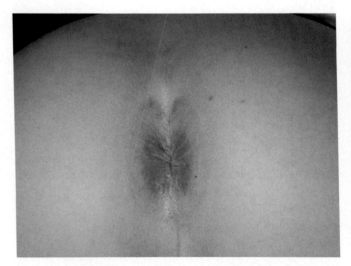

Figure 15.48 ■ Normal Anal Findings. The perianal skin often has increased pigmentation compared to the surrounding skin. Venous engorgement and skin irritation can mimic trauma. (Photo contributor: Cincinnati Children's Hospital Medical Center.)

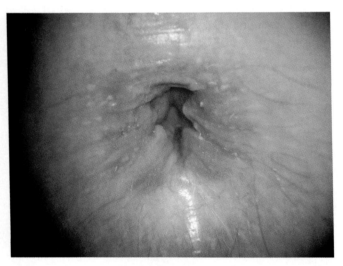

FIGURE 15.49 ■ Normal Anal Dilation and Venous Pooling. A relaxed external sphincter causes anal dilation in all children. Stool in the rectal vault contributes to dilation. Surrounding venous pooling may be mistaken for bruising. (Photo contributor: Cincinnati Children's Hospital Medical Center.)

Clinical Summary

Sexual abuse must be considered in any child with a genital or anal injury, a sexually transmitted infection, or a report of alleged abuse. Most abused children will have no examination findings that indicate abuse.

Acute injuries include lacerations, bruises, abrasions, and swelling. Most of these injuries heal quickly, often within a few days to a week. Nonacute examination findings caused by trauma are difficult to recognize and should be interpreted by a qualified child abuse expert.

Sexually transmitted infections diagnosed in a prepubertal child may indicate sexual abuse. *Neisseria gonorrhoeae, Chlamydia trachomatis, Trichomonas,* and syphilis are almost always transmitted by intimate sexual contact unless acquired perinatally. Condylomata acuminata (genital warts) and herpes simplex may be transmitted to the prepubertal child through sexual or nonsexual contact. False positive tests are not uncommon in this population with low disease prevalence.

Emergency Department Treatment and Disposition

See "The Child Sexual Abuse Examination."

Pearls

1. It is not necessary to measure the vaginal opening of prepubertal girls. The size of the introitus is dependent on examination technique, degree of patient relaxation, patient age, and other variables. There is no consensus on normal introitus size among experts.
2. Hymeneal notches at 3 and 9 o'clock can be a normal finding.
3. Changes to the posterior hymen, such as narrowing and notching, may be indicative of penetrating injury.

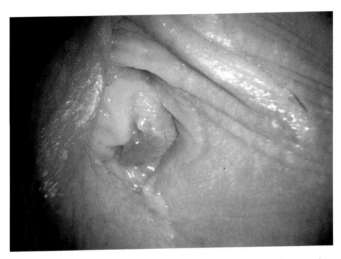

FIGURE 15.51 ■ Acute Bruise of the Hymen. The hymen has bruising from 3 o'clock to 5 o'clock after recent sexual assault. (Photo contributor: Cincinnati Children's Hospital Medical Center.)

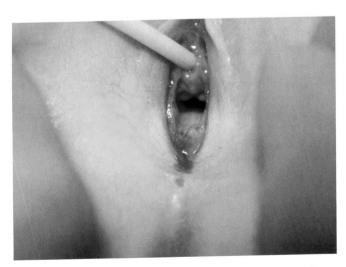

FIGURE 15.50 ■ Acute Laceration of the Hymen. An acute laceration with active bleeding is demonstrated. Injuries to the hymen are concerning for sexual abuse, and forensic specimens should be collected. (Photo contributor: Cincinnati Children's Hospital Medical Center.)

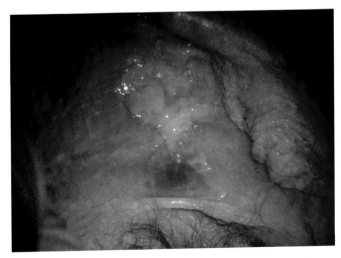

FIGURE 15.52 ■ Acute Trauma to the Posterior Fourchette. Bruising is present in the posterior fourchette after sexual assault. (Photo contributor: Cincinnati Children's Hospital Medical Center.)

4. Rectal abuse often causes no visible trauma. Consider sexual abuse if deep anal fissures are present.

5. The external anus is often darker in color than the surrounding skin and can be mistaken for erythema or bruising.

6. Condyloma lata (syphilis) can be mistaken for condylomata acuminata (warts).

7. Vaginal discharge in a prepubertal child should always be cultured for *N gonorrhoeae* and *Chlamydia*.

8. Eyelash nits are pubic lice. Sexual abuse must be considered.

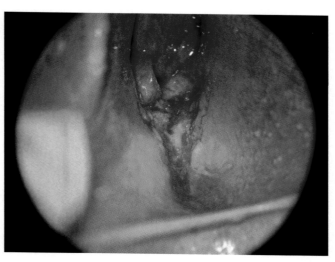

FIGURE 15.54 ▪ Deep Vaginal Tear. A laceration of the hymen is present at 6 o'clock and extends into the posterior fourchette. These injuries indicate penetrating trauma and are consistent with a history of acute sexual assault. (Photo contributor: Cincinnati Children's Hospital Medical Center.)

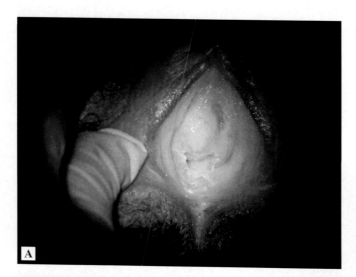

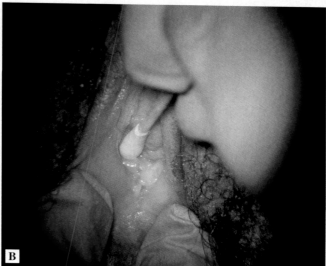

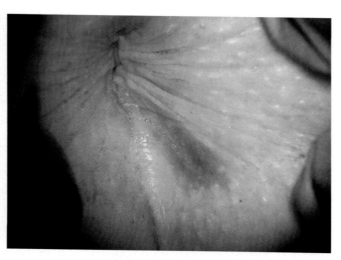

FIGURE 15.55 ▪ Bruise of the Perianal Skin. Bruising of the perianal area is noted at 5 o'clock. Bruising in the perianal area is concerning for sexual abuse, and forensic evidence should be obtained. (Photo contributor: Cincinnati Children's Hospital Medical Center.)

FIGURE 15.53 ▪ Cotton Swab Technique to Visualize Trauma. (**A**) Normally appearing adolescent hymen. (**B**) An acute hymenal injury at 7 o'clock seen with the cotton swab technique. Injuries can be missed if the hymen is not completely visualized. (Photo contributor: Cincinnati Children's Hospital Medical Center.)

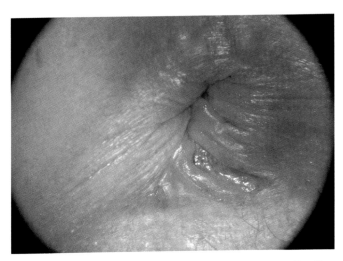

FIGURE 15.56 ■ Acute Perianal Lacerations with Venous Pooling. An acute perianal laceration is demonstrated. This laceration is deep and is concerning for sexual abuse. More superficial fissuring, commonly found on examinations, is nonspecific. Venous pooling is also present around the perianal area and can be confused with bruising. (Photo contributor: Cincinnati Children's Hospital Medical Center.)

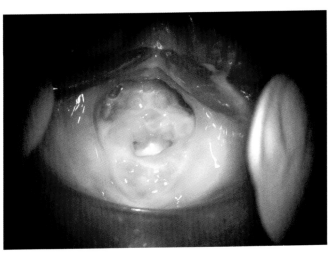

FIGURE 15.58 ■ Vaginal Discharge from *Neisseria gonorrhoea.* Vaginal discharge in a prepubertal child may be an indication of an STD even when a history of abuse is denied. All children with vaginal discharge should be cultured for *N gonorrhoeae* and *Chlamydia.* (Photo contributor: Cincinnati Children's Hospital Medical Center.)

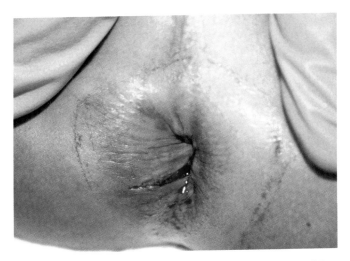

FIGURE 15.57 ■ Acute Deep Perianal Lacerations and Bruising. An acute rectal laceration is visible at 8 o'clock with bruising on the right side of the perianal area. (Photo contributor: Cincinnati Children's Hospital Medical Center.)

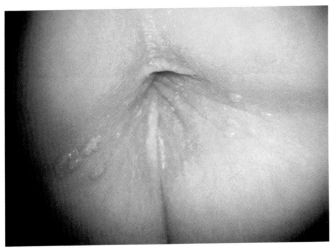

FIGURE 15.59 ■ Perianal Condyloma Acuminata. Several small perianal warts are visible. Warts can be transmitted sexually and nonsexually. Work up should include testing for other STDs as well as evaluation for sexual abuse. (Photo contributor: Cincinnati Children's Hospital Medical Center.)

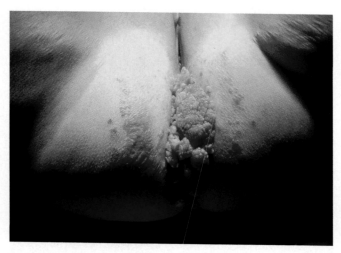

FIGURE 15.60 ■ Perianal Condyloma Acuminata. Extensive perianal warts are seen. (Photo contributor: Cincinnati Children's Hospital Medical Center.)

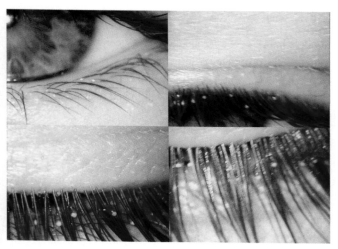

FIGURE 15.62 ■ Nits. Nits (the larval form of the louse) from *Phithirus pubis* are seen firmly adherent to the eyelashes in this child. Sexual abuse should be considered. (Photo contributor: Robert A. Shapiro, MD.)

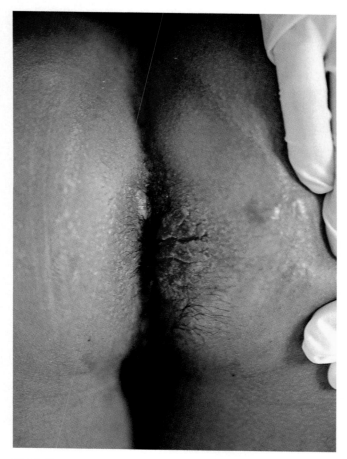

FIGURE 15.61 ■ Perianal Condyloma Lata (Secondary Syphilis). Perianal condyloma lata are visible around the rectum. (Photo contributor: Cincinnati Children's Hospital Medical Center.)

Clinical Summary

Straddle injuries are a frequent cause of genital trauma and most often result in unilateral abrasions, bruising, and hematomas of the labia majora and clitoral hood. In some instances the introitus will be injured, but trauma to and near the hymen are concerning for sexual abuse.

Emergency Department Treatment and Disposition

Check for urethral injury. Sitz baths and antibacterial ointment promote healing and minimize discomfort. If the child has difficulty voiding, she should be encouraged to void in a bath of warm water to reduce dysuria. Consider sexual abuse in all children with genital injuries.

Pearls

1. Straddle injuries usually present with a clear mechanism of injury and a physical examination that supports the history.
2. Straddle injuries do not typically involve the hymen or internal vaginal mucosa.

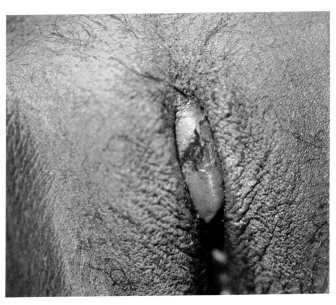

FIGURE 15.63 ■ Straddle Injury. Laceration of the clitoral hood due to a fall onto the bar of a bicycle. (Photo contributor: Robert A. Shapiro, MD.)

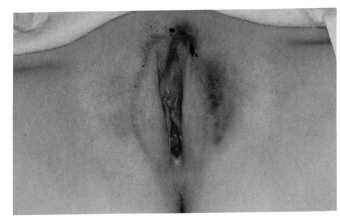

FIGURE 15.64 ■ Straddle Injury. Bruising to the left labia majora and clitoral hood following a fall onto the bicycle bar. (Photo contributor: Cincinnati Children's Hospital Medical Center.)

Clinical Summary

Adhesions of the labia minora occur in young girls and may persist until puberty. A thin translucent line is seen where the labia meet. Involvement is often limited to the posterior portion of the labia, but some children have more extensive adhesions that completely obscure the introitus.

Emergency Department Treatment and Disposition

Estrogen cream (Premarin) can be prescribed and applied gently over the adhesions twice daily for 2 to 4 weeks. Recurrence is not uncommon.

Pearls

1. Adhesions may be congenital or acquired.
2. It is postulated that vulvar irritation from sexual abuse may cause labial adhesions but supporting evidence is lacking.
3. Adhesions distort the vaginal anatomy and make identification of the hymen difficult.
4. Adhesions may be mistaken for scars.

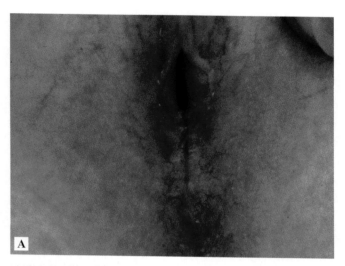

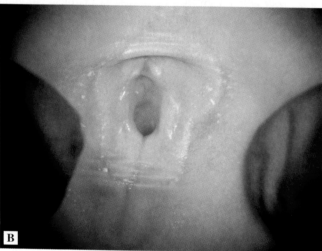

FIGURE 15.65A and B ■ Labial Adhesions. Labial adhesions obscure the hymen in these prepubertal girls. (Photo contributor: Cincinnati Children's Hospital Medical Center.)

Clinical Summary

The presenting signs of urethral prolapse are genital bleeding, vaginal mass, or urinary complaints. On examination, an annular erythematous vaginal mass is seen originating from the urethra. The mass may be friable and difficult to delineate from the surrounding genitalia. Urethral prolapse is commonly mistaken for vaginal injury.

Emergency Department Treatment and Disposition

The prolapse may resolve within a few weeks with conservative medical management consisting of daily sitz baths and topical estrogen cream. Antibiotic use is optional. Surgical repair may be needed when the prolapse is necrotic or when conservative management fails. Refer to urology if symptoms are severe or when conservative management has failed.

Pearls

1. Urethral prolapse often presents with painless genital bleeding of unknown etiology.
2. Prolapse is more common in African American girls aged 4 to 10 years.

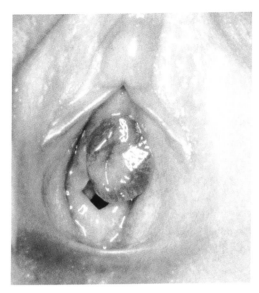

FIGURE 15.66 ■ Urethral Prolapse. A round reddish-purple mass is seen in this child's introitus. Careful examination reveals that the mass originates from the urethra. (Photo contributor: Michael P. Poirier, MD.)

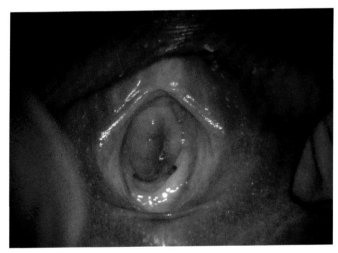

FIGURE 15.67 ■ Urethral Prolapse. A urethral prolapse seen in a dark-skinned child. (Photo contributor: Cincinnati Children's Hospital Medical Center.)

Clinical Summary

Acute bruising to the glans and corona of the penis can occur if the toilet seat falls onto the penis during voiding, trapping the penis between the seat and toilet bowl. This injury is not uncommon in boys of about 3 years of age whose height and development set the stage for this injury.

Emergency Department Treatment and Disposition

No specific treatment is needed unless the child is unable to void. Consult urology if the child cannot void. Consider sexual abuse in any child with a genital injury.

Pearl

1. Genital injuries are suspicious of sexual abuse if no appropriate history of accidental trauma is given.

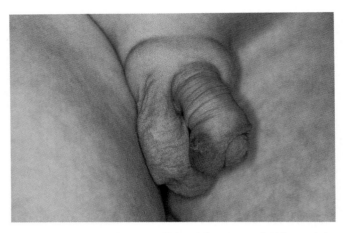

FIGURE 15.68 ■ Penile Injury. This toddler presented with a straightforward history of the toilet bowel falling onto his penis while voiding. He was able to void without difficulty. (Photo contributor: Kevin J. Knoop, MD, MS.)

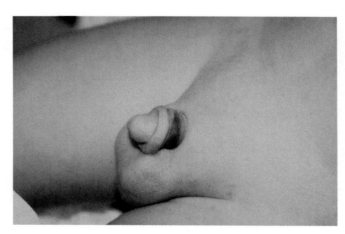

FIGURE 15.69 ■ Penile Injury. The toilet seat fell onto this toddler's penis and caused bruising to the penis. Discharge is appropriate if the child can void without difficulty. (Photo contributor: Charles J. Schubert.)

Clinical Summary

Perianal streptococcal infection causes rectal pain, itching, bleeding, and a tender erythematous rash around the anus. Anal fissures are common and constipation from voluntary stool retention may be present. Systemic symptoms are absent.

Emergency Department Treatment and Disposition

Culture the perianal skin for group A β-hemolytic streptococci. Treat with oral penicillin for 10 days. Substitute erythromycin for patients allergic to penicillin. Treatment failures should be treated with IM penicillin and/or oral clindamycin.

Pearls

1. Examine the pharynx and skin (desquamation) for streptococcal infection when considering perianal streptococcal infection.
2. Infection is unusual in children older than 10 years.
3. This infection may be mistaken for sexual abuse because of the overlap in clinical presentation: pain, redness, bleeding, and fissures without a recognized etiology.

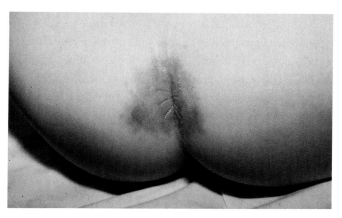

FIGURE 15.70 ■ Perianal Streptococcal Infection. Intense erythema around the anus consistent with perianal streptococcal infection. (Photo contributor: Raymond C. Baker, MD.)

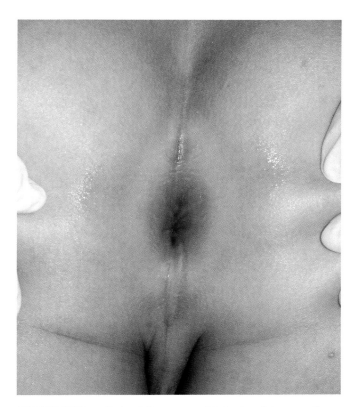

FIGURE 15.71 ■ Perianal Streptococcal Infection. Intense erythema around the anus consistent with perianal streptococcal infection. (Photo contributor: Kevin J. Knoop, MD, MS.)

Clinical Summary

Lichen sclerosus atrophicus (LSA) is an unusual dermatitis that affects the anogenital area. The diagnosis should be suspected whenever hypopigmented skin around the anus and genitalia are present. The hypopigmented area, in the shape of an hourglass, is caused by small white or yellowish papules that coalesce into large plaques. The affected skin is atrophic and bleeds easily after minor trauma. The hemorrhagic form of LSA includes subepithelial hemorrhagic lesions to the labia and affected skin, which can be mistaken for traumatic lesions. Children may complain of pruritus, dysuria, and bleeding.

Emergency Department Treatment and Disposition

Provide symptomatic care along with a high dose topical steroid cream and refer to a dermatologist for follow-up.

Pearl

1. Lichen sclerosus atrophicus is the most common dermatitis mistaken for sexual abuse.

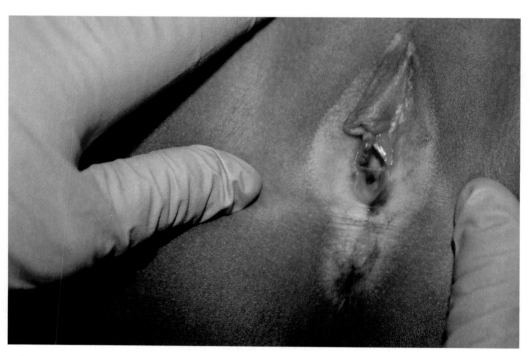

FIGURE 15.72 ■ Hemorrhagic Lichen Sclerosis Atrophicus. The perineum surrounding the vagina and anus is hypopigmented in an hourglass configuration. The hemorrhagic lesions are not traumatic in etiology. (Photo contributor: Cincinnati Children's Hospital Medical Center.)

Chapter 16

ENVIRONMENTAL CONDITIONS

Ken Zafren
R. Jason Thurman
Ian D. Jones

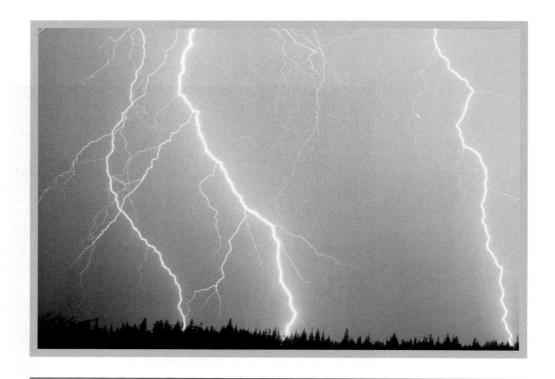

The authors acknowledge the special contributions of Peter Hackett, MD, The Institute for Altitude Medicine Telluride, Colorado; Edward Otten, MD, University of Cincinnati, Cincinnati, Ohio; James O'Malley, MD, Providence Alaska Medical Center, Anchorage, Alaska; Murray Hamlett, DVM and Kathy McCue, MD, Alaska Native Medical Center, Anchorage, Alaska; Sheryl Olson, RN, Monitou Springs, CO; Luanne Freer, MD, Yellowstone National Park, The Nashville Zoo, Nashville, TN; and the Nova Scotia Museum of Natural History, Halifax, Nova Scotia, Canada. The authors thank Joseph C. Schmidt, MD, Lawrence B. Stack, MD, and Alan B. Storrow, MD for their contributions to prior editions.

Clinical Summary

Retinal hemorrhages are common above 5200 m (17,060 ft) and are not always associated with acute mountain sickness (AMS). High-altitude retinal hemorrhages (HARH) are rarely symptomatic, but if found over the macula, these hemorrhages may cause temporary blindness. The diagnosis can be established by ophthalmoscopy. Without visualization of the lesion, the differential diagnosis of unilaterally decreased vision or blindness at high altitude includes migraine equivalent, cerebrovascular accident, and dry eye (often unilateral, due to strong winds), as well as all conditions found at sea level.

Emergency Department Treatment and Disposition

HARH generally resolve spontaneously after descent to lower altitudes. No treatment is necessary for asymptomatic HARH.

Patients with HARH associated with a decrease in vision should be referred to an ophthalmologist for follow-up.

Pearls

1. Patients with blurred vision and unilateral mydriasis at the high altitude should be asked about use of medications, including transdermal scopolamine patches.
2. As with almost all altitude-related problems, descent is the primary treatment. This is not emergent unless associated with severe altitude illness or progressive visual loss.
3. Although most symptomatic HARH resolve completely in 2 to 8 weeks, cases of permanent paracentral scotomata have been reported.

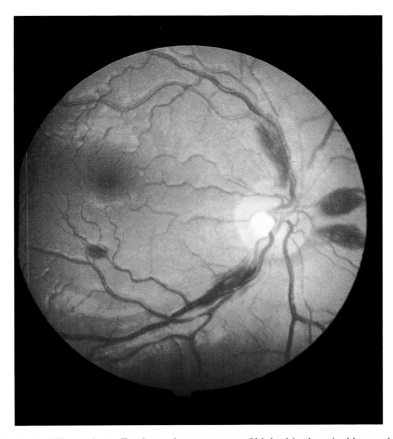

FIGURE 16.1 ■ High-Altitude Retinal Hemorrhage. Fundoscopic appearance of high-altitude retinal hemorrhage. (Photo contributor: Peter Hackett, MD.)

Clinical Summary

High-altitude pulmonary edema (HAPE) is a form of noncardiogenic pulmonary edema, generally beginning within the first 2 to 4 days after ascent above 2500 m (8202 ft). The earliest symptoms are fatigue, weakness, dyspnea on exertion, and decreased exercise performance. Symptoms of acute mountain sickness (AMS) such as headache, anorexia, and lassitude may also be present, but HAPE may develop without AMS. If untreated, a persistent dry cough develops, followed by tachycardia and tachypnea at rest with cyanosis. Patients suffering from HAPE generally experience nocturnal onset, and frequently report progressively worsening symptoms at night. Eventually the victim develops dyspnea at rest and orthopnea with audible crackles in the chest. Pink frothy sputum is a grave sign. Patients may experience concurrent mental status changes and ataxia due to hypoxemia or associated high-altitude cerebral edema (HACE).

Emergency Department Treatment and Disposition

Mild cases (oxygen saturation in the 90s on low-flow oxygen) at moderate altitudes (below 3500 m, 11,483 ft) may be treated at altitude with bed rest and oxygen. If supplemental oxygen and a reliable person are available, the patient may be discharged with oxygen therapy and bed rest at home or in lodgings. More severe cases should descend immediately and may require admission to a hospital at a lower altitude and, in extreme cases, intubation and mechanical ventilation. Nifedipine is of benefit but is not a substitute for descent. Some experts now use PDE-5 inhibitors such as sildenafil or tadalafil instead of nifedipine. Hyperbaric therapy, especially with a portable hyperbaric chamber (Gamow bag), has an efficacy equal to that of supplemental oxygen and is mainly helpful in prehospital settings where oxygen availability is limited.

Pearls

1. Crackles may be unilateral or bilateral but usually start in the right middle lobe and are heard first in the right axilla.
2. HAPE limited to the left lung in association with a small right hemothorax without pulmonary markings is pathognomonic for unilateral absent pulmonary artery syndrome. These patients develop HAPE at relatively low altitudes, sometimes below 2500 m.

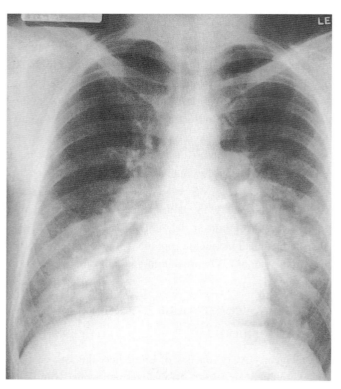

FIGURE 16.2 ■ High-Altitude Pulmonary Edema. Chest x-ray in patient with HAPE. Note normal heart size with bilateral "patchy" pulmonary infiltrates. (Photo contributor: Peter Hackett, MD.)

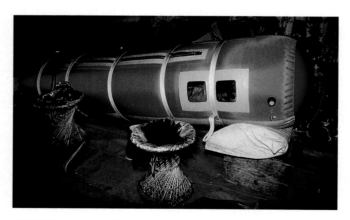

FIGURE 16.3 ■ "Gamow Bag." Portable hyperbaric chamber (Gamow bag). A HAPE patient is being treated at 4300 m at Pheriche, Nepal. Due to orthopnea, the patient was unable to tolerate lying flat, so the bag was propped up immediately after inflation. (Photo contributor: Ken Zafren, MD.)

3. Patients treated for HAPE may resume normal activities once they are asymptomatic and may ascend further during the same trip.

Clinical Summary

Acute mountain sickness (AMS) is a symptom complex which usually begins 12 to 24 hours after ascent to high altitude and consists of headache and one or more other symptoms, including gastrointestinal symptoms, fatigue and/or weakness, dizziness and/or lightheadedness, and difficulty sleeping. High-altitude cerebral edema (HACE) is a severe form of AMS and is defined by the presence of truncal ataxia or the presence of altered mental status. Usually this occurs as progression from AMS to HACE, but HACE may occur without antecedent AMS. If not effectively treated, HACE may progress to coma or death. Focal neurologic findings other than truncal ataxia are rare and should suggest another diagnosis, such as CVA or sagittal sinus thrombosis.

Emergency Department Treatment and Disposition

Treatment of HACE consists of immediate descent or evacuation, oxygen, and high dose dexamethasone. Simulated descent using a portable hyperbaric bag (Gamow bag) may be more effective than oxygen alone and may be used in place of oxygen in field settings. Actual descent may be complicated by the inability of the patient to walk unassisted or at all. Patients with HACE may not ascend during the same trip and probably should not reascend to altitude for several months.

Pearls

1. The first sign of HACE is truncal ataxia. This should be tested using tandem gait (heel-to-toe walking).
2. HACE may occur without symptoms of AMS.
3. HACE is often associated with some degree of HAPE.

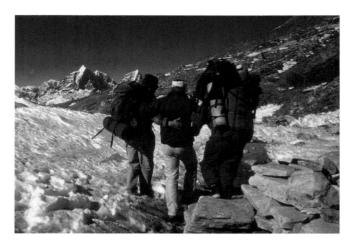

FIGURE 16.4 ■ HACE-Related Ataxia. Ataxia due to HACE in the Nepal Himalayas. The patient (middle) developed HAPE at 5600 m (18,400 ft) and severe truncal ataxia. Full ambulatory assistance was required, and immediate decent was undertaken. With decent, the patient's breathing improved, but he remained too ataxic to walk. (Photo contributor: Ken Zafren, MD.)

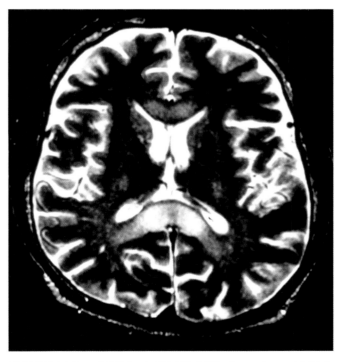

FIGURE 16.5 ■ MRI Brain-HACE. MRI of a patient with high-altitude cerebral edema. Note the increased white matter signal, especially in the splenium of the corpus callosum, in this T2-weighted image. (Photo contributor: Ken Zafren, MD.)

Clinical Summary

Accidental hypothermia is an unintentional decline in core temperature below 35°C (95°F). Presentation may be obvious or subtle, especially in urban settings. Symptoms vary from vague complaints to altered levels of consciousness. Physical findings include progressive abnormalities of every organ system. Following initial tachycardia, there is progressive bradycardia (50% decrease in heart rate at 28°C [82.4°F]) with decline in blood pressure and cardiac output. ECG intervals are prolonged, beginning with the PR interval followed by the QRS interval and finally the QT interval. A J wave (Osborn wave; hypothermic "hump") may be seen, but is neither pathognomonic nor prognostic. The J wave is present at the junction of the QRS complex and the ST segment. J waves may also be associated with central nervous system lesions, focal cardiac ischemia, young age, and sepsis. In mildly hypothermic patients, invisible preshivering muscle tone may obscure P waves.

Emergency Department Treatment and Disposition

Core temperature measurement is best made with an esophageal probe. Rectal temperature is less accurate without the use of a special low-reading thermometer. Gentle handling and appropriate warming methods are the mainstays of ED treatment. Cardiovascular instability often complicates rewarming; Advanced Cardiac Life Support (ACLS) guidelines for hypothermia provide guidance. If not obvious, a cause should be sought (eg, hypothyroidism, hypoglycemia, sepsis), as should associated pathology. Most patients require admission for observation or to treat associated injuries or comorbidities.

Pearls

1. The most common problems with the diagnosis of hypothermia in the ED stem from incomplete data on vital signs.
2. Low-reading thermometers, accurate core temperatures, averaging respirations over minutes, and Doppler pulse locations are crucial to appropriate management.
3. Atrial arrhythmias are generally benign and should not be treated. They resolve with rewarming.
4. Most cardiovascular drugs are inactive during hypothermia and should be given only once the body temperature is above 35°C (95°F).

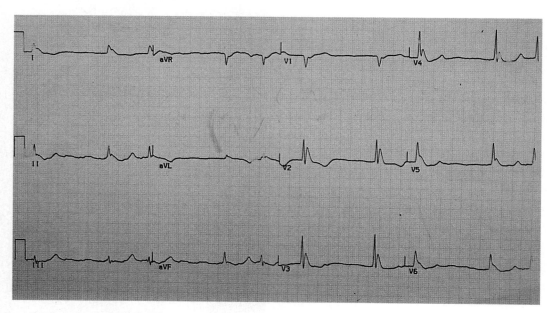

FIGURE 16.6 ■ J Waves. J waves in a hypothermic patient with core temperature (rectal probe) of 25.5°C. J waves may be seen at any temperature below 32.2°C, most frequently in leads II and V₆. Below a core temperature of 25°C, they are most commonly found in the precordial leads (especially V₃ and V₄) and their size increases. J waves are usually upright in aVL, aVF, and the left precordial leads (see also Fig. 23-43 "Hypothermia with Osborne Waves ("J" Waves) Present"). (Photo contributor: Alan B. Storrow, MD.)

Clinical Summary

Frostbite is true tissue freezing resulting from heat loss sufficient to cause ice crystal formation in superficial or deep tissue. Frostbite may affect the extremities, nose, or ears (and the scrotum and penis in joggers). Severity of symptoms is usually proportional to the severity of the injury. A sensation of numbness with accompanying sensory loss is the most common initial complaint. Often, by the time the patient arrives in the emergency department, the frozen tissue has thawed. The initial appearance of the overlying skin may be deceptively benign. Frozen tissue may appear mottled blue, violaceous, yellowish-white, or waxy. Following rapid rewarming, there is early hyperemia even in severe cases.

Favorable signs include return of normal sensation, color, and warmth. Edema should appear within 3 hours of thawing; lack of edema is an unfavorable sign. Vesicles and bullae appear in 6 to 24 hours. Early formation of large clear blebs that extend to the tips of affected digits is a good indicator. Small dark blebs that do not extend to the tips indicate damage to subdermal plexi and are a poor prognostic sign. When seen early or after rewarming occurs, frostbite may be indistinguishable from nonfreezing cold injury such as immersion foot. Mixed injuries are common.

Emergency Department Treatment and Disposition

If other injuries are ruled out by history and physical examination, rewarm frostbitten areas in warm water bath (37°C-39°C [98.6°F-102.2°F]). If associated with severe hypothermia, active core rewarming should precede frostbite rewarming. If swelling occurs, measure compartment pressures (including hands and feet) to determine the need for fasciotomy. Admit all patients with associated hypothermia or in whom swelling occurs. Superficial frostbite (minimal skin changes and erythema) may be treated by home care with nursing instructions. Deep superficial frostbite (clear, fluid-filled blebs, swelling, pain) may be treated by home care in a reliable patient. Deep frostbite (proximal hemorrhagic blebs, no swelling, no pulses) mandates hospital admission.

Pearls

1. Early transfer of the patient to a center experienced in the care of frostbite injuries (even if hundreds of miles away) should be considered. On the other hand, transfer of the patient to a major medical center that does not generally manage frostbite is seldom in the patient's best interest.

2. Treatment of clear versus hemorrhagic blisters is controversial; one approach is to debride clear blisters and use topical aloe vera while leaving hemorrhagic blisters intact.

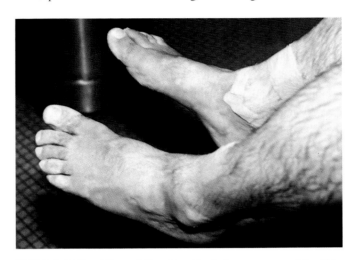

FIGURE 16.7 ■ Thawed Frostbite. Typical appearance of frostbite soon after rewarming. Deep frostbite was caused by wearing mountaineering boots that were too tight in extreme cold at high altitude. Note deceptively benign appearance of this devastating injury. (Photo contributor: James O'Malley, MD.)

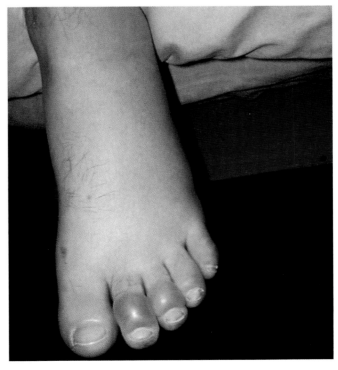

FIGURE 16.8 ■ Deep Superficial Frostbite. Clear blebs extending distally are indicators for favorable outcome. (Photo contributor: James O'Malley, MD.)

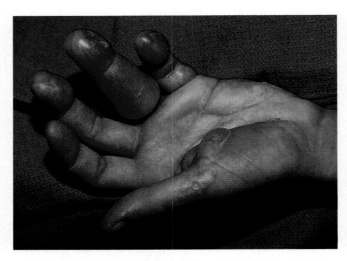

FIGURE 16.9 ■ Frostbite Blebs. Intact proximal blebs, both clear and hemorrhagic. (Photo contributor: Scott W. Zackowski, MD.)

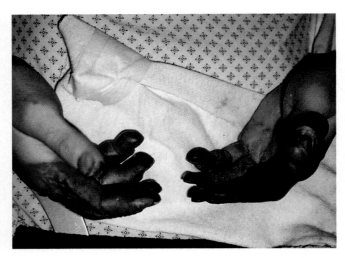

FIGURE 16.11 ■ Late Frostbite. Late appearance of frostbite with demarcation starting to occur. Early surgery should be avoided in favor of autoamputation unless infection supervenes. (Photo contributor: James O'Malley, MD.)

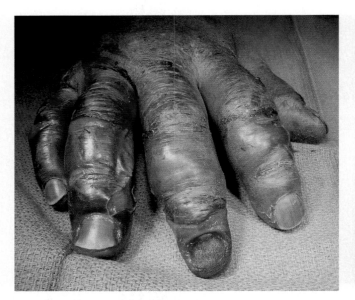

FIGURE 16.10 ■ Frostbite-Ruptured Blebs. Frostbite injury to the hand with ruptured blebs. (Photo contributor: R. Jason Thurman, MD.)

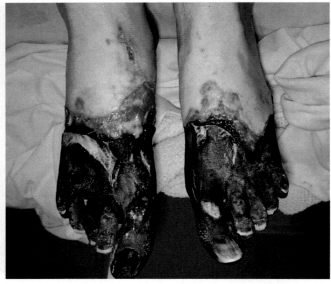

FIGURE 16.12 ■ Deep Frostbite. Late appearance of deep frostbite with clear demarcation. (Photo contributor: James O'Malley, MD.)

Clinical Summary

Pernio, also known as chilblain cold sores, is the result of nonfreezing cold exposure. Pernio appears within 24 hours of cold exposure, most frequently on the face, ears, hands, feet, and pretibial areas. A large range of lesions may be seen, with localized edema, erythema, cyanosis, plaques, and blue nodules occasionally progressing to more severe lesions including vesicles, bullae, and ulcerations. The lesions persist for up to 2 weeks and may become chronic. They are typically very pruritic and associated with burning paresthesias. Following rewarming, pernio often takes the form of blue nodules, which are quite tender. In the setting of recent cold exposure, pernio might be confused with the more severe syndrome of trench foot and its sequelae. If the history of cold exposure is not elicited, the differential diagnosis is potentially very broad.

Emergency Department Treatment and Disposition

Management is supportive. The skin should be warmed, washed, and dried. Affected extremities can be dressed in soft, dry, sterile dressings and elevated. Nifedipine (20-60 mg daily) may be helpful in chronic cases.

Pearls

1. Healing may be followed by hyperpigmentation.
2. Recurrences are possible following milder cold exposure.
3. Chilblains may be more frequent in young women, especially in association with Raynaud phenomenon, and may also be associated with underlying dermatologic or vascular disease.

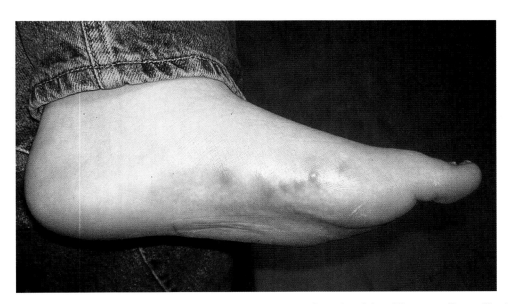

FIGURE 16.13 ■ Pernio. Pernio or chilblains with localized erythema, cyanosis, and nodules. (Photo contributor: Ken Zafren, MD.)

Clinical Summary

Immersion injury is a peripheral nonfreezing cold injury resulting from exposure to water, usually at temperatures just above freezing. However, the condition can occur during prolonged exposure to any wet environment cooler than body temperature. Dependency and immobility predispose to immersion injury. The degree of injury depends on exposure time and temperature. The first symptoms usually appear within hours; tissue loss may occur after many days of exposure. Prior to rewarming, the distal extremities are numb and swollen. The skin is first red, then changes to pale, mottled, or black. Cramping of the calves may occur. Immersion injury is distinct from tropical immersion foot or warm-water immersion foot as seen in the Vietnam War. Tropical immersion foot was typically seen after 3 to 7 days of exposure to water at 22°C to 32°C. Warm-water immersion foot was seen after 1 to 3 days at 15°C to 32°C. These syndromes were characterized by burning in the feet, pain on walking, pitting edema, and erythema, with wrinkling and hyperhydration of the skin. They resolved completely after rest and removal from the wet environment.

Emergency Department Treatment and Disposition

Hypovolemia, hypothermia, and associated injuries are the rule and should be treated first. General treatment of immersion foot (or hand) is the same as that for frostbite that has been rewarmed. Swelling may produce compartment syndrome and require fasciotomy. Most patients require admission to the hospital.

Pearls

1. Doppler may be useful to identify peripheral pulses, as pulses are often difficult to palpate in affected extremities.
2. Mixed injuries (frostbite and immersion) are common.

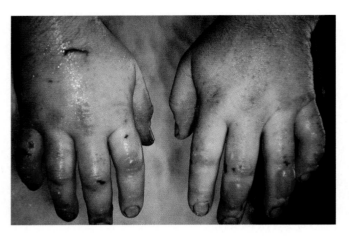

FIGURE 16.14 ■ Immersion Injury. Immersion injury to hands (unusual location) several hours after rewarming. The patient spent 18 hours bailing out a boat in waters just above freezing in Alaska. (Photo contributor: James O'Malley, MD.)

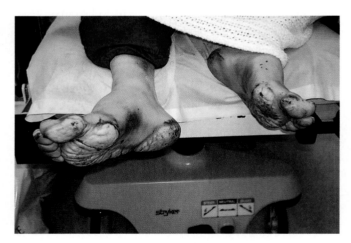

FIGURE 16.15 ■ Immersion Foot. Early appearance of immersion foot in a mentally ill homeless patient. (Photo contributor: Ken Zafren, MD.)

Clinical Summary

Ultraviolet (UV) radiation causes both acute and chronic skin changes. Sunburn is a partial-thickness burn, which may become a full-thickness injury if infected. "Sun poisoning" is a severe systemic reaction to UV radiation. Patients may complain of nausea, vomiting, headache, fever, chills, and prostration. Excessive UV radiation may cause injury to the cornea and conjunctiva, termed ultraviolet keratitis (photokeratitis, snow blindness). This painful condition may occur in skiers, welders, or tanning salon patrons who do not wear proper eye protection.

Photosensitivity reactions (photodermatoses) are of several types. Phototoxic reactions are an abnormal response to UV radiation caused by a substance that is ingested (eg, prescription or over-the-counter medications) or applied to the skin; there is a direct relation between the amount of UV exposure and severity. Photoallergic reactions are clinically similar to contact dermatitis and, like phototoxic reactions, may be precipitated by ingested or applied drugs. Unlike phototoxic reactions, photoallergies may be precipitated by a small amount of light. Phytophotodermatitis is precipitated by skin contact with certain plants followed by exposure to UV radiation.

Phototoxicity should be suspected in any patient with severe or exaggerated sunburn. Photoallergy is easily misdiagnosed as allergic eczema or contact dermatitis, especially since onset is often delayed up to 2 days after exposure. Phytophotodermatitis may mimic severe sunburn or contact dermatitis, especially rhus dermatitis. Endogenous photosensitizers (endogenous photodermatoses) include solar urticaria, porphyria cutanea tarda, polymorphous light eruption, and systemic lupus erythrematosus. These may be provoked by visible light as well as by UV radiation.

Emergency Department Treatment and Disposition

Treatment of sunburn and sun poisoning involves standard burn therapy and supportive care. Sunburn is usually a self-limited problem. Cool compresses and nonsteroidal anti-inflammatory drugs may be beneficial. Ultraviolet keratitis is treated with mydriatic-cycloplegic eyedrops to decrease pain; initial examination is made easier with topical anesthetics. Severe cases may require antibiotic ointment, narcotic analgesics, and bilateral eye patches for 12 to 24 hours, though the use of eye patches remains controversial. These patients require 24- to 48-hours follow-up; ophthalmology referral is indicated to rule out retinal damage.

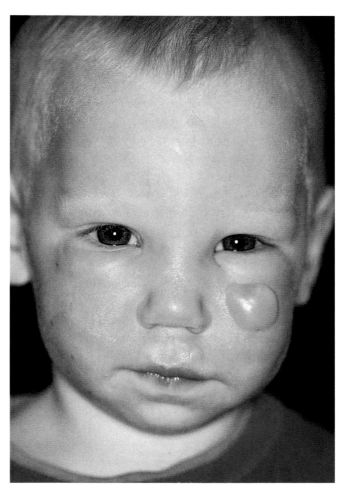

FIGURE 16.16 ■ Sunburn. Sunburn is characterized by erythema, edema, warmth, tenderness, and blisters. (Photo contributor: Kevin J. Knoop, MD, MS.)

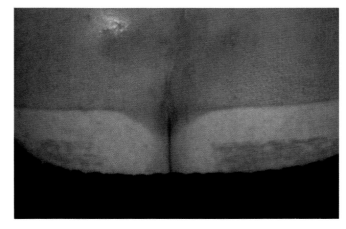

FIGURE 16.17 ■ Tanning Bed Burn. This patient suffered a severe diffuse partial thickness burn from prolonged UV exposure in a tanning bed. Note the sharp demarcation on the buttocks at the point where the patient was partially protected by his pants. (Photo contributor: R. Jason Thurman, MD.)

Treatment of photosensitivity reaction has two components: treatment of the sunburn and recognition of the sensitizing agent or endogenous medical condition. Topical steroids and oral analgesics and antipruritics may be helpful. Systemic steroids may be required. Patients with severe reactions should be referred to a dermatologist for possible photo patch testing.

Pearls

1. *Para*-aminobenzoic acid (PABA) in sunscreens may be a photosensitizer and can cause a photoallergic reaction.
2. The unique properties of individual skin types produce marked differences in response to UV radiation.
3. Victims of UV keratitis typically present 2 to 12 hours after exposure, thus many patients will present during the night with severe unexplained bilateral eye pain.

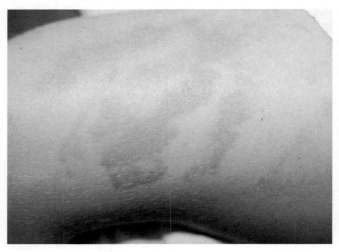

FIGURE 16.18 ■ Phytophotodermatitis. This reaction may require aggressive systemic steroid therapy. The case illustrated is a mild one caused by exposure to limes and UVA. A clue to the diagnosis is the patchy distribution with linear edges. More severe reactions resemble rhus dermatitis. (Photo contributor: Lee Kaplan, MD.)

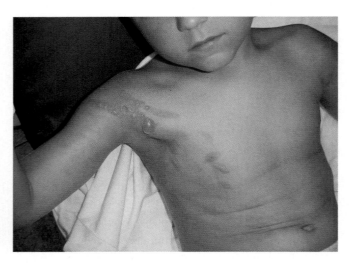

FIGURE 16.20 ■ Phytophotodermatitis—Lime. Phytophotodermatits caused by exposure to limes and UV radiation in Jamaica. The patient had been exposed while riding shirtless on a horse through a lime orchard. (Photo contributor: Stephan Russ, MD.)

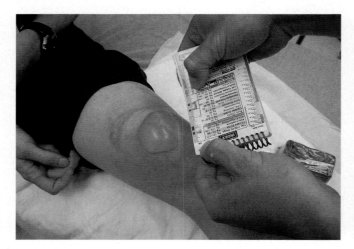

FIGURE 16.19 ■ Phytophotodermatitis—Cow Parsnip. Severe phytophotodermatitis caused by exposure to cow parsnip (*Heracleum lanatum*) in Alaska. Another name for cow parsnip is "pushkie," so this is also known locally as "pushkie burn." (Photo contributor: Kathy McCue, MD.)

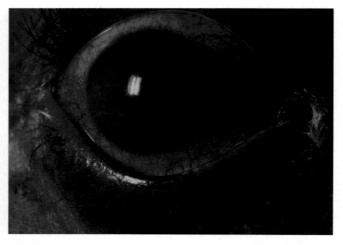

FIGURE 16.21 ■ Ultraviolet Keratitis. This patient presented with severe eye pain at 3 AM after a day of arc welding without proper eye protection. Notice the absence of flourescene uptake where the eyelids were protective. (Photo contributor: Lawrence B. Stack, MD.)

Clinical Summary

Lightning produces injury from high voltage, heat production, and explosive shock waves. Direct injuries include cardiopulmonary arrest, cardiac arrhythmias, and neurologic abnormalities such as seizures, deafness, confusion, amnesia, blindness, and paralysis. The patient may suffer contusions from the shock wave or from opisthotonic muscle contractions. Chest pain and muscle aches are common. One or both tympanic membranes rupture in more than 50% of victims. Cataracts are usually a delayed occurrence. Hematologic abnormalities including disseminated intravascular coagulation (DIC) have been described. Fetal demise may occur.

Burns may result from vaporization of sweat or moist clothing, heating of clothing and metal objects such as belt buckles or bra wiring, and direct effects of the strike. Linear burns and punctate burns are thermal burns. Feathering burns are not actually burns but rather skin markings caused by electron showers. They are pathognomonic of lightning injury. Diagnosis is straightforward when there is a thunderstorm, when there are witnesses to the strike, or when there are typical physical findings. Lightning on relatively sunny days (without loud thunder) striking a lone victim may produce a confusing picture. The scattering of clothing and belongings may mimic an assault. Side flashes from metal objects and wiring may produce indoor victims during storms.

Emergency Department Treatment and Disposition

History and physical examination to rule out associated injuries and standard emergency department care and workup for critical patients—including cardiac enzymes, urinalysis, and ECG, are necessary. All patients, even those apparently well, require admission for observation since their condition may change over several hours following the lightning strike.

Pearls

1. The amount of damage to the exterior of the body does not predict the amount of internal injury.
2. Since lightning most commonly produces cardiac standstill by means of massive direct current countershock, prompt, spontaneous return of normal heart rhythm (by virtue of cardiac automaticity) is the rule. However, respiratory arrest is often more prolonged. In a triage situation, the normal rules do not apply, since victims breathing spontaneously are already recovering. The rule

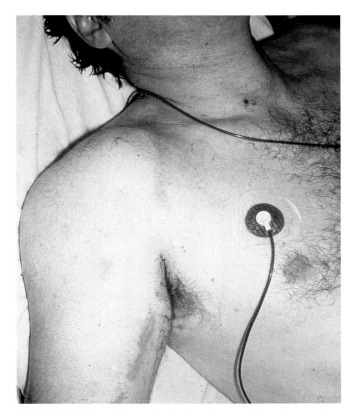

FIGURE 16.22 ■ Linear Lightning Burns. Linear burns from lightning are due to thermal effects. (Photo contributor: William Barsan, MD.)

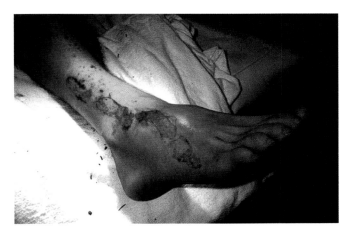

FIGURE 16.23 ■ Linear Lightning Burns. Linear lightning burns along the leg and foot of a strike victim. (Photo contributor: Sheryl Olson, RN.)

in lightning strikes is to resuscitate the "dead." Ventilatory support is often all that is required.
3. Psychological sequelae following lightning injuries are underreported and may include memory loss, difficulty with concentration, and depression.

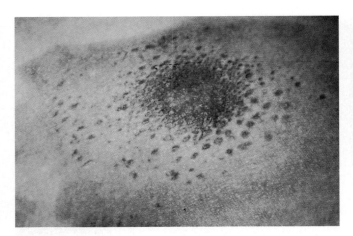

FIGURE 16.24 ■ Punctate Lightning Burns. Punctate burns due to lightning are partial or full-thickness thermal burns that range from a few millimeters to a centimeter in diameter. They are multiple and closely spaced. (Photo contributor: Arthur Kahn, MD.)

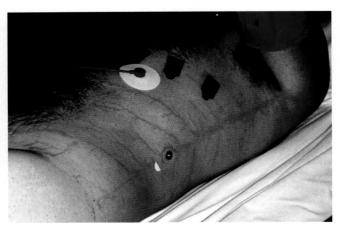

FIGURE 16.25 ■ Feathering. Feathering (ferning) on the left side of a lightning strike victim. (Photo contributor: Sheryl Olson, RN, BSN, CCRN.)

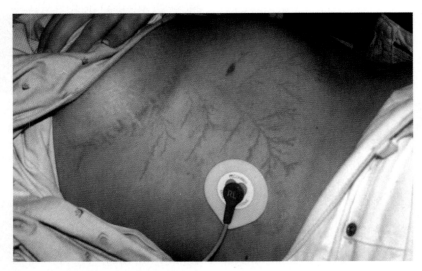

FIGURE 16.26 ■ Feathering from Underwire Bra. Feathering (ferning) burns are pathognomonic of lightning injury. These are not true burns but are imprints on the skin of electron showers. (Photo contributor: Sheryl Olson, RN, BSN, CCRN.)

Clinical Summary

Both domestic and wild animals are known to attack humans. Injuries are caused by combinations of penetrating and blunt trauma. Penetrating injuries can be inflicted by teeth, claws, and horns, while severe blunt injuries may result from the victim being knocked over, trampled or otherwise crushed, being thrown into the air, or being dragged. Injuries may involve massive tissue injury or avulsion often associated with neurovascular damage and long bone fractures.

Emergency Department Treatment and Disposition

Evaluation and treatment is the same as for any other multiple trauma victim with a high-energy mechanism. After attention to the ABCs, which may be complicated by injuries of the face, neck, or chest, victims should be evaluated for less obvious blunt traumatic injuries. Open fractures and injuries to internal organs may not be clinically apparent initially as with any multi-trauma victim.

Pearls

1. Wounds often require operative debridement and repair by appropriate specialists. Consider tetanus and rabies prophylaxis and antibiotic prophylaxis for high-risk wounds.
2. Bite wounds can penetrate the skull or joints. Evaluation should include x-rays and/or CT scanning along with appropriate surgical consultations.

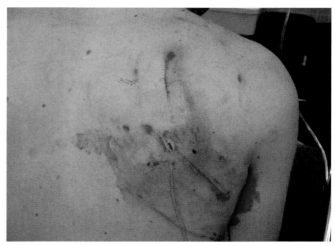

FIGURE 16.28 ■ Bear Attack—Open Scapula Fracture. Although grizzly claws aren't very sharp, they can exert considerable force. This innocuous appearing injury was complicated by an open scapula fracture. (Photo contributor: Luanne Freer, MD.)

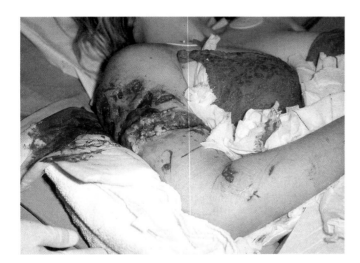

FIGURE 16.27 ■ Cougar Mauling. This patient has sustained large wounds as a result of a cougar attack. Here, the weight and force of this large animal has resulted in severe shearing injuries. Penetrating injuries from large animals may be deeper than they appear. (Photo contributor: Alan B. Storrow, MD.)

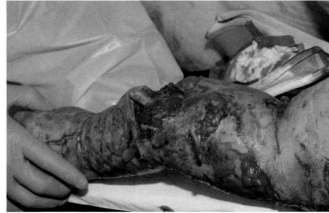

FIGURE 16.29 ■ Pit Bull Mauling. The left arm of a pit bull mauling victim. Note the open fracture of the radius. The patient sustained multiple severe defensive wounds to both arms resulting in extensive soft tissue and neurovascular injuries. (Photo contributor: R. Jason Thurman, MD.)

Clinical Summary

The most important species of coral snakes (Elapidae family) found in the United States are the eastern coral snake (*Micrurus fulvis*) and the Texas coral snake (*Micrurus tener*). Coral snakes have small mouths, and bites are usually limited to fingers, toes, or folds of skin. Due to a less efficient venom apparatus than their Crotalid colleagues, coral snakes generally need to hold on or chew to inflict a significant envenomation. The bite typically produces minimal local inflammation and pain, and paresthesias and muscle fasciculations are common. Systemic symptoms resulting from the powerful neurotoxic effects of the venom can include tremors, drowsiness, euphoria, marked salivation, and respiratory distress. Cranial nerve involvement, manifested by slurred speech and diplopia, may be followed by bulbar paralysis with dysphagia and dyspnea. Death may result from respiratory and cardiac arrest. Onset of severe symptoms may be delayed up to 12 hours, but may also be rapidly progressive.

Emergency Department Treatment and Disposition

In contrast to pit viper envenomation, prehospital application of a constrictive bandage may be of benefit in limiting the spread of neurotoxic coral snake venom. Severe systemic symptoms following envenomation by Elapidae may be delayed and cannot be accurately predicted by local wound reactions. It is therefore recommended that four to six vials of antivenom be administered for all suspected envenomations by eastern or Texas coral snakes. Treatment of western coral snake (*Micruroides euryxanthus*) bites is purely supportive. Tetanus prophylaxis should be addressed.

Pearls

1. Treatment with antivenom should be initiated early in cases of eastern coral snake bites, since symptoms are often delayed and severe.
2. The adage "red on yellow, kill a fellow; red on black, venom lack" applies to all coral snakes found in the United States but does not hold true in other parts of the world.
3. As many as 60% of North American coral snake bites do not result in envenomation of the victim.

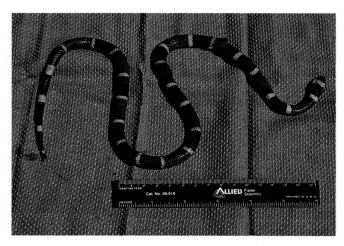

FIGURE 16.30 ■ Coral Snake. United States coral snake with typical coloring and red-on-yellow bands. (Photo contributor: Steven Holt, MD.)

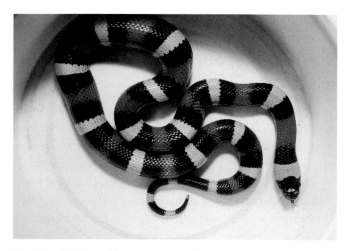

FIGURE 16.31 ■ Nonvenomous Milk Snake. As opposed to the red-on-yellow rings seen in the venomous US coral snake, these red-on-black rings indicate a nonvenomous snake. Unfortunately this applies only to animals native to the United States. (Photo contributor: Sean P. Bush, MD.)

Clinical Summary

The pit vipers (Crotalidae family) indigenous to the United States include rattlesnake species, cottonmouths, and copperheads. Physical characteristics of pit vipers include a triangular head, heat-sensing pits, elliptical pupils, and a single row of subcaudal ventral scales. Pit viper venom is complex and produces hematologic, cardiovascular, and neuromuscular effects. Clinically, pit viper envenomations are divided into four categories. Snakebites without envenomation are characterized only by the direct tissue damage caused by the strike. Minimal envenomations consist of fang marks and local swelling but no systemic symptoms. Moderate envenomations include progression of tissue changes beyond the immediate location of the bite and/or systemic symptoms and mild changes in coagulation parameters. Severe envenomations include marked local and progressive swelling and significant systemic symptoms and coagulopathy (eg, subcutaneous ecchymosis and/or signs of bleeding).

Emergency Department Treatment and Disposition

Prehospital management of pit viper bites should include immobilization and rapid transport without delay. Application of lymphatic constriction bands and use of extractor devices are controversial and may worsen focal complications of envenomation. Tourniquets and local incision are most likely ineffective and may do more harm than good. Electric shock, cryotherapy, and mouth suction are not recommended. Emergency department management includes resuscitation, establishing a physiologic baseline, and determining the need for antivenom. CroFab (Savage Labs), a recombinant antivenom effective in neutralizing venom toxins, eliminates the risk of horse serum allergy and should be used when available in patients requiring antivenom. Indications for antivenom administration include any progression of swelling, erythema, or ecchymosis beyond the immediate bite area, presence of any systemic signs of envenomation, or any coagulation abnormalities and/or bleeding complications associated with envenomation. Pit viper antivenom of horse serum derivation carries all the risks of any horse serum product. The dose of antivenom increases with the severity of envenomation. The package insert details the current recommendations for antivenom administration and allergy testing, but in general treatment is initiated with 4 to 6 vials of CroFab intravenously with further dosing regimen based on clinical course. Compartment syndrome is a possible complication of envenomation, and should initially be treated with antivenom. Fasciotomy should be performed only if compartment pressures are greater than 30 mm Hg in spite of antivenom treatment. Patients who do not develop evidence of envenomation after 8 hours of observation may be safely discharged home with close follow-up. Tetanus prophylaxis should be addressed and given when necessary.

Pearls

1. Up to half of all pit viper bites may be "dry" (without any injection of venom).
2. Subcutaneous epinephrine (0.3 mg) given prior to administration of horse serum antivenin may reduce the potential allergic response.

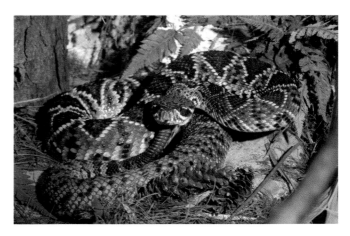

FIGURE 16.32 ■ Eastern Diamondback Rattlesnake. The eastern diamondback is the largest US rattlesnake and has a characteristic diamond-shaped pattern on its dorsal aspect. Note the triangular head, which is characteristic of pit vipers. (Photo contributor: R. Jason Thurman, MD.)

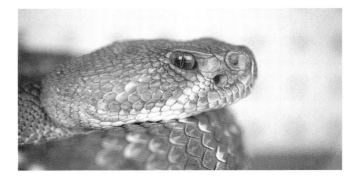

FIGURE 16.33 ■ Red Diamond Rattlesnake. The elliptical pupils and heat-sensing pits in this red diamond rattlesnake are characteristic of pit vipers. (Photo contributor: Sean P. Bush, MD.)

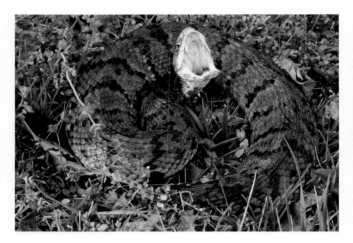

FIGURE 16.34 ■ Cottonmouth. The cottonmouth is a semiaquatic venomous pit viper that may crawl or swim with its head raised at an angle of 45 degrees. When disturbed, it may open its mouth wide to reveal a white lining. (Photo contributor: Stephen J. Knoop.)

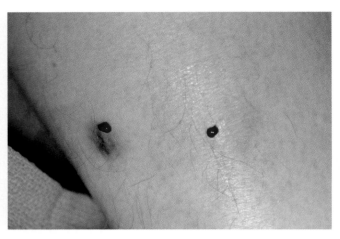

FIGURE 16.36 ■ Rattlesnake Envenomation, Minutes Old. Timber rattlesnake envenomation on the leg of an unsuspecting victim. The fang marks are 4 cm apart. (Photo contributor: R. Jason Thurman, MD.)

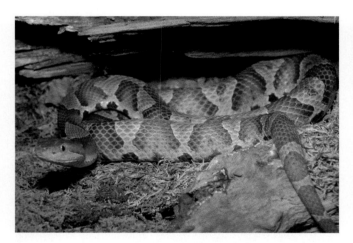

FIGURE 16.35 ■ Copperhead Snake. The Copperhead is frequently encountered in wooded mountains, abandoned buildings, and damp, grassy areas. It is able to climb low bushes and trees in search of food. (Photo contributor: R. Jason Thurman, MD.)

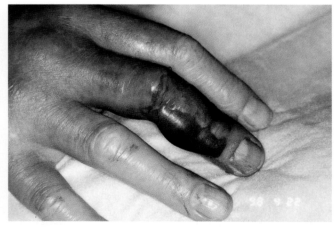

FIGURE 16.37 ■ Rattlesnake Envenomation, Day 1. This rattlesnake bite shows local swelling, some edema beyond the initial bite site, and a hemorrhagic bleb at 6 hours. It would be considered mild to moderate at this time. (Photo contributor: Sean P. Bush, MD.)

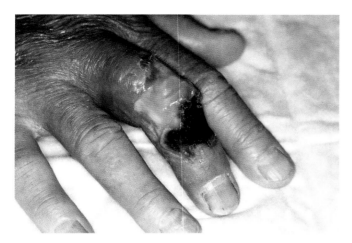

FIGURE 16.38 ■ Progression of Rattlesnake Envenomation 7 Weeks. Seven weeks later, the patient shown in Fig. 16.37 has progressed to tissue loss, eschar formation, and mild changes in coagulation parameters. (Photo contributor: Sean P. Bush, MD.)

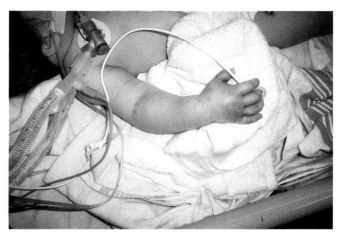

FIGURE 16.40 ■ Severe Rattlesnake Envenomation. This patient sustained a rattlesnake bite to his hand and presented with marked and progressive swelling, subcutaneous ecchymosis, and a significant coagulopathy. (Photo contributor: Sean P. Bush, MD.)

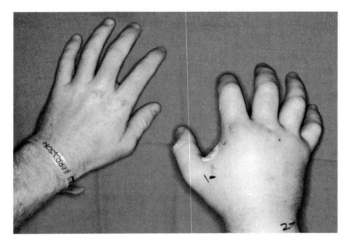

FIGURE 16.39 ■ Moderate Crotalid Envenomation. Patient was bitten by a rattlesnake on the dorsal aspect of the right hand who presented with edema extending to the wrist as well as nausea and vomiting. (Photo contributor: Edward J. Otten, MD.)

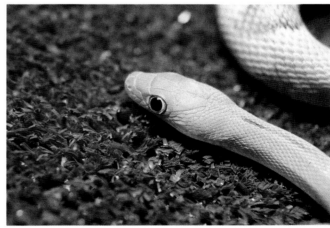

FIGURE 16.41 ■ Nonvenomous Snake. In contrast to the elliptical pupils and triangular head characteristic of pit vipers, this non-venomous rat snake has a rounded head and circular pupils. (Photo contributor: Sean P. Bush, MD.)

Clinical Summary

The black widow spider (*Latrodectus mactans*) is the prototype for the genus *Latrodectus*, several members of which cause human disease. The black widow spider is not particularly aggressive but will defend her web, which is often found in woodpiles, basements, and garages. Most envenomations occur between April and October, with bites most commonly located on the hand and forearm. The clinical presentation of severe and sustained muscle spasm is produced by a neurotoxic protein, which causes the release of acetylcholine and norepinephrine at the presynaptic neuromuscular junction. The initial bite may be mild to moderately painful and is often missed. Within approximately 1 hour, local erythema and muscle cramping begin, followed by generalized cramping involving large muscle groups such as the thighs, shoulders, abdomen, and back. Associated clinical features can include fasciculations, weakness, fever, salivation, vomiting, diaphoresis, localized sweating at the envenomation site, and a characteristic pattern of facial swelling called *Latrodectus* facies. Rare cases of seizures, uncontrolled hypertension, and respiratory arrest have occurred.

Emergency Department Treatment and Disposition

Treatment of the local wound should include cleansing and tetanus prophylaxis. Severe pain and spasm may require intravenous benzodiazepines and narcotics. Calcium gluconate infusion has long been recommended to reduce symptoms, although evidence for its efficacy is controversial. Antivenom exists and carries the same risk as all horse serum products. Antivenom should be strongly considered in cases of respiratory arrest, seizures, uncontrolled hypertension, and pregnancy.

Pearls

1. Of the five *Latrodectus* species indigenous to the United States, only three are black and only one has the orange-red hourglass marking.
2. Envenomations by *L mactans* can mimic an acute abdomen and should be considered in the differential diagnosis of patients presenting with severe acute abdominal pain.

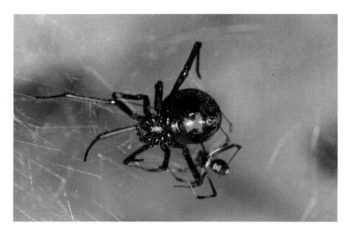

FIGURE 16.42 ■ Black Widow Spider (With Offspring). *Latrodectus mactans,* with characteristic hourglass marking on its abdomen. (Photo contributor: Lawrence B. Stack, MD.)

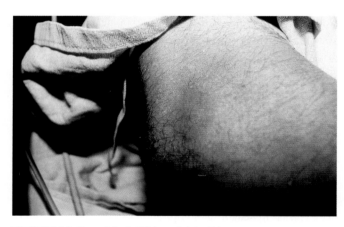

FIGURE 16.43 ■ Black Widow Spider Bite. The bite of the black widow spider is clinically subtle. Local reaction is usually trivial, as in this confirmed bite with a small patch of mild erythema. (Photo contributor: Gerald O'Malley, DO.)

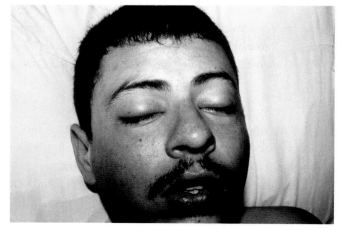

FIGURE 16.44 ■ Black Widow Facies. A pattern of facial swelling, known as *Latrodectus* facies, may occur several hours after envenomation. (Photo contributor: Gerald O'Malley, DO.)

Clinical Summary

The brown recluse spider (*Loxosceles reclusa*) is the prototypical member of the genus *Loxosceles*, which as a group can produce the typical necrotic arachnidism following envenomation. These small spiders (approximately 1 cm in body length and 3 cm in leg length) have a worldwide distribution and are identified by the striking fiddle-shaped markings on their anterodorsal cephalothorax. Initial envenomation may be painful, although patients often report no recollection of being bitten. Initial stinging gives way to aching and pruritus. The wound then may become edematous, with an erythematous halo surrounding a violaceous center. The erythematous margin often spreads in a pattern influenced by gravity, leaving the necrotic center near the superior aspect of the lesion. Bullae may erupt, and—over a period of 2 to 5 weeks—the eschar sloughs, leaving a deep, poorly healing ulcer. In approximately 10% of cases, systemic symptoms (loxoscelism) are present. Systemic features of brown recluse envenomation may include fever, nausea, vomiting, headache, morbilliform rash, arthralgias, and in severe cases, hemolytic anemia, coagulopathy, renal failure, and even death. Children are at higher risk of systemic disease.

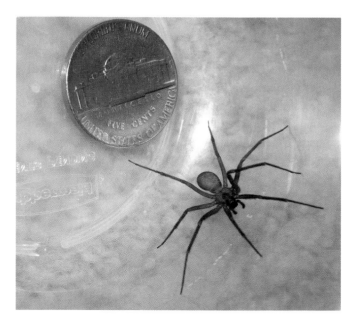

FIGURE 16.45 ■ Brown Recluse Spider. Brown recluse spider with characteristic "fiddle" marking on the anterodorsal aspect of the cephalothorax. (Photo contributor: R. Jason Thurman, MD.)

Emergency Department Treatment and Disposition

Most cutaneous lesions secondary to brown recluse spider bites can be managed with cold compresses, elevation, loose immobilization, and attention to tetanus immunization. Severe lesions may require reconstructive plastic surgery several weeks after wound stabilization. The use of dapsone to prevent lesion progression is controversial. Any systemic reaction with evidence of hemolysis, hemoglobinuria, or coagulopathy should prompt admission. Hyperbaric oxygen (HBO) therapy and antivenom have been suggested as possible adjuncts, but no clear consensus of preferred treatment has been established.

Pearls

1. The asymmetric spread of erythema, due to the local effects of gravity on the toxin, may help to distinguish a brown recluse spider bite from other arthropod envenomations.

2. If dapsone therapy is to be administered, screening for glucose-6-phosphate dehydrogenase (G6PD) deficiency should be considered.

3. Urinalysis may be helpful in identifying hemolysis early in the clinical course of system reactions.

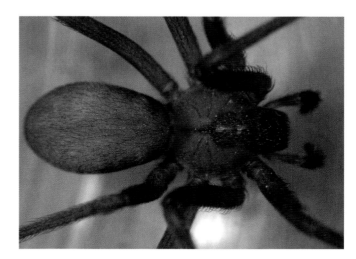

FIGURE 16.46 ■ Fiddle Back Marking. A close-up look at the characteristic fiddle back marking of the brown recluse spider. (Photo contributor: R. Jason Thurman, MD.)

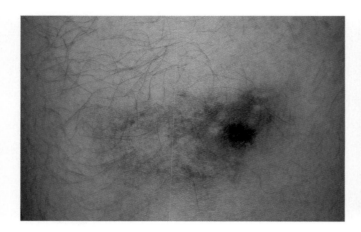

FIGURE 16.47 ■ Early Brown Recluse Spider Bite. Early brown recluse spider bite (approximately 8 hours) with a violaceous center surrounded by faint-spreading erythema. Note the "red, white, and blue" appearance. (Photo contributor: Lawrence B. Stack, MD.)

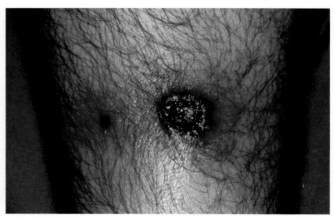

FIGURE 16.49A ■ Brown Recluse Spider Bite (4 days). Red, white, and blue appearance with significant asymmetric spread of erythema inferiorly down the leg beyond pen markings due to effect of gravity. (Photo contributor: R. Jason Thurman, MD.)

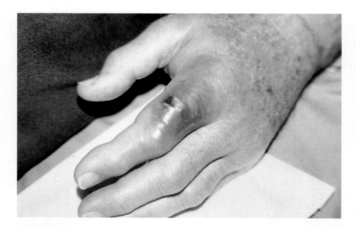

FIGURE 16.48 ■ Later Recluse Spider Bite (24 hours). Brown recluse spider bite at approximately 24 hours. Note asymmetric spread of erythema and early central ulcer formation. (Photo contributor: Edward Eitzen, MD, MPH.)

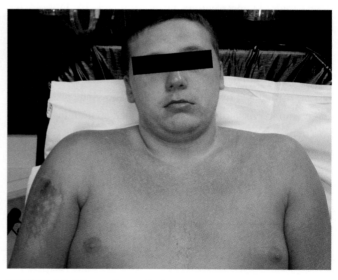

FIGURE 16.49B ■ Systemic Loxoscelism. This patient suffered fever, headache, and a diffuse erythematous rash as a result of systemic loxoscelism. Note the brown recluse envenomation on the patient's right arm. (Photo contributor: Shannon B. Snyder, MD.)

Clinical Summary

The most significant morbidity and mortality from scorpion stings is from the Buthidae family, characterized by a triangular central sternal plate. This family includes the venomous *Androctonus* genus in northern Africa, *Leiurus* in the Middle East, *Tityus* in South America, and *Centruroides* in North America.

Centruroides are found primarily in the southwestern United States and northern Mexico and are characterized by a variable subaculear tooth beneath the stinger, may be striped, and are yellow to brown in color. These scorpions tend to hide in crevices, woodpiles, bedding, clothing, and shoes. Envenomation produces a fairly mild local reaction of pain, swelling, burning, and ecchymosis.

Centruroides exilicauda (the bark scorpion) envenomation can lead to progressive symptoms and, very rarely, death. The venom of *C exilicauda* initially produces local paresthesias and pain (grade 1), which may be accentuated by tapping the involved area. More severe envenomations may produce remote paresthesias (grade II) and either somatic or autonomic nervous system dysfunction (grade III). Systemic symptoms may include tachycardia, nausea, wandering eye movements, blurred vision, difficulty breathing, trouble swallowing, restlessness, and involuntary shaking. Both somatic and autonomic dysfunction may be present (grade IV). Systemic reactions tend to be more severe in younger patients and may result in death, usually from respiratory arrest.

Emergency Department Treatment and Disposition

Treatment depends on the severity of envenomation. Grade I or II envenomations are treated with supportive care (ice, oral analgesia) and tetanus immunization. Envenomations that progress to grade III or IV must be treated aggressively and may require paralysis and intubation for severe spasms. Goat serum antivenom is available, but carries a risk of hypersensitivity reactions. Pain and paresthesias may persist for up to 2 weeks; but most systemic symptoms improve within 9 to 30 hours without antivenom treatment and usually peak at about 5 hours.

Pearls

1. Exercise caution when treating pain of *C exilicauda* envenomations with opioids, as synergistic respiratory depressive effects between venom and narcotics may occur.
2. If the scorpion is brought in, it should be examined for the presence of a triangular plate and subaculear tooth.
3. Almost all scorpions, including *C exilicauda,* fluoresce with intense brightness under cobalt light.

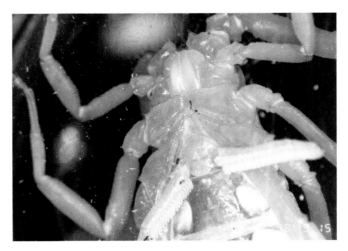

FIGURE 16.51 ■ Buthidae Sternal Plate. The triangular appearance of the sternal plate is well seen in this scorpion, a member of the Buthidae family. (Photo contributor: Sean P. Bush, MD.)

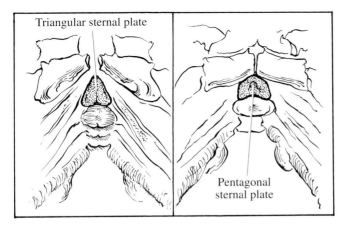

FIGURE 16.50 ■ Buthidae Sternal Plate. The Buthidae family is associated with the most significant envenomations and is characterized by triangular sternal plates (left). Members of the other scorpion families have pentagonal sternal plates (right).

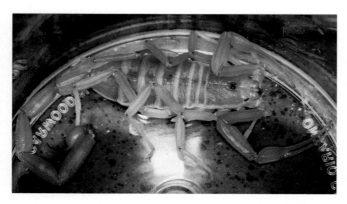

FIGURE 16.52 ■ *Centruroides exilicauda.* Members of this species are yellow to brown and usually less than 5 cm long. Below the stinger is the telson, within which are two glands containing venom. (Photo contributor: Sean P. Bush, MD.)

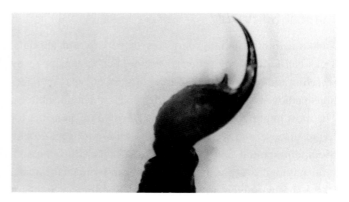

FIGURE 16.54 ■ *Centruroides limbatus.* Subaculear Tooth. A variable subaculear tooth is characteristic of *Centruroides.* This is an example of a large subaculear tooth on the telson from *C limbatus. Centruroides exilicauda* typically has a smaller, sometimes subtle "tooth." (Photo contributor: Sean P. Bush, MD.)

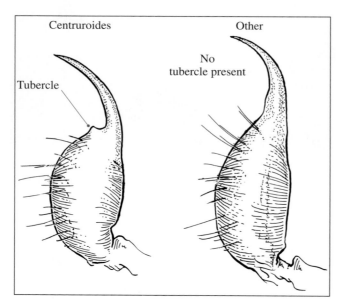

FIGURE 16.53 ■ Subaculear Tooth. The barb noted at the base of the stinger is variably present in *Centruroides* (left) and absent in other species (right).

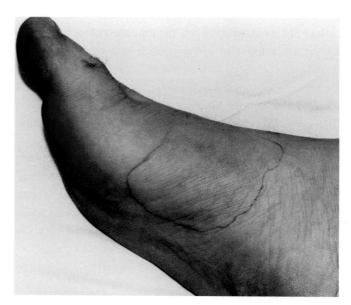

FIGURE 16.55 ■ Scorpion Sting. Most scorpion envenomations are mild and produce local pain, swelling, paresthesias, and mild ecchymosis. (Photo contributor: Stephen W. Corbett, MD.)

Clinical Summary

Ticks are blood-sucking parasites of people and animals. Ticks cause illness by acting as vectors for pathogens, or by secreting toxins or venoms. Ticks carry more types of infectious pathogens than any other arthropods except mosquitoes. The most important of these include *Borrelia* (responsible for Lyme disease and relapsing fever), *Rickettsia* (eg, Rocky Mountain spotted fever [RMSF]), *Ehrlichia* (Ehrlichiosis), viral pathogens (eg, Colorado tick fever), and babesiosis. Rashes are prominent in Lyme disease, RMSF, and Southern Tick Associated Rash Illness (STARI), sometimes present in relapsing fever, uncommon in Colorado tick fever, and absent in babesiosis.

Clinically important ticks in North America include *Ixodes dammini*, the deer tick (Lyme disease and babesiosis), *Dermacentor andersonii,* the wood tick (RMSF and Colorado tick fever), *D variabilis*, the dog tick (RMSF, Ehrlichiosis), and *Amblyomma americanum,* the lone star tick (a very widespread tick implicated in the transmission of Lyme disease outside of the range of *I dammini* as well as STARI and Erhlichiosis). More than 40 species of ticks can cause tick paralysis. In North America the most common cause is *D andersonii*, but *A americanum* and *Ixodes* species have also been associated with tick paralysis.

Tick paralysis develops 5 to 6 days after an adult female tick attaches. Over the next 24 to 48 hours, an ascending, symmetric, flaccid paralysis develops. Alternative presentations include ataxia and associated cerebellar findings without muscle weakness or isolated facial paralysis. Resolution of the paralysis after removal of the tick establishes the diagnosis.

Emergency Department Treatment and Disposition

If still embedded, the tick should be removed promptly by grasping it as close to the skin surface as possible, using blunt curved forceps or tweezers. The tick should be pulled out with slow, gentle traction, taking care not to crush or squeeze the body, which may result in injection of contaminated tick fluids. Other methods of tick removal—such as application of fingernail polish, isopropyl alcohol, or a hot match head—have not been proven to effect detachment and may induce regurgitation of tick contents into the wound.

Patients with tick paralysis may require supportive care, including mechanical ventilation. Patients with tick-borne illnesses may require admission for supportive care or intensive antibiotic treatment, but when clinically appropriate may be treated as an outpatient with appropriate antibiotic therapy.

Pearls

1. Prevention of tick bites includes the use of protective clothing containing *N,N*-diethylmetatoluamide (DEET).
2. A clear history of a tick bite is present in less than one-third of Lyme disease cases.
3. Unusual neurologic presentations, particularly bilateral peripheral seventh-nerve palsies, should prompt consideration of Lyme disease.

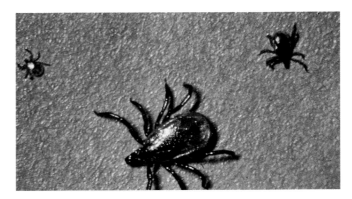

FIGURE 16.56 ■ Deer Tick. *Ixodes dammini*, the deer tick, is a vector of Lyme disease and babesiosis. (Photo contributor: the Centers for Disease Control and Prevention, Atlanta, GA.)

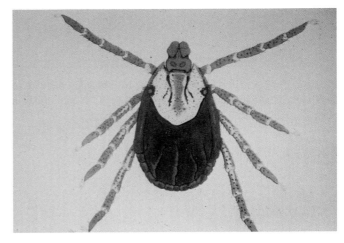

FIGURE 16.57 ■ Wood Tick. *Dermacentor andersonii*, the wood tick, is a vector of Rocky Mountain spotted fever and Colorado tick fever. (Photo contributor: the Centers for Disease Control and Prevention, Atlanta, GA.)

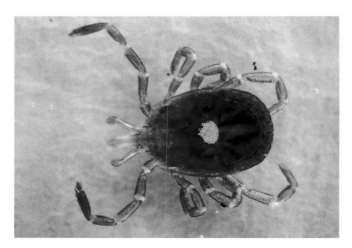

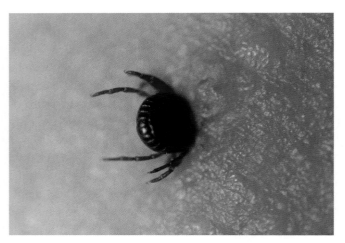

FIGURE 16.58 ■ Lone Star Tick. *Amblyomma americanum,* the lone star tick, has been implicated as a vector in Lyme disease. (Photo contributor: Sherman Minton, MD.)

FIGURE 16.59 ■ Imbedded Tick. This Lone Star tick was found imbedded into the patient's shoulder. It was easily removed intact with tweezers. (Photo contributor: R. Jason Thurman, MD.)

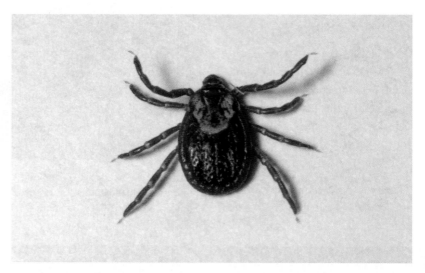

FIGURE 16.60 ■ American Dog Tick. *Dermacentor variabilis*, the dog tick, is a vector of Rocky Mountain spotted fever and ehrlichiosis. (Photo contributor: R. Jason Thurman, MD.)

Clinical Summary

The order Hymenoptera includes wasps, hornets, yellow jackets, bees, and ants. Envenomation usually results in local pain, mild erythema, swelling, and pruritus. Severe systemic or toxic reactions may occur from one or multiple stings, manifesting as gastrointestinal symptoms, headache, pyrexia, muscle spasms, or seizures. Anaphylaxis may occur within minutes from a single sting, and may cause death from airway obstruction and/or cardiovascular collapse. A serum sickness–type reaction may occur 7 to 14 days after envenomation.

Solenopsis invicta was imported from South America and is the most prominent fire ant in the United States. These ants are primarily found in the South and build mound nests in open grass settings, commonly in urban yards. Disturbing the nests may result in severe swarming attacks, a common occurrence in the unsuspecting barefoot victim. Bites are painful and produce sterile pustules that crust over in a few days.

Emergency Department Treatment and Disposition

Anaphylaxis is treated with conventional therapy with careful attention to airway management. Local reactions may be treated with ice packs, steroid cream, and oral antihistamines. Narcotics may be needed for severe pain.

Pearls

1. Honeybee stings are usually apparent since the stinger apparatus, including barb and venom sac, is often detached and present on the patient's skin. These should be removed by scraping them off, as grasping with tweezers may result in the release of more venom.

2. "Brazilian killer" or "Africanized" bees are present primarily in the southwestern United States. Their venom is not known to be more toxic; however, their aggressiveness, tendency to swarm in large numbers, and ability to travel long distances make them potentially more dangerous to humans.

3. Care should be taken to immediately remove any rings when envenomations are located on the hands or feet, as marked local swelling can occur, putting the distal digits at risk for ischemia.

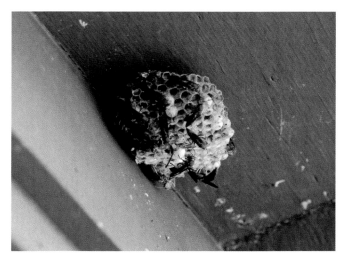

FIGURE 16.62 ■ Paper Wasp Nest. A typical paper wasp net in a roof corner. Disturbance of a nest may result in swarming attacks. (Photo contributor: Clay B. Smith, MD.)

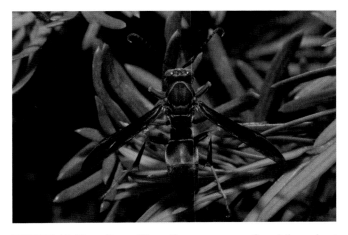

FIGURE 16.61 ■ Paper Wasp. Paper wasps are found throughout the world and often establish nests close to or within human dwellings. (Photo contributor: R. Jason Thurman, MD.)

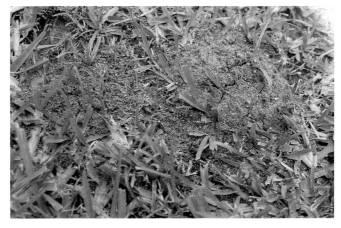

FIGURE 16.63 ■ Fire Ant Mound. This typical fire ant mound is a raised area of dirt in an urban yard. (Photo contributor: Alan B. Storrow, MD.)

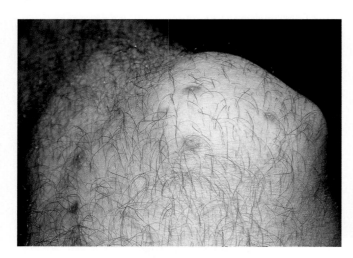

FIGURE 16.64 ■ Fire Ant Bites. These fire ant bites on the anterior knee occurred after this patient knelt on a mound. These bites are 3 days old; the initial sterile pustules have begun to crust over. (Photo contributor: Alan B. Storrow, MD.)

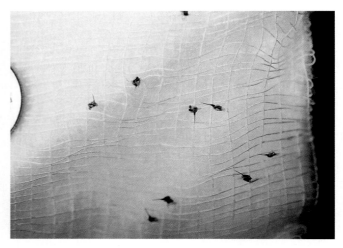

FIGURE 16.66 ■ Honeybee Stingers. The barbs and attached venom sacs (stinger apparatus) after removal from the patient. (Photo contributor: Alan B. Storrow, MD.)

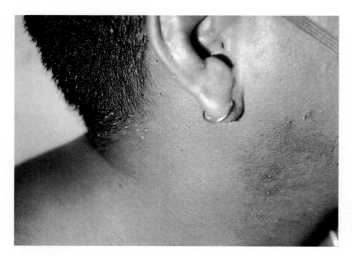

FIGURE 16.65 ■ Honeybee Envenomation. Many honeybee stingers (barbs and venom sacs) are seen on this patient's cheek and ear and along the hairline. (Photo contributor: Alan B. Storrow, MD.)

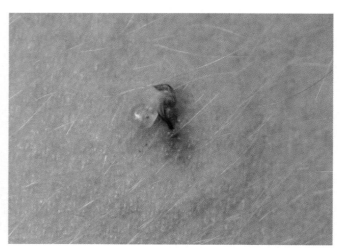

FIGURE 16.67 ■ Imbedded Honeybee Stinger. Note the venom sac, still pulsating and attached to the honeybee stinger imbedded in the victim. (Photo contributor: Lawrence B. Stack, MD.)

Clinical Summary

Caterpillar venom apparatus typically consists of barbed spines arranged in clumps or scattered about the dorsal surface of the insect. These are purely defensive in nature, and patients who are stung commonly have intentionally handled the insect or have had accidental skin contact while gardening. Envenomated patients typically present with acute pain followed by focal erythema and swelling. Caterpillars with a less sophisticated venom apparatus or low-potency venom may cause simple focal pruritus or urticaria, though some caterpillars are capable of producing a very painful sting requiring aggressive pharmacological pain control. Systemic symptoms are rare. The puss caterpillar, or wooly slug (*Megalopyge opercularis*) is perhaps the most famous and important venomous caterpillar in the United States. Found throughout the country, it appears hairy and flat and may reach a length of 4 cm.

Chiggers are the larvae of trombiculid mites and may inflict multiple intensely pruritic bites on their victims. They are parasitic only as larvae and infest humans by crawling onto them and latching on. Proper clothing precautions and repellents are usually effective in reducing unpleasant chigger infestations.

Centipedes are venomous arthropods that have one pair of legs per body segment. The first segment contains hollow curved "fangs" (really modified legs) bearing venom glands at the bases, which are capable of penetrating human skin. Centipedes generally use venom to kill prey, but when provoked, may envenomate humans and produce local intense burning pain, erythema, and swelling. Systemic reactions may occur but are uncommon.

Emergency Department Treatment and Disposition

Treatment of caterpillar, mite, and centipede envenomations is purely supportive and consists of pain control, antihistamines, topical antipruritic creams, and basic wound care.

Pearls

1. Infiltration with local anesthetics may be useful in markedly painful centipede envenomations or for the removal of retained "fang" fragments.
2. Attached caterpillar spines may be removed easily with adhesive tape.
3. The caudal appendages of centipedes are not associated with a venom apparatus.

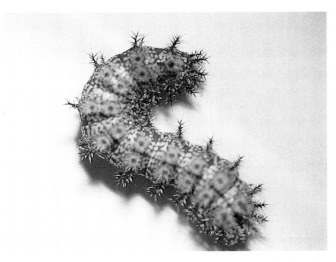

FIGURE 16.68 ■ Caterpillar with Barbed Spines. Typical garden caterpillar with barbed spines arranged in clumps. (Photo contributor: Alan B. Storrow, MD.)

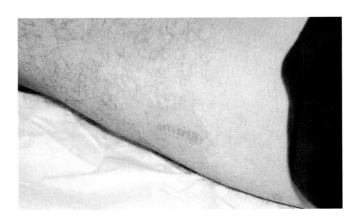

FIGURE 16.69 ■ Caterpillar Sting. Appearance of a caterpillar sting at 2 hours. The patient presented with moderate pain and severe itching. Note how the erythema follows the pattern of the caterpillar. (Photo contributor: Alan B. Storrow, MD.)

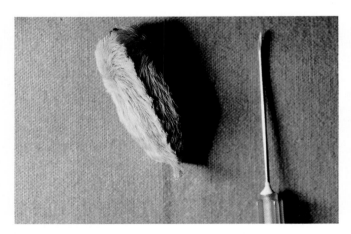

FIGURE 16.70 ▪ Puss Caterpillar. The "puss caterpillar" or "woolly slug" is likely the most important venomous caterpillar in the United States. The hairy appearance and small hair tail is characteristic. (Photo contributor: Alan B. Storrow, MD.)

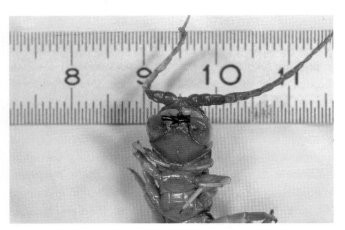

FIGURE 16.71 ▪ Centipede. Note the curved "fangs" (actually modified legs) on the first segment of this centipede from Texas. (Photo contributor: Alan B. Storrow, MD.)

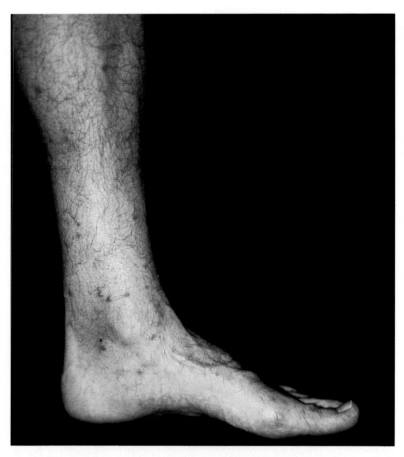

FIGURE 16.72 ▪ Chigger Bites. Chigger bites on a leg appear as puncta surrounded by erythema. (Photo contributor: Kevin J. Knoop, MD, MS.)

Clinical Summary

A middle ear squeeze (barotitis media) results from a decrease in pressure within the middle ear as an individual descends through water or is exposed to an increase in atmospheric pressure that can be seen in descending aircraft or while driving in mountainous terrain. According to Boyle's law, as pressure increases, volume must decrease proportionately. At a depth of approximately 4 ft, the pressure difference is great enough to collapse the eustachian tube and cause obstruction. If attempts to equalize the pressure (eg, Valsalva or Frenzel maneuver) fail, ascent is necessary or injury may ensue. If a diver continues to descend, hemorrhage and edema occur within the middle ear and rupture of the tympanic membrane (TM) may occur. The influx of water into the middle ear may cause extreme vertigo and lead to a diving disaster.

Barotitis media may present with pain only (grade 0), TM erythema (grade 1), erythema and mild TM hemorrhage (grade 2), gross TM hemorrhage (grade 3), free middle ear blood (grade 4), or free blood with TM perforation (grade 5).

Emergency Department Treatment and Disposition

Treatment includes decongestants and appropriate analgesia. Antihistamines may be of use for allergy-related eustachian tube dysfunction. Antibiotics are recommended for preexisting infections or for TM rupture. Most cases resolve spontaneously within hours to days. The patient should not resume diving until the condition has resolved or the TM is completely healed.

Pearls

1. Barotitis media is the most common medical problem associated with diving.
2. Associated barotraumatic injuries should be considered when the diagnosis of barotitis media is made.

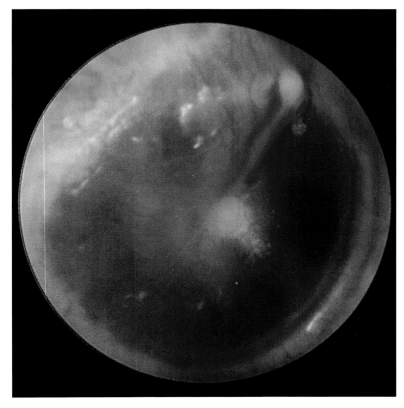

FIGURE 16.73 ■ Barotitis Media. Tympanic membrane erythema and mild hemorrhage consistent with barotitis media. (Photo contributor: Richard A. Chole, MD, PhD.)

Clinical Summary

Mask squeeze results when a diver fails to maintain the balance between the air pressure within his or her mask and the external water pressure during descent. If a diver descends without equalizing pressure by exhaling through the nose, significant negative air pressure will exist inside the mask. The net result may include rupture of capillary beds, leading to conjunctival hemorrhage and skin ecchymosis.

Emergency Department Treatment and Disposition

Treatment consists of ascent and essentially supportive care. A history of recent eye surgery or use of anticoagulant medication should be sought. A thorough eye examination should be performed and ophthalmologic consultation considered if warranted.

Pearls

1. Diver education and proper diving technique minimize the risk of mask squeeze.
2. Special consideration should be given to patients with anticoagulant use or recent keratotomy, as corneal incisions heal relatively slowly.

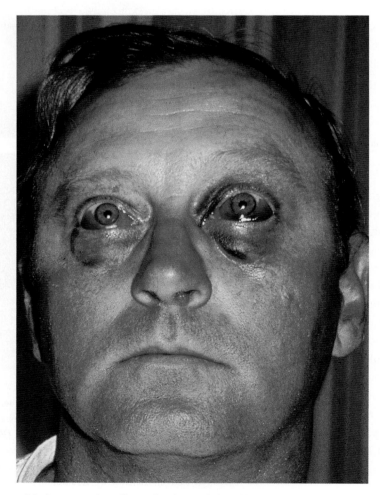

FIGURE 16.74 ■ Mask Squeeze. Mask squeeze in a diver who descended to 45 FSW without exhaling into his mask. (Photo contributor: Kenneth W. Kizer, MD; reprinted with permission from Auerbach PS (ed). *Wilderness Medicine: Management of Wilderness and Environmental Emergencies.* 3rd ed. St. Louis, MO: Mosby-Year Book; 1995.)

Clinical Summary

Stingrays are found throughout the oceans of the world. Stingrays are not typically aggressive and the majority of envenomations are defensive in nature. Injuries typically involve the lower extremity if the animal is stepped upon or upper extremity if the animal is handled. Fatal injuries have been reported from chest trauma, which may result in perforation of the myocardium. Stingray envenomation occurs when a reflexive and forceful forward thrust of the caudal spine or spines of the animal impacts the victim, producing a puncture wound or laceration. The force of injection causes the integumentary sheath covering the spine to be driven into the wound, fragmenting and potentially releasing venom, mucus, pieces of the sheath, and spine fragments deep within the wound. Envenomation typically produces immediate and intense pain, edema, and bleeding. The initially dusky or cyanotic wound may progress to erythema, with rapid fat and muscle hemorrhage. Systemic symptoms may include nausea, vomiting, diarrhea, diaphoresis, muscle cramps, fasciculations, weakness, headache, vertigo, paralysis, seizures, hypotension, and syncope.

Emergency Department Treatment and Disposition

The wound should be irrigated immediately and primary exploration accomplished to remove any visible debris. Pain relief should be initiated early, and narcotics may be needed. Stingray venom is made up of heat labile polypeptides that may be inactivated by immersion in hot water (43°C-46°C [110°F-115°F]) for 30 to 90 minutes. After soaking, wounds should be formally explored, debrided, and dressed for delayed primary closure or primary closure with drainage. Surgical consultation may be warranted in certain injury locations. A radiograph should be obtained after debridment to rule out retained foreign body. Broad-spectrum antibiotics covering marine organisms are recommended. Patients can usually be discharged home after a 3- to 4-hour observation period if no systemic symptoms arise. Tetanus prophylaxis should be given if indicated.

Pearls

1. Aggressive debridement is of primary importance in managing stingray wounds, as retained foreign bodies are a common problem.
2. Bacteria cultured from marine envenomations are extremely diverse. Antibiotics chosen should include coverage of staphylococci, streptococci, and *Vibrio* species.

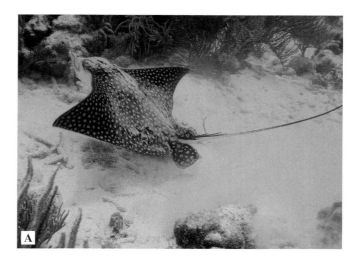

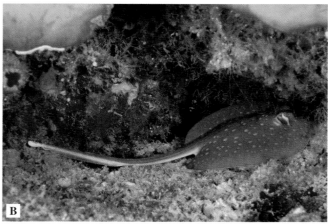

FIGURE 16.75 ■ Stingrays. (**A**) Spotted Eagle Stingray. This graceful stingray was photographed in waters off the coast of Bonaire. Note the three venomous spines at the base of the tail. (Courtesy of Lynne Bensten, RN); (**B**) Blue Spotted Stingray. This stingray was photographed in waters off Indonesia. Stingrays often dwell on the ocean floor and may burrow into the sand, leading to envenomation by accidentally stepping on the animal. (Photo contributor: Ian D. Jones, MD.)

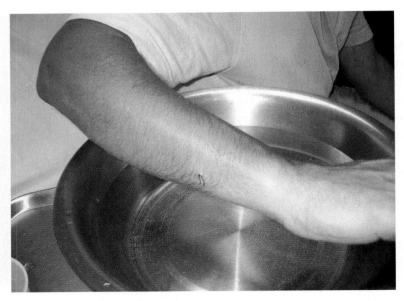

FIGURE 16.76 ▪ Stingray Barb in Forearm. This envenomation occurred after the fisherman inadvertently caught a stingray and was envenonmated taking the animal off the hook. The barb is imbedded in the patients forearm. (Photo contributor: John Meade, MD.)

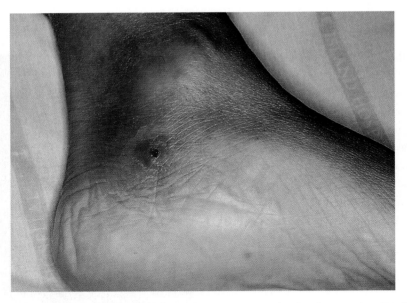

FIGURE 16.77 ▪ Stingray Envenomation. Puncture wound from stingray envenomation in a lower extremity. (Photo contributor: Daniel L. Savitt, MD.)

Clinical Summary

Sea urchins belong to the phylum Echinodermata and are nonaggressive, slow-moving creatures. Envenomation usually occurs after accidental contact with the organism. Long, brittle, venom-filled spines or specialized jaw-like appendages (pedicellariae) are responsible for the injury. Other echinoderms, notably the crown of thorns starfish, may also cause injury via similar mechanisms. The spines frequently break and pedicellariae can remain attached and active for several hours. They may advance into muscle or joint spaces and cause infection or injury from the venom itself. The usual presentation is burning pain progressing to localized muscle aches. Erythema and edema may be present. Multiple envenomations may produce systemic symptoms including nausea, vomiting, abdominal pain, paresthesias, numbness, paralysis, hypotension, syncope, or respiratory distress. While the envenomation causes a reaction that may be quite painful, deaths, though reported, are exceedingly rare.

Emergency Department Treatment and Disposition

Following envenomation, the affected area should be submersed in hot water (43°C-46°C [110°F-115°F]) for 30 to 90 minutes. Pedicellariae may be removed by applying shaving cream and gently scraping with a razor. Obvious embedded spines should be removed. An x-ray should be performed to rule out retained foreign body. In certain cases, CT, ultrasound, or MRI may be considered. Hand wounds often require surgical debridement. Retained spines often dissolve spontaneously; however, granulomas may form, producing locally destructive inflammation. Antibiotics may be useful in certain cases, and tetanus prophylaxis should be addressed.

Pearls

1. Sea urchin envenomation involving a joint may produce severe synovitis.
2. Some species of sea urchin contain dye, which may give the false impression of a retained spine.
3. Sea urchins known to be hazardous to humans are generally found in the Indian Ocean, Pacific Ocean, and Red Sea.

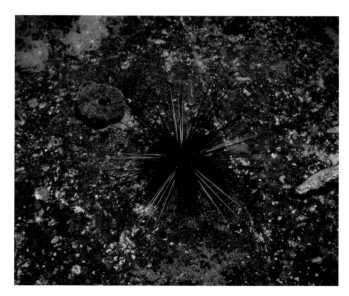

FIGURE 16.78 ■ Long Spined Sea Urchin. The majority of urchins are nonvenomous and only cause injury from puncture wounds. Their spines may break off in the victim, resulting in a high likelihood of infection. (Photo contributor: Ian D. Jones, MD.)

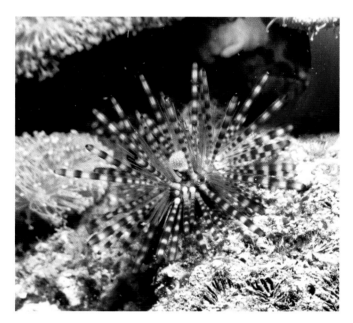

FIGURE 16.79 ■ Fire Urchin. Fire urchins are venomous sea urchins. Envenomations from fire urchins, while extremely painful, are seldom if ever fatal. (Photo contributor: Ian D. Jones, MD.)

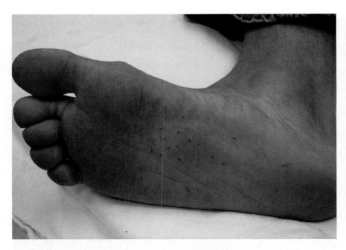

FIGURE 16.80 ■ Sea Urchin Envenomation. Note the multiple puncture wounds on the foot of a patient who accidentally stepped on a sea urchin in shallow water. (Photo contributor: Saralyn R. Williams, MD.)

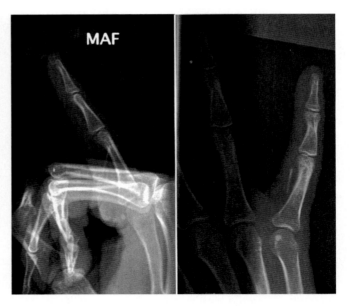

FIGURE 16.82 ■ Sea Urchin Spine on X-Ray. This x-ray is of a patient who was reaching into a rock crevasse in the ocean and experienced sudden sharp pain. Note the retained sea urchin spine in the fifth digit adjacent to the proximal phalynx. (Photo contributor: Marion Berg, MD.)

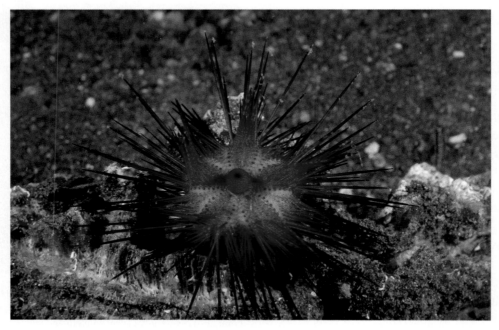

FIGURE 16.81 ■ Fire Urchin. A beautiful fire urchin, found in the Indo-Pacific. (Photo contributor: Ian D. Jones, MD.)

COELENTERATE ENVENOMATION

Clinical Summary

The phylum Coelenterata contains approximately 10,000 different species, of which several hundred are a danger to humans. This diverse group includes hydrozoans (eg, Portuguese man-of-war, stinging hydrozoans, and fire coral), scyphozoans (ie, "true" jellyfish), and anthozoans (ie, soft corals, stony corals, and anemones). They account for more marine envenomations than any other phylum. The important species involved in human injuries have stinging cells called nematocysts. Nematocysts are enclosed in venom sacs and are present in tentacles that hang from air-filled structures. After external contact, the nematocysts are discharged from their sacs, often penetrating the skin, and release their venom. Nematocyst venom is an extremely complex substance containing numerous proteins and enzymes. Clinical presentation following envenomation ranges from the mild dermatitis to cardiovascular and pulmonary collapse. Mild envenomations usually result in a self-limited papular inflammatory eruption associated with burning and limited to areas of contact. Moderate to severe envenomations produce a spectrum of neurologic, cardiovascular, respiratory, and gastrointestinal symptoms. Anaphylactoid reactions—including hypotension, dysrhythmias, bronchospasm, and cardiovascular collapse—may occur, resulting in unexplained drownings.

Emergency Department Treatment and Disposition

Concurrently with primary resuscitation, nematocyst decontamination should be accomplished beginning with seawater flushing. The hypotonic nature of fresh water, as well as isopropyl alcohol, may cause additional nematocysts to fire and should be avoided. A 5% solution of acetic acid (vinegar) applied for at least 30 minutes is the most widely accepted mechanism for inactivating nematocysts. It has been suggested to remove tentacles with the application of shaving cream, followed in 5 minutes by a careful scraping with a firm, dull object (eg, tongue blade, credit card). Pruritus may be treated with antihistamines. Pain may be addressed with immersion in hot water or with systemic analgesics. Any victim with systemic symptoms requires at least 6 to 8 hours of observation because rebound phenomena are common.

Pearls

1. The box jellyfish (*Chironex fleckeri*) is generally considered the most deadly of marine animals and is most predominant in Australian and Southeast Asian waters.
2. The detached tentacles of some species may contain active nematocysts for months, even when fragmented on the beach or floating in water.
3. The Portuguese man-of-war is present in the Floridian Atlantic coast and the Gulf of Mexico. It is known to have a neurotoxin that may cause severe pain. Death, while reported, is extremely rare.

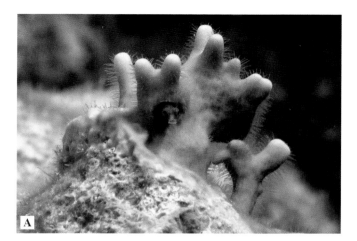

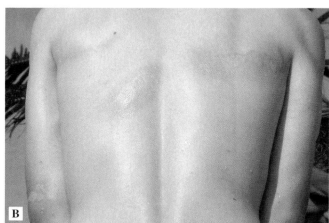

FIGURE 16.83 ■ Fire Coral. (**A**) Fire coral. (Photo contributor: Ian D. Jones, MD); (**B**) Fire coral envenomation. After contact, fire coral most commonly causes immediate local burning pain, followed by erythematous papules or urticarial eruptions. Pruritus may last for several days. (Photo contributor: Emily R. Stack.)

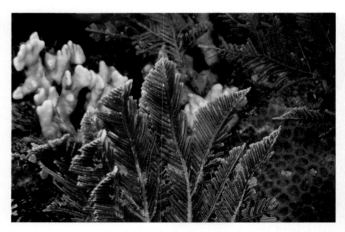

FIGURE 16.84 ▪ Stinging Hydrozoan. Similar to fire coral, contact with stinging hydrozoan results in local burning pain followed by erythematous papules or urticarial eruptions and blisters. (Photo contributor: Ian D. Jones, MD.)

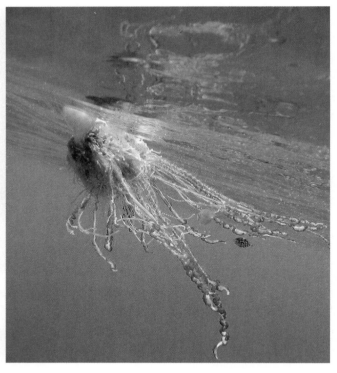

FIGURE 16.86 ▪ Portuguese Man-O-War. The beautiful Portuguese Man-O-War with multiple tentacles dangling in the water. The tentacles, filled with venomous nematocysts, can extend several meters in length. (Photo contributor: Adam Laverty)

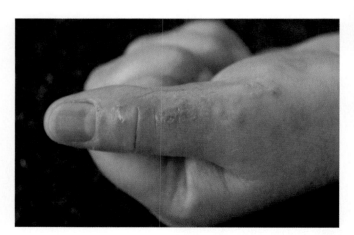

FIGURE 16.85 ▪ Hydrozoan Envenomation. This hydrozoan sting resulted from accidental direct contact with the diver's finger while taking an underwater photograph. (Photo contributor: Ian D. Jones, MD.)

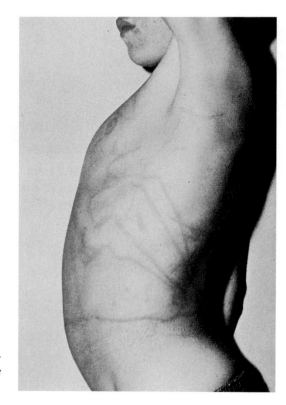

FIGURE 16.87 ▪ Coelenterate Envenomation. The sharp angulations and undulations characteristic of jellyfish envenomation. (From Halstead BH. *Venomous Marine Animals of the World*. Washington, DC: US Government Printing Office; 1965.)

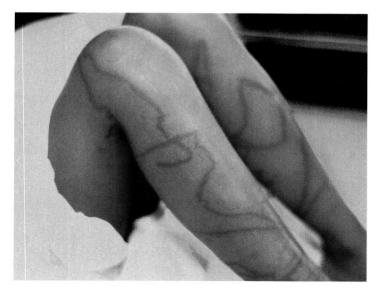

FIGURE 16.88 ■ Coelenterate Envenomation. Jellyfish envenomation on the lower extremities. (Photo contributor: the Department of Dermatology, Naval Medical Center, Portsmouth, VA.)

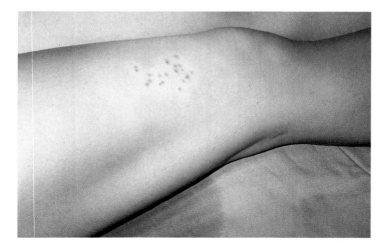

FIGURE 16.89 ■ Sea Anemone Tattooing. Contact with sea anemones results mainly in local skin irritation, initially manifest as pruritus, burning, throbbing, and, sometimes radiation of pain to other areas. The area involved may reveal blistering, local edema, and violaceous petechial hemorrhages. The skin papules are confined to the areas of contact and may persist for 7 to 10 days. (Photo contributor: Gerald O'Malley, DO.)

Clinical Summary

Marine dermatitis, also known as "sea bather's eruption," is a pruritic condition commonly mislabelled *sea lice.* Symptoms usually occur a few minutes to 12 hours after exposure. The offending organisms are probably numerous and include the larval form of the thimble jellyfish and the planula form of the sea anemone *Edwardsiella lineata.* The rash consists of erythematous wheals and papules, which may be extremely pruritic. Systemic manifestations include fever, malaise, headache, conjunctivitis, and urethritis. Unlike cercarial dermatitis, marine dermatitis primarily affects areas of the body covered by caps, fins, and bathing suits.

Cercarial dermatitis, or "swimmer's itch," occurs when humans become accidental hosts of nonhuman schistosomes. This causes an immune response that results in itching, erythema, and mild edema. After 60 minutes, the classic signs are red macules that become pruritic papules 3 to 5 cm in diameter and surrounded by erythema.

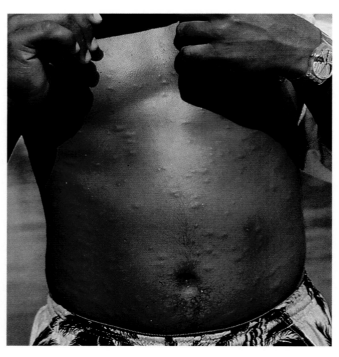

FIGURE 16.90 ■ Marine Dermatitis. Typical appearance of marine dermatitis. (Photo contributor: Richard A. Clinchy III, PhD.)

Emergency Department Treatment and Disposition

Marine dermatitis is self-limited, rarely persisting beyond 2 weeks. The dermatitis may be partially prevented by a vigorous soap-and-water scrub after saltwater bathing. Treatment is symptomatic, and calamine lotion with 1% menthol may bring relief. Topical steroids may provide additional relief. In severe cases, oral antihistamines and corticosteroids may be necessary.

Cercarial dermatitis is treated with isopropyl alcohol or calamine lotion. Severe cases may require systemic corticosteroids, whereas bacterial infection may require topical or oral antibiotics.

Pearls

1. Marine dermatitis primarily affects areas covered by caps, fins, and bathing suits.
2. During late spring and summer, incidence increases along the US east coast. In one reported outbreak, 25% of individuals entering the water were affected.

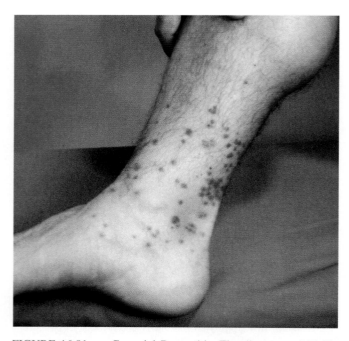

FIGURE 16.91 ■ Cercarial Dermatitis. The discrete and highly pruritic papules of cercarial dermatitis commonly occur on exposed body areas. (Photo contributor: David O. Parrish, MD. Used with permission from Parrish DO. Seabather's eruption or diver's dermatitis. *JAMA.* 1993;270:2300-2301.)

Clinical Summary

Scorpion fish are colorful venomous marine animals found primarily in tropical waters. Their exotic beautiful appearance has made them increasingly popular among marine aquarists in the United States. Many envenomations have resulted from mishandling. They are well camouflaged in the wild and stings are usually caused by accidentally stepping on them. Scorpion fish are grouped into the genera *Pterois* (lion fish), *Scorpaena* (scorpion fish proper), and *Synanceja* (stone fish), with the severity of envenomation progressing respectively. All have multiple spines associated with venom glands; envenomation results from skin puncture followed by venom release. Immediately following a sting, the victim experiences intense pain that, if untreated, lasts for hours. The site may become warm, erythematous, and edematous and vesicles may arise. Lion fish stings are painful but relatively mild, usually limited to localized pain and tissue responses. Severe systemic effects are more common with stone fish stings and may produce a constellation of cardiovascular, pulmonary, neurologic, and gastrointestinal sequelae. Death has been reported from stone fish stings.

Emergency Department Treatment and Disposition

Hot water immersion (43°C-46°C [110°F-115°F]) for 30 to 90 minutes is initiated as soon as possible. Rebound pain is common and is treated with repeated hot water immersion. The wound should be inspected for pieces of spine and sheath. Thorough warm saline irrigation should be performed along with wound exploration. Severe pain is treated with local injection of lidocaine without epinephrine and with narcotic analgesia. Antibiotic prophylaxis should be considered in high-risk wounds and tetanus status addressed.

Pearls

1. Stone fish stings are the most dangerous. Severe systemic reactions may occur. Antivenin (Commonwealth Serum Labs, Australia) is available.
2. Scorpion fish venom is heat-labile. Hot water immersion is effective in treating pain and inactivating venom.
3. Since 2002, Indo-Pacific lionfish have been reported in increasing numbers from New York to the Bahamas.

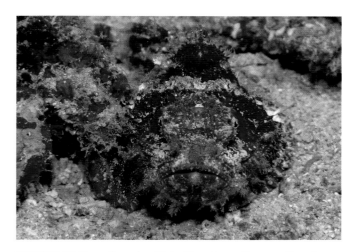

FIGURE 16.93 ■ Scorpion Fish. Note the well-camouflaged scorpion fish, leading to accidental contact and envenomation in unsuspecting divers. (Photo contributor: Ian D. Jones, MD.)

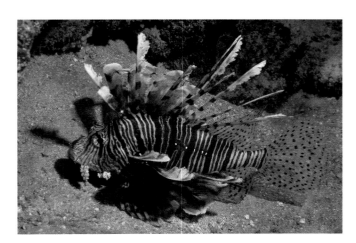

FIGURE 16.92 ■ Lion Fish *(Pterois volitans)*. Envenomations occur by contact with the erectile spines on the dorsal, pelvic, and anal fins of the fish. (Photo contributor: Ian D. Jones, MD.)

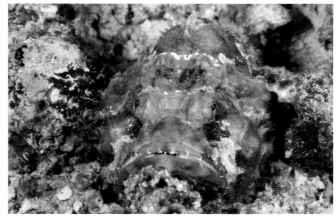

FIGURE 16.94 ■ Stonefish. The extremely venomous stonefish is spectacularly camouflaged. Envenomation usually results when the unsuspecting victim steps on the fish. (Photo contributor: Ian D. Jones, MD.)

Clinical Summary

Sea snakes are members of the elapid family of snakes which have evolved to survive in a variety of ocean habitats. There are over 70 species of sea snakes with the majority found in the tropical portions of the Indian and Pacific Oceans. Sea snakes are not found in the Atlantic or Carribean. Most species of sea snakes live close to the coast although there is a pelagic species, *Pelamis platurus* that is found across a large swath of the Pacific Ocean. Reports vary regarding the docile nature of sea snakes, although it is well reported that some species have a much higher propensity to bite. Bites occur when the animal is disturbed or inadvertently handled. There are many reports of bites occurring as fishermen are removing the snake from their nets. Because of the small size of the organism's fangs, bites may be inconspicuous and are often painless. The majority of bites do not result in envenomation.

The most potent toxin in sea snake venoms, similar to other elapids, is a neurotoxin that competes for acetylcholine at the neuromuscular junction. Severe envenomations may ultimately lead to paralysis and respiratory failure. Additional components of the venom are myotoxic and may result in rhabdomyolysis and renal failure.

The symptoms of sea snake envenomation generally occur within 30 minutes of envenomation and may be quite variable. Common symptoms include confusion, headache, myalgias, weakness of the facial muscles, followed by an ascending flaccid paralysis and ultimately respiratory arrest.

Emergency Department Treatment and Disposition

Treatment for a sea snake bite includes a combination of supportive care and the immediate administration of polyvalent sea snake antivenom. Supportive care should include intubation if indicated. The patient should also be carefully observed for signs of rhabdomyolysis and hyperkalemia. The patient should be aggressively hydrated to avoid further complications such as renal failure. Consultation with a toxicologist or individual experienced in managing sea snake envenomations should be considered.

Pearls

1. An effective polyvalent antivenom exists and is effective against envenomation from all species of sea snakes.
2. In addition to respiratory support, victims of sea snake envenomation should be observed for the development of rhabdomyolysis and hyperkalemia.

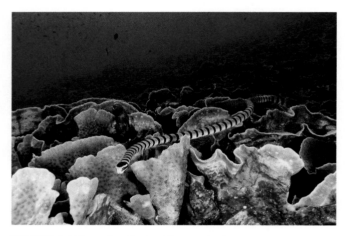

FIGURE 16.95 ■ Sea Snake. The sea krait, seen here swimming free in the ocean, is very docile and rarely bites humans unless provoked. (Photo contributor: Ian D. Jones, MD.)

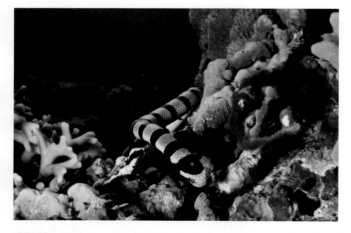

FIGURE 16.96 ■ Sea Snake. A close-up of a sea snake found feeding on a reef. (Photo contributor: Ian D. Jones, MD.)

CEPHALOPOD ENVENOMATION

Clinical Summary

There are over 750 species of cephalopods found throughout the world's oceans. Cephalopods are members of the phylum mollusca and include cuttlefish, squid, octopuses, and the nautilus. Several species of cephalopods are known or thought to be venomous but only the blue-ringed octopus, genus *Hapalochlaena*, poses a significant threat to humans.

Four separate species of blue-ringed octopus are known to exist. All are small and none exceed a few inches in size. The animal is found in tide pools and shallow reefs across a wide area of the Indo-Pacific ranging from Japan to Australia. The blue-ringed octopus is generally not aggressive and is relatively nondescript when left in peace. When threatened, however, the animal will flash or pulsate with striking iridescent blue rings. Bites occur when the animal is disturbed or inadvertently handled. It may be found hiding in old bottles or shells in tidal pools and in this way poses a hazard to collectors. Like other cephalopods, the blue-ringed octopus has a beak that can be powerful enough to penetrate a wet suit. Some bites may be relatively painless.

Blue-ringed octopus venom has several identified components. The most powerful component of the venom, tetrodotoxin, is a potent sodium channel blocker that is identical to the toxin found in pufferfish. Once bitten, symptoms may develop in as few as 10 minutes and include perioral paresthesias, facial weakness, and nausea and vomiting. In some patients, especially children, hypotension may be present. As symptoms progress, flaccid paralysis and respiratory arrest may result.

Emergency Department Treatment and Disposition

Treatment for a blue-ringed octopus bite is entirely supportive, as no antivenin currently exists. The patient almost always has a normal sensorium unless profoundly hypoxic or hypercarbic. Primary management of severe envenomations includes management of hypotension and prolonged ventilatory support until the toxin can be degraded and excreted.

Pearls

1. No antivenin exists for a blue-ringed octopus envenomation.
2. The patient's mental status is usually normal and a victim may be fully conscious despite being paralyzed and apneic.

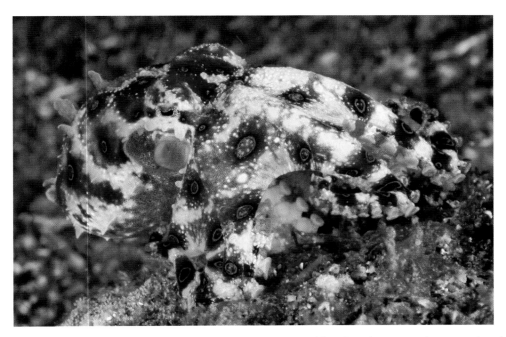

FIGURE 16.97 ■ Blue-Ringed Octopus. The beautiful but highly venomous blue-ringed octopus, demonstrating the iridescent blue colorations seen when the animal is threatened. (Photo contributor: Ian D. Jones, MD.)

Clinical Summary

Erysipeloid, also known as "fish handler's disease," is a bacterial skin infection caused by *Erysipelothrix rhusiopathiae*. This condition is frequently seen in those who handle raw meat, fish, and shellfish. The offending organism enters the body through a break in the skin and causes a local infection within 2 to 7 days. Lesions are characterized by an edematous central purplish-red area, surrounded first by central clearing and then circumscribed by an advancing raised, erythematous ring. The area is usually pruritic and painful and may be associated with fever, malaise, and regional lymphadenopathy.

Emergency Department Treatment and Disposition

If left untreated, erysipeloid will usually resolve spontaneously in about 3 weeks. Skin infections may be treated with penicillin VK, cephalexin, or erythromycin. If severe infection occurs, it should be treated with appropriate broad-spectrum antibiotics.

Pearls

1. A history of occupational or recreational exposure to fish or shellfish is the key to diagnosis.
2. *Erysipelothrix rhusiopathiae* is usually resistant to aminoglycoside antibiotics, thus these should be avoided.

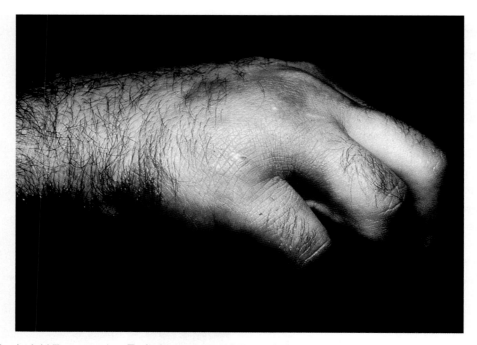

FIGURE 16.98 ■ Erysipeloid Envenomation. Typical appearance of *Erysipelothrix rhusiopathiae* skin infection. (Photo contributor: Paul S. Auerbach, MD; Reprinted with permission from Auerbach PS (ed). *Wilderness Medicine: Management of Wilderness and Environmental Emergencies.* 3rd ed. St. Louis, MO: Mosby-Year Book; 1995.)

Clinical Summary

Poison ivy, oak, and sumac cause more cases of allergic contact dermatitis than all other allergens combined. At least 70% of the US population is sensitive to the *Toxicodendron* species.

The dermatitis begins as pruritus and redness usually within 2 days of exposure in susceptible persons. The degree of dermatitis depends on the patient's degree of sensitivity, amount of allergen exposure, and the reactivity of the skin at the exposed body location. The dermatitis may vary from erythema to erythema with papules to erythema with vesicles and bullae. A linear distribution of the cutaneous lesions is strongly suggestive of *toxicodendron* dermatitis. This distribution occurs after contaminated fingernails have scratched the skin or plant parts rubbed against it.

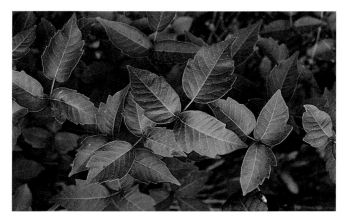

FIGURE 16.99 ■ Poison Ivy. *Toxicodendron radicans* (poison ivy—shrub or climbing vine). Note that the leaves of poison ivy have three leaflets and the stems are commonly reddish orange. Poison ivy occurs throughout the United States. (Photo contributor: Lawrence B. Stack, MD.)

Emergency Department Treatment and Disposition

An immediate rinse or shower with warm water and soap may minimize the reaction. If symptoms are limited to erythema and papules and a small surface area, calamine lotion or topical steroid sprays may provide adequate symptomatic relief. Pruritus may be decreased with oral antihistamines (eg, diphenhydramine or cyproheptadine) and oatmeal baths. Vesicles and bullae may require Domeboro compresses (for 60 minutes three times daily) to help dry these lesions and relieve pruritus. Systemic corticosteroids tapered over 3 weeks are used in severe reactions. Secondary infection should be treated with systemic antibiotics against staphylococcal and streptococcal species.

Pearls

1. Fluid from the vesicles or bullae does not contain any allergen.
2. Removal of the allergen from the skin within 30 minutes of exposure may prevent dermatitis.
3. Deliberate removal of allergen from under the fingernails may prevent spreading.
4. Treatment with systemic steroids for less than 2 or 3 weeks may result in rebound exacerbations of the dermatitis.

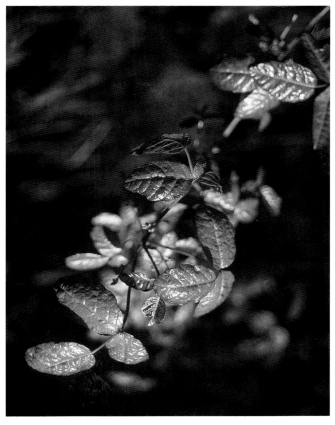

FIGURE 16.100 ■ Poison Oak. *Toxicodendron diversiloba* (poison oak). Like poison ivy, the terminal part of the branch has a cluster of three shiny leaves. It grows as a tree or woody shrub and occurs west of the Rocky Mountains. (Photo contributor: Ken Zafren, MD.)

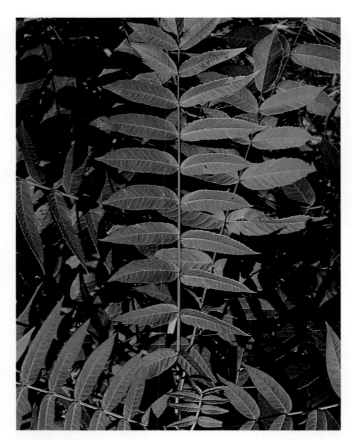

FIGURE 16.101 ■ Poison Sumac. *Toxicodendron vernix* (poison sumac). Note that the leaves of poison sumac have 7 to 13 leaflets. It grows as a tree or woody coarse shrub. Only one species of poison sumac is found in the United States. (Photo contributor: Lawrence B. Stack, MD.)

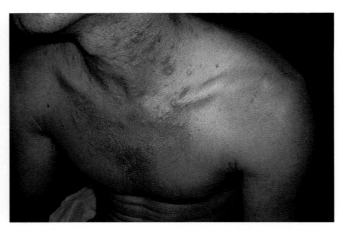

FIGURE 16.103 ■ Poison Oak Dermatitis. Erythematous papules and vesicles. This fire-fighter was exposed to urushiol, the allergen of poison oak, ivy, and sumac, in smoke from burning poison oak. (Photo contributor: Ken Zafren, MD.)

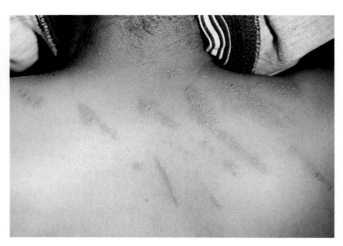

FIGURE 16.104 ■ Poison Ivy. Erythematous papules and vesicles in a linear distribution consistent with *Toxicodendron* dermatitis. (Photo contributor: Alan B. Storrow, MD.)

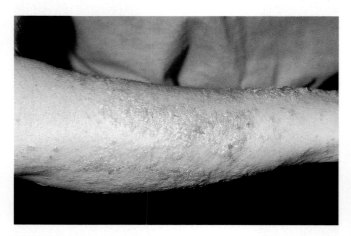

FIGURE 16.102 ■ Poison Sumac Dermatitis. A moderately severe local reaction to poison sumac. Note the vesicles, bullae, and exudates characteristic of a contact dermatitis. (Photo contributor: Alan B. Storrow, MD.)

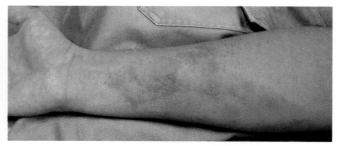

FIGURE 16.105 ■ Poison Ivy. A highly pruritic vesicular eruption of *Toxicodendron* dermatitis on the patient's forearm. (Photo contributor: R. Jason Thurman, MD.)

Clinical Summary

Sporotrichosis is a fungal skin infection caused by *Sporothrix schenckii*, an organism primarily found on plants and flowers and in soil; the problem is common among gardeners and florists. It also affects those who handle animals, since the fungus may inhabit animals' claws. Infection arises as contaminated thorns, spines, or claws penetrate the victim's skin. After an average incubation period of 3 weeks, localized infections become apparent. "Fixed" cutaneous infections are localized to the inoculation site and are manifest as 2- to 4-mm papules or nodules. They may ulcerate, become surrounded by raised erythema, and are typically painless. Progression to lymphocutaneous infections occurs in about 70% of cases. Patients present with a nodule at the site of penetration, with appearance of subcutaneous nodules and skip areas along lymphatic tracks later. The lesions may wax and wane over months to years. Patients with cutaneous sporotrichosis typically lack systemic symptoms.

Emergency Department Treatment and Disposition

Sporotrichosis may be successfully treated with oral potassium iodide for 1 month after clinical manifestations have resolved. Alternative therapy includes oral itraconazole, ketoconazole, or terbinafine, while disseminated infections may require intravenous amphotericin B. Outpatient therapy is appropriate for nondisseminated infections. Tetanus status should be addressed.

Pearls

1. Fungal cultures and tissue biopsy cultures are somewhat useful to confirm the diagnosis.
2. Treatment must be continued for 1 month following clinical resolution to eradicate *S schenckii*.
3. Although rare, a pulmonary form of sporotrichosis after inhalation exposure has been reported.

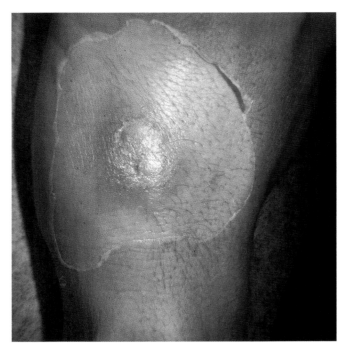

FIGURE 16.106 ■ Fixed Sporotrichosis. The ulcer and surrounding erythema of fixed cutaneous sporotrichosis could be confused with a brown recluse spider bite. (Photo contributor: Edward J. Otten, MD.)

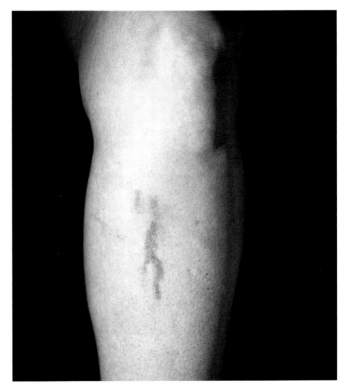

FIGURE 16.107 ■ Lymphocutaneous Sporotrichosis. Lymphatic spread is common in cutaneous sporotrichosis. (Photo contributor: Kevin J. Knoop, MD, MS.)

Chapter 17

TOXICOLOGICAL CONDITIONS

Saralyn R. Williams
Matthew D. Sztajnkrycer
R. Jason Thurman

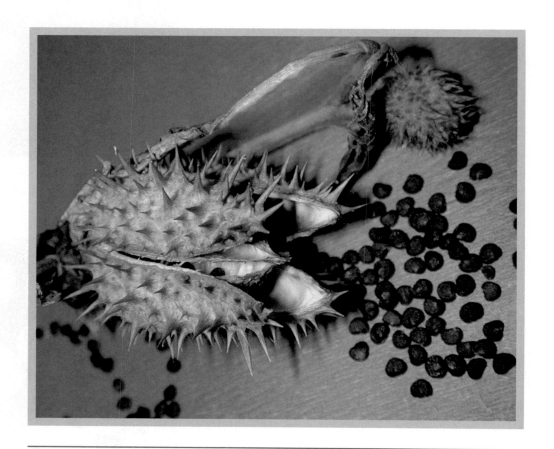

Clinical Summary

A white powder easily dissolved in water, methamphetamine may be abused by ingestion, insufflation ("snorting"), parenteral injection, and smoking. "Ice" refers to a pure preparation of methamphetamine hydrochloride in large crystalline form.

Clinical effects of methamphetamine use are similar to those noted with cocaine use, manifesting as a sympathomimetic toxidrome. Although clinically indistinguishable from cocaine toxicity, the duration of effects is appreciably longer. Habituated users may use methamphetamine every few hours around the clock, for periods of 3 to 6 days, a use pattern typically referred to as a "run." The initial euphoric stimulant "rush" degenerates during the course of the run into a series of repetitive activities, often referred to as "tweaking." During the period of tweaking, paranoia and hallucinations may appear. After the run, a depressive phase referred to as a "crash" occurs.

The most common cardiovascular manifestations of toxicity are tachycardia and hypertension, although myocardial ischemia has been reported. Despite the cardiovascular effects, central nervous system (CNS) toxicity is the primary reason most methamphetamine users present for medical care. Patients are typically anxious and aggressive, and life-threatening agitation may occur. Visual and tactile hallucinations and psychoses are common. Poor dentition is common among chronic users ("meth mouth"), and appears multifactorial in nature.

3,4-Methylenedioxymethamphetamine (MDMA, "ecstasy") is a synthetic blend of methamphetamine and mescaline, resulting in promotion of serotonin release and inhibition of reuptake. In addition to signs and symptoms of methamphetamine toxicity, MDMA may result in syndrome of inappropriate antidiuretic hormone (SIADH) with subsequent hyponatremia and cerebral edema.

Emergency Department Treatment and Disposition

Treatment is primarily supportive, and is focused upon the signs and symptoms of toxicity. Cardiac monitoring is indicated for symptomatic patients. As with other causes of sympathomimetic toxicity, initial management focuses upon control of agitation and hyperthermia and prevention of complications (eg, rhabdomyolysis). Benzodiazepines are the first line of therapy for agitation. Hypertonic sodium may be indicated for MDMA-associated cerebral edema and seizures.

Pearls

1. As with cocaine, the use of β-blockers and neuroleptic agents is contraindicated in the setting of acute toxicity.
2. In addition to the medical complications associated with methamphetamine use, the manufacture of methamphetamine is associated with exposure to a number of toxic chemicals.
3. The hyperthermia associated with acute amphetamine poisoning may result in end-organ damage similar to patients with heat-stroke-like illness.

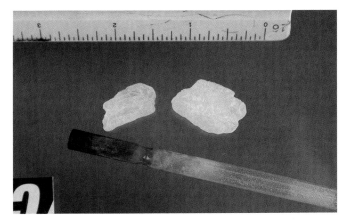

FIGURE 17.1 ■ "Ice" Methamphetamine. An example of the "ice" form of amphetamines with a pipe. (Photo contributor: US Drug Enforcement Administration.)

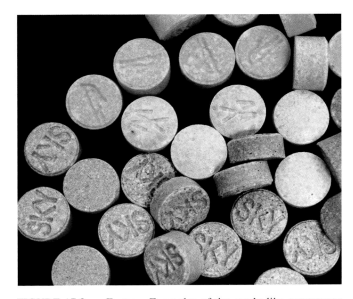

FIGURE 17.2 ■ Ecstasy. Examples of the candy-like appearance of ecstasy tablets. (Photo contributor: US Drug Enforcement Administration.)

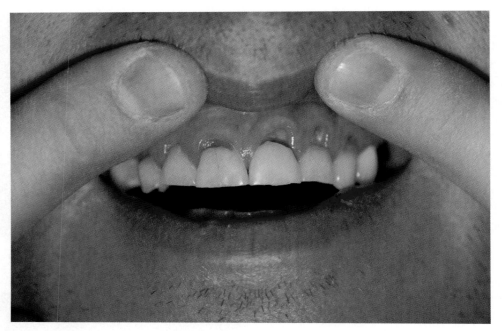

FIGURE 17.3 ■ Early "Meth Mouth." "Meth mouth," the extensive and accelerated dental caries associated with chronic methamphetamine abuse. (Photo contributor: R. Jason Thurman, MD.)

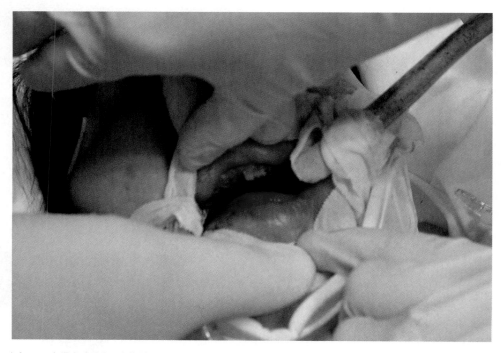

FIGURE 17.4 ■ Advanced "Meth Mouth." Note the severe dental decay in this chronic methamphetamine abuser. (Photo contributor: Carson Harris, MD.)

Clinical Summary

Cocaine is a natural alkaloid derived from the leaves of *Erythroxylum coca*. Cocaine hydrochloride (powder cocaine) is a crystalline white powder. "Crack," the free-base of cocaine hydrochloride, is an off-white substance named both for its rock-like appearance ("rock") and due to the sound it makes when heated. In contrast to powder cocaine, crack may be smoked as it vaporizes instead of burning.

Cocaine intoxication manifests as a sympathomimetic toxidrome, with tachycardia, hypertension, diaphoresis, mydriasis, delirium, and hyperthermia. Cocaine use increases psychomotor activity, which causes anxiety and agitation and increases heat production. Increased muscular activity may result in rhabdomyolysis. Numerous neurological complications have been reported after cocaine use, including subarachnoid hemorrhage, intracerebral hemorrhage, cerebral infarction, and seizures. Toxicity most commonly results from recreational overdose, but may also occur due to the rupture of smuggled ingested packets of large quantities of cocaine due to the practice of cocaine "body-packing."

Cardiovascular toxicity, including acute myocardial infarction, is well described after cocaine use. Dysrhythmias, including supraventricular tachycardia, atrial fibrillation and flutter, ventricular tachycardia, ventricular fibrillation, and torsades de pointes have been reported. Cocaine is a sodium channel blocker and may cause QRS widening on the ECG. Chronic cocaine use predisposes to development of a dilated cardiomyopathy. Aortic dissection and rupture have been associated with cocaine use.

Pulmonary effects of cocaine use include reactive airway disease exacerbation, pneumothorax, pneumomediastinum, and cardiogenic and noncardiogenic pulmonary edema (NCPE). "Crack-lung" refers to an acute pulmonary syndrome of dyspnea, hypoxia, and diffuse pulmonary alveolar infiltrates.

Emergency Department Treatment and Disposition

Treatment is primarily supportive, and focused upon the signs and symptoms of toxicity. No specific antidote exists. Serum cocaine levels are not clinically useful. Cardiac monitoring is indicated for symptomatic patients. Initial management focuses upon control of agitation and hyperthermia, and prevention of complications (eg, rhabdomyolysis). The use of neuroleptic agents is relatively contraindicated for cocaine-associated psychomotor agitation due to the negative effects of these

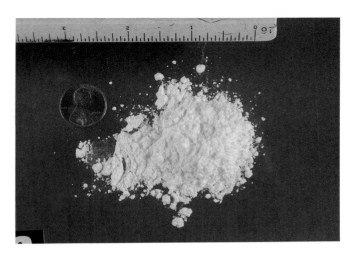

FIGURE 17.5 ■ Cocaine Powder. Cocaine powder. (Photo contributor: US Drug Enforcement Administration.)

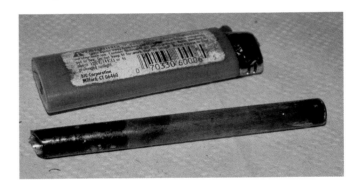

FIGURE 17.6 ■ Drug Paraphernalia. Crack pipe sequestered in the rectum during a patient's arrest, resulting in laceration of the hemorrhoidal venous plexus and massive hemorrhage. (Photo contributor: Matthew D. Sztajnkrycer, MD, PhD.)

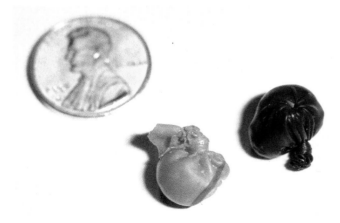

FIGURE 17.7 ■ Cocaine Body-Packing. Cocaine-filled balloon packets from the stool of a cocaine "body-packer" (penny used for scale). Radiopaque packets are often visible on KUB radiograph in the left upper quadrant. Severe toxicity may result in the event of a ruptured packet. (Photo contributor: Alan B. Storrow, MD.)

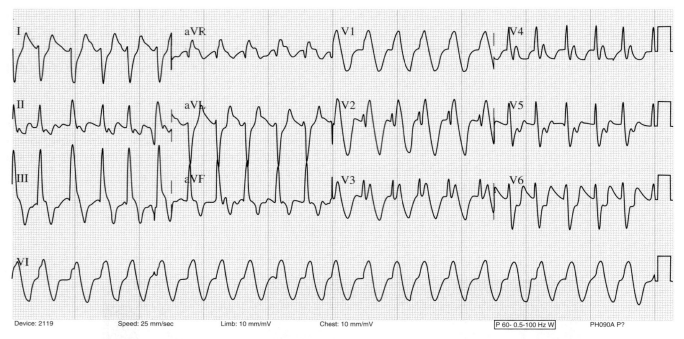

FIGURE 17.8 ■ Cocaine Cardiotoxicity. The initial 12-lead EKG of a patient with acute cocaine and cocaethylene poisoning. His initial serum pH was 6.8. (Photo contributors: Thomas Babcock, MD and Laurie Lawrence, MD.)

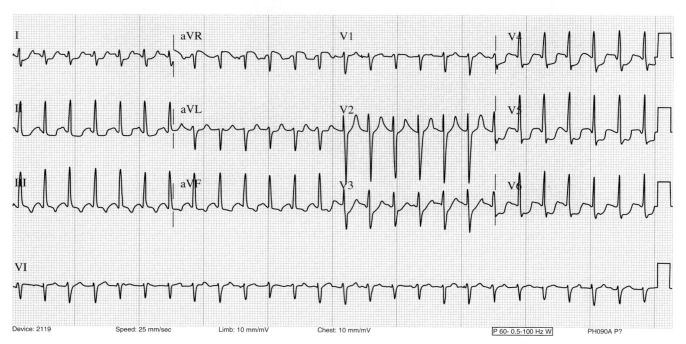

FIGURE 17.9 ■ Treated Cocaine Cardiotoxicity. The 12-lead EKG of the same patient in Fig. 17.8, 68 minutes later after aggressive treatment with sodium bicarbonate to a serum pH of 7.26. (Photo contributors: Thomas Babcock, MD and Laurie Lawrence, MD.)

agents on thermoregulation, seizure threshold, and the potential for dysrhythmias. Benzodiazepines are the first line of therapy for agitation. They also appear beneficial in the management of cocaine-associated chest pain. Sodium bicarbonate administration should be considered for QRS widening in the setting of acute cocaine poisoning.

Pearls

1. The use of β-blockers is contraindicated in the management of cocaine-associated chest pain and myocardial ischemia due to the potential for vasospasm and hypertensive crisis ("unopposed α-effect").

2. Although the risk of myocardial infarction is greatest immediately after use, myocardial ischemia may occur up to 6 weeks after last use.

3. Cocaethylene may form in vivo after the use of cocaine and ethanol. Cocaethylene is more cardiotoxic than cocaine and has a longer half-life.

4. The rupture of a cocaine packet in a body-packer may result in fatal toxicity. Emergent surgical intervention should be considered for immediate removal of the packets as a life-saving maneuver.

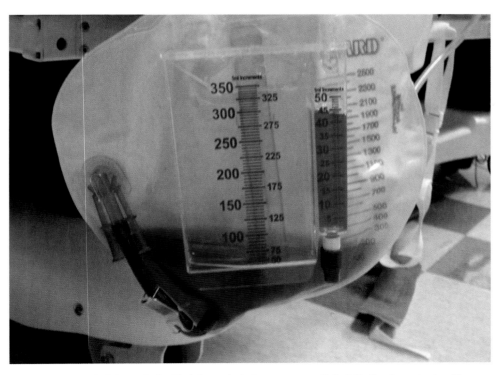

FIGURE 17.10 ■ Cocaine-Induced Rhabdomyolysis. Rhabdomyolysis is a common clinical finding in patients with severe cocaine poisoning. (Photo contributor: Mohamud Daya, MD.)

Clinical Summary

Anticholinergic toxidrome is best illustrated by the mnemonic: hot as a hare, blind as a bat, mad as a hatter, red as a beet, and dry as a bone. As the etiology reflects central and peripheral muscarinic receptor blockade, it is more accurately termed an antimuscarinic toxidrome. A centrally mediated delirium may occur, but is typically not violent but rather is associated with mumbling speech and persistent "picking" behaviors. Other manifestations include hyperthermia, mydriasis, dry mucus membranes and axillae, tachycardia, decreased gastrointestinal motility, and urinary retention.

Many xenobiotics are antimuscarinic. One of the more common is diphenhydramine. Tricyclic antidepressants, phenothiazines, cyclobenzaprine, carbamazepine, atropine, scopolamine, glycopyrrolate, and belladonna alkaloids all have antimuscarinic properties. Plants such as jimson weed contain belladonna alkaloids and may be used recreationally.

Emergency Department Treatment and Disposition

Initial assessments of the vital signs and the duration of the QRS on electrocardiogram are important. Since many antimuscarinic xenobiotics are also sodium channel blockers, QRS interval should be monitored. Hyperthermia occasionally occurs and is treated with evaporative cooling. Most of these patients require supportive care, with the administration of benzodiazepines for agitation. A Foley catheter may be needed for treatment of the urinary retention. Occasionally, physostigmine is used as a diagnostic reversal agent for antimuscarinic poisoning, but its risks versus benefits must be considered. The half-life of physostigmine is only about 20 minutes.

Pearls

1. Diphenhydramine is a sodium channel-blocking agent and may cause QRS widening.
2. Physostigmine crosses the blood-brain barrier so an improvement in antimuscarinic delirium can be elicited.
3. Glycopyrrolate is an antimuscarinic that does not cross the blood-brain barrier so delirium does not occur.

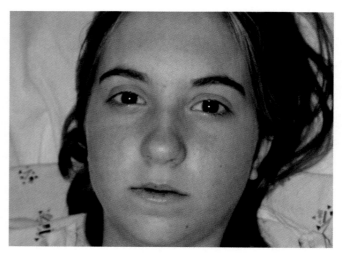

FIGURE 17.11 ■ Anticholinergic Mydriasis. Mydriasis and flushing are some of the characteristic findings of anticholinergic toxidrome. (Photo contributor: Matthew D. Sztajnkrycer, MD, PhD.)

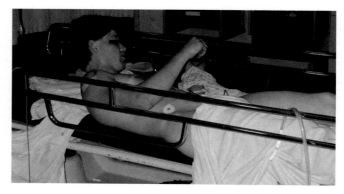

FIGURE 17.12 ■ Anticholinergic Delirium. Anticholinergic delirium is manifested by agitation, confusion, and a "picking" behavior. (Photo contributor: Matthew D. Sztajnkrycer, MD, PhD.)

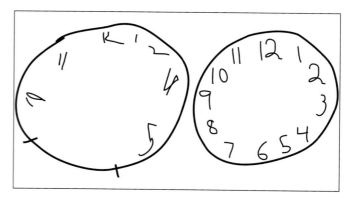

FIGURE 17.13 ■ Anticholinergic Delirium. Prior to treatment with physostigmine, a patient suffering acute anticholinergic delirium drew the clock on the left. Following physostigmine administration, the patient drew the clock on the right. (Photo contributor: Division of Medical Toxicology, University of California, San Diego.)

Clinical Summary

Opium is derived from the poppy plant, *Papaver somniferum.* Opiates are naturally occurring drugs derived from opium, and include morphine, codeine, and paregoric. The term opioid refers to drugs with opium-like activity. Heroin is a semisynthetic derivative of morphine, containing two acetyl groups (diacetyl-morphine). Pure heroin is a bitter-tasting white powder. Most street-grade heroin varies in color from white to dark brown, depending upon purity and additives. Mexican "black tar" heroin may be sticky like roofing tar or hard like coal, and appears dark brown to black in color. In addition to heroin, opioid toxicity may occur through diversion of legal narcotic agents. Time-released oxycodone preparations can be abused by chewing the tablets, snorting crushed tablets, or dissolving and parenterally administering the tablets. All these methods bypass the sustained release mechanism of legitimate use, resulting in an immediate release of large amounts of oxycodone.

The classic opioid toxidrome is a clinical triad of coma, respiratory depression, and miosis. However, opioid-related CNS depression can range from mild sedation to coma. Normal or dilated pupils may occur after overdose of meperidine, propoxyphene, or pentazocine, or in the setting of CNS hypoxia. Death is typically due to respiratory depression, which in turn is related to central and peripheral toxicity. Noncardiogenic pulmonary edema (NCPE) is associated with the use of certain opioids, including heroin, methadone, morphine, and propoxyphene.

Emergency Department Treatment and Disposition

Care of these patients focuses upon airway management and antidotal therapy. Whole bowel irrigation has been advocated after ingestion of sustained release formulations, or in the setting of body-packing and body-stuffing. In the latter, abdominal x-rays are indicated to look for evidence of foreign bodies. Chest radiographs are indicated for assessment of NCPE. Specific drug levels do not assist in patient management. Rhabdomyolysis and cerebral hypoxia may occur after prolonged periods of respiratory and CNS depression. Naloxone is the antidote of choice for significant opioid toxicity. Indications include respiratory or CNS depression after known or suspected opioid overdose. In administering naloxone, care should be taken not to precipitate acute opioid withdrawal.

Pearls

1. The presence of adulterants such as scopolamine or clenbuterol may mask or alter the appearance of the classic opioid toxidrome.
2. Recurrent toxicity and life-threatening respiratory depression may occur following short-term reversal with naloxone administration, especially in body-stuffers or after ingestion of sustained release formulations.

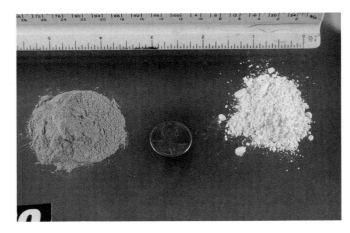

FIGURE 17.14 ■ Asian Heroin. (Photo contributor: US Drug Enforcement Administration.)

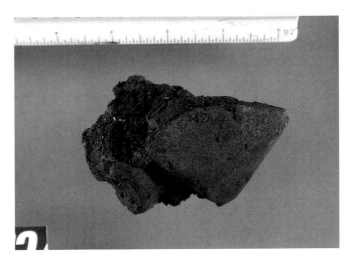

FIGURE 17.15 ■ Black Tar Heroin. Black tar heroin has a different appearance and texture than the South American and Asian heroin. Because it has a "gummier" texture, it is usually injected or smoked. Black tar heroin is associated with wound botulism. (Photo contributor: US Drug Enforcement Administration.)

3. The use of naloxone in the setting of tramadol toxicity is relatively contraindicated due to the occurrence of seizures.

4. Propoxyphene has sodium channel—blocking effects like type 1A antidysrhythmics. Evidence of widening of the QRS interval in the setting of propoxyphene poisoning should be treated with administration of intravenous sodium bicarbonate solution.

5. The use of black tar heroin has been associated with wound botulism.

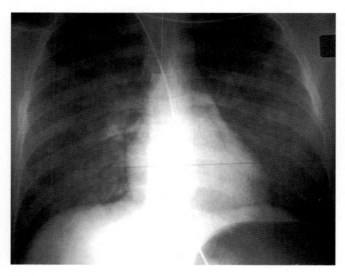

FIGURE 17.16 ■ Heroin-Related Noncardiogenic Pulmonary Edema. Noncardiogenic pulmonary edema may occur in the setting of opioid poisoning. The radiograph demonstrates the bilateral airspace opacities and the normal-sized cardiac silhouette. (Photo contributor: Division of Medical Toxicology, University of California, San Diego.)

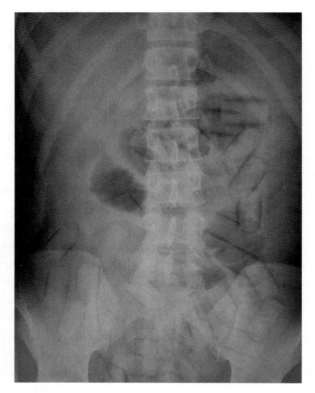

FIGURE 17.17 ■ Heroin Body-Packing. KUB radiograph of a "packer" demonstrating the presence of radiopaque foreign bodies. Rupture of a packet may result in severe opioid toxicity. (Photo contributor: Jason Chu, MD.)

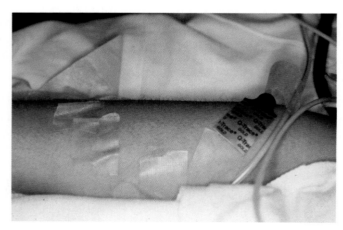

FIGURE 17.18 ■ Piloerection. Piloerection may be noted with acute opioid withdrawal. (Photo contributor: Division of Medical Toxicology, University of California, San Diego.)

Clinical Summary

Despite the advent of the newer antidepressant agents (eg, serotonin-specific reuptake inhibitors), tricyclic antidepressant (TCA) toxicity remains a significant cause of poisoning morbidity and mortality in the United States. TCAs exert effects on multiple systems, including voltage-gated sodium channels, potassium channels, H_1-histamine receptors, D_2-dopamine receptors, M_1-muscarinic receptors, α_1-adrenergic receptors, and the GABA-A receptor complex.

TCA toxicity is related to pharmacological effects on the myocardium, CNS, and vasculature. M_1-muscarinic receptor blockade may result in an anticholinergic toxidrome. CNS toxicity may range from sedation to coma. Seizures, agitation, and delirium may occur. Inhibition of voltage-gated sodium channels results in characteristic widening of the QRS complex. A limb-lead QRS duration greater than 120 msec is associated with an increased incidence of seizures, while a limb-lead QRS duration greater than 160 msec is associated with an increased incidence of ventricular dysrhythmias. Similarly, in adults, a terminal R wave in lead aVR greater than or equal to 3 mm is associated with increased risk of seizure or dysrhythmias.

Emergency Department Treatment and Disposition

Signs and symptoms of significant overdose typically occur early. All patients presenting after TCA overdose should receive continuous cardiac monitoring and an ECG. Aggressive airway management may be indicated. No specific antidote exists for TCA poisoning. Benzodiazepines are the agent of choice for seizures. Management of QRS widening involves intravenous administration of sodium bicarbonate; controversy exists regarding optimal method of administration (intermittent dosing versus continuous infusion). Symptomatic patients should be admitted to the ICU due to the potential for rapid deterioration.

Pearls

1. In one study, half of all patients presenting to emergency department with trivial signs of poisoning had catastrophic deterioration within 1 hour.
2. The use of flumazenil and physostigmine is contraindicated in the management of patients with ECG evidence of TCA poisoning.
3. The cyclic antidepressant amoxapine is associated with an increased risk of seizures and status epilepticus in the absence of ECG warning signs.

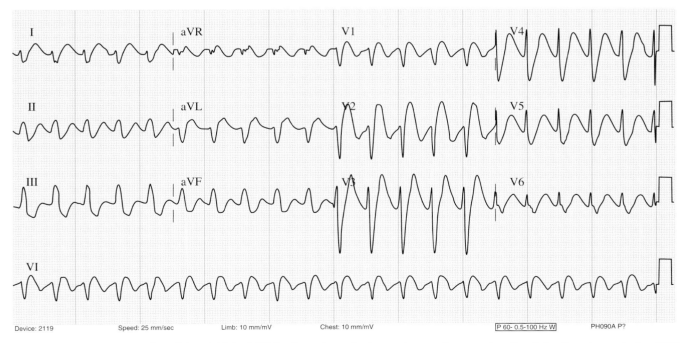

Device: 2119   Speed: 25 mm/sec   Limb: 10 mm/mV   Chest: 10 mm/mV   P 60- 0.5-100 Hz W   PH090A P?

FIGURE 17.19 ■ TCA Cardiotoxicity. A 12-lead EKG of a patient who ingested a massive quantity of amitriptyline, demonstrating QRS widening. The patient presented awake and alert, but rapidly became obtunded. (Photo contributor: Thomas Babcock, MD and Clay Smith, MD.)

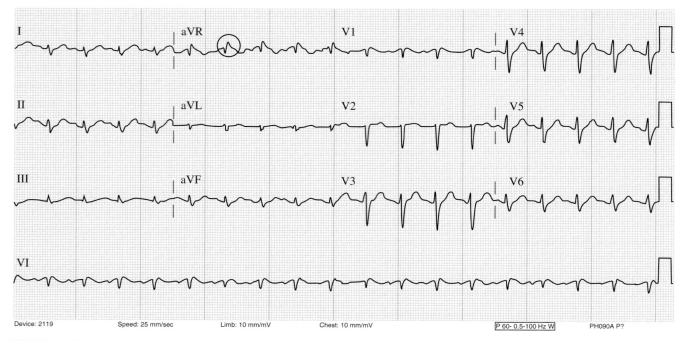

FIGURE 17.20 ■ TCA Cardiotoxicity-Treated. Repeat 12-lead EKG of the patient from Fig. 17.19 approximately 2 hours and 45 minutes after the first EKG. A total of 12 amperes of sodium bicarbonate had been administered intravenously. This EKG demonstrates the terminal R wave changes in aVR associated with sodium channel—blocking effects (circle). (Photo contributors: Thomas Babcock, MD and Clay Smith, MD.)

Clinical Summary

β-Blockers and calcium channel blockers are indicated for the management of angina, hypertension, myocardial infarction, and cardiac dysrhythmias, as well as the treatment of noncardiovascular conditions (eg, glaucoma, thyrotoxicosis, migraine headache prophylaxis). β-Blocking agents may be selective for B_1-adrenergic receptors, or nonselective. With therapeutic use, the commonly available calcium channel blockers are selective for the membrane-bound L-type calcium channel. Inhibition of this channel prevents influx of extracellular calcium.

Toxicity presents as an exaggeration of clinical effects, with significant toxicity manifesting predominantly as bradycardia and hypotension. β-Blocker toxicity may result in hypoglycemia, especially in children. Certain agents, such as propranolol, are associated with CNS toxicity (including seizures and CNS depression) and fast sodium channel blockade (analogous to tricyclic antidepressant toxicity). Calcium channel blocker toxicity is associated with hyperglycemia, believed to be secondary to impaired insulin release (a calcium-dependent process) and impaired peripheral utilization.

Emergency Department Treatment and Disposition

The use of aggressive gastrointestinal decontamination (eg, whole bowel irrigation) has been advocated for sustained release preparations. In addition to standard ACLS measures, glucagon has been used as a specific antidote for β-blocker toxicity. No treatment has been universally successful in the management of severe calcium channel blocker toxicity. Calcium, high-dose insulin, and glucagon have all been tried with variable success. Management of these patients should involve early consultation with a poison control center or toxicologist.

Pearls

1. Topical β-adrenergic blocker administration (eg, for glaucoma) can result in significant systemic toxicity.
2. Development of toxicity may be appreciably delayed after ingestion of sustained-release formulations.
3. The presence of hyperglycemia versus hypoglycemia may help differentiate calcium channel blocker poisoning from β-blocker poisoning respectively.
4. Due to the potential for significant local tissue toxicity, calcium chloride therapy should optimally be administered through a central venous catheter.

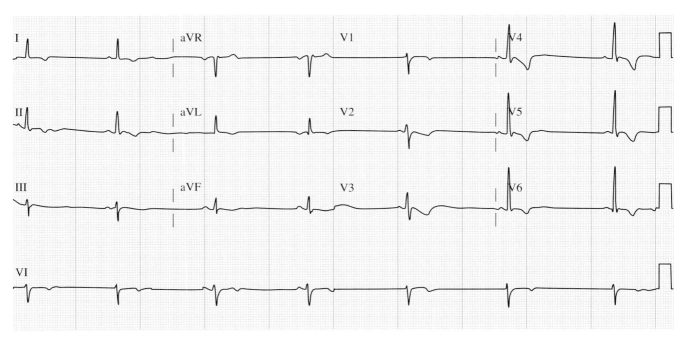

FIGURE 17.21 ■ β-Blocker Overdose. Atenolol poisoning resulting in severe bradycardia. The patient had also ingested digoxin but remained bradycardic after treatment with Fab fragments. (Photo contributor: Saralyn R. Williams, MD.)

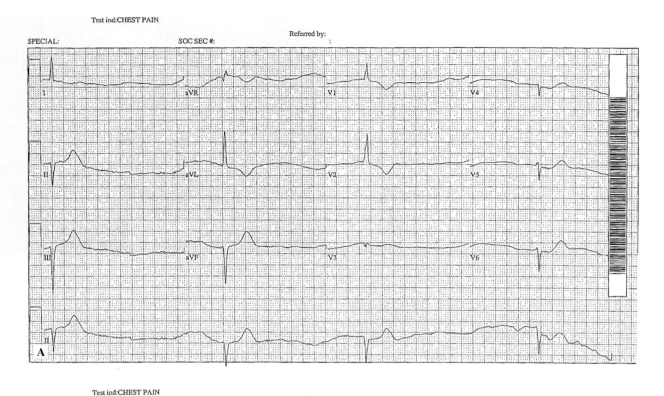

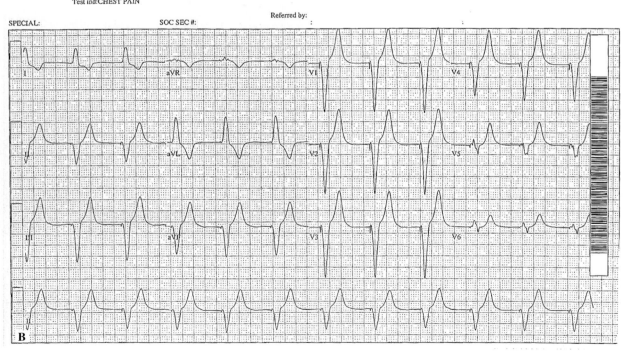

FIGURE 22A and B ▪ Calcium Channel Blocker Overdose. (**A**) Verapamil poisoning causes profound negative inotropy and chronotropy. The 12-lead EKG demonstrates the bradycardia that may occur. (**B**) The same patient after transvenous pacing was initiated. (Photo contributor: Matthew D. Sztajnkrycer, MD, PhD.)

Clinical Summary

Salicylates are a common cause of analgesic poisoning. Many preparations are available including immediate-release and enteric-coated formulations. Acute ingestions of large quantities of aspirin may have delayed absorption due to the formulation of the drug or the formation of bezoars. Poisoning may occur with chronic ingestions as well, particularly in older patients.

Salicylates are a weak acid and this dictates much of their absorption in the stomach and distribution in the body. Early effects after ingestion include gastrointestinal irritation which may lead to nausea and vomiting. Classically, salicylate-poisoned patients present with a mixed acid-base picture. Central stimulation of the respiratory drive results in a primary respiratory alkalosis. As a result of disrupted energy mechanics and decreased ATP production, metabolic acidosis and lactate accumulation occur. Ketonuria may also be noted. As a consequence, the initial pH of the patient's serum may be acidemic or alkalemic depending on the predominant acid-base disorder at the time of blood sampling. Hyperthermia occurs due to the generation and release of heat secondary to uncoupling of oxidative phosphorylation. Coma and seizures demonstrate severe nervous system toxicity and are associated with poor outcomes. Increased capillary permeability may result in noncardiogenic pulmonary edema (NCPE) and cerebral edema.

Emergency Department Treatment and Disposition

Fluid resuscitation to replace volume depletion is paramount early in the presentation. Since salicylate is a weak acid, pH manipulation by maintaining the serum pH in the 7.45 to 7.55 range reduces the volume of distribution of the drug and allows for alkalinization of the urine which enhances the renal elimination of the salicylic acid. Potassium replacement is usually needed. Hemodialysis should be considered for deterioration in the acid-base status of the patient, renal failure, NCPE, or cerebral edema. A serum salicylate concentration greater than 100 mg/dL is another consideration for dialysis, as is an increasing level in the setting of adequate decontamination. However, the level is not the sole criterion. Patients with serum salicylate levels much less than 100 mg/dL, particularly patients with chronic ingestions, may meet clinical criteria for extracorporeal elimination. Admission should be strongly considered for most of these ingestions.

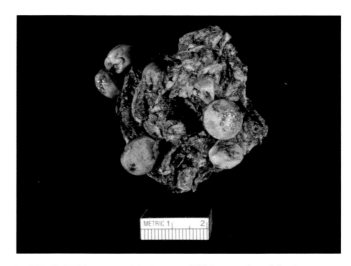

FIGURE 17.23 ■ Aspirin Bezoar. Pill bezoar found in the gastrointestinal tract of a patient who ingested approximately 750 adult formulation enteric-coated aspirin tablets. At the time of death, approximately 13 hours after ingestion, the serum salicylate level was 128 mg/dL. More than 300 partially digested pills remained in the GI tract on postmortem. (Photo contributor: Jared M. Orrock, MD.)

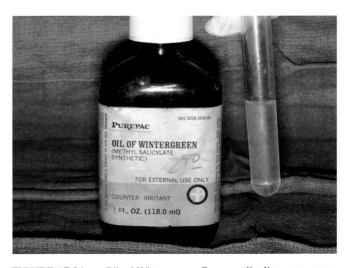

FIGURE 17.24 ■ Oil of Wintergreen. Severe salicylism may occur from ingestion of products that contain a high concentration of oil of wintergreen (methylsalicylate). This bottle of oil of wintergreen is a 98% solution, which contains the equivalent of 7000 mg of salicylate per teaspoon. (Photo contributor: R. Jason Thurman, MD.)

Pearls

1. Methyl salicylate in a 98% concentration (oil of wintergreen) translates into 1400 mg/mL. One teaspoon (5 mL) provides the equivalent 7000 mg of salicylic acid.

2. If a patient with severe salicylism must be intubated, careful attention should be made to mimic the minute ventilation of the nonparalyzed patient. If a respiratory acidosis is allowed to occur, the patient will become severely acidemic which allows the salicylate to further distribute into the tissues and poison the mitochondria.

3. While acetazolamide administration results in alkalinization of the urine, the excretion of the bicarbonate into the urine comes at the expense of promoting acidemia, which could further drive the salicylate into the central nervous system, enhancing toxicity.

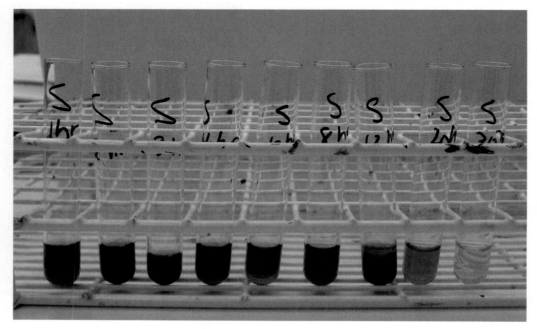

FIGURE 17.25 ■ Trinder Reagent. In the presence of salicylates, the addition of Trinder reagent to urine specimen will yield a purple color. This picture demonstrates the reaction to Trinder reagent from urine samples collected serially 1 hour to 30 hours after ingestion of 650 mg aspirin. (Photo contributor: Sheila Dawling, PhD.)

Clinical Summary

Acetaminophen is a widely available analgesic and antipyretic agent. It is commonly found in combination with opioids, decongestants, antihistamines, and other over-the-counter and prescription products. Patients may complain of nausea and vomiting shortly after a toxic ingestion, but may also be asymptomatic. Signs and symptoms of acute liver injury occur within 36 hours after ingestion. Occasionally, patients present to the emergency department when they develop the signs of hepatotoxicity, not realizing that the large ingestion of an acetaminophen-based product is the etiology.

In the overdose setting, acetaminophen exerts its toxic effects via a metabolite that is created via the P-450 enzyme system. The metabolite causes centrilobular necrosis of the liver which may lead to fulminant hepatic failure. Renal failure may also occur. Fatalities from hepatic failure usually occur 3 to 5 days after the ingestion. Treatment includes the administration of *N*-acetylcysteine (NAC), which can prevent acetaminophen-induced hepatotoxicity if initiated within 8 hours of the acute ingestion.

Emergency Department Treatment and Disposition

Activated charcoal may be considered in patients who present within 2 hours of acetaminophen overdose. A serum acetaminophen level (mcg/mL) drawn at 4 hours after a single acute ingestion can be plotted on the Rumack-Matthew nomogram to determine the need for treatment. If the serum level is at or above the treatment line, the patient should be treated with a standard course of oral or intravenously administered NAC. Patients who require administration of NAC should be admitted to the hospital.

Pearls

1. Acetaminophen is a common agent in many over-the-counter medications. Patients who overdose on these medications require routine checking of a serum acetaminophen level to identify those who may need treatment with NAC.

2. The formulation of oral NAC is available in a 20% solution. The 20% solution comprises 20 g of NAC per 100 mL of solution. For the average 70 kg adult, the initial oral loading dose of 140 mg/kg would be 9.8 g, or approximately 50 mL of the 20% solution.

3. Massive ingestions of acetaminophen may result in an anion gap metabolic acidosis.

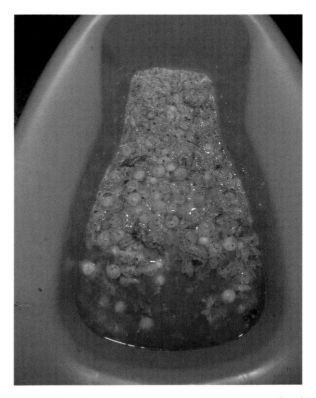

FIGURE 17.26 ■ Acetaminophen Overdose. Multiple acetaminophen-containing pills are seen in the vomit of an overdose patient. The patient had ingested the pills a few hours prior to presentation in a suicide attempt. (Photo contributor: Alan B. Storrow, MD.)

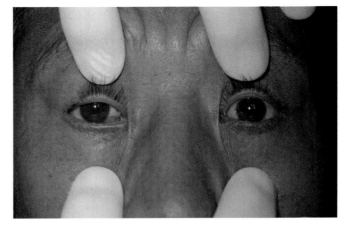

FIGURE 17.27 ■ Acetaminophen Overdose. This patient developed hepatic failure with marked jaundice as a result of an intentional acetaminophen overdose. (Photo contributor: R. Jason Thurman, MD.)

Clinical Summary

Caustics are a diverse group of household and industrial products and pharmaceutical agents that cause functional and histological tissue damage through direct contact. They represent the second most common toxic exposure for children 5 years of age or under. These agents are frequently described in terms of pH, with acids typically having a pH less than 3 and alkali (bases) typically having a pH greater than 11.

Alkali exposure results in a liquefactive necrosis, with deep and progressive tissue damage, predominantly to the esophagus. Endoscopic grading of esophageal burns is similar to thermal burns, ranging from mucosal hyperemia and edema (grade I) to full-thickness burns (grade III). Acid ingestion results in coagulative necrosis, which limits the depth of penetration. Damage is predominantly localized to the gastric mucosa, with pooling of the caustic agent in the antrum.

Emergency Department Treatment and Disposition

The primary goal of management is airway assessment and stabilization. Hypotension is a grave finding. A serum pH less than 7.20 may indicate the need for surgical exploration. Activated charcoal decontamination is relatively contraindicated. Endoscopy is recommended after large or deliberate caustic ingestion, presence of oral burns, or persistent refusal to take oral liquids. Steroids are occasionally used as an effort to prevention of esophageal strictures in selected patients, but the decision to administer is made based upon endoscopic grading.

Pearls

1. The absence of oropharyngeal burns is a poor predictor of distal esophageal injury. The presence of vomiting, drooling, or stridor is more predictive of significant esophageal injury on endoscopy.
2. Analogous to thermal burns after smoke inhalation, upper airway edema and airway obstruction may occur abruptly.
3. Ingestion of muriatic acid (HCl) results in an initial nonanion gap metabolic acidosis.

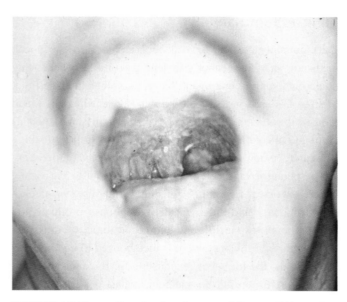

FIGURE 17.28 ■ Caustic Oropharyngeal Burns. This patient suffered caustic burns from drinking brake fluids in a suicide attempt. (Photo contributor: Saralyn R. Williams, MD.)

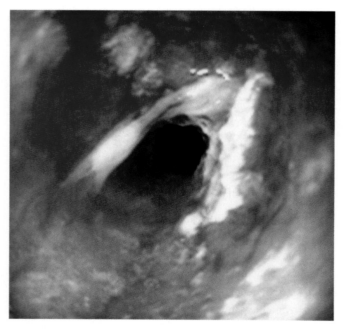

FIGURE 17.29 ■ Caustic Esophageal Burns. These esophageal burns were caused by an accidental ingestion of Lye in a pediatric patient. (Photo contributor: Philip E. Stack, MD.)

Clinical Summary

The commonly available toxic alcohols include ethylene glycol, methanol, and isopropanol. Ethylene glycol is a sweet-tasting liquid commonly found in antifreeze, as well as in brake fluid. Methanol is used in lock deicers, windshield wiper fluid, and industrial solvents. Isopropanol is commonly marketed as "rubbing" alcohol, although it is also found in nonstreaking glass and window cleaners, soaps, cosmetics, and antifreezes.

The parent toxic alcohols have the potential to intoxicate, but are not otherwise toxic. Sequential metabolism via alcohol dehydrogenase and aldehyde dehydrogenase produces the organic acids responsible for end-organ toxicity and metabolic acidosis. Ethylene glycol is metabolized to glycolic and oxalic acids; the former is responsible for the acidosis while the latter is responsible for calcium oxalate deposition in the renal tubules and delayed acute renal failure (24-72 hours post-ingestion). Hypocalcemia may occur with severe intoxication. Cranial nerve palsies may also occur 5 to 20 days after ingestion. Although less intoxicating than ethanol, methanol is metabolized to formic acid, which is responsible for both acidosis and direct retinal toxicity. Symptoms may develop after only a few hours. Patients often report blurred or dim vision ("snowstorm") prior to development of objective signs, including optic disc hyperemia, pupillary dilation, and poor accommodation. Pancreatitis and delayed basal ganglia lesions may occur. Isopropanol metabolism is limited to ketone formation and does not result in significant acidosis.

Emergency Department Treatment and Disposition

Decontamination options are limited, as activated charcoal does not bind alcohol and gastrointestinal absorption is rapid. Emergency management is directed toward supportive care, diagnosis of the agent, and prevention of further metabolism. Methanol, ethylene glycol, and isopropanol levels may not be readily available. However, care should be taken in interpreting ancillary data, such as urinary fluorescence and the osmolar gap. Inhibition of alcohol dehydrogenase by either ethanol (the preferred substrate) or fomepizole is the mainstay of initial therapy. Administration of folate (methanol) or pyridoxine and thiamine (ethylene glycol) may inhibit organic acid production or increase degradation. Hemodialysis is indicated for signs of end-organ toxicity (eg, anion gap acidosis, renal failure, mental status changes) and possibly for elevated toxic alcohol levels.

Pearls

1. Provided adequate metabolism has occurred, isopropanol ingestion will demonstrate the presence of large amounts of ketones on a urine dipstick assay.
2. Only a few sips of concentrated methanol or ethylene glycol are required to produce toxicity in a toddler; these ingestions should be viewed as a "one pill can kill" exposure.
3. Coingestion of ethanol may delay development of eventual toxicity due to competitive blockade of alcohol dehydrogenase.

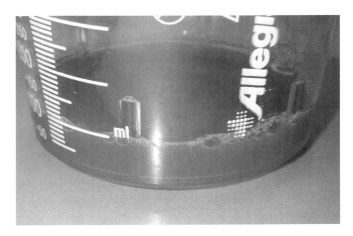

FIGURE 17.30 ■ Antifreeze. Addition of fluorescein to antifreeze gives colorless ethylene glycol its green appearance. (Photo contributor: Matthew D. Sztajnkrycer, MD, PhD.)

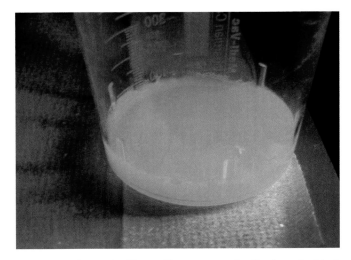

FIGURE 17.31 ■ Antifreeze Fluorescence. Application of a black light to antifreeze will demonstrate the fluorescence in body fluids, provided fluorescein has been added. This sample was obtained from the emesis of an overdose patient. (Photo contributor: Matthew D. Sztajnkrycer, MD, PhD.)

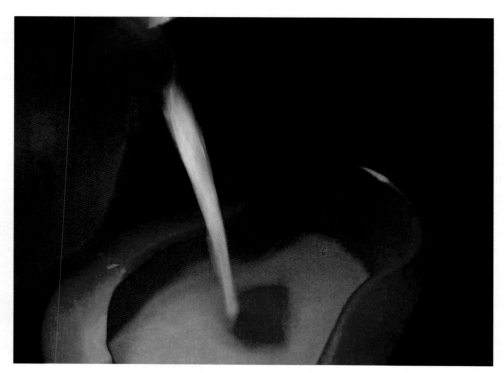

FIGURE 17.32 ▪ Urine Fluorescence. Under black light, the urine of this ethylene glycol overdose patient shows a bright fluorescence. (Photo contributor: Matthew D. Sztajnkrycer, MD, PhD.)

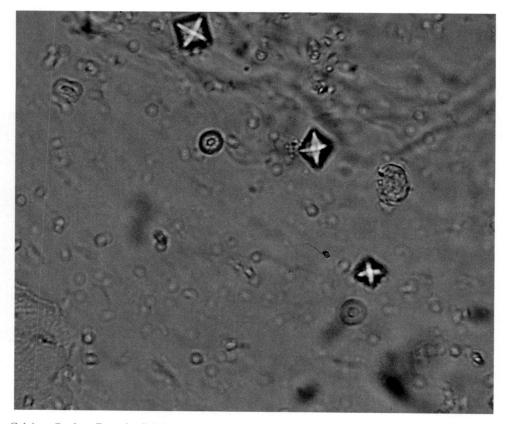

FIGURE 17.33 ▪ Calcium Oxalate Crystals. Calcium oxalate crystals may be seen in the urine of the patient who ingested ethylene glycol and metabolized the parent compound to create oxalic acid. (Photo contributor: Susan K. Strasinger. *Urinalysis and Body Fluids*, 3rd ed. Philadelphia: Davis; 1994.)

Clinical Summary

The cellular asphyxiants are a diverse group of substances including carbon monoxide, cyanide, sodium azide, nitrites and other methemoglobin-producing oxidizing agents, and hydrogen sulfide, all of which interfere with the cellular utilization of oxygen. Depending on the substance, the interference may occur at the level of hemoglobin, the electron transport chain, or both. In contrast with the simple asphyxiants, ambient oxygen concentrations are not affected.

Carbon monoxide is a colorless and odorless gas generated from the incomplete combustion of carbonaceous compounds. Carbon monoxide remains a leading cause of poisoning morbidity and mortality. The affinity of carbon monoxide for hemoglobin is 250 times greater than that of oxygen. Binding of carbon monoxide to hemoglobin shifts the oxyhemoglobin dissociation curve to the left, further impairing tissue oxygen delivery. Symptoms of acute poisoning may range from headache to ischemic chest pain, seizures, and CNS depression. Up to 40% of poisoned patients develop delayed neurologic sequelae (DNS); most cases of DNS are associated with an initial loss of consciousness.

Although a nonspecific enzyme inhibitor, cyanide is classically described as inhibiting the mitochondrial cytochrome a-a₃ complex, thereby interfering with oxidative phosphorylation. The interaction between cyanide and the cytochrome a-a₃ complex is reversible. Sources of cyanide include industrial and household chemicals, plants, and structure fires. Clinical manifestations reflect dysfunction of oxygen-sensitive organs, including the CNS and cardiovascular systems. A cyanide toxidrome has been described, consisting of altered mental status, mydriasis, respiratory depression, hypotension, tachycardia, and metabolic (lactic) acidosis.

Emergency Department Treatment and Disposition

Immediate management focuses upon airway stabilization and antidotal therapy. Carboxyhemoglobin levels should be obtained in patients with suspected carbon monoxide poisoning. Pregnancy status should be determined in females presenting with suspected carbon monoxide poisoning. Blood cyanide levels are not typically available in the immediate care setting. While 100% oxygen is the accepted antidote for acute carbon monoxide poisoning, controversy persists regarding the mode of administration (normobaric oxygen versus hyperbaric oxygen).

Potential indications for hyperbaric oxygen include syncope, altered mental status (especially with evidence of cerebellar dysfunction), acidosis, and pregnancy. Specific therapies for cyanide poisoning include the cyanide antidote kit which contains amyl nitrite, sodium nitrite, and sodium thiosulfate. Hydroxocobalamin was approved for treatment of suspected cyanide poisoning in December 2006.

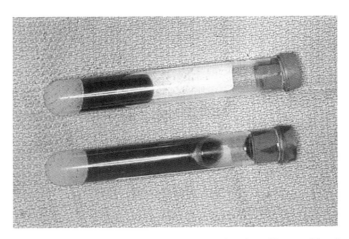

FIGURE 17.34 ■ Carbon Monoxide Poisoning. Venous blood samples with the bright red one (bottom sample) taken from a patient with acute carbon monoxide poisoning. The dark red venous blood (top sample) is a control sample from a patient with no carboxyhemoglobin. (Photo contributor: Daniel L. Savitt, MD.)

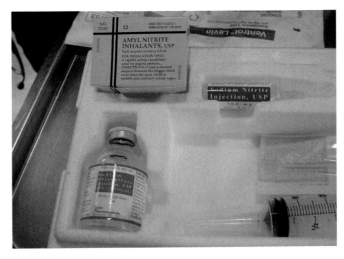

FIGURE 17.35 ■ Cyanide Antidote Kit. Three components of the original cyanide antidote kit included an amyl nitrite pearl, sodium nitrite, and sodium thiosulfate. The nitrites are used to induce methemoglobinemia and the sodium thiosulfate to enhance elimination of the cyanide. (Photo contributor: Matthew D. Sztajnkrycer, MD, PhD.)

Pearls

1. The decision to treat acute carbon monoxide poisoning is based upon history and physical examination, and not solely upon carbon monoxide level.
2. Maternal carboxyhemoglobin levels fail to accurately reflect fetal carboxyhemoglobin levels.
3. Methylene chloride and nickel carbonyl are metabolized to carbon monoxide, resulting in on-going exposure and potential for toxicity.
4. In victims of structure fires who present without severe burns, a plasma lactate greater than 10 mmol/L correlates with cyanide level greater than 40 mol/L.
5. Empiric therapy with sodium thiosulfate may be considered for victims of structure fires in whom suspicion exists for cyanide poisoning.

Clinical Summary

Methemoglobin occurs when the iron atom in deoxyhemoglobin loses an electron, resulting in a ferric (Fe^{3+}) ion instead of the usual ferrous (Fe^{2+}) state. Ferric iron can no longer bind to oxygen, thereby reducing the oxygen-carrying capacity of hemoglobin. The presence of methemoglobin also shifts the oxygen hemoglobin dissociation curve to the left which results in decreased release of oxygen to the tissues. Infants may be more susceptible to the development of methemoglobinemia due to reduced activity of their NADH methemoglobin reductase. Illnesses in infants such as diarrhea, dehydration, and acidosis may also induce methemoglobin.

The most common causes of methemoglobin are acquired rather than congenital. Common pharmaceutical agents that cause methemoglobin include sulfonamides, dapsone, phenazopyridine, chloroquine, benzocaine, prilocaine, and more rarely lidocaine. Nitrites, which are used in the older cyanide antidote kit, induce methemoglobin.

Clues to the diagnosis include the patient who appears cyanotic and does not improve with the administration of oxygen. The pulse oximeter reading will drop to the mid 80% range but does not correlate with the percent of methemoglobin. The blood may appear chocolate in color and does not become red with exposure to oxygen. The arterial blood gas will demonstrate an overall normal partial pressure of oxygen with a resulting normal calculated arterial saturation. Methemoglobin may be measured via a co-oximeter using either arterial or venous heparinized blood.

Emergency Department Treatment and Disposition

Any patient who appears cyanotic should initially be treated with administration of supplemental oxygen, and advanced airway management as appropriate. In general, any patient who is symptomatic from methemoglobinemia or has a level exceeding 25% to 30% should be treated with methylene blue.

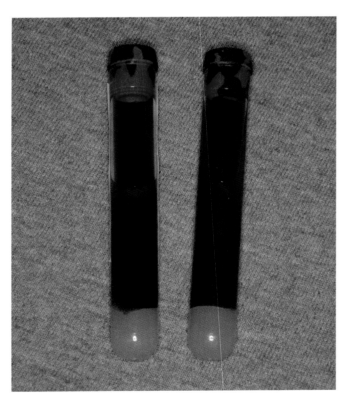

FIGURE 17.36 ■ Methemoglobinemia—"Chocolate Blood." "Chocolate blood" from an arterial sample of a patient with methemoglobinemia (left) compared to the normal bright red arterial blood (right). (Photo contributor: Kevin J. Knoop, MD, MS.)

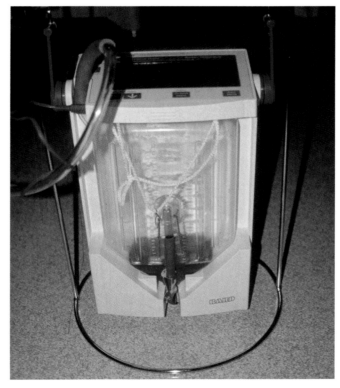

FIGURE 17.37 ■ Methylene Blue Urine. Methylene blue is excreted renally and gives a blue-green color to the urine. (Photo contributor: Division of Medical Toxicology, University of California, San Diego.)

Methylene blue is available in a 1% solution and is administered as a 1 to 2 mg/kg dose intravenously over 5 minutes. This may be repeated if there is no initial response in 20 to 30 minutes. Patients who have methemoglobinemia from dapsone or aniline dyes may have recurrence and require additional dosing of methylene blue.

Pearls

1. High doses of methylene blue (5-7 mg/kg) may cause paradoxical methemoglobinemia and hemolysis.

2. The intravenous administration of methylene blue may interfere with the reading of the pulse oximeter and cause the reading to decrease transiently.

3. Methylene blue accelerates the ability of NADPH methemoglobin reductase to reduce the ferric iron of methemoglobin back to a ferrous iron.

4. Methylene blue may not reverse methemoglobin in a patient with G6PD deficiency due to the absence of NADPH and may increase the risk of hemolysis.

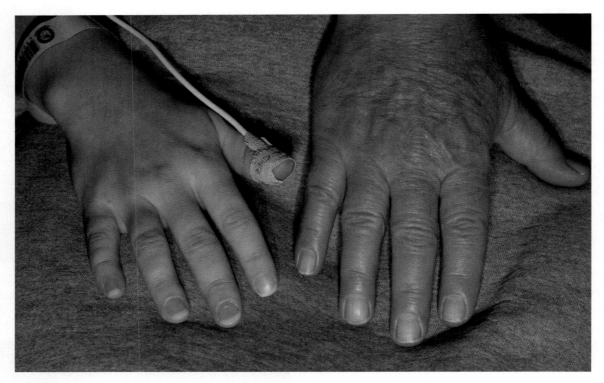

FIGURE 17.38 ▪ Methemoglobinemia—Cyanosis. Methemoglobinemia resulted in the cyanotic appearance of this pediatric patient as noted on the hand on the left side of the image compared with the normal adult control on the right. (Photo contributor: Kevin J. Knoop, MD, MS.)

Clinical Summary

Inhalant abuse is the intentional inhalation of vapors for the purpose of becoming "high." More common among adolescents, the median age of first use is around 13 years of age. Sniffing refers to the inhalation of the agent directly from a container, such as airplane glue. Huffing involves placing solvent on some type of fabric and inhaling the vapors from the fabric. Bagging is the name given to the technique of spraying the solvent into a bag and then rebreathing from the bag. Occasionally the bag is placed over the head, potentially resulting in asphyxiant death. Inhalants are rapidly absorbed via the lungs and cross into the brain. Initial effects include euphoria and occasional hallucinations. CNS depression may occur. Acute cardiotoxicity may also occur and is thought to be the cause of "sudden sniffing death." The cause of death is thought to be due to increased myocardial sensitization that promotes dysrhythmogenesis in the setting of a catecholamine surge such as running. Chronic effects from inhalant abuse include leukoencephalopathy, cardiomyopathy, cerebellar degeneration, and neuropathy.

Emergency Department Treatment and Disposition

Clues to the diagnosis of inhalant abuse are the presence of spray paint on the fingers or the face. Due to the increased solvent content in metallic-colored paints, gold and silver spray paint are particularly popular. Cardiac dysrhythmias tend to have a poor prognosis. Current recommendations suggest the use of β-blockers to treat ventricular dysrhythmias. Consider electrolyte abnormalities and acid-base status, particularly with toluene-based products. Carbon monoxide poisoning may occur after methylene chloride inhalation. Benzodiazepines may be used for treatment of agitation.

Pearls

1. Chronic abuse of nitrous oxide (N_2O) may result in a megaloblastic anemia and distal axonal sensorimotor neuropathy that may be a result of irreversible oxidation of cobalamin (vitamin B_{12}). In addition to being used medicinally as "laughing gas," nitrous is abused from "whippets," which are the cartridges of compressed air used for whipping cream canisters.
2. Chronic abuse of toluene may result in potassium wasting renal tubular acidosis. Some of the carburetor cleaners that contain toluene also contain methanol.

3. Amyl, butyl, and isobutyl nitrites are strong oxidizers and may produce methemoglobinemia. These may be sold as "poppers."
4. Iatrogenic toxicity may occur after administration of the sedative chloral hydrate.

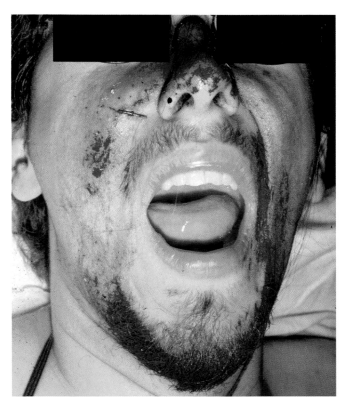

FIGURE 17.39 ■ "Huffing." Patients who huff spray paints may present with the paint on their face and hands. (Photo contributor: Alan B. Storrow, MD.)

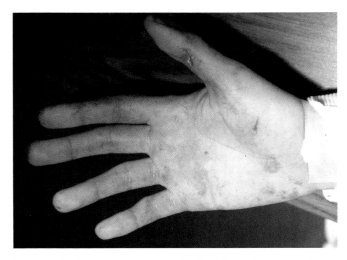

FIGURE 17.40 ■ "Huffing." The hand of the patient in Fig. 17.39. (Photo contributor: Alan B. Storrow, MD.)

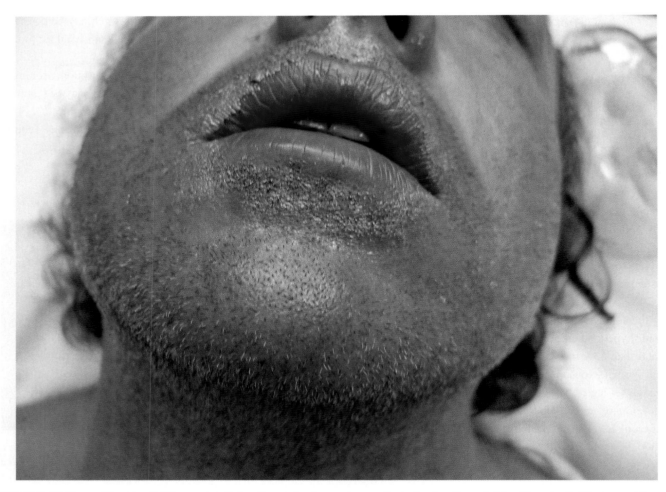

FIGURE 17.41 ■ "Bagging." Silver paint lining the perioral area in a patient abusing the paint by "bagging." (Photo contributor: R. Jason Thurman, MD.)

Clinical Summary

Hydrofluoric acid (HF) is a colorless, corrosive liquid available in both commercial (>20%) and household (<20%, typically 6%-12%) formulations. Commercially, HF is used in glass etching, electroplating, and semiconductor manufacturing. Consumer products are typically marketed as rust removers and chrome cleaners. Although toxic via the dermal, ocular, pulmonary, and gastrointestinal routes, the majority of patients present after dermal exposure, typically to the hands and fingers. The severity of local injury depends upon the HF concentration and the extent of exposure.

Symptoms and tissue effects may be appreciably delayed, especially with household formulations. In addition to the coagulative necrosis noted with other inorganic acids, HF causes toxicity by the binding and precipitation of calcium ions. In addition to local effects, significant and potentially life-threatening systemic effects may occur including hypocalcemia, hyperkalemia, and hypomagnesemia. Concentrations greater than 50% may cause rapid decompensation with even small dermal exposures (1% total body surface area).

In the setting of hand exposure, pain is typically described as developing gradually into a severe unremitting deep burning sensation. Early local erythema is variable. Especially with higher HF concentrations, a pale blanched appearance may develop.

Emergency Department Treatment and Disposition

Treatment varies depending upon the route of exposure, but is directed toward decontamination, neutralization of the fluoride ion, and pain control. In the setting of ingestion or significant dermal exposure (more than 5% TBSA of a household HF formulation), serum electrolytes, including calcium and magnesium, should be determined. In addition to pain control, management options for hand burns include commercially available calcium gluconate gel, subcutaneous calcium gluconate infiltration, and regional intravenous and intra-arterial calcium gluconate infusion.

Pearls

1. An expedient 2.5% calcium gluconate gel can be made by adding 3.5 g calcium gluconate powder to 5 oz (150 mL) of water-based lubricant. Alternatively, 10 crushed 1 g calcium carbonate antacid tablets may be added to 20 mL water-based lubricant. The resultant gel may be placed in a rubber glove and placed on the patient's hand for topical treatment.

2. With significant dermal exposure or ingestion, prolonged cardiac and serum electrolyte monitoring may be required; sudden, delayed cardiac arrest has occurred.

3. Replacement of calcium and magnesium may require substantially larger doses than typically required.

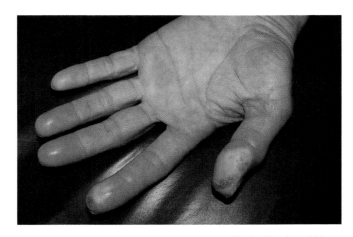

FIGURE 17.42 ■ Hydrofluoric Acid Burns. Hydrofluoric acid burn due to application of a rust remover agent. The patient presented hours later after initial use with severe, deep pain in the thumb and index finger. (Photo contributor: Karen Rogers, MD.)

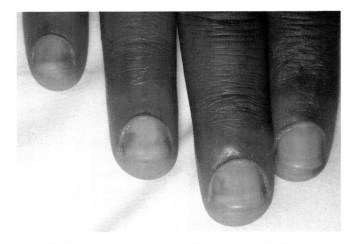

FIGURE 17.43 ■ Hydrofluoric Acid Burn—Nailbeds. Hydrofluoric acid can seep underneath the nailbeds, resulting in blanched discoloration. (Photo contributor: Lawrence B. Stack, MD)

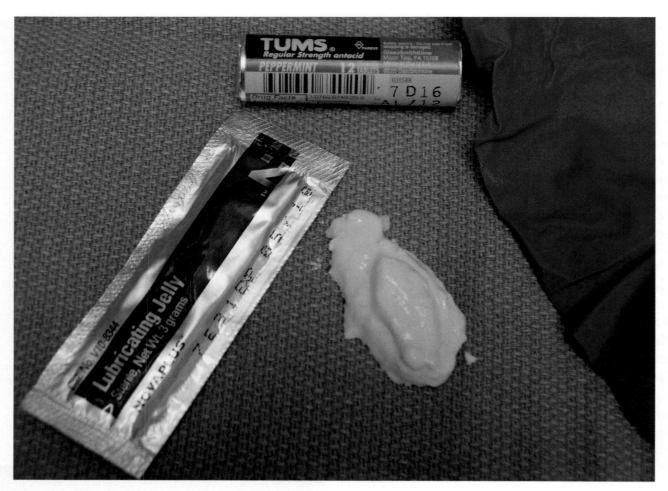

FIGURE 17.44 ■ Hydrofluoric Acid Burn Treatment. Expedient topical therapy for hydrofluoric acid burns can be made using crushed calcium containing antacids mixed with surgical jelly. The jelly may be placed in a rubber glove, then the glove on the patient's hand. (Photo contributor: Matthew D. Sztajnkrycer, MD, PhD.)

Clinical Summary

Botulinum is a potent neurotoxin that blocks the release of acetylcholine. It is derived primarily from *Clostridium botulinum*, although a few other clostridial species produce a homologous neurotoxin that results in clinical botulism. Botulinum toxin blocks release of acetylcholine which results in decreased activation of muscarinic and nicotinic receptors. Initial effects may include nonspecific findings such as nausea and vomiting, constipation, and throat complaints. The classic neurologic findings are due to the lack of receptor activation of the nicotinic receptor at the neuromuscular junction. Dysarthria, dysphagia, diplopia, and mydriasis progress to a descending symmetric paralysis.

The common types of botulism include foodborne (ingestion of preformed toxin), infantile (*in vivo* production of toxin), and wound botulism (*in vivo* production of toxin). While foodborne has the features classically described, infantile botulism manifests as the constipated, floppy baby. Wound botulism is most commonly associated with "skin popping," a technique of subcutaneous injection of an illicit drug, usually black tar heroin. Diagnosis is initially a clinical one, with subsequent verification via a murine assay of the presence of botulinum toxin in a patient sample. This assay is performed through either the state department of health or the Centers for Disease Control and Prevention.

Emergency Department Treatment and Disposition

Any patient in whom botulism is suspected should be admitted to the hospital. Careful monitoring of the airway status is important to ensure that the patient has adequate ventilatory capacity. The local health department should be notified to assist with the procurement of botulinum antitoxin for foodborne and wound botulism patients. Human botulinum immune globulin is available through the California Department of Health for the treatment of infantile botulism.

Pearls

1. The initial chief complaint of a patient with wound botulism may be "sore throat" since the patient has dry mucus membranes and difficulty swallowing.
2. Since botulinum toxin does not cross the blood-brain barrier, the mental status should not be affected unless the patient has respiratory insufficiency.

3. Early signs of infantile botulism may be difficulty with feeding since feeding for an infant requires use of the cranial nerves.

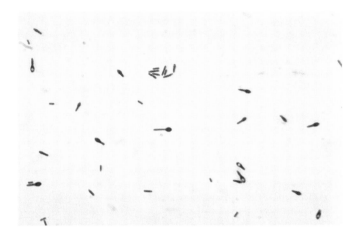

FIGURE 17.45 ■ *Clostridium botulinum. Clostridium botulinum* is a gram-positive rod that will have terminal or subterminal spores. These spores are heat resistant. (Photo contributor: the Centers for Disease Control and Prevention.)

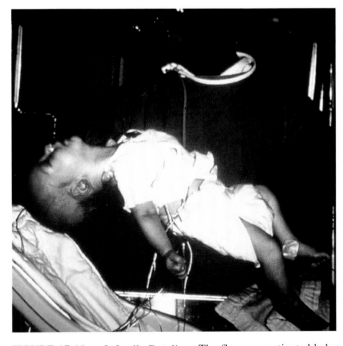

FIGURE 17.46 ■ Infantile Botulism. The floppy-constipated baby is a classic presentation of infantile botulism. (Photo contributor: the Centers for Disease Control and Prevention.)

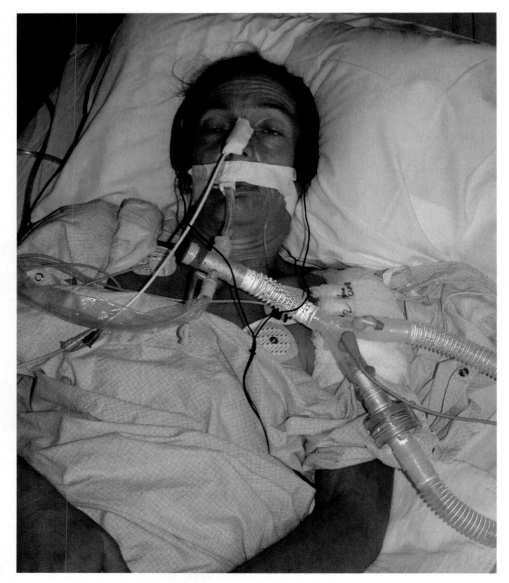

FIGURE 17.47 ■ Wound Botulism. Wound botulism occurs from the *in vivo* production of botulinum toxin. It manifests the same neurotoxicity with the ptosis, bulbar paralysis, and respiratory compromise as foodborne botulism. Note the profound ptosis in this patient. (Photo contributor: William H. Richardson, III, MD.)

Clinical Summary

Arsenic, a tasteless and odorless metalloid, is well absorbed by multiple routes of administration. Although arsenic exists in both inorganic and organic species, only the inorganic form is responsible for toxicity. Contaminated soil and water with inorganic arsenic are the primary sources of exposure to the general population. Chronic arsenic poisoning due to contaminated water continues to be a global health issue.

Arsenic inhibits multiple enzymes critical to the production of ATP. It inhibits pyruvate dehydrogenase complex, decreases the citric acid cycle, and decreases gluconeogenesis. Acute arsenic poisoning typically starts with acute onset of nausea, vomiting, abdominal pain, and "rice water" diarrhea. Acute encephalopathy, acute renal failure, lung injury, and death may occur. Later findings in survivors include alopecia, rash, Mees lines, and neuropathy. Chronic toxicity results in dermatologic changes such as hyperpigmentation or hypopigmentation. Hyperkeratosis may occur on the skin, particularly the palms and soles. Peripheral vascular disease (Blackfoot disease) may occur. Arsenic is a known carcinogen and is associated with skin and lung cancers.

Emergency Department Treatment and Disposition

After an acute ingestion, an abdominal radiograph may demonstrate radiopaque material in the gastrointestinal tract. Supportive care with maintenance of electrolytes is important. A 24-hour urine collection in a metal-free container is the optimal method for determining arsenic burden. However, the acutely ill patient will likely require chelation before urine results are available. Chelation is usually initiated with intramuscular dimercaprol (British Antilewisite, BAL). Succimer, an oral analogue of the BAL, may be useful in subacute poisoning. Patients with suspected acute arsenic poisoning should be admitted to an intensive care unit.

Pearls

1. When a nonselective heavy metal urine test is performed for possible arsenic exposure, the measured arsenic typically reflects the presence of nontoxic organic species from dietary sources such as seafood, rather than toxic inorganic species. As such, urine should either be speciated, or the patient advised to refrain from seafood prior to urine collection.

2. Intravenous arsenic trioxide is approved by the Food and Drug Administration for treatment of acute promyelocytic leukemia unresponsive to other therapies.

3. Acute arsenic poisoning is one of the few heavy metals that is directly cardiotoxic as it blocks delayed rectifier channels. Torsades de pointes has been described in the setting of acute arsenic poisoning.

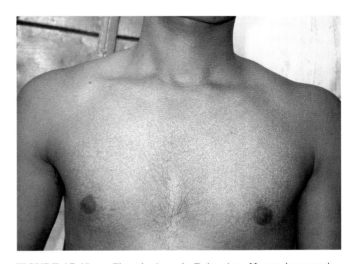

FIGURE 17.48 ■ Chronic Arsenic Poisoning. Hyperpigmentation of the skin is a clinical finding from chronic arsenic poisoning. (Photo contributor: Lawrence B. Stack, MD.)

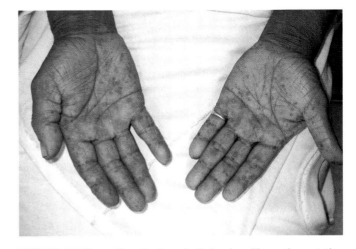

FIGURE 17.49 ■ Chronic Arsenic Poisoning. Hyperpigmentation and hypopigmentation along with hyperkeratosis are findings on the palms of patients with chronic arsenic poisoning. (Photo contributor: Lawrence B. Stack, MD.)

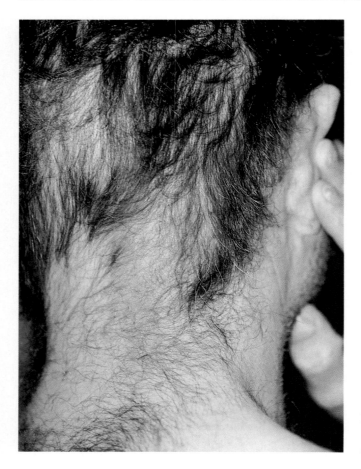

FIGURE 17.50 ■ Chronic Arsenic Poisoning. The patchy hair loss seen in this photograph is from chronic arsenic poisoning. (Photo contributor: Selim Suner, MD, MS.)

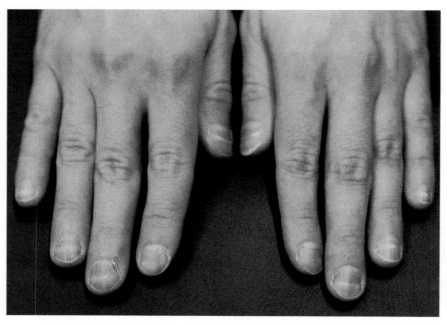

FIGURE 17.51 ■ Mees Lines. Characteristic Mees lines of chronic arsenic poisoning. Note the transverse white lines on all the nails of both hands. Mees lines are often seen in conjunction with polyneuropathy of arsenic poisoning. (Photo contributor: Robert Hoffman, MD.)

Clinical Summary

Mercury occurs in three different forms (elemental, inorganic, and organic), each with its own clinical pattern of poisoning. Elemental mercury ("quicksilver") is found in thermometers and sphygmomanometers. Elemental mercury poisoning is associated with inhalation of volatilized mercurial ions, which may occur after vacuuming or heating. Manifestations include cough, fevers, chills, and dyspnea. Acute interstitial pneumonitis may occur and may progress to severe lung injury and death. Inorganic mercury poisoning usually occurs from the ingestion of the mercurial salts. Initial presentation is acute caustic gastroenteritis that may be hemorrhagic. Renal failure is a prominent finding in these patients. Organic mercury poisoning occurs from ingestion of short chain alkyl mercurial compounds. Methylmercury distributes into brain tissue and causes neurologic disease such as ataxia, paresthesias, visual difficulties, movement disorders, and speech difficulties. Methylmercury is also a known teratogen.

Emergency Department Treatment and Disposition

After an ingestion of a mercurial substance, a radiograph may demonstrate radiopaque material in the gastrointestinal tract. If elemental mercury was injected intravenously, mercurial emboli may be seen in the lungs. Local injection in the skin may demonstrate mercury deposition in the soft tissues. Ingestion of elemental mercury rarely results in significant absorption. For inhalational injury due to elemental mercury, respiratory support may be required. Ingestion of inorganic mercury may lead to early cardiovascular collapse as a result of the severe volume depletion. Fluid resuscitation and electrolyte management are critical. Chelation with dimercaprol (BAL) may be initiated early and when the patient is able to take oral medications, the chelator may be switched to succimer. For organic mercury poisoning, oral succimer may be the firstline agent.

Pearls

1. Elemental mercury toxicity has occurred when it is heated and used to extract gold from jewelry.
2. "Mad as a hatter" is a term used to describe the delirium for anticholinergic poisoning; however, the term is derived from the erethism and hatter's shakes from mercury exposure during the felt-hat manufacturing process in the late 19th and early 20th century.

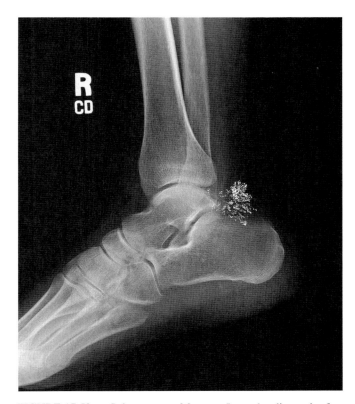

FIGURE 17.52 ■ Subcutaneous Mercury. Lateral radiograph of an ankle demonstrating elemental mercury in the tissues. The patient had a barometer break into his skin. (Photo contributor: Saralyn R. Williams, MD.)

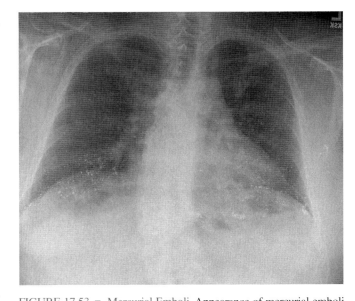

FIGURE 17.53 ■ Mercurial Emboli. Appearance of mercurial emboli in the pulmonary vascular tree on chest x-ray. Though this may be seen from intentional intravenous mercury injection, this patient absorbed the mercury intravenously following an accident involving multiple shattered thermometers. (Photo contributor: John Worrell, MD.)

3. Organic mercury is eliminated via the fecal route, so urine samples for methylmercury will not be reflective of the body burden.

4. BAL is suspended in peanut oil, and so can only be administered as an intramuscular injection, and to non-peanut-sensitive individuals.

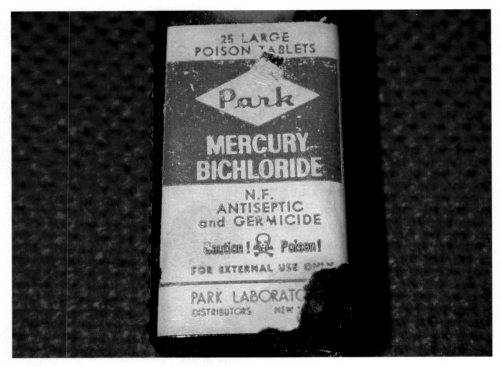

FIGURE 17.54 ■ Mercury Salts. Mercury salts were used as topical antiseptics. Ingestion of inorganic mercury is caustic to the gastrointestinal tract and causes rapid renal failure. (Photo contributor: Matthew D. Sztajnkrycer, MD, PhD.)

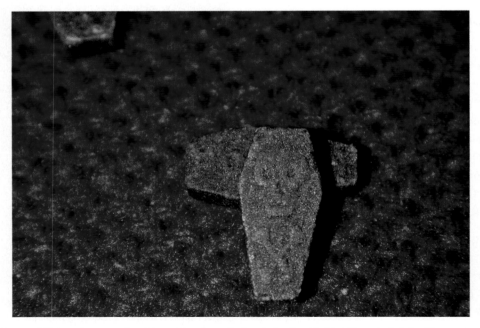

FIGURE 17.55 ■ Mercury Tablets. An example of the tablets from the bottle in Fig. 17.54. Although faded with age, the coffin-shaped tablets contain the word "poison" on one side and the "skull-and-crossbones" on the other. (Photo contributor: Matthew D. Sztajnkrycer, MD, PhD.)

Clinical Summary

Although the prevalence of markedly elevated lead levels in the population has been declining, acute and chronic lead poisoning still occur. Lead is well absorbed by the lungs and less well via the gastrointestinal tract. Lead paint in older homes is a continued source of lead exposure. Other possible exposures may occur from occupational exposures, retained lead bullets in synovial fluid, jewelry, lead-painted toys, fishing weights, ceramic glazes, and cosmetics. Severe lead poisoning in adults has also been associated with ingestion of contaminated moonshine.

Lead poisoning affects multiple organ systems. Neurotoxicity may range from subtle personality changes to encephalopathy and cerebral edema. At the societal level, even small lead burdens are associated with statistically significant decreases in intelligence quotient. Motor neuropathy such as foot drop and wrist drop may be seen in adult patients, especially after occupational exposure. Microcytic anemia may occur and basophilic stippling of the red cells may be seen. Hypertension and an acute nephropathy may occur. Abdominal pain may be described by patients but unlike other heavy metal poisonings, constipation is more likely than diarrhea. Radiographic "lead lines," bands of increased density on long bones metaphyses, may be seen in young children. These densities are not due to deposition of lead but rather increased calcium deposition.

Emergency Department Treatment and Disposition

Whole blood lead level is the primary measure of lead exposure, but is not usually available in real time. Radiographic studies may demonstrate radiopaque substances from ingested jewelry or paint chips in children. Lead encephalopathy must be aggressively managed. Dimercaprol (BAL) is administered intramuscularly and CaNa$_2$EDTA is later given intravenously. Chelation with oral therapy of succimer is currently recommended in asymptomatic children with levels between 45 and 70 mcg/dL. Reducing the exposure in children is paramount to treatment and the source of the lead may be elusive.

Pearls

1. One source of lead exposure in children is through the occupation of the parent. Workers in a lead dust environment will bring home the lead dust on their clothes and shoes.

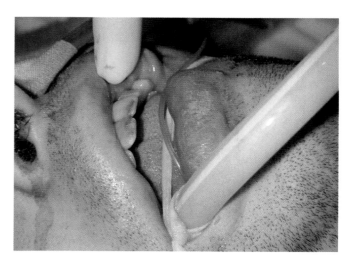

FIGURE 17.56 ■ Acute Lead Poisoning. This patient presented with acute encephalopathy after ingesting lead-based, Tangerine-scented gloss glaze used for making pottery. The substance is present on the teeth, lips, and nose (from vomiting). (Photo contributor: Matthew D. Sztajnkrycer, MD, PhD.)

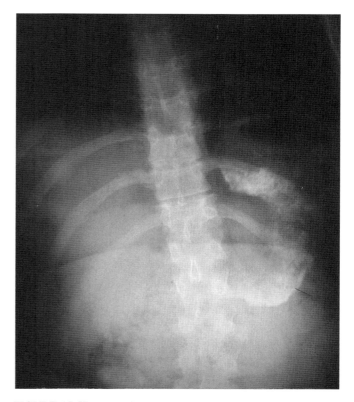

FIGURE 17.57 ■ Radiopaque Lead. The abdominal x-ray of the patient in Fig. 17.56. Lead is radiopaque when ingested. (Photo contributor: Matthew D. Sztajnkrycer, MD, PhD.)

2. Imported eye cosmetics with lead have been a source of pediatric exposures in certain ethnic groups.

3. Azarcon and greta are lead-based remedies that are used to treat diarrheal illnesses.

4. Adults usually require much higher blood lead levels than children before encephalopathy occurs.

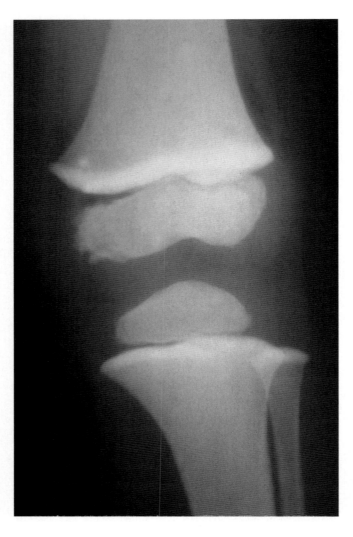

FIGURE 17.58 ▪ Lead Lines. Lead lines seen in a pediatric patient with chronic lead poisoning. The increased radiographic densities on the metaphyseal growth plates demonstrate radiological growth retardation and increased calcium deposition. (Photo contributor: David Effron, MD.)

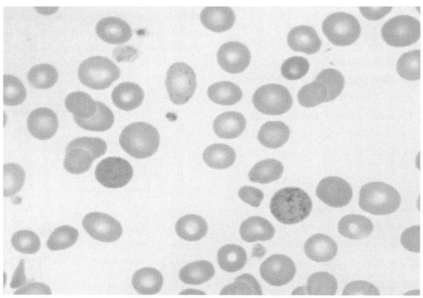

FIGURE 17.59 ▪ Basophilic Stippling. Basophilic stippling along with a microcytic anemia may be seen in patients with chronic lead poisoning. (Photo contributor: Debbie Bennes, BS, MLT, ASCP.)

Clinical Summary

Iron is a commonly used pharmaceutical agent and supplement found in prenatal and multivitamins. Although the incidence has declined, acute iron poisoning remains a significant cause of pediatric morbidity and mortality. The toxic dose depends upon the quantity of elemental iron in the preparation, which in turn depends upon the iron formulation. While the minimum toxic dose remains controversial, ingestion of more than 40 mg/kg elemental iron may result in toxicity, while ingestion of more than 60 mg/kg elemental iron is associated with severe morbidity and possible mortality.

Iron toxicity is classically described as a four-stage process. Stage I develops within the first few hours of ingestion and reflects the direct caustic effects of iron on the gastrointestinal tract. Signs and symptoms may include abdominal pain and GI bleeding. Stage II, variably present, is a redistributive or quiescent phase; although the initial GI symptoms resolve during this phase, acidosis and end-organ toxicity may still develop. With significant toxicity, individuals may progress directly from Stage I to Stage III. Stage III is the phase of overt shock, metabolic acidosis, and end-organ dysfunction (including delayed hepatic failure). Individuals who survive Stage III may rarely progress to Stage IV, gastric outlet obstruction secondary to the initial caustic insult of Stage I.

Emergency Department Treatment and Disposition

Activated charcoal does not bind iron. Whole bowel irrigation has been advocated for substantial ingestions and for patients with evidence of iron tablets on abdominal radiographs. Serum iron levels peak between 2 and 6 hours post-ingestion. Levels obtained more than 6 hours after ingestion are unreliable due to tissue redistribution. Patients with evidence of iron toxicity (eg, persistent vomiting, acidosis, altered mental status, and hypotension) or a 4- to 6-hour post-ingestion serum level more than 500 mcg/dL should receive chelation with deferoxamine.

Pearls

1. Acute iron ingestion and the risk for toxicity must be assessed based upon the quantity of elemental iron ingested, not the total amount ingested.

2. The absence of radiopaque materials on abdominal radiographs is not a reliable indicator to exclude potential iron toxicity; liquid and pediatric (chewable) formulations are not typically radiopaque.

3. Despite the potential for anaphylactoid reactions and hypotension, patients requiring chelation therapy should receive deferoxamine via the intravenous route.

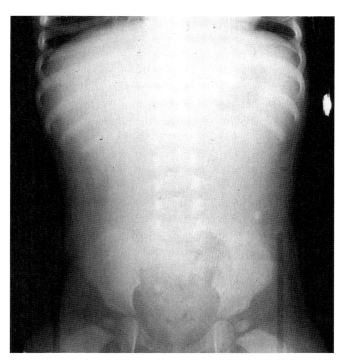

FIGURE 17.60 ■ Radiopaque Iron. KUB radiograph of a patient with an acute iron ingestion, demonstrating radiopaque foreign bodies as noted in the left mid-quadrant and right lower pelvis. (Photo contributor: Saralyn R. Williams, MD.)

Iron formulation	Percent elemental iron
Ferrous fumurate	33%
Ferrous chloride	28%
Ferrous sulfate	20%
Ferrous lactate	19%
Ferrous gluconate	12%

FIGURE 17.61 ■ Elemental Iron. This table compares the percent elemental iron between the different iron formulations. The percent elemental iron tells what percent of the weight of the tablet is actually iron. (Photo contributor: Saralyn R. Williams, MD.)

Clinical Summary

Mushrooms are the fruits of certain fungi. *Amanita phalloides* (the "death cap") and *Amanita ocreata* (the "destroying angel") species produce amatoxins and account for most fatalities attributed to mushroom ingestion. Mushroom poisoning commonly occurs in the early fall, when wild mushrooms are abundant and amateur foragers mistake poisonous mushrooms for edible ones.

Amatoxin poisoning results in severe symptoms of gastroenteritis including nausea, vomiting, profuse watery diarrhea, and abdominal pain at least 6 to 24 hours after ingestion. Hematemesis, hematochezia, and severe dehydration resulting in hypotension may occur. Metabolic acidosis and electrolyte losses may be found in severe poisoning. Gastrointestinal symptoms may last 12 to 24 hours and are followed by a latent period of apparent improvement. This period is followed by a rise in liver enzymes and bilirubin and elevations in the PT and PTT. Fulminant hepatic failure and renal failure may become apparent.

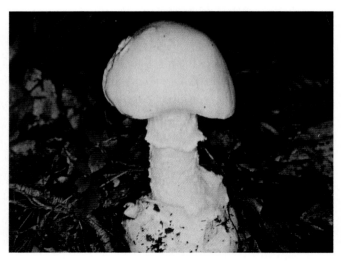

FIGURE 17.62 ■ *Amanita phalloides.* The "death cap" produces amatoxins and accounts for most of the fatalities due to mushroom ingestion. (Photo contributor: Edward J. Otten, MD.)

Emergency Department Treatment and Disposition

Administration of activated charcoal may be recommended depending on the time since ingestion. Specific interventions that may be helpful but are yet unproved include charcoal hemoperfusion, high-dose cimetidine, high-dose penicillin, high-dose ascorbic acid, *N*-acetylcysteine, and hyperbaric oxygen therapy. Vitamin K may be helpful to improve coagulopathy resulting from hepatic failure.

Pearls

1. A single "death cap" may contain enough amatoxin to kill an adult.
2. Cooking these mushrooms does not substantially alter their toxicity.
3. Not all *Amanita* species of mushrooms cause hepatotoxicity when ingested. Some *Amanita* species are hallucinogens and one causes renal failure.

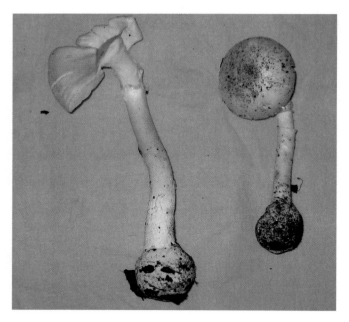

FIGURE 17.63 ■ *Amanita ocreata.* These mushrooms were samples of *Amanita ocreata* provided by a family who had ingested them and subsequently developed significant hepatotoxicity. (Photo contributor: Division of Medical Toxicology, University of California, San Diego.)

Clinical Summary

Cardiac glycosides (CG) are found in the leaves, flowers, and seeds of *Nerium oleander* (common oleander), *Thevetia peruviana* (yellow oleander), *Digitalis purpurea* (foxglove), *Strophanthus gratus* (ouabain), *Convallaria majalis* (lily of the valley), *Apocynum cannabinum* (dogbane), *Urginea maritima* and *Urginea indica* (squill), and *Cheiranthus cheiri* (wallflower). If ingested, they produce clinical findings similar to digoxin toxicity. The drinking of foxglove and oleander tea may be a cause of CG toxicity. Therapeutic effects occur from inhibition of the cardiac cell membrane sodium-potassium adenosine triphosphate pump, resulting in increased automaticity, decreased conduction through the AV node, and improved inotropy.

Toxic effects are an exaggeration of therapeutic effects. Bradydysrhythmias may result from impaired pacemaker function. Tachydysrhythmias may occur from increased automaticity. Nausea, vomiting, abdominal pain, confusion, depression, and fatigue may be present. Headaches, paresthesias, weakness, scotomas, and visual color disturbances (yellow halos around lights) may also be seen.

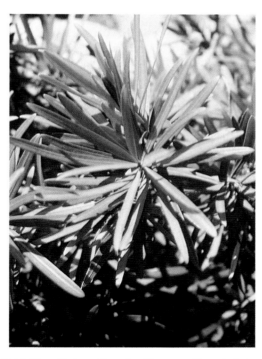

FIGURE 17.64 ■ Nerium Oleander (Common Oleander). A common decorative plant in subtropical climates often seen lining roads and highways. Flowers may be white, yellow, red, or purple. Plants may grow to a height of 15 ft. (Photo contributor: Lawrence B. Stack, MD.)

Emergency Department Treatment and Disposition

Atropine may be initially given for bradydysrhythmias. Refractory bradydysrhythmias require pacing. Ventricular tachydysrhythmias have been treated with phenytoin or lidocaine when digoxin-specific Fab fragments are not available. Activated charcoal is the preferred method of decontamination. Cardioversion should be avoided in CG toxicity. Digoxin-specific Fab fragments are the treatment of choice for life-threatening dysrhythmias or CG-induced hyperkalemia.

Pearls

1. Treat CG overdose from plant exposure in the same way as an acute digoxin overdose. Higher doses of digoxin-specific Fab fragments may be required.
2. Calcium should be avoided in treating CG-associated hyperkalemia, as it may worsen ventricular arrhythmias.
3. Dysrhythmias characterized by increased automaticity coupled with the presence of conduction disturbances are highly suggestive of cardiac glycoside toxicity.

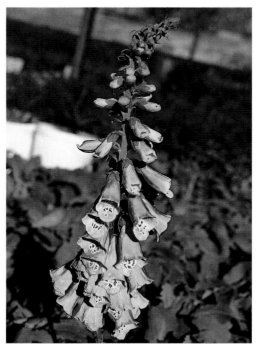

FIGURE 17.65 ■ *Digitalis purpurea* (Purple Foxglove). The ornamental plant. (Photo contributor: Lawrence B. Stack, MD.)

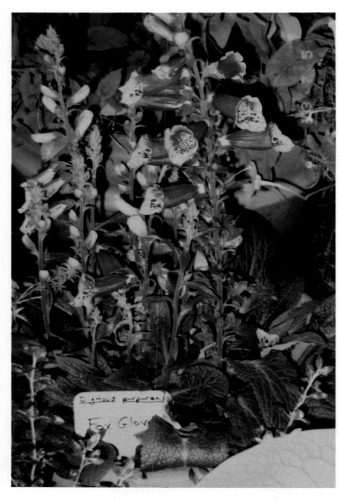

FIGURE 17.66 ■ *Digitalis purpurea.* A potted plant of *Digitalis purpurae.* When the stalks of flowers stop blooming, the leaves of the remaining plant are fairly nondescript. (Photo contributor: Saralyn R. Williams, MD.)

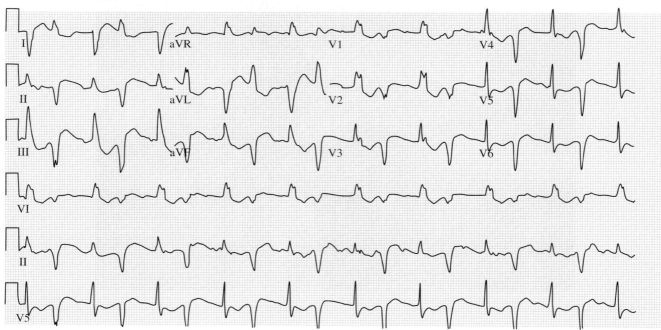

FIGURE 17.67 ■ Bidirectional Ventricular Tachycardia. An example of bidirectional ventricular tachycardia that occurred in a patient with digoxin toxicity. (Photo contributor: Binh Ly, MD.)

Clinical Summary

Dieffenbachia (dumb cane) is a common houseplant that causes toxic effects when ingested owing to large amounts of insoluble oxalate crystals in its leaves. The oxalate crystals are highly irritating, and those who ingest the leaves experience painful burning of the lips, tongue, mouth, and esophagus. Marked swelling of the tongue, lips, and oropharynx can occur, and airway patency may become a major issue in managing these patients. Ocular exposures may occur as well, resulting in painful burning, erythema, and eyelid swelling. Fortunately, calcium oxalate crystals are not absorbed and the profound hypocalcemia associated with soluble oxalates is not seen with Dieffenbachia poisoning.

Emergency Department Treatment and Disposition

Topical anesthetics are helpful in controlling severe pain from burning mucous membranes. Management is largely supportive, as the painful oral burns experienced with Dieffenbachia exposure usually limit ingestion. As with any oropharyngeal burn, airway issues must be addressed. A period of observation is appropriate to make sure that airway compromise does not occur with continued swelling. If leaves are swallowed and the patients are symptomatic, GI consultation should be considered to assess the extent of esophageal injury. Decontamination is usually not necessary, as the plant is rarely swallowed in significant amounts.

Pearls

1. Performance of nasopharyngoscopy may be helpful in assessment of airway patency for more posterior burns.
2. Patients should be instructed not to swallow topical anesthetics, as toxicity may result with extensive use.

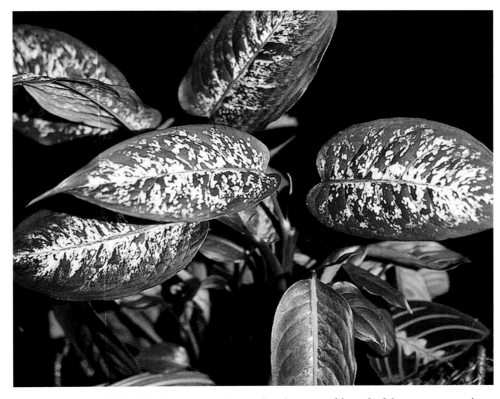

FIGURE 17.68 ■ *Dieffenbachia. Dieffenbachia* is a common houseplant because of its colorful appearance and ease of indoor growth. (Photo contributor: Kevin J. Knoop, MD, MS.)

Clinical Summary

Jimsonweed (*Datura stramonium*) is a toxic plant that contains tropane alkaloids consisting of atropine, scopolamine, and hyoscyamine compounds. Ingestion may occur through the drinking of tea made from the leaves or flowers of jimsonweed or from eating the plant's seeds or leaves. Poisoned victims demonstrate an anticholinergic toxidrome resulting from the antimuscarinic receptor effects of atropine and scopolamine. Patients may exhibit altered mental status, xerostomia, xeroderma, xerophthalmia, blurred vision, mydriasis, tachycardia, decreased bowel and bladder motility, and hyperthermia.

Emergency Department Treatment and Disposition

Treatment initially consists of assessing the ABCs (airway, breathing, circulation) and stabilization measures. Hypotension resulting from tropane alkaloid ingestion usually responds to fluid boluses. Vasopressor agents are rarely necessary. Activated charcoal may be recommended early after ingestion but may not change outcome as the toxins are absorbed rapidly. Whole-bowel irrigation is contraindicated with intestinal ileus and must be considered with great caution in jimsonweed ingestion due to decreased bowel motility. Physostigmine may be of benefit to treat severe anticholinergic toxicity, but may be better utilized as a diagnostic agent after consultation with the poison center. Severe agitation and psychosis may be treated with benzodiazepines and carefully administered properly dosed physostigmine.

Pearls

1. Examination of the axillae for xeroderma may be helpful to detect peripheral anticholinergic syndrome and distinguish between anticholinergic and sympathomimetic toxidromes.
2. Administering 1% pilocarpine drops does not reverse anticholinergic mydriasis.

3. Jimsonweed toxicity should be considered in the differential diagnosis of children and adolescents presenting with acute altered mental status, especially when accompanied by signs of anticholinergic toxicity.

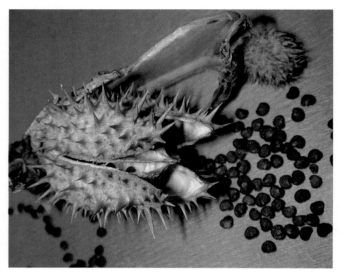

FIGURE 17.69 ■ Jimsonweed. Jimsonweed plant with seeds. (Photo contributor: Matthew D. Sztajnkrycer, MD, PhD.)

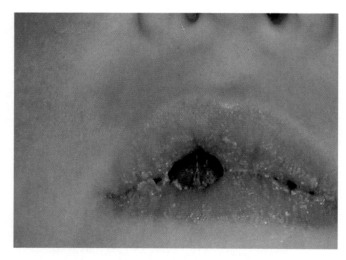

FIGURE 17.70 ■ Jimsonweed-Induced Xerostomia. A severe case of xerostomia from the antimuscarinic effects of Jimsonweed ingestion. Note the associated erythema on the patient's cheek. (Photo contributor: R. Jason Thurman, MD.)

Clinical Summary

Peyote (*Lophophora williamsii*) is a cactus plant found primarily in the southwestern United States. The cactus contains a significant amount of mescaline, a potent hallucinogen with structural similarities to norepinephrine. Peyote buttons and seeds are frequently ingested for recreational use, but are also used in the religious ceremonies of some Native American groups. Toxicity of peyote is generally mild and self-limited, but hypotension and respiratory depression can occur. Mescaline induces some sympathomimetic effects due to its similarity to norepinephrine, and marked visual hallucinations and a sense of depersonalization follow. These effects are often accompanied by unpleasant GI symptoms such as severe nausea and vomiting. Full recovery from these symptoms usually occurs within a few hours.

Emergency Department Treatment and Disposition

Treatment of peyote ingestion is largely supportive; severe toxic effects are uncommon. Marked agitation may be managed with benzodiazepines.

Pearls

1. An individual peyote button contains about 45 mg of mescaline; a mescaline dose of 5 mg/kg usually produces psychotropic effects.
2. Botulism poisoning has been reported from the ingestion of dried peyote buttons.

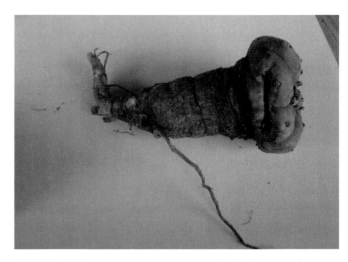

FIGURE 17.72 ■ Peyote Cactus. An individual crown of peyote. (Photo contributor: Martin Terry, PhD.)

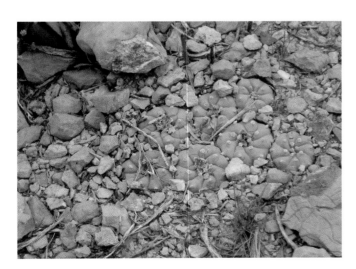

FIGURE 17.71 ■ Peyote Cactus Patch. Patch of peyote crowns growing in the desert. (Photo contributor: Martin Terry, PhD.)

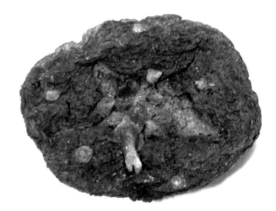

FIGURE 17.73 ■ Peyote Button. This desiccated button of peyote is the form that is ingested for recreational or religious purposes. (Photo contributor: Martin Terry, PhD.)

Clinical Summary

The jequirity pea (*Abrus precatorius*) and castor bean (*Ricinus communis*) belong to a family of poisonous plants that contain toxalbumins. The chief toxin of the jequirity pea is abrin, which is structurally very similar to the toxin ricin of the castor bean. Ingestion of jequirity peas and castor beans rarely results in toxicity, as a majority of the plant toxin is concentrated within the hard shell of the seeds. However, when these seeds are chewed or the shell is digested, symptoms of severe gastroenteritis follow within 1 to 3 days. Nausea, vomiting, abdominal pain, and diarrhea are common but in severe cases may be accompanied by hemorrhagic gastritis and hematemesis, seizures, arrhythmias, marked dehydration, CNS depression, and even death. Unfortunately, because of the colorful attractive nature of jequirity peas and castor beans, most cases of ingestion occur in the pediatric age group. Because of the very high potency of these toxins, they are occasionally used for homicidal purposes and growing concern exists for their potential utilization as an agent of bioterrorism.

Emergency Department Treatment and Disposition

Treatment of jequirity pea and castor bean ingestions is largely supportive, as there is no specific antidote for abrin or ricin. Gastric decontamination may be considered and may include activated charcoal and whole bowel irrigation. In asymptomatic patients, decontamination, careful observation, and close follow-up are adequate. With symptoms of toxicity, however, admission is recommended, as the potential for marked clinical worsening is present.

Pearls

1. Most jequirity pea and castor bean ingestions are benign, as the vast majority of abrin toxin resides within the undigested shell of the plant.
2. The toxalbumins abrin and ricin are structurally similar to botulinum toxin, cholera toxin, diphtheria toxin, and insulin.
3. Severe allergic reactions with anaphylaxis have been reported with handling of the seeds of castor bean and are also seen among workers in factories where castor oil is produced.
4. Castor bean plant is commercially cultivated as a source of castor oil. Such oil has been used for centuries as a purgative and as a lubricant for machines.

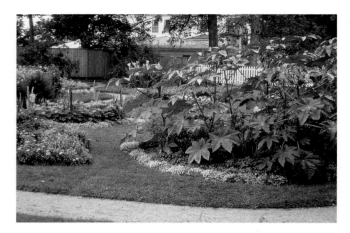

FIGURE 17.74 ■ Castor Bean Plant. The castor bean plant is large and leafy; it may reach a height of 10 to 12 ft. (Photo contributor: Alex Wilson.)

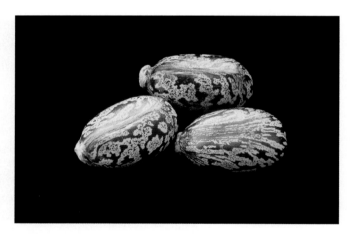

FIGURE 17.75 ■ Castor Bean. Typical appearance of the castor bean. (Photo contributor: Alex Wilson.)

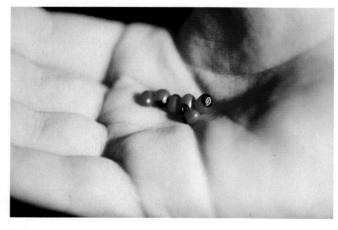

FIGURE 17.76 ■ Jequirity Pea. Jequirity peas are also known as rosary peas, Indian beans, Buddhist's beads, crab's eyes, and prayer beads. They are about 5 mm in diameter and have a colorful glossy shell, usually red with a black center, although black and white may also be seen. (Photo contributor: Kevin J. Knoop, MD, MS.)

Clinical Summary

Vancomycin is a glycopeptide antibiotic that has activity against gram-positive bacteria. It has little to no activity against gram-negative bacteria or mycobacteria. It is poorly absorbed after oral administration, although it may be used orally for treatment of pseudomembranous colitis. Intravenous administration is the most common route. This is well tolerated with minimal burning at the site of the IV; however, rapid infusion may occasionally cause degranulation of mast cells and basophils. As a result, the patient experiences erythematous flushing, particularly of the face and neck; hence the name "red man syndrome." Tachycardia and hypotension may occasionally be seen.

Emergency Department Treatment and Disposition

Slowing the intravenous infusion usually resolves the flushing. Increasing the dilution of vancomycin in solution may also assist with preventing the flushing. Diphenhydramine has been used for treatment and may be used as a pretreatment.

Pearls

1. Other syndromes known to causing flushing include scombroid poisoning, disulfiram reactions, and hydroxocobalamin infusions.
2. Concomitant administration of aminoglycoside with vancomycin may increase the risk of nephrotoxicity.

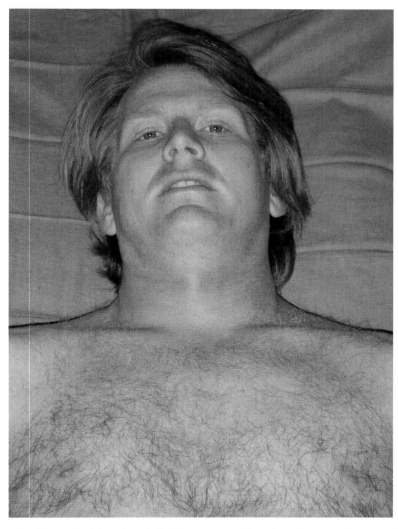

FIGURE 17.77 ■ Red Man Syndrome. Facial and neck flushing are manifestations that may be seen with red man syndrome from intravenous vancomycin infusion. (Photo contributor: R. Jason Thurman, MD.)

Chapter 18

WOUNDS AND SOFT TISSUE INJURIES

Chan W. Park
Michael L. Juliano
Dana Woodhall

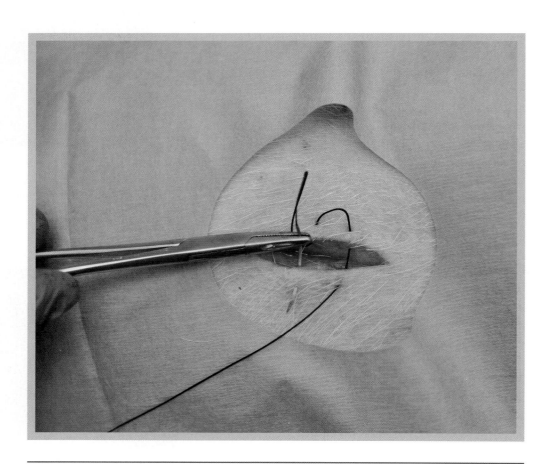

Clinical Summary

The goals of minor wound care are to achieve optimal wound aesthetics and infection prevention. Preliminary wound management begins with assessment, adequate hemostasis, foreign body removal, and irrigation. For most uncomplicated wounds, irrigation is the most effective means of reducing bacterial count. However, debridement may be necessary in contaminated wounds because devitalized tissue may impair the wound's ability to resist infection.

Emergency Department Treatment and Disposition

Rendering appropriate analgesia is important prior to initiating any wound cleansing or irrigation. While normal saline and sterile water are often used for irrigation, running tap water has been shown to be equally efficacious in simple well-vascularized wounds. In contaminated wounds, antiseptic solutions, such as povidone-iodine diluted in a 1:10 ratio using normal saline as the diluent, may help in disinfecting the wound. Bacterial-static solution cleaners, such as nonionic surfactant cleaner, may also help in reducing the bacterial inoculum. Solutions containing ionic detergents such as Betadine surgical scrub should not be used for this purpose as it is toxic to the wound tissue. If necessary, scrubbing of wounds should be done carefully as to avoid damaging viable tissue.

Irrigation remains the most effective means of reducing the bacterial inoculum; Five hundred to 1000 mL of irrigation fluid or 60 mL/cm of wound length is usually adequate for most uncomplicated wounds. The recommended irrigation pressure of 5 to 8 lb per square inch (PSI) can easily be accomplished by attaching an 18- or 19-gauge intravenous catheter sheath, or a commercially available splash shield, to a 20 or 30 mL syringe. A typical bulb system is suboptimal as it generates only 0.5 to 1 PSI. Debris that cannot be irrigated from the wound should either be scrubbed or sharply debrided using iris scissors or a scalpel. The tissue should appear pink and viable, with a scant amount of fresh bleeding indicating good vascular supply. High-pressure irrigation (ie, >25 PSI) may be necessary in highly contaminated wounds or complicated wounds that require operating room wash out. However, it offers no advantage for routine wounds cared for in the emergency department.

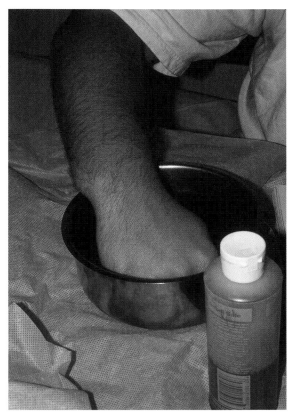

FIGURE 18.1 ■ Wound Soaking. Soaking is an appropriate method for loosening debris and coagulated blood but is not a substitute for irrigation. (Photo contributor: Matthew D. Sztajnkrycer, MD, PhD.)

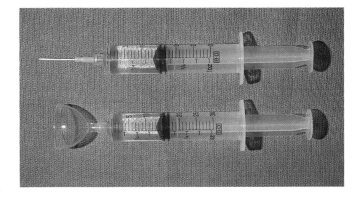

FIGURE 18.2 ■ High-Pressure Irrigation Devices. The ideal pressure for routine wound irrigation is 5 to 8 PSI. This can be easily achieved through the use of a 30 syringe attached to a commercially available device with an 18- or 19-gauge intravenous catheter sheath (top) or splash shield (bottom) (Photo contributor: Matthew D. Sztajnkrycer, MD, PhD.)

Pearls

1. Universal precautions, including gloves and face shield, should always be observed during wound cleaning and irrigation.

2. Antibiotics are no substitute for thorough wound cleansing and irrigation.

3. Shaving the eyebrow for wound repair is contraindicated due to the unpredictable pattern of hair regeneration.

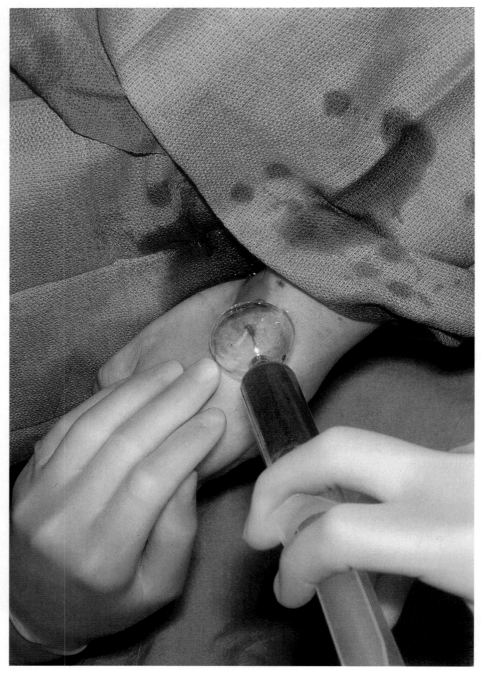

FIGURE 18.3 ▪ Wound Irrigation. After adequate anesthesia, an infected animal bite is opened and thoroughly irrigated using a 30 cc syringe and commercial splash shield. Note that even with the attached splash shield, there can be significant splatter and potential for body fluid exposure. Universal precautions should be followed at all times. (Photo contributor: Matthew D. Sztajnkrycer, MD, PhD.)

Clinical Summary

Proper wound assessment and preparation are essential to good wound management. This involves consideration of age and mechanism of injury, risk for contamination or foreign body, risk to the nerve, blood vessel and tendon, tetanus status and identifying comorbid conditions that may affect wound healing.

Emergency Department Treatment and Disposition

To achieve adequate wound exploration, the patient must be compliant. The use of local or regional anesthesia is usually sufficient in making the patient comfortable. However, conscious sedation may be required in uncooperative patients. A good neurovascular check should be documented prior to any anesthetic administration. The simplest way to control bleeding is by applying direct pressure. Other methods include the use of blood pressure cuff or tourniquet to achieve temporary hemostasis. Anesthetic solution containing epinephrine (1:100,000 dilution) may help constrict small vessels; however, prior to injection, one must first draw back the syringe to avoid direct cannulation of a vessel. Moreover, caution should be exercised when using any vasoconstrictors in areas of end arterial circulation such as in fingers, nose, toes, ears, and penis.

While hemostats or other self-restraining devices such retractors may help achieve adequate wound exposure, care must be exercised to avoid damaging the dermis and the tissue's vascular integrity. If exposure is still not adequate despite hemostasis and separation, the wound margins may be slightly extended to allow better visualization. Extension is performed by using a scalpel or a fine iris scissor. The wound is extended from one end, through the epidermis and dermis only, to avoid further injury to underlying structures. Once the superficial fascia has been exposed, it may be carefully and bluntly dissected using forceps or scissors.

Pearls

1. For scalp lacerations, carefully inspect the wound for sharp objects (ie, foreign body or bone fragment) prior to palpating it to assess for depressed skull fracture.
2. Never probe a wound blindly or blindly attempt to control bleeding with hemostats.

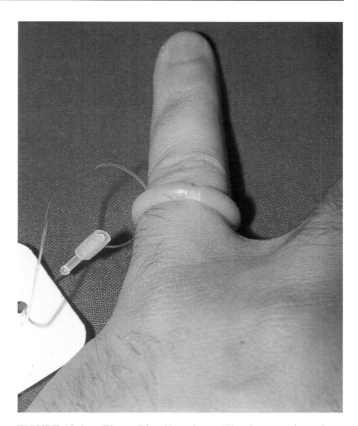

FIGURE 18.4 ■ Finger Ring Tourniquet. The ring tourniquet is an effective means of hemostasis. Removal after the procedure is important to prevent finger ischemia and necrosis. Another effective method of hemostasis involves using a Penrose drain tightened with hemostats. (Photo contributor: Matthew D. Sztajnkrycer, MD, PhD.)

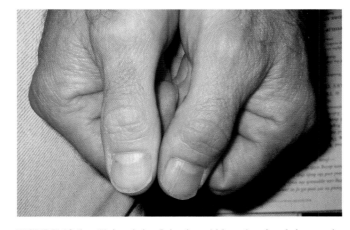

FIGURE 18.5 ■ Epinephrine Injection. Although epinephrine can be used to help achieve hemostasis, it should be used with caution on areas with poor collateral blood supply. Epinephrine has been injected into the right thumb which shows the pallor of finger ischemia. (Photo contributor: Selim Suner, MD, MS.)

3. At 1:100,000 dilution, epinephrine-containing anesthetic solution may be used with caution in areas of end arterial circulation such as the ear, fingers, nose, toes, and penis.

4. If epinephrine-induced tissue ischemia occurs, injection of phentolamine around the area of ischemia may help restore flow.

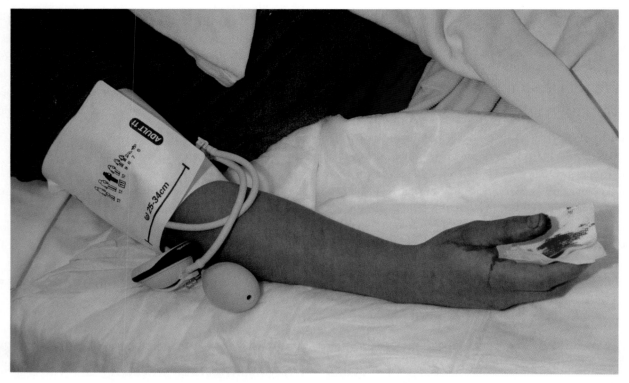

FIGURE 18.6 ■ Wound Exploration. A blood pressure cuff is an alternative means to obtain hemostasis before sterile preparation and wound exploration. (Photo contributor: Alan B. Storrow, MD.)

Clinical Summary

All foreign bodies can become a nidus for delayed infection. All reasonable attempts should be made to remove it when possible. Radiographic evaluation may assist in locating foreign bodies that cannot be directly visualized. Foreign bodies are characterized as being either *reactive* (eg, organic materials such as wood, bone, and soil) or *nonreactive* (eg, glass and metal).

Emergency Department Treatment and Disposition

A high level of clinical suspicion should accompany any injury pattern at risk for foreign body penetration. The patient is often unaware that a foreign body was present in their wound. Wounds at increased risk for foreign body include laceration caused by broken glass, perioral injuries with loss of dentition, and injuries to the hands and feet involving needles, nails, or splinters.

Suspicion of a retained foreign body mandates local wound exploration and the consideration of radiographic or ultrasound evaluation. Nearly 80% of objects can be identified on plain radiographs. More specifically, approximately 90% of glass fragments greater than 2 mm in size can be identified through the use of plain radiographs; fragments as small as 0.5 mm can be identified in 50% to 60% of cases. In situation where plain radiograph is poor, ultrasound may help locate the object.

Due to their increased risk for delayed infection and poor wound healing, reactive material must be removed. Nonreactive objects, however, may be left in place if reasonable effort to remove it has been unsuccessful and no potential for harm to a vital structure exists. Glass, however, has the potential for significant irritation and a removal attempt should be considered.

Pearls

1. The base of the wound must be visualized as many foreign bodies hide there.
2. In descending order of frequency, common foreign bodies retained in hand wounds are wood splinters, glass fragments, metallic objects, and needles.
3. Missed retained foreign bodies are a very common source of litigation in emergency medicine.

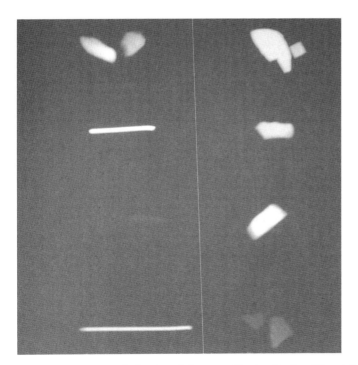
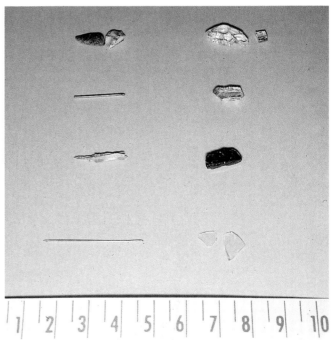

FIGURE 18.7 ■ Radiodensity of Common Foreign Bodies. The plain radiograph (left) demonstrates the radiodensity of common foreign bodies. Counterclockwise from top left: pebbles, paper clip fragment, wood splinter, hollow needle, light bulb glass, dark ("beer bottle") glass, transparent glass, and automobile windshield glass. Note that, although faint, the wood splinter is visible on the plain radiograph. Ruler markings (right) for the photograph of the corresponding objects are in centimeters. (Photo contributor: Matthew D. Sztajnkrycer, MD, PhD.)

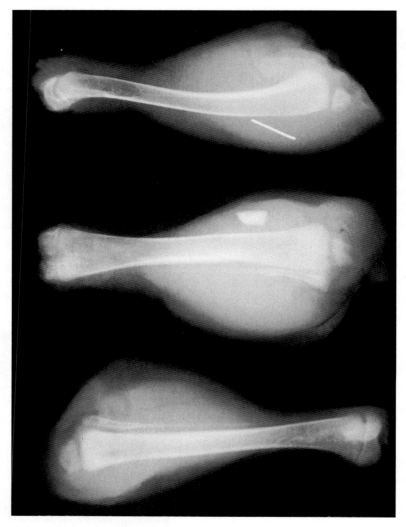

FIGURE 18.8 ▪ Radiodensity of Common Foreign Bodies in Tissues. The paper clip, dark glass, and wood splinter (*top to bottom*) imaged in Fig.18.7 were inserted into chicken legs and radiographs taken. The wood splinter is no longer clearly visible within the soft tissue. For purposes of foreign-body localization, a minimum of two radiographic views at 90 degrees to one another are obtained, and the site of the foreign body entry clearly marked. (Photo contributor: Matthew D. Sztajnkrycer, MD, PhD.)

Clinical Summary

Traumatic surface wounds are caused by one of three mechanisms: shearing, tension, or compression. Such a division helps to guide management decisions involving infection risk and scar formation.

Shearing Injuries

These types of injury are caused by sharp objects, such as glass shards or knives, which impart low-energy injury and minimal tissue destruction. A majority of uncomplicated shearing injuries (ie, those not involving neurovascular or anatomically important structures) are repaired primarily in the emergency department. The risk of infection is low and scar formation is typically cosmetically acceptable. Puncture wounds are typically due to sharp objects that pierce the skin and penetrate into deeper tissues. Such wounds are at a higher risk for infection, foreign-body retention, and underlying structure injury.

Tension or Partial Avulsion Injuries

These types of injuries occur when an object strikes the skin at a sharp angle creating a triangular flap. A flap of this type results in potential vascular disruption, greater tissue destruction, and a higher risk for infection and tissue ischemia. During the repair, vascular supply to the flap must be meticulously preserved; otherwise the flap may become ischemic.

Crush or Compression Injuries

These occur when a blunt object strikes tissue at a right angle, imparting a high degree of kinetic energy. This force results in significant tissue destruction of the skin and its underlying supportive fascial layers. Crush injuries are typically ragged, with irregular wound edges and a complex laceration pattern. Despite meticulous wound care and careful primary closure, the resulting scars may be cosmetically poor.

Emergency Department Treatment and Disposition

All patients requiring wound management should have their tetanus status adequately updated. Careful documentation of functional and neurovascular status at the time of initial evaluation is very important as the examination may change over time. Upon optimizing wound preparation, appropriate closure tension must be achieved. If open fracture is suspected or confirmed, intravenous antibiotics are administered and a consultation with an orthopedic surgeon should be obtained. Repair of traumatic wounds depends on the depth, complexity, and location. Deep wounds are closed in layers or by using a vertical mattress technique to remove dead space and relieve tension. Superficial wounds may be repaired with staples, simple interrupted sutures, or running sutures. In certain circumstances, the use of adhesive skin closures or adhesive glues may be adequate.

Pearls

1. Shearing injury is the most common wound mechanism seen in the emergency department.
2. Simple, uncontaminated, and uncomplicated wounds caused by clean, sharp objects may undergo primary closure up to 18 hours from the time of injury with good cosmetic result (see Simple Wound Closures).

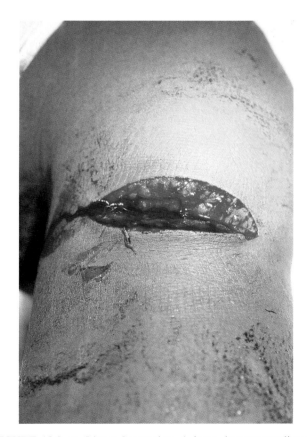

FIGURE 18.9 ■ Linear Laceration. A large, but uncomplicated, linear leg laceration is demonstrated. Given the depth and gaping nature of the wound, it can be closed using a layered closure to remove surface tension at the wound edges and promote a more cosmetically acceptable outcome. (Photo contributor: Alan B. Storrow, MD.)

3. The vascular supply to a flap is often tenuous; improper closure may further compromise the tissue, especially at the tip. A repair using a corner stitch will help minimize further ischemia (see Complex Wound Closures).

4. Crush injuries have an increased susceptibility to infection. Thorough cleansing, copious irrigation, and judicious debridement are required.

5. High-pressure injection injury (eg, paint or grease gun, see Chapter 11, Extremity Trauma) require orthopedic consultation.

6. The need for aggressive debridement and deep irrigation of puncture wounds, as well as the role of prophylactic antibiotics, is controversial. Uncomplicated clean punctures presenting less than 6 hours after injury should be superficially cleaned and irrigated.

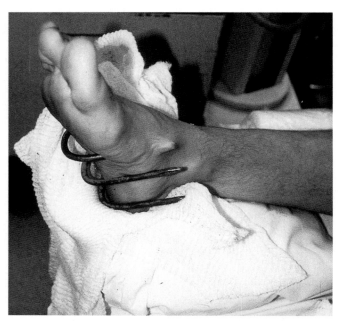

FIGURE 18.11 ■ Puncture Wound. A puncture wound to the foot with a contaminated garden instrument. Tetanus status must be carefully addressed in such an injury. A radiograph of the foot demonstrated no associated bony injuries. (Photo contributor: Matthew D. Sztajnkrycer, MD, PhD.)

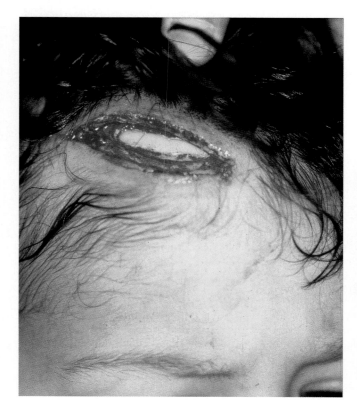

FIGURE 18.10 ■ Linear Laceration. A long, linear shearing laceration involving the forehead and scalp, with exposed galea. The wound is explored and palpated for evidence of a depressed or open skull fracture. Closure of large galeal lacerations is recommended to prevent spread of infection. Large frontal galeal lacerations are also repaired to prevent a cosmetic deformity of the frontalis muscle. (Photo contributor: Kevin J. Knoop, MD, MS.)

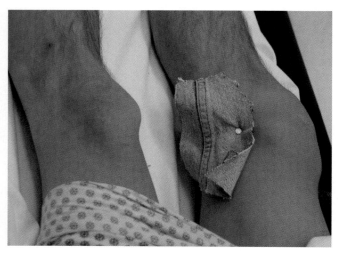

FIGURE 18.12 ■ Nail Gun Puncture Wound. Nail gun use may result in deep-puncture wounds. Radiographic evaluation is mandatory to assess for bone and joint involvement. (Photo contributor: R. Jason Thurman, MD.)

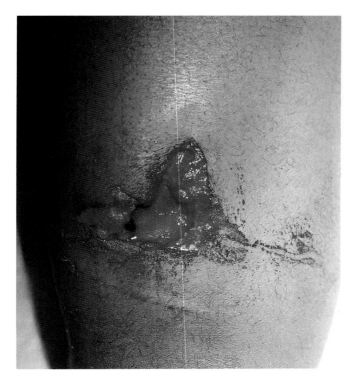

FIGURE 18.13 ■ Partial Avulsion Injury. This patient has sustained a typical partial avulsion laceration from a fall onto the edge of a staircase. Note the triangular "flap" in the upper left quadrant of the wound. Closure of partial avulsion injuries must be particularly meticulous to reduce any further compromise of the flap tip's vascular supply. (Photo contributor: Alan B. Storrow, MD.)

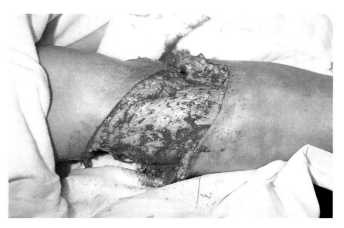

FIGURE 18.14 ■ Lower Extremity Degloving Avulsion. The patient sustained a complex degloving injury after her lower extremity became tangled in a rope while she was water-skiing. (Photo contributor: Alan B. Storrow, MD.)

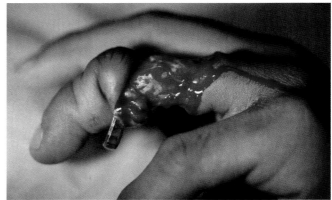

FIGURE 18.15 ■ Finger Degloving Avulsion. Rings being caught and forced proximally are a common cause of finger degloving. (Photo contributor: Selim Suner, MD, MS.)

TABLE 18.1 ■ RECOMMENDATIONS FOR TETANUS PROPHYLAXIS

Vaccination History	Clean, Minor Wounds	All Other Wounds
Unknown or <3 doses	Td or Tdap (Tdap preferred for ages 11-18)	Td or Tdap (Tdap preferred for ages 11-18), *plus* TIG
3 or more doses and ≤5 years since last dose	None	None
3 or more doses and 6-10 years since last dose	None	Td or Tdap (Tdap preferred for ages 11-18)
3 or more doses and >10 years since last dose	Td or Tdap (Tdap preferred for ages 11-18)	Td or Tdap (Tdap preferred for ages 11-18)

Table courtesy of the Centers for Disease Control and Prevention. Please go to www.cdc.gov for the most current information.
All other wounds can include: contaminated with dirt, feces, soil, and saliva; puncture wounds; avulsions; and wounds caused by missiles, crushing, burns, and frostbite.
Td = tetanus, diphtheria.
Tdap = tetanus, reduced diphtheria, and pertussis.
TIG = tetanus immune globulin.

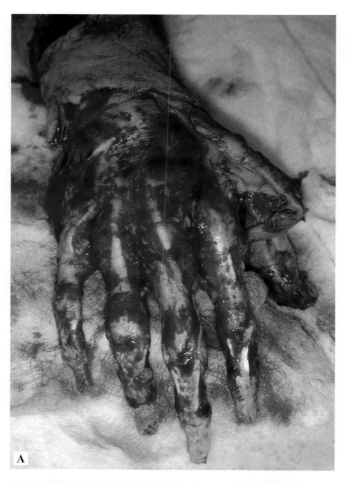

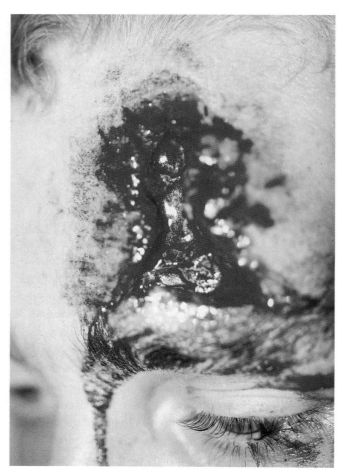

FIGURE 18.17 ■ Crush (Compression) Injury. A fall from a bicycle has resulted in a complex stellate laceration, characterized by ragged, irregular wound edges. The potentially high forces involved in producing a crush wound may be sufficient to cause deeper damage. Computed tomography of the head unfortunately demonstrated a left frontal hemorrhagic contusion. (Photo contributor: Matthew D. Sztajnkrycer, MD, PhD.)

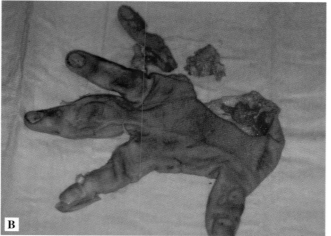

FIGURE 18.16 ■ Hand Degloving Avulsion. This extensive degloving (**A**) was caused by an industrial accident and resulted in near complete removal of the skin of the hand (**B**). (Photo contributor: Lawrence B. Stack, MD.)

Clinical Summary

The ear is composed of a poorly vascularized cartilaginous skeleton covered by tightly adherent skin. Given the paucity of subcutaneous tissue, ear injury that results in hematoma formation can cause pressure necrosis of the cartilage. The goal of repairing an ear laceration involves completely covering the exposed cartilage and preventing hematoma formation.

Emergency Department Treatment and Disposition

Prior to repair, the area is examined for signs of acute hematoma formation or other associated traumatic injuries. Hemotympanum or Battle sign suggests the presence of a more serious closed head injury, especially basilar skull fracture. Blunt trauma may result in barotrauma to the ear resulting in perforation of the tympanic membrane. Examination can be facilitated by local anesthesia infiltration or, in the case of larger or more complex lacerations, a regional nerve block.

Simple lacerations through the earlobe or the helix can be repaired with interrupted 6-0 nonabsorbable monofilament sutures if the cartilage is not exposed. Simple lacerations that involve the cartilage are primarily repaired by ensuring complete coverage of the exposed cartilage by careful apposition of the overlying skin. The skin generally provides sufficient support so that sutures are not required for the cartilage itself. If the wound is sufficiently irregular and cartilage debridement becomes necessary to avoid undue wound tension, the debridement should be kept to a minimum.

A perichondral hematoma must be drained within 72 hours to prevent potential pressure necrosis which can result in a "cauliflower" ear. Ear wounds are best dressed with a mastoid pressure dressing either primarily or after later hematoma drainage. Such a dressing reduces the chances for future hematoma formation and its complications. Ear sutures are removed in 3 to 5 days in children, 4 to 5 days in adults.

Pearls

1. Epinephrine-containing anesthetic at a 1:100,000 dilution may be used in ear laceration repair.
2. Hematoma evacuation needs to be rechecked in 24 hours to evaluate for reaccumulation.
3. If cartilage has been exposed or a hematoma drained, antistaphylococcal antibiotic coverage is recommended.
4. Complex lacerations and hematomas of the ear are best cared for in conjunction with a consultant.

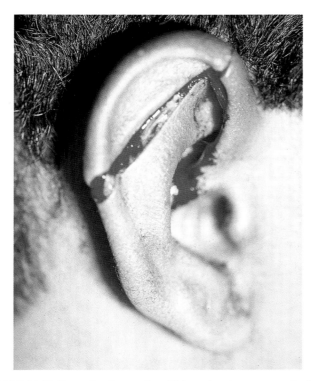

FIGURE 18.18 ■ Ear Laceration. This patient has presented after sustaining an uncomplicated, linear laceration to the pinna. Closure must cover all exposed cartilage. (Photo contributor: Alan B. Storrow, MD.)

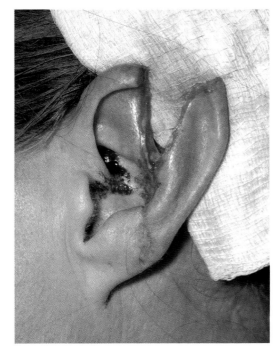

FIGURE 18.19 ■ Ear Laceration. Complex ear laceration through the helix down through the anti-helix. (Photo contributor: Lawrence B. Stack, MD)

Clinical Summary

Lip lacerations may result in significant cosmetic defects if not properly repaired. The lip has two significant anatomic landmarks: the mucosal border, which divides intraoral and external portions of the lip, and the vermilion border, which separates the lip mucosa from the skin of the face. Meticulous alignment of the vermilion border and its associated "white line" is the cornerstone of cosmetic repair. Lip anatomy may be distorted by the kinetic energy of the impact as well as the resultant edema surrounding the wound. Lacerations of the lip's vermilion border may be partial- or full-thickness, compromising the underlying orbicularis oris.

Emergency Department Treatment and Disposition

Given the high bacterial content of the oral cavity, lip lacerations will not remain clean during repair. The goal of irrigation is to remove clotted blood and gross contaminants such as tooth fragments or dirt. If a fractured tooth is noted, the wound must be explored for fragments. If the tooth or fragment is unaccounted for, then a panorex or soft tissue radiograph of the face and a chest radiograph should be obtained. Anesthesia for laceration repair is best performed using either an infraorbital (upper lip) or mental (lower lip) nerve block since local infiltration often distorts the tissue and impairs proper alignment of the vermilion border.

If the vermilion border is violated by a superficial laceration, then the first suture, typically 6-0 in size, is placed at the border to reestablish anatomic relationships. Once alignment is judged adequate, simple interrupted sutures are used for completion. If the laceration extends within the oral cavity, absorbable 5-0 sutures are used to close the intraoral component.

With deep or "through and through" lacerations involving the orbicularis oris, the muscle layers are initially approximated with deep, usually 5-0, absorbable sutures. Once the muscle is approximated, the first skin suture is again placed at the vermilion border.

Sutures are removed in 3 to 5 days in children, 4 to 5 days in adults. The patient is advised to eat soft foods, not to apply excessive force to the suture line, and to rinse after eating to prevent the accumulation of food particles.

Pearls

1. Misalignment of the vermilion border by as little as 1 mm may result in a cosmetically noticeable defect.
2. A marking pen may be used to identify landmarks prior to placing the sutures, as suturing itself causes some tissue edema, bleeding, and distortion.
3. Any patient with a lip laceration requires a thorough inspection of the oral cavity for associated trauma, including dental fractures, oral lacerations, and mandibular injuries.

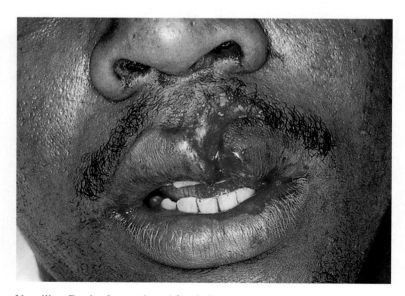

FIGURE 18.20 ■ Complex Vermilion Border Laceration. After being assaulted, this patient sustained a large laceration through the vermilion border and the orbicularis oris muscle. Examination of the wound demonstrated an underlying fracture of the alveolar ridge with subluxation of the number 10 tooth. (Photo contributor: Matthew D. Sztajnkrycer, MD, PhD.)

Clinical Summary

Tendon injuries are often associated with lacerations to the hand or wrist. A thorough neurovascular examination is critical; accurate assessment requires documentation of both motor function and strength. Partial tendon ruptures, including near complete, may still result in normal function.

Emergency Department Treatment and Disposition

Prior to wound examination, a thorough examination of the extremity is performed to assess neurovascular and motor function. All individual flexor and extensor tendons are assessed, including deep and superficial flexor digitorum tendons. Abnormal resting posture of the involved extremity can also indicate tendon injury. Tendons are taken through a full range of motion, including re-creation of limb position at the time of insult, in order to detect injuries along the length of the tendon. Adequate tendon exploration requires excellent hemostasis, which can be achieved through direct pressure, or the brief use of a blood pressure cuff or other tourniquet. Initial wound care should include irrigation, exploration for foreign bodies, debridement, antibiotics, and tetanus prophylaxis if indicated.

Partial tendon lacerations are treated conservatively, with splinting in neutral position and appropriate follow-up. Isolated extensor tendon lacerations may be repaired in the emergency department upon arranging follow-up with the appropriate specialist. Flexor tendon lacerations generally require emergent consultation with a hand surgeon or orthopedic surgeon.

Pearls

1. While extensor tendon repair may be accomplished by an emergency department physician with appropriate training and experience, flexor tendon lacerations are a challenging orthopaedic surgery problem and require referral.

2. Flexor tendons are weakest approximately 3 weeks after repair.

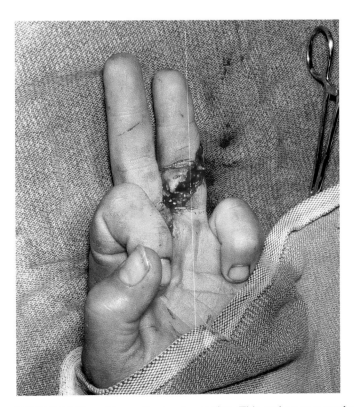 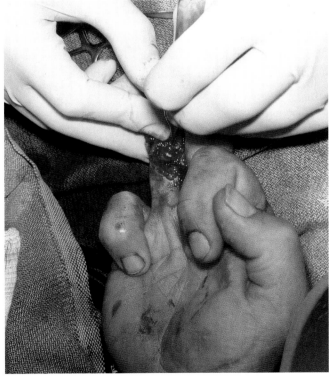

FIGURE 18.21 ■ Flexor Tendon Laceration. This patient presented to the emergency department after sustaining a laceration to his third and fourth digits (left). The injury was associated with an inability to flex these two digits. Wound exploration revealed the distal segment of the transected flexor tendon apparatus (right). (Photo contributor: Matthew D. Sztajnkrycer, MD, PhD.)

3. Kanavel's four cardinal sign of infectious tenosynovitis (a potential complication) are: (1) intense pain on attempts to extend the flexed finger, (2) flexion posture of the finger, (3) sausage digit, and (4) tenderness on palpation over the tendon sheath. Infectious tenosynovitis requires immediate consultation with a hand specialist (see Chapter 12, Extremity Conditions).

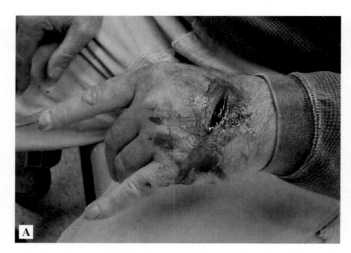 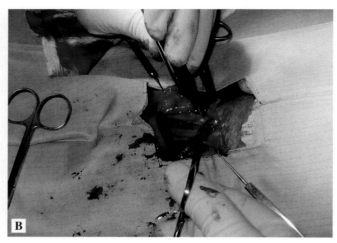

FIGURE 18.22 ■ Extensor Tendon Laceration. Note the laceration over the third and forth metacarpals (**A**). Inability to extend the long fingers is strong clinical evidence of complete disruption of the extensor tendon. Wound exploration and repair of the extensor tendon was completed under sterile conditions (**B**). (Photo contributor: Selim Suner, MD, MS.)

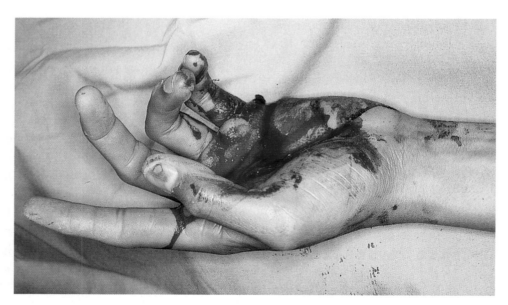

FIGURE 18.23 ■ Flexor Tendon Laceration. This patient with a palmar laceration is unable to flex his index finger secondary to complete disruption of the flexor tendon. (Photo contributor: Daniel L. Savitt, MD.)

Clinical Summary

Bite wounds (abrasions, lacerations, and punctures) account for approximately 1% to 2% of all emergency department visits in the United States. The majority of animal bites are minor. Statistics on the true incidence of mammalian bites is not known because many people do not seek emergency care. Dog bites predominate, at 80% to 90%, with cat bites accounting for another 5% to 15%. Human bites rank third in emergency department statistics; bites from other animals (raccoons, foxes, etc) are rare.

The microbiology of bite wounds is frequently polymicrobial with mixed aerobic and anaerobic bacteria. *Pasteurella multocida* (a gram-negative anaerobe) has been cultured from up to 80% of cat bites and 25% of dog bites. Other clinically relevant bacterial species include different *Pasteurella* species (*P canis*, *P dagmatis*), *Streptococcus, Staphylococcus, Moraxella, Corynebacterium, Neisseria, Enterococcus, Fusobacterium, Bacteroides, Porphyromonas, Prevotella*, and *Peptostreptococcus*. *Eikenella corrodens* has been recovered from human bites. *Capnocytophaga canimorsus* (formerly known as DF-2), a virulent organism which can be normal oral flora in dogs (16%) and cats (18%), can lead to sepsis, disseminated intravascular coagulation, gangrene, or death in susceptible individuals (immunocompromised, asplenic, or diabetic).

A number of risk factors are predictive of bite wound complications and influence wound management. In the United States, dog bites cause approximately 20 deaths per year, commonly in children bitten on the face and neck with exsanguination. The primary site of a bite wound in adults is on the extremities. The hand is at highest risk for developing infection (30%). The most infection-resistant location is the face, owing to its generous blood supply. Puncture wounds, especially from cats, are at the highest risk of infection (incidence between 30% and 50%). Abrasions, regardless of animal, are unlikely to become infected with proper wound care.

Emergency Department Treatment and Disposition

The management of bite wounds depends on location, animal involved, time elapsed before presentation and type of wound. All wounds should be thoroughly cleaned and debrided. Radiographs may be obtained to exclude bony injury or retained dentition. Contusions and superficial abrasions can be treated with local wound care.

Recommendations vary regarding the timing of wound closure. Closure of bite wounds to the face and head can be performed up to 12 hours (and in some reports up to 24 hours) after copious wound cleaning if there are no signs of infection. Puncture wounds, hand lacerations, or high-risk wounds (wounds > 12 hours or clinically infected) should not be closed. Delayed primary closure should be considered. Cat bites are best left open and treated with thorough irrigation. While a linear incision over the puncture wound may facilitate cleaning and exploration, efficacy of this is questioned. Radiographs of cat bite sites are recommended to look for retained teeth. Large, easily irrigated human bites less than 12 hours old on the trunk or a proximal extremity may be sutured. Human bites to areas other than the face and head should generally be left open and considered for delayed primary closure. Hand injuries caused by human bites are left open and managed in consultation with a hand specialist (see Chapter 11, Extremity Trauma, Clenched Fist Injury). The emergency physician should maintain a high index of suspicion for human bite in any laceration near the metacarpals.

All sutured bite wounds should be reevaluated by a healthcare provider within 24 hours. Closed wounds which appear infected (exudate, erythema) on reevaluation should be opened, irrigated, and allowed to close by secondary intention. Cyanoacrylate adhesives should never be used to close a bite wound.

Antibiotic therapy recommendations for bite wounds differ widely. Antibiotics are not recommended for minor wounds (where proper local wound care should be sufficient). Antibiotics are recommended for all cat bites, all hand wounds, and in persons with chronic diseases (eg, diabetes). Empiric antibiotic therapy is started with broad-spectrum antibiotics such as ampicillin-sulbactam, cefoxitin, or ceftriaxone. Alternatively, ciprofloxacin (or trimethoprim-sulfamethoxazole in children) and clindamycin can be used. Infection by *P multocida* classically becomes apparent within 24 hours of the bite and is marked by prominent pain, erythema, and swelling. Amoxicillin-clavulanate is the suggested regimen to cover polymicrobial infections and infections caused by *P multocida* or *C canimorsus*. Cultures are not recommended for initial treatment. However, cultures should be obtained in purulent wounds or any wound worsening during antibiotic therapy. Tetanus immunization status should be determined and appropriately updated.

Rabies infection is rare in the United States; worldwide, dogs are the number one reservoir (see Chapter 21, Tropical Medicine, Rabies). Carnivorous animals (eg, raccoons,

skunks, foxes, dogs, or bats) are more likely to be infected. If an animal is suspected as rabid, it should be detained and observed for any signs of rabies; occasionally this requires euthanasia and necropsy. Bats require special attention as many people do not recall being bitten. Healthcare professionals should have a low threshold for instituting rabies prophylaxis in persons with a bat exposure or in whom the animal is not available. Local animal control offices can be contacted for recommendations on appropriate rabies prophylaxis measures.

Pearls

1. All patients with bite wounds from susceptible animals (especially bats) should be assessed for rabies exposure as well as tetanus status.
2. Given cosmetic concerns and low infection risk, dog bites to the head and face can generally be sutured up to 24 hours after appropriate irrigation.
3. Although rare, a potentially fatal cause of dog-bite infection is *C canimorsus*, a gram-negative rod. Patients with this infection are often immunocompromised (neutropenia), asplenic, or diabetic and may present with sepsis, disseminated intravascular coagulation, and gangrene. The recommended antibiotic for treatment is amoxicillin-clavulanate. Penicillin-allergic patients can be treated with fluoroquinolones or clindamycin.
4. Bites which become infected within 24 hours, especially from cats, should be assumed to be caused by *P multocida*.

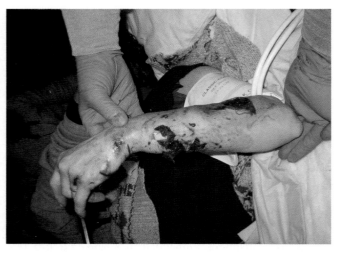

FIGURE 18.25 ■ Dog Bite. This patient sustained multiple avulsion injuries to her arm from a pit bull attack. Note the injuries to both the hand and forearm. (Photo contributor: Selim Suner, MD, MS.)

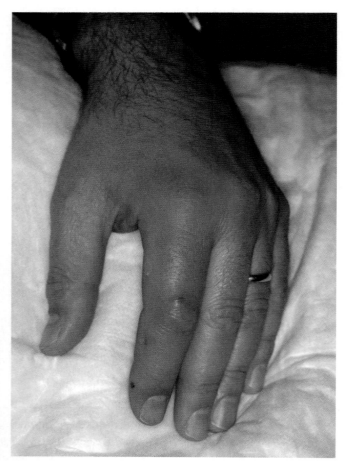

FIGURE 18.26 ■ Cat Bite. This patient was bitten by a cat. Note the swelling and erythema to the index finger indicating infection, possibly with *P multocida* (a prominent and fastidious organism seen commonly with feline bites). (Photo contributor: Kevin J. Knoop, MD, MS.)

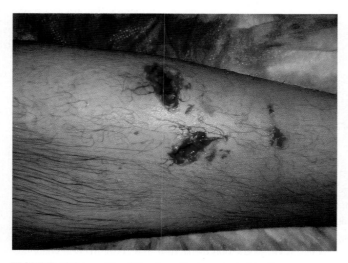

FIGURE 18.24 ■ Dog Bite. A patient presented to the emergency department after being bitten by a dog. He sustained lacerations to his lower leg. (Photo contributor: Selim Suner, MD, MS.)

Clinical Summary

Fishhooks are designed to catch fish and remain in place. The barb(s) of the fishhook prevent backing the hook out of the puncture site. Several different methods have been described for removal.

Emergency Department Treatment and Disposition

The wound is thoroughly cleaned and irrigated; tetanus status is addressed. Adequate anesthesia, usually local, is essential for removal. However, procedural sedation may be needed if a child has a fishhook embedded in a sensitive area (eg, eyelid).

The method used to remove the hook depends primarily on the location of the barb relative to the skin surface and the body part in which the fishhook is embedded. The most common removal technique is the "push-through and cut" technique. This is recommended when the tip of the fishhook is close to breaking through the skin surface after being embedded (see figures). Care should be taken when performing this maneuver in the hand or face as pushing the fishhook forward may damage nearby structures.

Superficially embedded hooks or hooks with small barbs may be removed in a retrograde fashion, by exerting pressure on the fishhook shaft toward the barb and backing the hook out through the original site of penetration. This technique can be performed manually or with the use of a string (see figure).

Another method uses an 18-gauge needle which can be inserted in line with the curve of the fishhook to cover the barb, then the hook and needle are removed together. For difficult retrograde removal, a small incision may be required in line with the concavity of the fishhook. Treble hooks should be separated above the skin and removed individually.

Once fishhooks are removed, the wound should be cleaned, irrigated, and left open. Antibiotics are usually not necessary; however, treatment for *Vibrio* species (noncholera, especially *Vibro parahaemolyticus*) should be considered in wounds contaminated with saltwater. The antibiotic of choice is doxycycline.

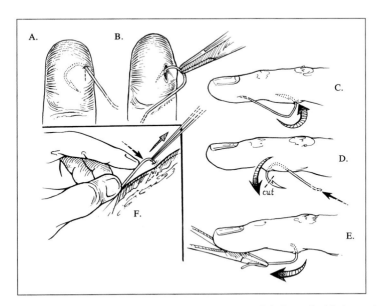

FIGURE 18.27 ■ Fishhook Removal. Hooks with small barbs that are only superficially embedded may be carefully backed out through the original puncture site (**A** and **B**). This may require a small incision, made in line with the concavity of the curve of the hook. The push-through technique is useful for hooks with large barbs or those more deeply embedded. The hook is pushed out through the skin, the barb removed, and the remainder of the hook subsequently removed through the original penetration site (**C, D,** and **E**). The traction (string) technique provides an alternative for removing hooks with small barbs. While pressing down on the shaft of the hook, traction is applied with 0 silk or umbilical tape. A swift yank of the cord in the direction opposite the barb will dislodge the hook (**F**). Care is taken to warn bystanders of the potential for the fishhook to fly across the room.

Pearls

1. Thorough irrigation and debridement of devitalized tissue is necessary after removal of a fishhook.
2. Hooks embedded in cartilaginous structures, such as the ear or nose, are best managed with the push-through methods.
3. Hooks that penetrate joint spaces or bone should be managed in consultation with an orthopedic surgeon.

4. Fishhooks that penetrate the globe of the eye are left in place and emergent ophthalmologic consultation is obtained. The patient is placed in the semi-recumbent position to decrease intraocular pressure and the globe is protected with an eye shield. Pressure patches are contraindicated, as they may extrude intraocular contents.

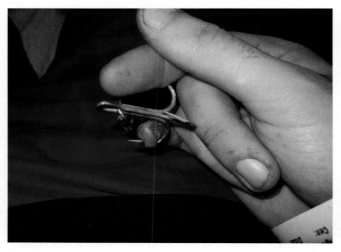

FIGURE 18.28 ■ Multiple Pronged Fishhook. This patient had an injury involving a three-pronged fishhook. Care must be taken when removing this hook due to the multiple sharp tips and potential for damaging surrounding structures. (Photo contributor: Selim Suner, MD, MS.)

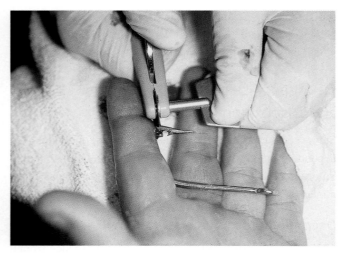

FIGURE 18.29 ■ Fishhook Injury and Removal. A patient presented to the emergency department with a fishhook embedded in his finger. The push-through technique was used to remove the hook. Use of a ring cutter proved unsuccessful; a bolt cutter was eventually required to remove the distal portion of this large hook. (Photo contributor: Alan B. Storrow, MD.)

Clinical Summary

The majority of wounds seen in the emergency department (ED) are uncomplicated lacerations which can be repaired primarily. Complications of wound closure (dehiscence, infection, improper healing) can be minimized by proper suturing techniques. It is important for the emergency physician to stress to the patient, or patient's caretakers, that scar formation is certain to occur with any wound closure.

Proper suturing technique approximates the wound edges and decreases wound tension. Wound edge eversion is essential for proper healing as the edge will flatten with time. Noneverted wound edges will depress after the initial repair, which can lead to poor cosmetic result.

Emergency Department Treatment and Disposition

Suture techniques utilized in the ED must be individualized depending on physician's skill, type, and laceration location. Suture material, size, and duration before removal are determined by the anatomic site of the wound.

Deep Interrupted Sutures

Use deep, absorbable sutures, if necessary, to reduce wound tension before superficial repair. It is important to remember to start the deep suture from the bottom of the wound, continue across the top (subdermally), and return to the bottom in finishing. This will leave the knot at the bottom of the wound, decreasing the chance that suture material will exit the wound at the surface.

Simple Interrupted Closures

This closure involves single nonabsorbable sutures, each independently tied. The needle should penetrate the skin at a 90 degree angle and the needle should exit the other side of the wound at a 90 degree angle.

Staples

Staples are a rapid means of closing linear wounds. Staples should not used on the hands, feet, face, or over joints. Wound edge eversion is also critical for staple closure to obtain the best outcome.

Running Closure

This rapid closure technique involves taking several bites along the length of a wound without tying individual knots. Knots are tied only at the beginning and end.

Liquid Wound Adhesives

Cyanoacrylate adhesives have advantages in wound closure because of closure speed and lack of a repeat visit for suture removal. Anesthesia may not be required. Small linear lacerations are ideal for this closure. The wound must be dry and free of active bleeding for proper adhesion. Practice is required to gain the necessary skill in using this technique. Antibiotic ointment should not be applied to the wound as this will dissolve the adhesive.

Elastic Wound Closure Strips

Elastic wound closures strips have the same advantages and indications as adhesives. Wound closure strips can be used alone or in conjunction with a tissue adhesive such as benzoin resin. This can be applied to the normal skin on either side of the wound and used as an anchor point for the strip. The edges of strip will curl up over time and can be trimmed by the patient as needed. Closure strips usually fall off completely in 2 to 3 weeks. Wound closure strips are not recommended in children as they have a tendency to remove them prematurely. Wound closure strips can also be used after suture removal to give the wound more time to gain tensile strength.

Pearls

1. The bites on both sides of a wound should be equidistant for both optimum wound healing and cosmetic outcome.
2. In gaping wounds, surface tension must be reduced with the use of deep sutures.
3. Use of cyanoacrylate wound adhesives or elastic wound closure strips does not obviate the need for good wound care, including thorough irrigation and exploration. Local or regional anesthesia may still be required.
4. Cyanoacrylate can be dissolved with antibiotic ointment, which may be used to remove the adhesive from areas that were nonintentionally glued together.

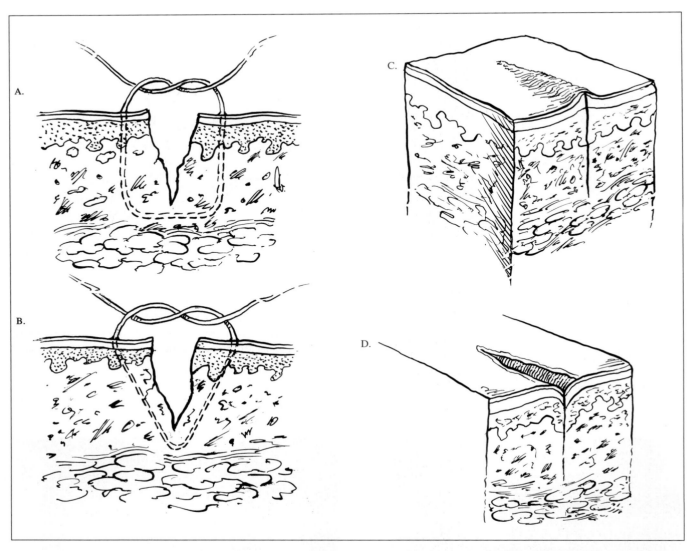

FIGURE 18.30 ■ Wound Edge Eversion. Eversion of wound edges is critical for optimal wound healing. For proper eversion, the needle point should enter the epidermis at a 90-degree angle, generating a square or bottle-shaped suture configuration (**A**). This results in a slight rise of the skin edges above the skin plane (right). Such eversion will flatten at the level of the skin plane during healing. Entry at a shallower angle (**B**) often leads to wound edge inversion, eventual contraction of the wound edges below the skin plane, and subsequent scar formation (right).

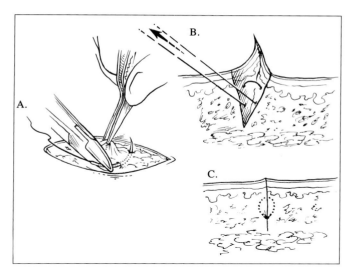

FIGURE 18.31 ■ Deep Sutures. Judicious placement of deep sutures allows approximation of the dermis, reduces tension on the wound edges, and may facilitate final superficial closure. The needle is driven from deep within the wound to a superficial level (**A**). On the opposite side of the wound, the needle is driven from superficial to deep (**B**). By having the leading and trailing suture come out on the deep and same side of the superficial cross suture, the knot is buried within the wound (**C**).

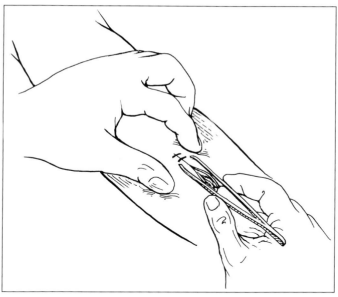

FIGURE 18.33 ■ Staple Closure. Meticulous care must be taken when using staples to properly approximate and evert wound edges. This can be facilitated through the use of forceps during staple closure.

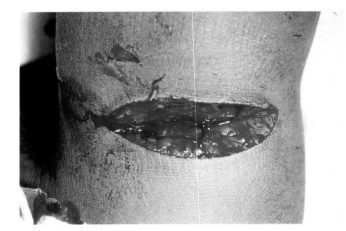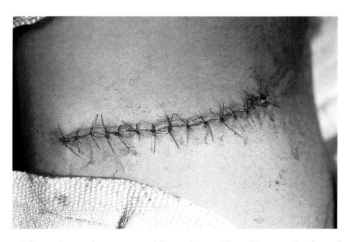

FIGURE 18.32 ■ Simple Interrupted Wound Closure. An uncomplicated linear laceration generated by a sharp object. For anesthesia and hemostasis, the wound edges are infiltrated with lidocaine-containing epinephrine. The wound is subsequently closed with simple interrupted sutures. Attention is paid to obtaining a degree of wound edge eversion. (Photo contributor: Alan B. Storrow, MD.)

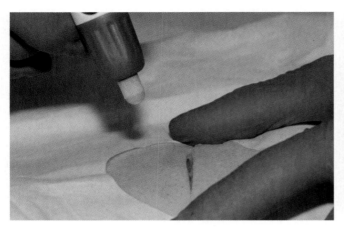
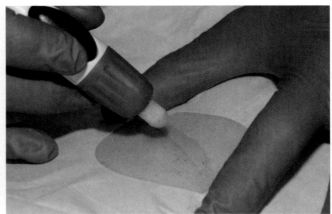

FIGURE 18.34 ■ Liquid Wound Adhesive Closure. Wounds that are ideal for this type of closure are small, linear, and hemostatic. Care must be taken to ensure the wound edges are correctly approximated before applying the adhesive. (Photo contributor: Michael L. Juliano, MD.)

TABLE 18.2 ■ SUTURE MATERIALS, SIZE, AND DURATION BY ANATOMIC SITE			
Anatomic Site	**Skin**	**Deep**	**Duration**
Scalp	5-0, 4-0 monofilament	4-0 absorbable	6-8 days
Ear	6-0 monofilament	N/A	4-5 days
Eyelid	7-0, 6-0 monofilament	N/A	4-5 days
Eyebrow	6-0, 5-0 monofilament	5-0 absorbable	4-5 days
Nose	6-0 monofilament	5-0 absorbable	4-5 days
Lip	6-0 monofilament	5-0 absorbable	4-5 days
Oral mucosa	N/A[a]	5-0 absorbable	N/A
Face/forehead	6-0 monofilament	5-0 absorbable	4-5 days
Chest/abdomen	5-0, 4-0 monofilament	3-0 absorbable	8-10 days
Back	5-0, 4-0 monofilament	3-0 absorbable	12-14 days
Arm/leg	5-0, 4-0 monofilament	4-0 absorbable	8-10 days
Hand	5-0 monofilament	5-0 absorbable	8-10 days[b]
Extensor tendon	4-0 monofilament	N/A	N/A
Foot/sole	4-0, 3-0 monofilament	4-0 absorbable	12-14 days

[a]Not applicable.
[b]Add 2 to 3 days for joint extensor surfaces.
Source: Adapted from Trott AT: *Wounds and Lacerations: Emergency Care and Closure.* 2nd ed. St. Louis, MO: Mosby–Year Book; 1997.

Clinical Summary

The horizontal and vertical mattress sutures and the corner stitch may be used in the emergency department to manage wounds that cannot be closed with simple techniques.

Emergency Department Treatment and Disposition

Vertical Mattress Suture

The vertical mattress suture is a useful technique for deep wounds. It acts as both a deep and superficial closure, thereby reducing wound tension. The suture is performed by first taking a large tissue bite through the fascial layer approximately 1 cm from the wound edge and crossing equidistant to the other wound edge. The needle is then reversed and a second small bite through the epidermal-dermal junction 1 to 2 mm from the wound edge is taken.

Horizontal Mattress

The horizontal mattress suture is best used for wide, gaping wounds with a risk of increased wound tension after closure (eg, lacerations overlying a joint). The first step in this closure is a simple untied interrupted suture. Rather than tying the knot at this point, a second simple interrupted suture is placed in the reverse direction approximately 5 mm from the first. The knot is finally tied on the side of the initial bite.

Corner Stitch

A corner stitch is used to close triangular wounds or flaps. A simple interrupted suture cannot be placed to approximate the point of the flap. If this is done the wound will not approximate

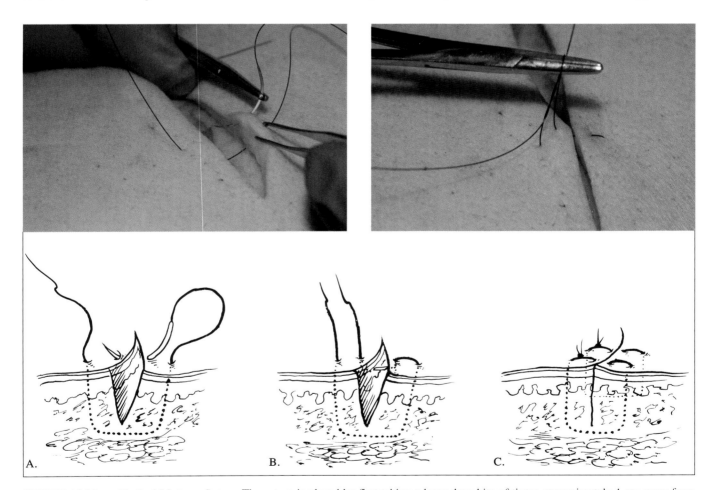

FIGURE 18.35. ■ Vertical Mattress Suture. The suture is placed by first taking a large deep bite of tissue approximately 1 cm away from the wound edge and exiting at the same location on the other side of the wound. A second small superficial bite is then performed in the reverse direction (**A**). When the bites are complete (**B**), tying results in nice apposition of the wound edges (**C**). This technique is especially useful in areas of lax skin, such as the elbow or dorsum of the hand. (Photo contributor: Michael L. Juliano, MD.)

correctly and the chances of dehiscence are higher due to the already tenuous blood supply to the flap. The technique is effectively a half-buried horizontal mattress suture, where the needle is initially introduced through the skin in the noncorner area of the wound. The needle is brought out through the dermis and then passed horizontally through the dermis of the triangular portion of the wound. It is then brought through the dermis on the other portion of the wound and out through the opposite noncorner area, where the knot is tied. Once the corner is secured, simple sutures are used to repair the rest of the wound, with care taken to place the sutures far enough from the tip to optimize circulation.

Pearls

1. Utilization of a mattress suture can aid in wound edge eversion and tension reduction. They are particularly useful in areas where the deep subcutaneous tissues are too fragile for deep sutures (eg, over a joint or shin).
2. *Excessive* wound edge eversion and strangulation are potential disadvantages of mattress sutures.
3. A single corner stitch may be used to close several corners of a stellate wound.

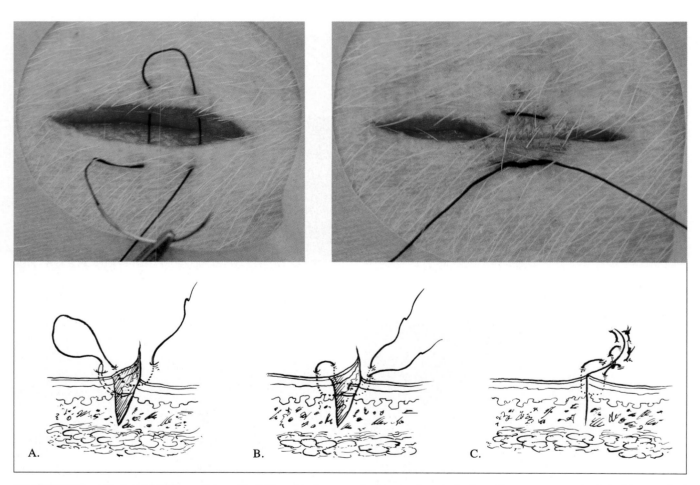

FIGURE 18.36 ▪ Horizontal Mattress Suture. Useful in achieving wound edge eversion, the horizontal mattress suture begins with a standard suture throw. A second bite is taken approximately half a centimeter from the first exit (**A**) and brought through at the original starting edge, half a centimeter from the original entry point (**B** and **C**). (Photo contributor: Michael L. Juliano, MD.)

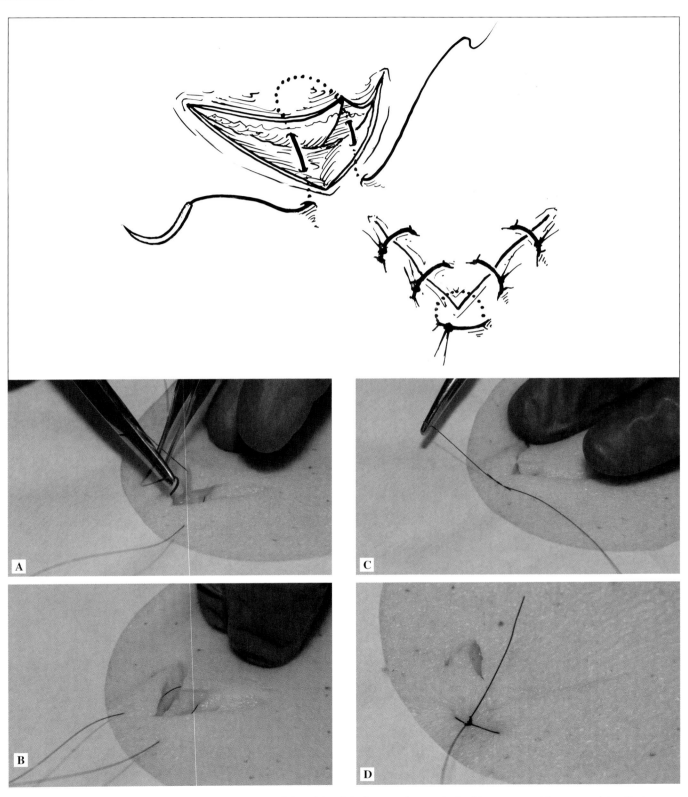

FIGURE 18.37 ■ Corner Stitch. Flaps generated by partial avulsion injuries must be repaired with care to avoid compromising the tenuous blood supply of the flap. The corner stitch is performed through the use of a half-buried horizontal mattress suture. The suture begins percutaneously away from the wound corner. The suture needle is then brought horizontally through the corner at the level of the dermis and back out through the epidermis at the opposite noncorner portion of the wound (**A**). This technique avoids placing suture material near the apex of the flap (**B**). Tying (**C**) results in approximation of the corner (**D**). (Photo contributor: Michael L. Juliano, MD).

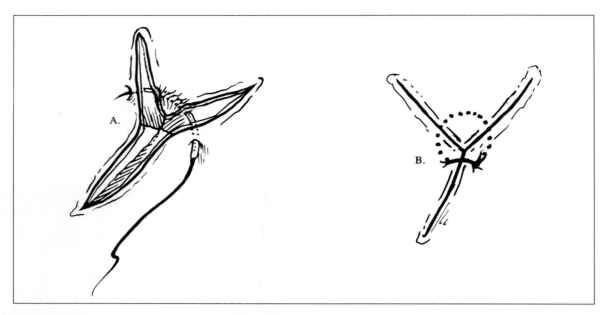

FIGURE 18.38 ▪ Corner Stitch for Stellate Wounds. The corner stitch may also be used to close stellate lacerations.

Clinical Summary

All wounds are subject to two main complications: infection and dehiscence. All wounds evaluated in the emergency department are assumed to be contaminated. Contamination of a wound occurs either at the time of the injury or through direct migration of normal skin flora. A key factor in determining bacterial concentration in the wound is time elapsed until presentation. Wounds should therefore be thoroughly cleaned and irrigated in a timely manner following presentation. Wound infection is suggested by pain, warmth, erythema, edema, and purulent drainage.

Wounds are at risk for dehiscence at any time after suturing; however, at 7 to 10 days after repair, a wound is at its weakest (this also closely coincides with suture removal). Factors that contribute most to wound dehiscence are those that impair wound healing, primarily: infection, medications (especially corticosteroids), foreign bodies, advanced age, poor nutritional status, diabetes mellitus, and peripheral vascular disease. Elastic wound closure strips can be applied after suture removal and may reduce the incidence of wound dehiscence.

Scarring is not considered a complication of wound repair. However, some individuals can produce hypertrophic scars or keloids. Hypertrophic scars are the result of excessive collagen deposition within the borders of the original wound. Keloids represent inappropriate scarring that extends beyond the boundaries of the original wound. While keloids are most commonly described in the Africa American population, they may occur in any ethnic group. Wound myiasis is infestation by fly larvae (maggots, see Chapter 21, Tropical Medicine, Myiasis) that invade necrotic tissue.

Emergency Department Treatment and Disposition

Local wound infections are treated with suture removal, thorough irrigation, and possible radiographic or visual wound exploration for missed foreign bodies. A 7-day course of a first-generation cephalosporin or antistaphylococcal penicillin is appropriate for most infections; however if *Methicillin-resistant Staphylococcus Aureus* (MRSA) is suspected, the antibiotic choice should be adjusted (eg, trimethoprim-sulfamethoxazole). For animal bites, other antibiotics (eg, amoxicillin/clavulanate) may be more appropriate. Sepsis, advanced infections, or infections in persons with chronic medical problems (eg, diabetes, immunocompromised) should be managed with parenteral antibiotics and possible inpatient admission.

Wound dehiscence is managed conservatively by treating the underlying causes and allowing healing via secondary intention. Dehiscence of wounds in cosmetically sensitive areas is best managed in conjunction with a consultant. Myiasis is treated with wound cleaning and irrigation.

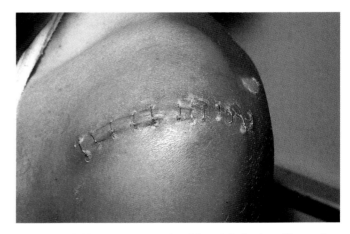

FIGURE 18.39 ■ Postoperative Wound Infection. The patient presented to the emergency department with increasing pain and redness at the site of his staple closure. The area was erythematous, tender, and warm and had scant purulent drainage around some of the staples. (Photo contributor: Matthew D. Sztajnkrycer, MD, PhD.)

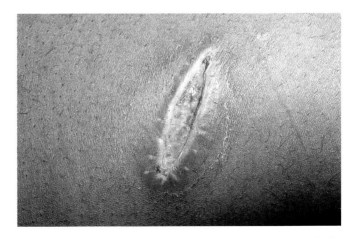

FIGURE 18.40 ■ Wound Dehiscence. After suture removal, the patient returned to the emergency department. The wound had dehisced but had a clean base of granulation tissue. The wound was allowed to close by secondary intention. (Photo contributor: Alan B. Storrow, MD.)

Pearls

1. All accidental wounds are considered contaminated and treated as such. Thorough irrigation and cleansing is of paramount importance in preventing wound infection.
2. Expedient ED wound care is important, since bacterial contamination increases over time.
3. The tensile strength of the wound is at its weakest between 7 to 10 days.
4. MRSA skin infections are becoming more commonplace in the emergency department. They should be treated with appropriate antibiotics, such as trimethoprim-sulfamethoxazole.

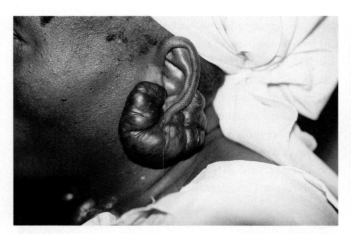

FIGURE 18.41 ■ Keloid. The degree of excessive scar bulk extending beyond the original wound margins may be dramatic and cosmetically significant. (Photo contributor: Thea James, MD.)

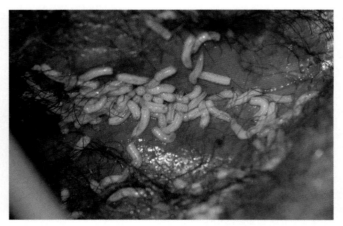

FIGURE 18.42 ■ Wound Myiasis. Necrotic tissue can be invaded by fly larvae (maggots). (Photo contributor: Lawrence B. Stack, MD.)

Clinical Summary

Burns can be caused by heat, electricity, chemicals, friction, or radiation exposure. Damage to the skin barrier can leave the patient susceptible to infection, fluid loss, and electrolyte abnormalities. Long-term consequences of burns include permanent scarring, loss of sensation to the affected area, and in severe cases loss of extremities due to inadequate circulation.

Emergency Department Treatment and Disposition

Burns are assessed by determining the percentage of body surface area (BSA) involved, the depth of the burn, and the area of the body involved. A common system used to estimate BSA is following the "rule of nines." This system breaks up the body into zones that each equate to nine percent of BSA. Some clinicians use the palm of their hand as an equivalent to 1% BSA and measure the area involved by using this method.

First-degree burns only involve the epidermal layer of skin. These burns are red, painful, and heal in approximately 1 week. Second-degree burns are subdivided into two categories, superficial partial thickness and deep partial thickness. Superficial second-degree burns extend from the epidermis to the superficial dermis. Pain, skin blistering, and intact capillary refill are characteristics of these burns. Deep partial thickness burns are painless, white in color, and do not blanch. At this depth there is damage to hair follicles and sweat glands. The entire thickness of the skin is compromised in third-degree burns. They appear pale, feel leathery, and are painless. Fourth-degree burns extend through the layers of the skin and involve muscle or bone.

Pain control, adequate cleansing of the area, debridement of large blisters, and application of topical antimicrobials to minor burns are part of emergency department management. One percent silver sulfadiazine, bacitracin, or triple-antibiotic ointment are antimicrobial options. Dressing changes should occur daily and patients must be instructed to watch for signs of infection. Follow-up with a burn-care expert needs be arranged within a few days of discharge for deep partial thickness or third-degree burns.

Patients with major burns must be assessed for airway protection and adequate circulation. Clinicians should also remember to cover the burned areas with a clean, dry sheet; administer aggressive pain control to patients; and aggressively address fluid resuscitation. The Parkland formula is commonly used to estimate fluid requirements. The patient's weight in kilograms is multiplied by the percent BSA involved; this number is multiplied by 4 mL of lactated Ringers solution. Half of this amount is given during the first 8 hours and the remaining amount is given over the next 16 hours of resuscitation. It is recommended to keep urine output approximately 0.5 to 1.0 mL/kg/h. In order to monitor for effects of cell breakdown, urinalysis, creatine kinase, and an EKG should be obtained. Circumferential burns of the extremities may compromise circulation. If distal pulses are decreased, an escharotomy should be considered to prevent compartment syndrome.

Referral to a burn unit should be planned in cases that include partial thickness burns that involve greater than 10% BSA, third-degree burns, or involvement of the hands, feet, face, or perineum. Electrical burns, chemical burns, inhalation injuries, and patients with significant comorbidities should also be considered for a burn unit.

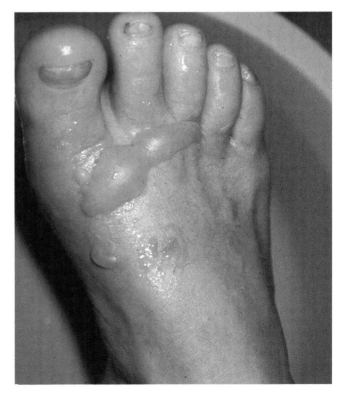

FIGURE 18.43 ■ Second-Degree Burn. This patient has sustained a second-degree burn to his foot. After cleansing the area, the blisters should be debrided and antimicrobial ointment should be applied. (Photo contributor: Alan B. Storrow, MD.)

Pearls

1. Evaluation of burns includes noting the amount of BSA involved and the depth of the burn.

2. Minor burns can be managed in the emergency department. Pain control, irrigation, debridement, antimicrobial ointments, and dressing changes are the mainstays of therapy.

3. Adherent tar should be cooled; mayonnaise, polysporin ointment, mineral oil, commercially available cream or oil-based solvents have been suggested to aid in removal.

4. Cleaning of tar burns can be assisted by the use of topical mayonnaise or butter.

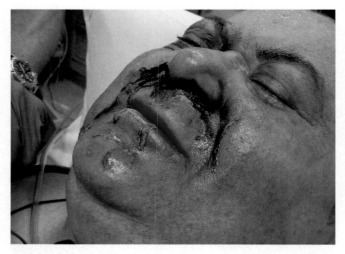

FIGURE 18.44 ■ Facial Burn. This patient's injury was a result of an explosion of his oxygen cannula. Ensuring that the patient has a protected airway in this type of injury is crucial. (Photo contributor: Chan W. Park, MD.)

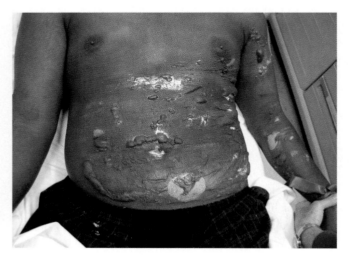

FIGURE 18.46 ■ Abdominal Burn. Mostly second-degree abdominal burn. (Photo contributor: Chan W. Park, MD.)

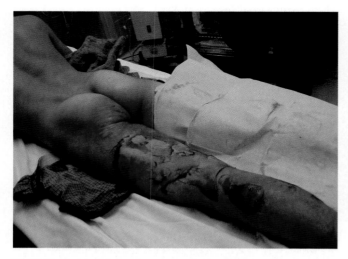

FIGURE 18.45 ■ Extensive Burn Injury. Burns can be of varying depths; this patient has both second- and third-degree burns to his lower extremity. Distal pulses should be closely monitored to guarantee that there is adequate circulation. (Photo contributor: Chan W. Park, MD.)

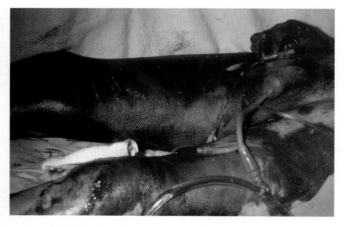

FIGURE 18.47 ■ Tar Burn. Tar burn after initial cleaning. (Photo contributor: Lawrence B. Stack, MD.)

Clinical Summary

Decubitus ulcers develop when soft tissue is compressed between a bony prominence and a hard external surface. Compression of the tissue results in decreased blood flow, which promotes tissue ischemia and cell death. Pressure, shearing forces, friction, and excessive moisture are all contributing factors to the formation of pressure ulcers. Areas commonly affected include the sacrum, heels, and posterior scalp. All patients may develop decubitus ulcers, but those at higher risk include immunocompromised patients, nursing home tenants, patients with underlying neurologic conditions, and immobilized trauma patients.

Decubitus ulcers are typically divided into four stages. *Stage one* ulcers are characterized by an area of nonblanchable erythema over intact skin. A *stage two* pressure sore appears as a shallow, open sore with a pink wound base. When the wound is full thickness with no muscle, tendon, or bone exposed, it is defined as a *stage three* ulcer. If muscle, tendon, or bone is exposed it is described as *stage four*. Some wounds may have an area of black eschar over them; these wounds cannot be categorized since the depth of the injury cannot be determined.

Emergency Department Treatment and Disposition

Prevention is key in caring for decubitus ulcers. All patients who have decreased mobility, such as trauma and nursing home patients, should have their entire skin surface regularly checked for skin breakdown. Backboards, c-collars, and other immobilizing devices should be removed as soon as possible. If medical necessity dictates that these devices can not be removed, blankets and pillows may be used to pad hard surfaces. High-risk patients should also be repositioned frequently to prevent ulcer formation.

Once a decubitus ulcer has formed, treatment includes pain relief, keeping the affected area moist, and keeping pressure off the area to prevent further tissue destruction. There are multiple commercial products available to use for the treatment of pressure ulcers. A few examples include hydrocolloid dressings, Silvadene, or vacuum-assisted closing (VAC) sponges. If there is dead tissue present, it must be debrided; if the area is large and has progressed to a stage three or four ulcer, surgical intervention to construct a skin flap may be necessary. The main complications of decubitus ulcer formation include infection and skin dehiscence. All decubitus ulcers must be frequently monitored for healing and potential complications.

Pearls

1. Physicians should perform a full skin examination on all hospitalized patients.
2. Decubitus ulcers are divided into four stages. If an eschar is present, the ulcer cannot be categorized.
3. Remove hard external surfaces and immobilizing devices as soon as possible.
4. Treatment of decubitus ulcers includes pain control, proper wound care, and prevention of further tissue destruction.

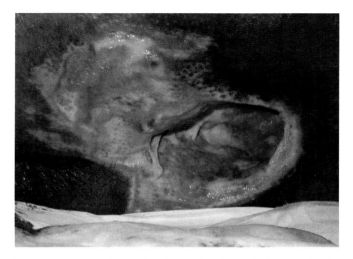

FIGURE 18.48 ■ Stage Three Decubitus Ulcer. This example of a stage three decubitus ulcer extends into the subcutaneous tissue. (Photo contributor: Lawrence B. Stack, MD.)

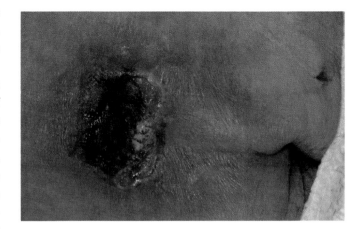

FIGURE 18.49 ■ Unstageable Decubitus Ulcer. Because this pressure sore is covered by an eschar, the stage can not be determined. This wound will need to be debrided. (Photo contributor: Lawrence B. Stack, MD.)

Clinical Summary

Electricity may cause harm by heat generated through tissue resistance or directly by the current on cells. Skin, nerves, vessels, and muscles usually sustain the greatest damage. Many factors affect the severity of injury: type of current (DC or AC), current intensity, contact duration, tissue resistance, and current pathway through the body. Those at high risk for electrical injury are toddlers, and people who work with electricity.

When electricity traverses the tissues, it may cause a host of injuries: contact burns, thermal injury, arc burns, muscular tetany, or blunt trauma due to severe muscle contraction. Sudden death (asystole, respiratory arrest, ventricular fibrillation), myocardial damage, cerebral edema, neuropathies, disseminated intravascular coagulation, myoglobinuria, compartment syndrome, and various metabolic disorders have been described.

High-voltage DC or AC current typically causes a single violent muscular contraction that throws the victim from the source. As a result, blunt trauma and blast injuries may occur. Low-voltage AC currents (as from a household outlet) typically cause muscular tetany, forcing the victim to continue contact with the source.

Emergency Department Treatment and Disposition

After initial stabilization, consider cervical spine immobilization, oxygen administration, cardiac monitoring, and intravenous crystalloid infusion. A Foley catheter will help monitor urine output and is especially important if rhabdomyolysis is suspected.

Diagnostic testing to consider includes: ECG, CBC, urinalysis, CPK, CPK-MB, electrolytes, BUN, creatinine, and coagulation profile. Radiographic assessment is important for those with a suspicion of trauma.

Severe or high-risk injuries should be admitted to a burn unit, or trauma center with burn consultation. Patients with minor, brief, low-intensity exposures, with a normal ECG, normal urinalysis, and no significant burns or trauma may be considered for discharge after 6 to 8 hours of observation.

Pearls

1. The low resistance of water makes its association with electricity particularly dangerous.

2. High-risk features include high-voltage exposure (>600 V), deep burns, neurologic injury, dysrhythmias, abnormal electrocardiogram, evidence of rhabdomyolysis, suicidal intent, or significant associated trauma.

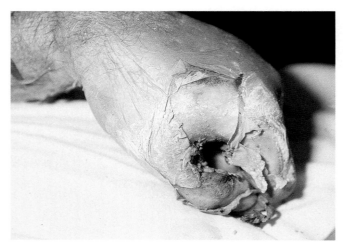

FIGURE 18.50 ■ Electrical Burn. This patient grabbed a high-voltage power line with his hand. Exit wounds occur where the patient is grounded, often through the feet when standing. This patient with transthoracic injury should have cardiac monitoring. (Photo contributor: Alan B. Storrow, MD.)

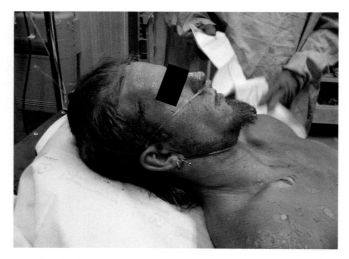

FIGURE 18.51 ■ Electrical Flash-Over Burn. A patient struck by flash over electricity while repairing urban outdoor electric lines. (Photo contributor: Selim Suner, MD, MS.)

Chapter 19

FORENSIC MEDICINE

William S. Smock
Lawrence B. Stack

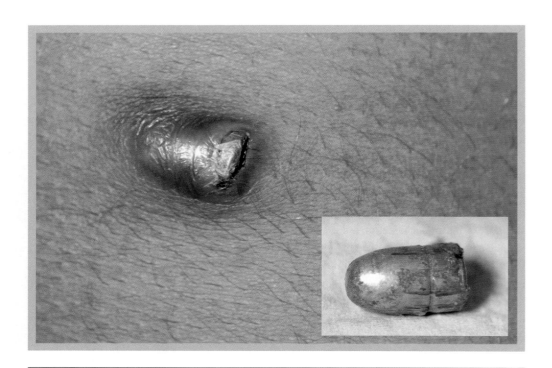

Clinical Summary

Gunshot injuries are classified as entrance, exit, or atypical (grazing) wounds. Physical findings in and around these wounds may offer evidence as to the actual mechanism, supporting or refuting the initial history given to the provider. As these findings may be transient, the emergency physician must be diligent in recognizing and documenting them at the time of presentation.

Entrance Wounds

Gunshot wounds of entrance are divided into four categories based on their range of fire: *distant, intermediate, close,* and *contact.* Range-of-fire is the distance from the gun's muzzle to the victim.

The size of the entrance wound bears no relation to the caliber of the inflicting bullet. Entrance wounds over elastic tissue will contract around the tissue defect and have a diameter much less than the caliber of the bullet.

Distant Wounds: The distant wound is inflicted from a range sufficiently distant that the bullet is the only projectile expelled from the muzzle that reaches the skin. There is no tattooing or soot deposition associated with a distant entrance wound. As the bullet penetrates the skin, friction between it and the epithelium results in the creation of an "abrasion collar" (Fig. 19.1). The width of the abrasion collar will vary with the angle of impact. Elongated abrasion collars from projectiles that enter on an angle may produce a collar with a "comet tail" (Fig. 19.2). Most entrance wounds will have an abrasion collar; however, gunshot wounds to the palms and soles are exceptions—their entrance wounds appear slit-like (Fig. 19.3).

Intermediate-Range Wounds: Tattooing is pathognomonic for an intermediate-range gunshot wound and presents as punctate abrasions from contact with partially burned or unburned grains of gunpowder (Fig. 19.4). This tattooing cannot be wiped away. Clothing and hair, as intermediate objects, may prevent the gunpowder grains from making contact with the skin. Tattooing can, but rarely does, occur on the palms and soles owing to the thickness of their epithelium.

Tattooing has been reported with a range of fire as close as 1 cm and as far away as 4 ft. The density of the abrasions and the associated pattern will depend on the barrel length, muzzle-to-skin distance, type of gunpowder (ball, flattened ball, or flake), presence of intermediate objects, and caliber of the weapon. Spherical powder travels farther and has greater penetration than flattened ball or flake powder.

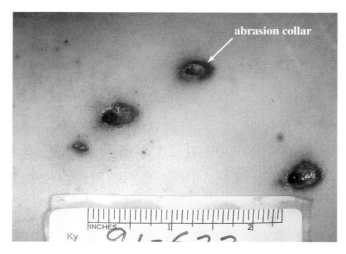

FIGURE 19.1 ■ Distant Gunshot Wound. The elliptical abrasion collars associated with these gunshot wounds of entrance indicate that the projectile passed from right to left. The range of fire is classified as distant or indeterminate based on the lack of carbonaceous material or gunpowder tattooing. (Photo contributor: William S. Smock, MD.)

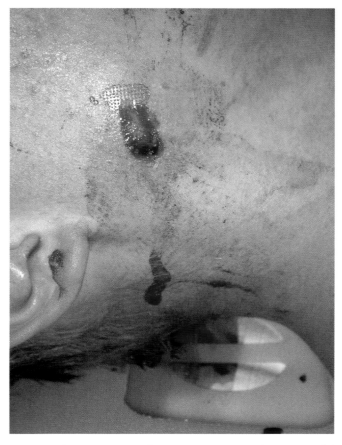

FIGURE 19.2 ■ "Comet-Tailed" Abrasion Collar. The "comet tail," abrasion collar located at the superior aspect of the wound indicates the bullet entered the wound at an angle. The "comet tail" also indicates the bullet's direction of travel; anterior to posterior. (Photo contributor: William S. Smock, MD.)

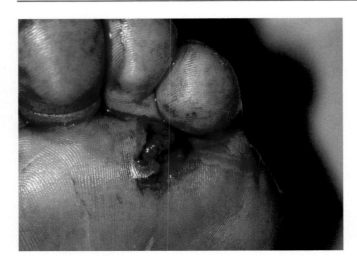

FIGURE 19.3 ▪ Entrance Wound on Sole. Entrance wounds on the soles of the feet do not generate abrasion collars due to the thickness of the skin. (Photo contributor: William S. Smock, MD.)

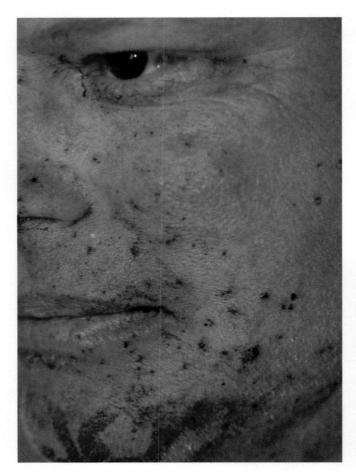

FIGURE 19.4 ▪ Intermediate-Range Gunshot Wound. Punctate abrasions present on the cheek are the result of impact with unburned or partially burned gunpowder. This phenomenon is termed *tattooing or stippling*. Tattooing is pathognomonic for intermediate-range gunshot wounds. (Photo contributor: William S. Smock, MD.)

Close-Range (Near-Contact) Wounds: "Close range" is defined as the maximum range at which soot is deposited on the clothing (Fig. 19.5) or wound (Fig. 19.6) and typically is a muzzle-to-victim distance of 6 in or less. On rare occasions, however, soot has been found on victims as far as 12 in from the offending weapon. The concentration of soot will vary inversely with the muzzle-to-victim distance and its appearance will be affected by the type of gunpowder and ammunition used, the barrel length, the caliber, and the type of weapon.

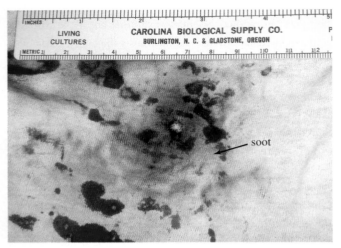

FIGURE 19.5 ▪ Close-Range Gunshot Wound. The deposition of carbonaceous material or soot is seen on a T-shirt from a close-range gunshot wound. Clothing should be collected and placed in separate paper bags for transport to the crime laboratory. (Photo contributor: William S. Smock, MD.)

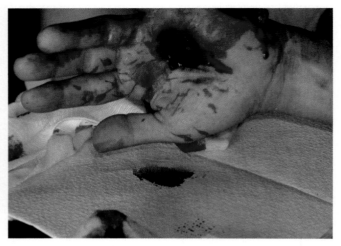

FIGURE 19.6 ▪ Close-Range Gunshot Wound. Soot is seen on this patient's hand suggesting a close-range or near-contact wound. (Photo contributor: William S. Smock, MD.)

Contact Wounds: A contact wound occurs when the barrel or muzzle is in contact with the skin or clothing as the weapon is discharged. Contact wounds can be described as tight, where the muzzle is pushed hard against the skin, or loose, where the muzzle is incompletely or loosely in contact with the skin or clothing. Wounds sustained from tight contact with the barrel can vary in appearance from a small hole with seared, blackened edges (from the discharge of hot gases and an actual flame) (Fig. 19.7), to a gaping, stellate wound (from the expansion of the skin from gases). Large stellate wounds are often misinterpreted as exit wounds based solely upon their size and without adequate examination of the wound.

In a tight-contact wound, all materials—the bullet, gases, soot, incompletely combusted gunpowder, and metal fragments—are driven into the wound. If the wound is over thin or bony tissue, the hot gases will cause the skin to expand to such an extent that it stretches and tears. These tears will have a triangular shape, with the base of the tear overlying the entrance wound. Larger tears are associated with ammunition of .32 caliber or greater, or magnum loads.

Stellate tears are not pathognomonic for contact wounds. Tangential wounds, ricochet or tumbling bullets, and some exit wounds may also be stellate in appearance. These wounds are distinguished from tight-contact wounds by the absence of soot and powder within the wound. In some tight-contact wounds, expanding skin is forced back against the muzzle of the gun, causing a characteristic pattern contusion called a *muzzle contusion* (Fig. 19.8). These patterns are helpful in determining the type of weapon (revolver or semiautomatic)

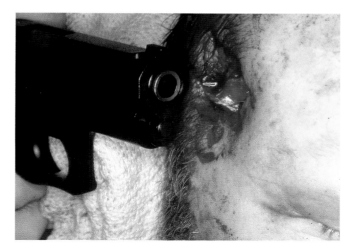

FIGURE 19.8 ■ Contact Gunshot Wound with Muzzle Abrasion. A contact gunshot wound to the right temple with stellate tears, seared skin, soot deposition, and muzzle imprint. A muzzle abrasion or muzzle imprint on the patient's right temple was the result of the injection of gases into the skin, causing a rapid and forceful expansion of the skin against the barrel of this 9-mm semiautomatic pistol. (Photo contributor: William S. Smock, MD.)

used to inflict the injury and should be documented prior to wound debridement or surgery.

With a loose-contact wound, where the muzzle is angled or held loosely against the skin, soot and gunpowder residue will be present in and around the wound (Fig. 19.9). The angle between the muzzle and skin will determine the soot pattern. A perpendicular, loose-contact or near-contact injury

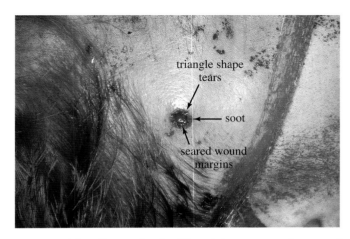

FIGURE 19.7 ■ Contact Gunshot Wound. A contact gunshot wound from a .22-caliber handgun. Note the small, triangle-shaped tear, soot, and seared wound margins. (Photo contributor: William S. Smock, MD.)

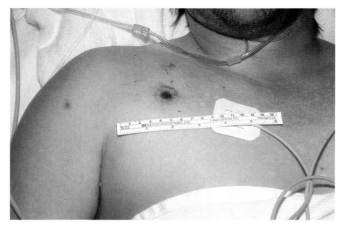

FIGURE 19.9 ■ Loose-Contact Gunshot Wound. Self-inflicted contact wound to the right upper chest with a 9-mm handgun. The wound margins display searing and soot deposition. (Photo contributor: William S. Smock, MD.)

results in searing of the skin and deposition of the soot evenly around the wound. A tangential loose or near-contact injury produces an elongated searing pattern and deposit of soot around the wound.

"Bullet wipe" is soot residue, soft lead, or lubricant, which may leave a gray rim or streak on the skin or clothing overlying an entrance wound (Fig. 19.10). This gray discoloration may also be found around the abrasion collar but is usually more prominent on clothing.

Exit Wounds

Determining whether a wound is an entrance or an exit wound should be based on the physical characteristics and physical evidence associated with the wound and *never upon the size* of the wound. Exit wounds are the result of a bullet pushing and stretching the skin from inside outward. The skin edges are generally everted, with sharp but irregular margins (Figs. 19.11 to 19.13). Abrasion collars, soot, searing, and tattooing are not associated with exit wounds. Soot can be seen at an atypical exit wound site if the entrance wound is close to the associated exit wound. Soot is propelled through the short wound tract and appears faintly on the exit wound surface.

Exit wounds assume a variety of shapes and appearances and are *not* consistently larger than their corresponding entrance wounds. The size of an exit wound is determined primarily by the amount of energy possessed by the bullet as it exits the skin and by the bullet's size, shape, attitude, and energy transmitted to underlying tissue that is extruded from the wound, for example, bone. A bullet's usual nose-first attitude will change upon entering the skin to a tumbling and yawing one. A bullet with sufficient energy to exit the skin in a sideways attitude or one that has increased its surface area by mushrooming may produce an exit wound larger than its entrance wound. Energy transferred to bone, with resultant ballistic fracture, may also result in an exit larger than the entrance wound. A "false abrasion collar" or "shored exit" wound may mimic an entrance wound. This occurs when the epithelium is pressed against a supporting surface such as a floor, wall, chair, firm mattress, or wallet (Figs. 19.14 and 19.15).

Graze Wounds

Graze wounds are considered atypical and result from tangential contact with a passing bullet. The direction of the bullet's path may be determined by careful wound examination. The bullet produces a trough and may cause the formation of skin

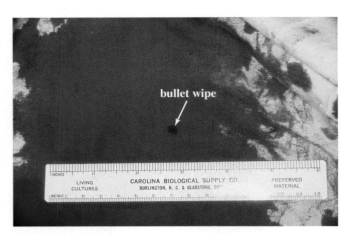

FIGURE 19.10 ■ Bullet Wipe. "Bullet wipe" is residue and lead deposited on clothing or skin. The presence of this residue on clothing may help to determine whether the wound is an entrance wound. (Photo contributor: William S. Smock, MD.)

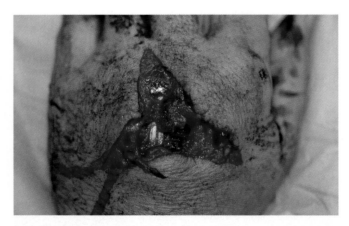

FIGURE 19.11 ■ Stellate Tears from Exit Wound. Stellate tears in an exit wound from a .45-caliber handgun. (Photo contributor: William S. Smock, MD.)

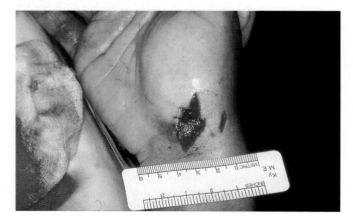

FIGURE 19.12 ■ Exit Gunshot Wound. A stellate exit wound. Exit wounds may take on a variety of appearances. Stellate exit wounds should not be confused with contact wounds. The lack of soot and seared skin tells the physician that this is an exit wound. (Photo contributor: William S. Smock, MD.)

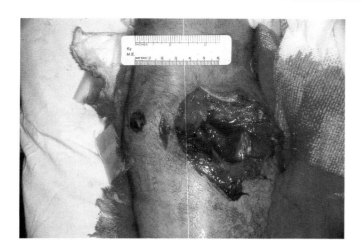

FIGURE 19.13 ■ High-Velocity Gunshot Wound. A perforating high-velocity gunshot wound to a lower extremity. The gaping exit wound resulted from the transfer of energy from the projectile to the tibia. The impact propelled multiple bony fragments through the skin. (Photo contributor: William S. Smock, MD.)

tags on the lateral wound margins (Figs. 19.16 and 19.17). The base of these tags point toward the weapon and away from the direction of bullet travel.

Pearls

1. Distant-range gunshot wounds are inflicted from a distance greater than 4 ft and typically there is no tattooing, soot, or searing associated with the wound.

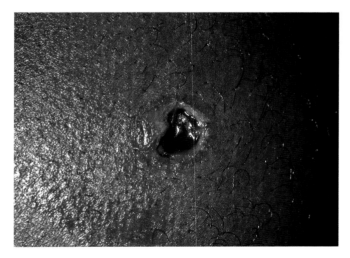

FIGURE 19.14 ■ Shored Gunshot Exit Wound. A "shored exit" or "false abrasion collar" associated with a gunshot wound of exit. The false abrasion collar results when the skin is supported by a firm surface as the bullet exits. Shored exits occur when epithelium is pressed against a supporting surface (ie, floor, wall, chair, firm mattress, or wallet in this case). (Photo contributor: William S. Smock, MD.)

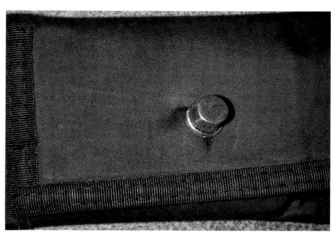

FIGURE 19.15 ■ Wallet Causing Shored Gunshot Exit Wound. The wound seen in Fig. 19.14 occurred as a result of this wallet against the exit site. (Photo contributor: William S. Smock, MD.)

2. Intermediate-range gunshot wounds are inflicted at a distances up to 4 ft and characteristically are associated with tattooing from partially burned and unburned gunpowder imbedded in the skin.

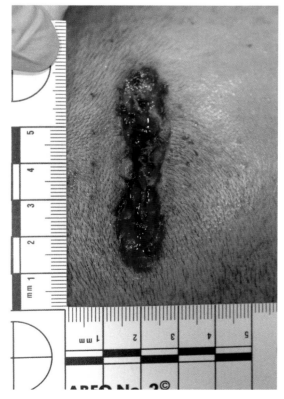

FIGURE 19.16 ■ Graze Gunshot Wound. A superficial graze wound from a 9-mm projectile. Determining the directionality of a graze wound is difficult. (Photo contributor: William S. Smock, MD.)

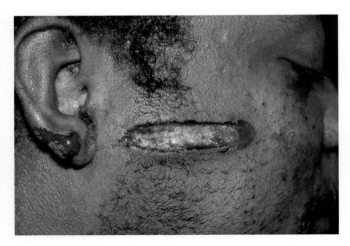

FIGURE 19.17 ■ Graze Gunshot Wound. A deep graze wound from a handgun is seen. The dark wound margins are the result of drying artifact and should not be confused with the deposition of soot. (Photo contributor: Lawrence B. Stack, MD.)

3. Near or close-contact gunshot wounds are defined as the maximum range at which soot is deposited on the wound or clothing and typically occur at a distance of 6 in or less.

4. Contact gunshot wounds (barrel is in contact with the skin or clothing at time of discharge) vary in size but will include triangular tears, searing, and soot within or around the wound.

5. Abrasion collars, soot, searing, and tattooing are not associated with exit wounds.

6. Determination of whether a wound is an entrance or exit wound should **only** be based on the physical characteristics of the wound and clothing and not on the size of the wound.

7. Emergency physicians should attempt to recognize, preserve, and collect short-lived evidence whenever the clinical situation allows.

Every "weapon" (hand, belt, hot iron, knife, electrical cord, baseball bat, tire iron) can leave a mark, design, or pattern stamped or imprinted upon or just below the level of the epithelium. The imprints of these weapons are called *pattern injuries*, which are considerably reproducible. These injuries can be categorized into three major classifications according to their source: sharp-force, blunt-force, and thermal-pattern injuries.

SHARP-FORCE-PATTERN INJURIES

Clinical Summary

There are two types of sharp-force injuries: incised and stabbed. The incised wound is longer than it is deep. The stab wound is defined as a puncture wound that is deeper than it is wide. The wound margins of sharp-force injuries are clean and lack the abraded edges of injuries from blunt forces. Forensic information can be gathered during the examination of a stab wound. Some characteristics of a knife blade, single- or double-edged, can be determined by visual inspection. Characteristics such as serrated versus sharp can be determined if the blade was drawn across the skin during insertion or withdraw from the victim. Serrated blades do not always leave these characteristic marks.

Pearls

1. Incised wounds are longer than they are deep.
2. Stab wounds are puncture wounds that are deeper than they are long.
3. Knife-blade characteristics (single or dual edged, serrated or smooth) can frequently be determined by visual inspection of the wound.

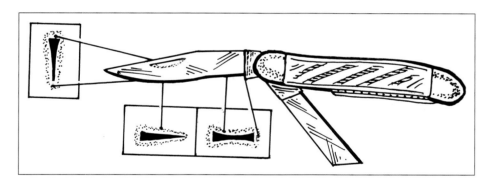

FIGURE 19.18 ■ Stab Wound. A stab wound from a single-edged knife blade will impart a sharp edge and a dull edge to the wound. If the blade penetrates to the proximal portion of the blade, a contusion may result from contact with the hilt of the knife.

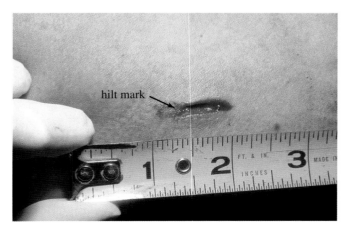

FIGURE 19.19 ■ Single-Edge Stab Wound with Hilt Mark. A single-edged stab wound with a small hilt mark associated with the dull edge of the blade. (Photo contributor: William S. Smock, MD.)

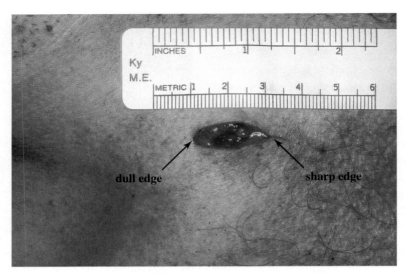

FIGURE 19.20 ■ Single-Edge Stab Wound. A stab wound from a single-edged knife blade. The left side of the wound corresponds with the dull edge of the blade and the right side with the sharp edge of the blade. (Photo contributor: William S. Smock, MD.)

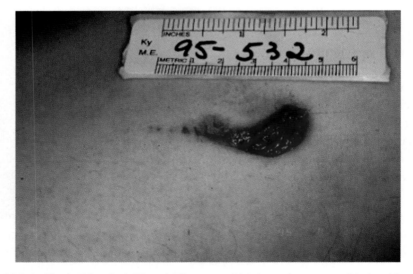

FIGURE 19.21 ■ Serrated Blade Single-Edge Stab Wound. The serrated blade made contact with the skin either on entry or exit from the wound. (Photo contributor: William S. Smock, MD.)

Clinical Summary

The most common blunt force is the contusion (Fig. 19.22). The *pattern contusion* is a common injury that helps identify the causative weapon. A blow from a linear object leaves a contusion that is characterized by a set of parallel lines separated by an area of central clearing. The blood underlying the striking object is forcibly displaced to the sides, which accounts for the pattern's appearance. Pattern injuries that an emergency physician should recognize include those caused by the hand (slap marks, fingertip contusions, grab marks, choke holds, fingernail abrasions), solid objects (baseball bat, tire iron, 2 by 4, belt, shoe, comb), and bite marks.

Other manifestations of blunt-force trauma to the skin are the abrasion and the laceration. A weapon with a unique shape or configuration may stamp a mirror image of itself on the skin. The presence of a subconjunctival hemorrhage may be suggestive of choking, strangulation, or suffocation.

Pearls

1. A contusion is the most common blunt-force injury pattern.
2. Blood underlying the force of the contusion is displaced to either side of the object, causing a *pattern contusion* in the shape of that object. This pattern is recognized by the central clearing surrounded by parallel contusions.
3. Emergency physicians must be able to recognize the pattern injuries caused by the hand, solid objects, and bites.

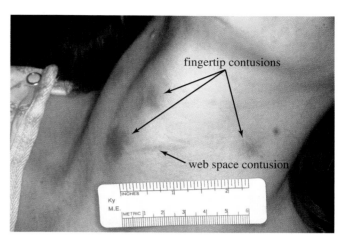

FIGURE 19.22 ■ Fingertip Contusion Pattern. This patient exhibits fingertip contusions as well as a web-space contusion. These injuries are the result of being choked by her assailant's left hand. (Photo contributor: William S. Smock, MD.)

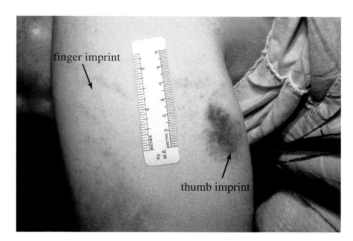

FIGURE 19.23 ■ Grab-Mark Pattern Contusions. This victim of domestic assault has two patterns of injury present over the outer aspect of her upper arm. The contusion on the left reveals a central clearing bordered by two parallel lines, which is the result of forceful contact with an extended finger. The contusion on the right is the result of fingertip pressure applied by the thumb of her assailant. (Photo contributor: William S. Smock, MD.)

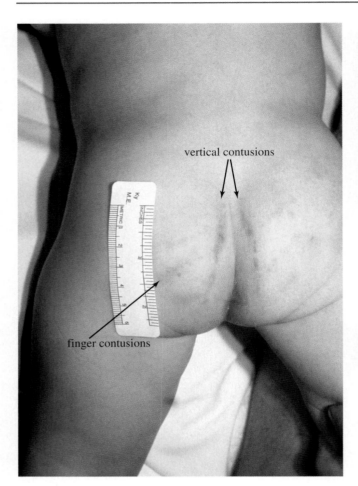

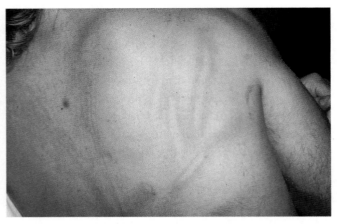

FIGURE 19.25 ■ Police Baton Contusions. This patient sustained multiple blows from a police baton during his arrest. The central clearing bordered by two parallel contusions is indicative of impact with a rounded linear object. (Photo contributor: William S. Smock, MD.)

FIGURE 19.24 ■ Slap-Mark Pattern Contusions. This victim of assault presents with two pattern injuries. Diagonally oriented across both buttocks are pattern contusions with central clearing as well as parallel contusions. The vertically oriented contusions are the result of forceful contact as a blow was delivered with an open hand. The presence of these vertical contusions is virtually pathognomonic of inflicted injury. (Photo contributor: William S. Smock, MD.)

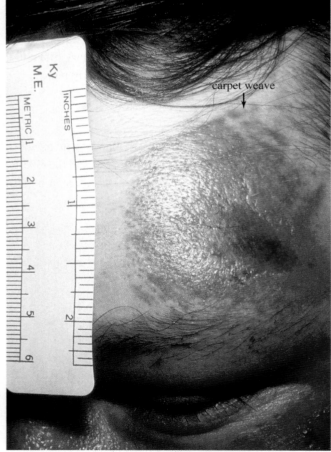

FIGURE 19.26 ■ Carpet-Weave Pattern Abrasion. A pattern abrasion of the forehead from a domestic assault. The weave of the carpet is appreciated on the outer margins of the abrasions. This injury occurred when the patient's forehead was slammed into the carpet. (Photo contributor: William S. Smock, MD.)

Clinical Summary

A thermal-pattern injury is a common form of abuse or assault, especially in children and the elderly. The detailed history of the incident should include the position of the patient relative to the thermal source. This will help determine whether the injury was inflicted or accidental. Pattern of thermal injuries commonly encountered in the emergency department include *flatiron burns, curling-iron burns, immersion burns,* and *splash burns.* A sharp or clear line of demarcation between burned and unburned tissue characterizes immersion or dipping burns. In contrast, splash burns are characterized by an irregular or undulating line or by isolated areas of thermal injury, usually round or oval in shape, caused by droplets of hot liquid. The severity of the scald injury depends upon the length of the time the skin was in contact with the offending substance and the temperature of the substance itself. Tap or faucet water causes full-thickness thermal damage in 1 second at 70°C, and 180 seconds at 48.9°C. Law-enforcement agency should routinely measure the household's or institution's water temperature in any investigation involving a scald injury of a child, a developmentally delayed person, or an elderly patient.

Pearls

1. A thermal-pattern injury is a common form of abuse seen in infants, institutionalized patients, and the elderly.
2. Emergency physicians must recognize thermal-pattern injuries of abuse.

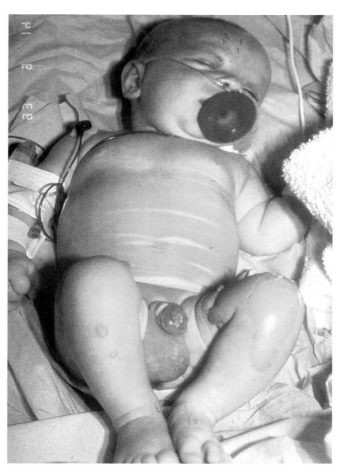

FIGURE 19.28 ■ Scald Burn Thermal Injury Pattern. Superficial and partial-thickness burns were noted on the patient's anterior surface only. The areas of abdominal sparing indicate that the victim was flexed and curled at the time of injury. The child's caretaker, the mother's boyfriend, admitted to holding the child under a running hot-water tap. Partial-thickness burns on the penis and medial thighs are indicative of pooling of the liquid in those areas, resulting in a time-dependent injury. (Photo contributor: William S. Smock, MD.)

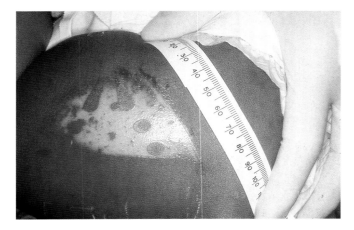

FIGURE 19.27 ■ Clothes-Iron Thermal Injury Pattern. A thermal injury inflicted by an iron. The areas of sparing are associated with the iron's steam holes. (Photo contributor: William S. Smock, MD.)

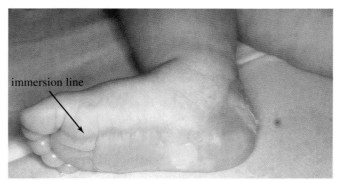

FIGURE 19.29 ■ Immersion-Line Thermal Injury Pattern. A classic "immersion line" is seen in a thermal-pattern injury. The line of demarcation is associated with the depth of the immersion. (Photo contributor: William S. Smock, MD.)

Chapter 20

HIV CONDITIONS

J. Michael Ballester
Roderick Morrison

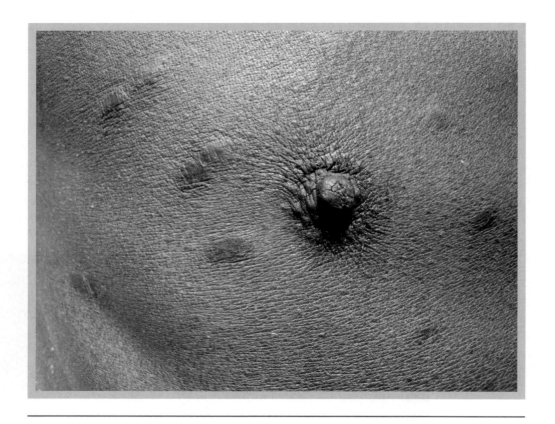

The authors would like to acknowledge the special contributions of Shane Cline, MD and Michael Krentz, MD for their excellent work on prior editions of this chapter.

Clinical Summary

Establishing the diagnosis of primary HIV infection is very important from a public health perspective. Patients are highly infectious during acute HIV secondary to an enormous viral load in both blood and genital secretions. Such patients may be unaware that they are infected and therefore may put others at risk. Clinical illness accompanies primary HIV infection in approximately two-thirds of patients. The usual time from HIV exposure to the development of symptoms is approximately 10 to 20 days, with average symptom duration of 1.5 to 2 weeks. The most common symptoms following seroconversion include fever, swollen lymph nodes, sore throat, myalgias/arthralgias, diarrhea, nausea/vomiting, weight loss, headache, mucocutaneous lesions, and a generalized maculopapular rash located over the face, neck, and trunk. This rash is seen in over 50% of persons with symptomatic primary HIV infection. The lesions are typically small, well-circumscribed, erythematous, nonpruritic and nontender. Less frequently, patients may demonstrate neurologic signs and symptoms consistent with meningoencephalitis, myelopathy, and peripheral neuropathy. If obtained, laboratory studies may show lymphopenia and thrombocytopenia.

Emergency Department Treatment and Disposition

Historically, HIV testing has rarely been performed in the emergency department setting owing to the difficulty of obtaining consent, lack of resource availability, lack of time for counseling and most importantly, uncertain follow-up for linking infected patients to treatment and long-term care. However, there are presently multiple examples of emergency department screening programs that have shown promise in the early detection of HIV infection. Emergency physicians should take a careful history for HIV risk factors and should be cautious but honest in entertaining this diagnosis. Patients should be educated about disease transmission and referred for prompt follow up and further outpatient testing and evaluation.

Pearls

1. Maintain a high degree of clinical suspicion for acute HIV infection, especially when patients present with mononucleosis-like symptoms, unexplained rash, mucocutaneous ulcers or lymphadenopathy, and aseptic meningitis.
2. Ensure proper follow up for patients in whom the diagnosis of acute HIV infection is entertained.

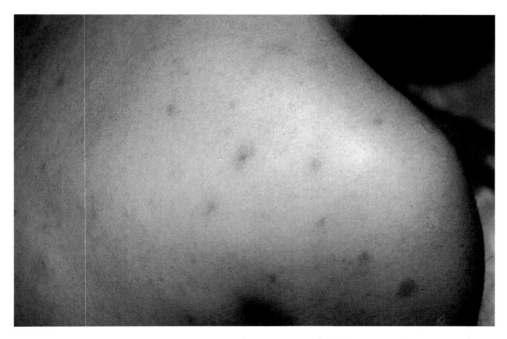

FIGURE 20.1 ■ Primary HIV Infection. A maculopapular rash is seen in over half of persons with symptomatic acute HIV infection. This less typical papular/vesicular rash was present in a patient with primary HIV infection. (Photo contributor: Gregory K. Robbins, MD, MPH.)

Clinical Summary

Oral hairy leukoplakia (OHL) is a disease of the lingual squamous epithelium caused by the Epstein-Barr virus. OHL generally affects the lateral portion of the tongue, although the floor of the mouth, palate, or buccal mucosa may also be involved. The lesions are described as white corrugated plaques that, unlike *Candida*, cannot be scraped from the surface to which they adhere. Most often OHL is asymptomatic, although occasionally this condition can cause pain. Diagnosis is usually clinical, though definitive diagnosis can be made by biopsy characteristically revealing acanthosis and parakeratosis.

Emergency Department Treatment and Disposition

Patients who are known to be HIV-seropositive can be educated to the disease and reassured. OHL is not considered to be a premalignant lesion. If the patient happens to be symptomatic, Zidovudine, oral acyclovir, ganciclovir, foscarnet, and/or topical podophyllin may be prescribed in consultation with an infectious disease specialist.

Pearls

1. Oral candidiasis can be distinguished from OHL by utilizing a swab in an attempt to remove the exudate characteristic of thrush and by observing pseudohyphal elements microscopically.
2. OHL is fairly specific for HIV infection, rarely observed in patients with other immunodeficiencies. There are however other mucocutaneous lesions seen in HIV patients that might be easily mistaken for OHL—these include oral candidiasis, geographic tongue, oral herpes simplex virus, cytomegalovirus, and idiopathic aphthous ulcerations.

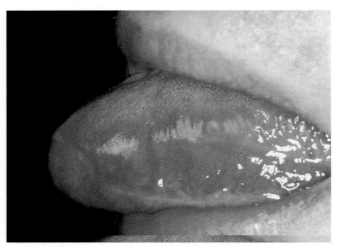

FIGURE 20.2 ■ Oral Hairy Leukoplakia. Typical-appearing lesions on side of tongue in this patient with HIV. (Photo contributor: Robert Brandt, MD.)

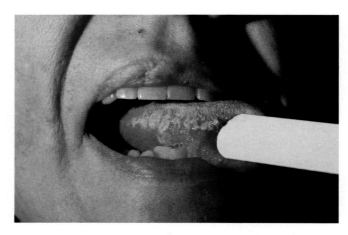

FIGURE 20.3 ■ Oral Hairy Leukoplakia. Exudate does not scrap off the tongue in oral hairy leukoplakia, differentiating it clinically from oral thrush. (Photo contributor: Kevin J. Knoop, MD, MS.)

Clinical Summary

Oral infections are seen in over half of all HIV patients, with the severity of infection often correlating with the degree of immunosuppression. Oral candidiasis can occur at all stages of HIV disease. The usual causative agent is *Candida albicans*, but over 150 other species of *Candida* have become more prevalent and resistant in recent years due to chronic antifungal use. Oral candidiasis, or "thrush," can be classified as pseudomembranous, angular, or erythematous. Pseudomembranous candidiasis can be diagnosed by identifying removable whitish plaques on the tongue, uvula, and buccal mucosa. Erythematous thrush appears as smooth red patches along the soft and hard palate.

As in other conditions associated with immunocompromised patients, vaginal candidiasis is common and can cause a severe whitish discharge with vulvar erythema. It is not uncommon for women to present to the emergency department for evaluation of vaginal candidiasis as their first clinical manifestation of the HIV infection.

Emergency Department Treatment and Disposition

Poor oral intake secondary to pain associated with severe oral or esophageal candidal infections can cause dehydration and malnutrition, often requiring intravenous hydration and hospitalization. There is no "standard" therapy for candidiasis in the HIV patient. Both oral and vaginal candida infections can be treated with nystatin or clotrimazole troches. Alternatively, systemic treatment with either ketoconazole or fluconazole is usually effective. For severe or refractory cases, amphotericin B or caspofungin remain the drugs of choice.

Pearls

1. Oral candidiasis is a poor prognostic sign, indicative of the progression to AIDS in the seropositive patient.
2. Esophageal candidiasis frequently accompanies oral candidiasis and any history of dysphagia or odynophagia should prompt concerns regarding possible esophagitis. Endoscopy with biopsy may be the only way to definitively establish a specific diagnosis. Ensure follow up in 3 to 5 days when treating empirically for presumptive esophageal candidiasis.
3. Popular one-dose oral treatments for oral and vaginal candidal infections are associated with a high rate of relapse in HIV patients.
4. HAART therapy has resulted in a dramatic decrease in the prevalence of oral, esophageal candidiasis and in refractory disease.

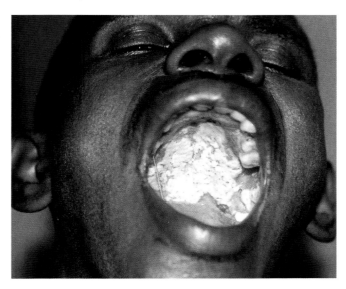

FIGURE 20.4 ■ Oral Candidiasis. Removable whitish plaques on the palate are seen in this HIV patient with pseudomembranous candidiasis. (Photo contributor: Thea James, MD.)

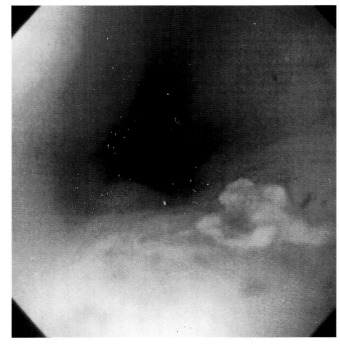

FIGURE 20.5 ■ Esophageal Candidiasis. Endoscopy demonstrating esophageal candidiasis in this HIV patient. (Photo contributor: Edward C. Oldfield III, MD.)

5. Consider possible drug interactions when prescribing anti-fungal medications. For example, the absorption of keto-conazole is impaired by the simultaneous administration of antacids and cimetidine. Because of these interactions, many clinicians favor fluconazole, since lack of gastric acid or the presence of food does not affect the affect its absorption. Fluconazole however, does raise serum levels of warfarin and sulfonylureas.

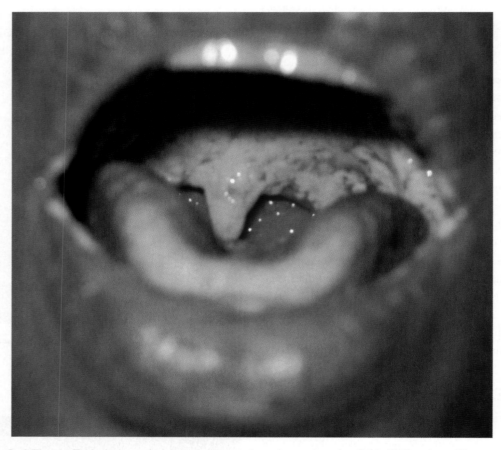

FIGURE 20.6 ▪ Oral Thrush. Typical plaque lesions are seen on the palate and uvula of this HIV patient. (Photo contributor: Seth W. Wright, MD.)

Clinical Summary

Kaposi sarcoma (KS) is a low-grade vascular tumor associated with human herpesvirus 8. Since the introduction of HAART, the incidence of KS in HIV-infected persons has declined. Kaposi sarcoma can demonstrate a variable clinical course, ranging from minimal disease to explosive growth resulting in significant morbidity and mortality. Skin involvement is characteristic but extracutaneous spread of KS is common, particularly to the oral cavity, GI tract, and the respiratory tract. The skin lesions appear most often on the lower extremities, face (especially the nose), oral mucosa, and genitalia. Most commonly, the lesions are papular, ranging in size from several millimeters to centimeters in diameter. Less commonly, the lesions may be plaque-like, especially on the soles of the feet or exophytic and fungating with breakdown of overlying skin.

Oral lesions occur in one-third of KS patients with the most common site being the palate, followed by the gingiva and tongue. GI lesions are present in approximately 40% of patients with KS at initial diagnosis and 80% at autopsy. Lesions may be asymptomatic or cause one or more of the following symptoms: weight loss, abdominal pain, nausea/vomiting, upper or lower GI bleeding, malabsorption, obstruction, and diarrhea.

Pulmonary involvement is common in AIDS-related KS. Affected persons may present with shortness of breath, fever, cough, hemoptysis, or chest pain or as an asymptomatic finding on chest x-ray. Diagnosis can be confirmed via bronchoscopy.

Emergency Department Treatment and Disposition

Most, if not all, patients with KS should receive HAART. In addition, there are a variety of other therapies directed at the tumors. Local therapy may be useful for cosmesis or symptom control of individual lesions. Options include topical gels, external beam irradiation, and/or intralesional chemotherapy. Systemic chemotherapy and newer immunomodulator therapy (interleukin-12, angiogenesis inhibitors) are reserved for more extensive disease, especially visceral involvement.

Pearls

1. HIV patients who present with persistent raised purple lesions warrant biopsy.
2. Perform a careful skin and oral examination in HIV patients.
3. Note that half of patients with oral involvement have other GI tract involvement as well. Heme testing of stool is a good preliminary screen.
4. KS is the most common tumor arising in the HIV-infected patient, and is considered an AIDS-defining illness.
5. Corticosteroid therapy has been associated with the induction of KS and with the exacerbation of preexisting KS disease in HIV-infected persons. This is important, given the frequent use of steroids in HIV-infected persons with a variety of disorders including PCP pneumonia and ITP.

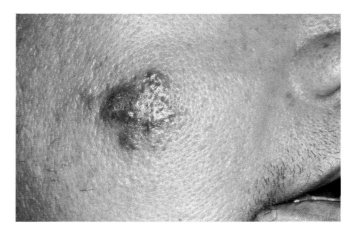

FIGURE 20.7 ■ Kaposi Sarcoma. A single violaceous patch is seen on the face of an HIV-positive patient. (Photo contributor: George Turiansky, MD.)

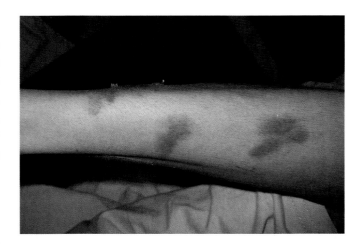

FIGURE 20.8 ■ Cutaneous Kaposi Sarcoma. Characteristic nonraised violaceous Kaposi sarcoma lesions on the arm of this Caucasian patient with HIV. (Photo contributors: Seth W. Wright, MD and Universidad Peruana Cayetano Heredia, Lima, Peru.)

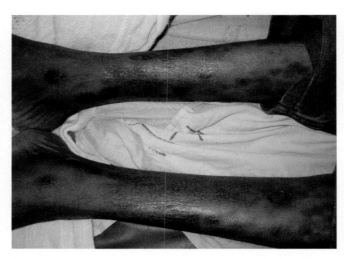

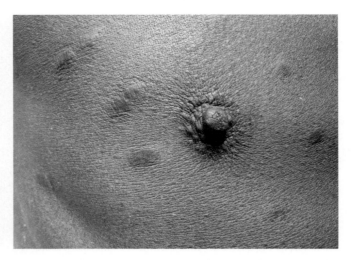

FIGURE 20.9 ■ Kaposi Sarcoma. Multiple black KS lesions, as typically seen in darker skinned patients. (Photo contributor: Seth W. Wright, MD.)

FIGURE 20.10 ■ Kaposi Sarcoma. Multiple KS lesions surrounding the nipple of this patient with advanced HIV. (Photo contributor: Seth W. Wright, MD.)

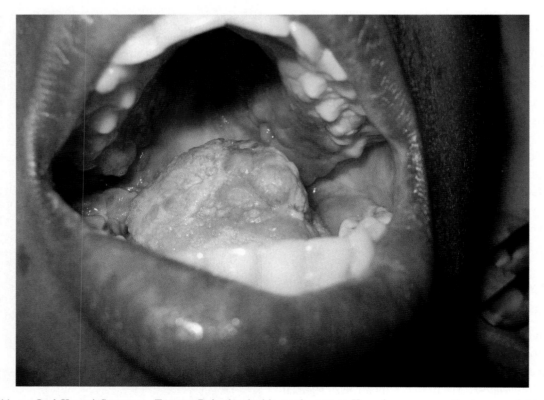

FIGURE 20.11 ■ Oral Kaposi Sarcoma—Tongue. Raised palpable erythematous Kaposi sarcoma on the tongue of this HIV patient. (Photo contributor: Seth W. Wright, MD.)

Clinical Summary

Toxoplasmosis gondii is a widespread intracellular protozoan parasite with a definitive host stage in cats. Ingestion of oocysts from the cat litter or soil, ingestion of bradyzoites from undercooked meat (especially pork), or transplacental migration of tachyzoites is thought to spread the disease. Immunocompetent persons are usually asymptomatic, but immunocompromised persons (especially HIV-positive persons with <100 CD4 cells/μL) are subjected to reactivation of latent disease with considerable morbidity and mortality.

Patients with CNS toxoplasmosis most often present with symptoms consistent with intracranial mass lesions (headache, focal neurologic deficit, nausea/emesis, and/or seizure) or encephalitis (fever, confusion, altered mental status). Contrasted computed tomography (CT) of the head typically reveals ring-enhancing lesions with a predilection for the basal ganglia. Magnetic resonance imaging (MRI) of the head is more sensitive than CT for identifying these lesions. Serological tests can be unreliable; however cerebrospinal fluid (CSF) detection of *T gondii* antibodies can be helpful. Definitive diagnosis of cerebral pathology is obtained by open or stereotactic brain biopsy.

Ocular toxoplasmosis is a common complication of HIV disease. Patients typically present with eye pain and decreased visual acuity. Retinitis may be diagnosed by ophthalmoscopic evaluation revealing characteristic exudates and hemorrhage. Toxoplasmosis retinitis appears as raised yellow-white, cottony lesions in a nonvascular distribution, unlike the edematous perivascular exudates of CMV retinitis.

Patients with pulmonary toxoplasmosis infections typically present with fever, dyspnea, and a nonproductive cough. Chest x-ray typically reveals reticulonodular infiltrates. Definitive diagnosis can be made via detection of tachyzoites in broncho-alveolar lavage (BAL) fluid.

Emergency Department Treatment and Disposition

If the patient presents with seizures, loading doses of antiepileptics such as fosphenytoin should be administered. There are two combination regimens considered to be first choice for the treatment of toxoplasmosis. The most commonly used regimen is pyrimethamine and sulfadiazine for 6 weeks or until neurological findings have resolved; however, for those with sulfa allergies, pyrimethamine and clindamycin is the alternative. HIV patients who are seropositive for *T gondii* should receive prophylaxis or chronic suppressive therapy. This is most commonly achieved using trimethoprim-sulfamethoxazole—the dose is the same as for *Pneumocystis* pneumonia.

In cases of suspected ocular toxoplasmosis, a complete eye examination, including slit-lamp examination and measurements of intraocular pressure, should be performed before consulting ophthalmology.

Pearls

1. Space-occupying lesions due to toxoplasmosis can lead to increased intracranial pressure. Head CT with contrast to rule out these lesions should be considered prior to attempting a lumbar puncture to prevent iatrogenic herniation.

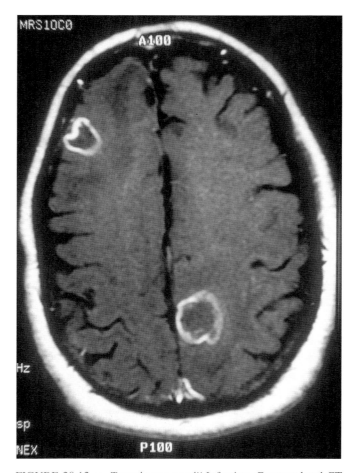

FIGURE 20.12 ■ *Toxoplasma gondii* Infection. Contrast head CT showing typical multiple ring-enhancing lesions seen in *T gondii* CNS infection. (Photo contributor: Edward C. Oldfield III, MD.)

2. Consider steroids and seizure prophylaxis for patients with severe cerebral edema as evidenced by confusion, lethargy, coma, and/or papilledema.

3. Patients with HIV should be counseled to avoid eating undercooked meats and to use gloves when handling soiled cat litter.

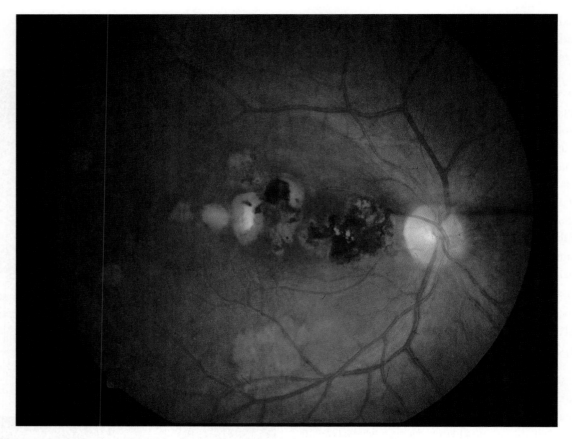

FIGURE 20.13 ■ Toxoplasmosis Retinitis. Ocular toxoplasmosis is a common complication of HIV disease. The lesion is a focal destructive chorioretinitis which leaves well-defined, heavily pigmented scars, especially in the macular area. (Photo contributor: Department of Ophthalmology; Naval Medical Center, San Diego, CA.)

Clinical Summary

The most common presentation of *Cryptococcus* in the context of HIV is meningitis, although pulmonary, disseminated, and cutaneous infections occur. The organism *Cryptococcus neoformans* is widely distributed—often in bird droppings—and is usually acquired via inhalation. It typically manifests itself in patients whose CD4 cell counts are less than 50/μL. The onset tends to be insidious with fairly nonspecific symptoms such as fever, nausea, and headache. As the infection progresses, the patient's level of consciousness may decline and significant changes in affect may be noted. Seizures or focal neurological presentations are rare and neck stiffness and/or photophobia may be absent. Diagnosis is usually made on examination of CSF. Opening pressures may be quite elevated on lumbar puncture, and CSF values usually reveal a normal CSF glucose concentration, a mildly elevated CSF protein concentration, and a CSF leukocyte count of less than 20/mL. India ink staining shows the organisms directly with an approximate sensitivity of 50%, while cryptococcal latex antigen testing has a sensitivity approaching 90%. Definitive diagnosis is made via blood and/or CSF culture.

Emergency Department Treatment and Disposition

Treatment should begin with the timely institution of broad-spectrum antibiotics when acute CNS infection is suspected or if the patient appears "toxic" and/or has unstable vital signs. Most often, the decision to treat for cryptococcal meningitis will be based on the results of the lumbar puncture (LP) results, along with consultation with infectious disease specialists. If the results are suggestive of *Cryptococcus*, standard treatment consists of amphotericin B with flucytosine for approximately 4 to 6 weeks. Fluconazole can be substituted if side effects of the above-stated drugs become too disabling. Fluconazole is also considered the maintenance drug of choice for *Cryptococcus* in HIV-positive patients after the initial 6 weeks is finished—treatment is for life.

Pearls

1. Perform the LP only after CT with contrast rules out space-occupying lesions, and do so with the patient in a lateral decubitus position so as to obtain an accurate opening pressure.

2. "False-positive" India ink stains can occur with other encapsulated organisms such as *Klebsiella pneumoniae, Rhodotorula, Candida,* and *Proteus.*

3. Blood cultures are positive in more than three-quarters of patients with cryptococcal meningitis.

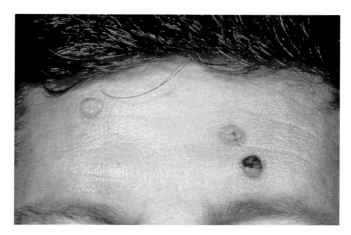

FIGURE 20.14 ■ Cryptococcal Infection. Cryptococcal skin lesions in disseminated form. Note that the umbilicated centers give a similar appearance to that of molluscum contagiosum. (Photo contributor: Briana Hill, MD.)

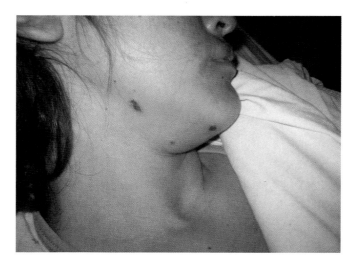

FIGURE 20.15 ■ Cryptococcal Infection. Cutaneous cryptococcal lesions are often clinically difficult to distinguish from other cutaneous eruptions. (Photo contributors: Seth W. Wright, MD and Universidad Peruana Cayetano Heredia, Lima, Peru.)

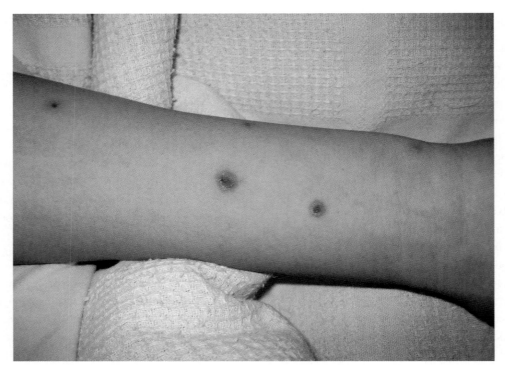

FIGURE 20.16 ■ Cryptococcal Infection. This patient had extensive cutaneous involvement with disseminated cryptococcal infection. (Photo contributors: Seth W. Wright, MD and Universidad Peruana Cayetano Heredia, Lima, Peru.)

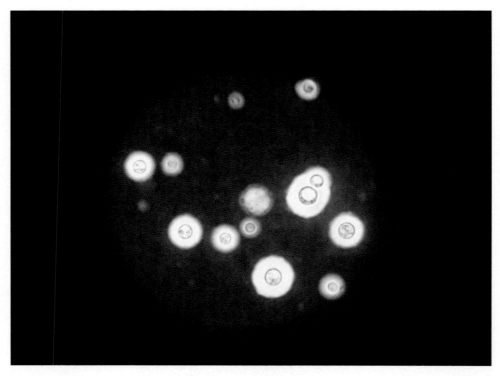

FIGURE 20.17 ■ India Ink Preparation. *Cryptococcus neoformans* seen as encapsulated yeast on India ink preparation of the CSF from an HIV patient with cryptococcal meningitis. (Photo contributor: Seth W. Wright, MD.)

Clinical Summary

Cytomegalovirus (CMV) can be a cause of considerable morbidity in HIV-infected individuals, especially in the later stages of disease. It is thought that CMV infects over three-quarters of HIV patients, usually resulting from a latent infection. Most types of CMV infections occur once the CD4 count is below 100 cells/μL. The major problems encountered are, in order of frequency, retinitis, colitis, esophageal ulceration, encephalitis, and pneumonitis.

CMV retinitis is the most common cause of blindness and eye disease in HIV patients. Although usually unilateral to begin with, the infection frequently spreads to involve both eyes. Patients typically present with loss of vision, floaters, scotomata, visual field loss, orbital pain, and/or headache. Funduscopic examination reveals exudates and hemorrhages, which follow the vasculature of the retina, giving it the typical "pizza pie" or "cottage cheese and ketchup" appearance.

CMV colitis is an uncommon but serious complication of HIV. The usual presenting features include generalized abdominal pain, diarrhea which may be bloody, and a low-grade fever. Loops of dilated large bowel may be seen on abdominal x-ray, but definitive diagnosis is via sigmoidoscopy and mucosal biopsy, revealing the characteristic "owls eye" inclusion bodies.

Emergency Department Treatment and Disposition

Treatment for all forms of CMV infections should be started as soon as possible with either ganciclovir or foscarnet given intravenously for at least 3 weeks and up to 6 weeks in cases of CMV encephalitis. Cidofovir is available for use when the above drugs are contraindicated. Relapse is common with CMV retinitis and if left untreated can progress to complete blindness.

Pearls

1. Ocular complaints in HIV patients require a comprehensive eye examination along with ophthalmology involvement.
2. Patients with CMV esophagitis often complain of odynophagia and/or substernal chest pain, but very infrequently of dysphagia; this is a key clinical distinction from candidal esophagitis.
3. Myelosuppression is a major toxic effect of ganciclovir, while foscarnet/cidofovir may cause nephrotoxicity.

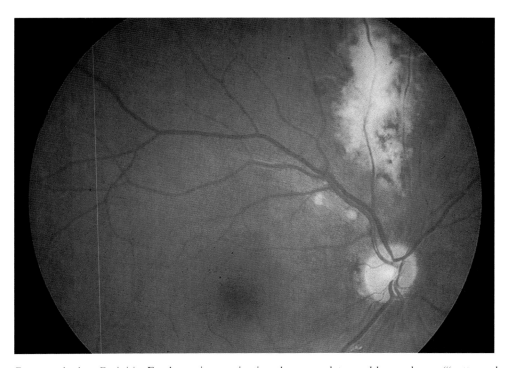

FIGURE 20.18 ■ Cytomegalovirus Retinitis. Funduscopic examination shows exudates and hemorrhages ("cottage cheese and ketchup" appearance) seen with CMV retinitis. (Photo contributor: Edward C. Oldfield III, MD.)

Clinical Summary

Leishmaniasis is a protozoan parasite that is spread by the bite of the female sand fly. The protozoan is endemic in over 80 countries with over 20 species being identified. The infection begins when flagellated forms of the parasite are injected into the skin, are taken up by macrophages, and then multiply. Resulting disease is either manifested as cutaneous disease, mucocutaneous disease, or disseminated disease, with a high rate of individual variability in presentation. The coinfection of HIV and *Leishmania* causes synergistic immunologic disturbances, due to the inability of the advanced HIV patient to mount a critical CD+ T-cell response. Cutaneous lesions tend to occur on exposed areas of skin, often without recollection of a sand fly bite. Lesions begin as a papule that enlarges to form an ulcer with granulomatous tissue at the base, with raised erythematous heaped up margins. In immunocompetent hosts, resolution can occur spontaneously, however this may take several weeks. Visceral leishmaniasis (kala azar, black fever) is caused by rapid spread to all organs of the body throughout the reticuloendothelial system. Often seen as a disease of adolescence in endemic countries, characteristic clinical signs and symptoms include organomegaly, fever, severe weight loss, pancytopenia, and hypergammaglobulinemia. Progression to GI involvement leads to severe diarrhea, malabsorption, cachexia, and death. HIV-infected patients are particularly susceptible to severe GI involvement, including hemorrhage.

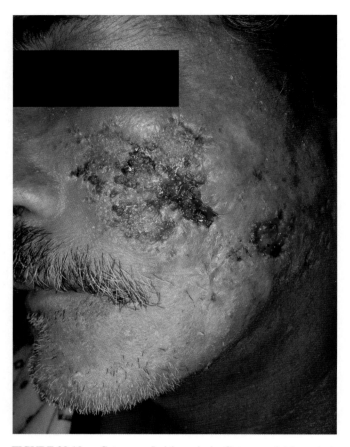

FIGURE 20.19 ■ Cutaneous Leishmaniasis. Cutaneous leishmaniasis involving the face of an HIV-infected patient. (Photo contributors: Seth W. Wright, MD and Universidad Peruana Cayetano Heredia, Lima, Peru.)

Emergency Department Treatment and Disposition

Treatment for the disease is rarely initiated in the emergency department, but close referral to a dermatologist and infectious disease specialist should be arranged. Often the ulcers seen can become superinfected, requiring antibiotic therapy. Many ulcers spontaneously heal, and do not require therapy.

Pearls

1. Maintain a high index of suspicion for this disease, especially in travelers, military personnel, or immigrants.
2. Leishmanial organisms are abundant in skin lesions, and can be demonstrated by stained smears of ulcer scrapings. Advice for treatment is also available through the CDC's Division of Parasitic Diseases.

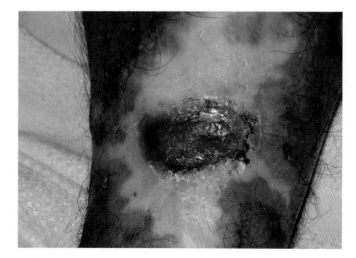

FIGURE 20.20 ■ Cutaneous Leishmaniasis. Recurrent cutaneous leishmaniasis on the same patient's arm. (Photo contributors: Seth W. Wright, MD and Universidad Peruana Cayetano Heredia, Lima, Peru.)

Clinical Summary

Following primary infection with varicella zoster virus, the virus migrates to the dorsal root sensory ganglia where it becomes latent. Reactivation of the virus, known as shingles, is characterized as a painful vesicular eruption in a dermatomal distribution or less commonly, multiple dermatomal distributions. Many patients will experience a prodrome of lancinating pain and hyperalgesias over the skin surface from days to weeks preceding the painful eruptions. Approximately 5% of patients will develop "zoster paresis," characterized by focal motor weakness following the rash.

Dissemination of the virus in HIV patients is common, often leading to meningoencephalitis, retinitis, and pneumonitis. Herpes zoster oticus (Ramsay Hunt syndrome) includes ipsilateral facial paralysis, ear pain, and vesicles in the auricle and auditory canal. Herpes zoster ophthalmicus occurs from the spread of virus from the trigeminal ganglion along the ophthalmic division of the trigeminal nerve, resulting in facial and potentially eye involvement. Cerebral angiitis is a complication of herpes zoster involving the ipsilateral carotid or middle cerebral artery, with subsequent contralateral aphasia or focal deficits.

The diagnosis of herpes zoster in the emergency department is often made clinically, by either recognizing the pain syndrome or visualizing the rash. Immunocompromised patients may demonstrate multidermatomal distribution, or scattered vesicles at a distant site. Approximately 20% of patients will have systemic symptoms such as malaise, fever, headache, or fatigue. Culture, serologic testing, or PCR confirms the diagnosis. A Tzanck test can be obtained by scraping the base of a lesion in an attempt to demonstrate multinucleated giant cells.

Emergency Department Treatment and Disposition

Three antiviral drugs are used to treat herpes zoster infections; acyclovir, famciclovir, and valacyclovir. Patients with disseminated disease, disease in more than one dermatome, or ophthalmic zoster should receive intravenous acyclovir (10-12.5 mg/kg IV q 8 h for 10-14 days). Moreover, treatment of zoster ophthalmicus should include topical antibiotics and an immediate referral to ophthalmologist. For uncomplicated mild cases of herpes zoster, acyclovir (800 mg five times a day for 10 days) or famciclovir (500 mg tid for 7 days) is recommended. Providing treatment of the disease within 72 hours of rash onset will result in a more rapid resolution of cutaneous lesions and decrease viral shedding, but will not change the incidence of postherpetic neuralgia. Immunocompromised patients should not be placed on glucocorticoids. Narcotics, capsaicin cream, and tricyclic antidepressants can be used for pain control.

From a preventive standpoint, the Centers for Disease Control and Prevention (CDC) recommends that immunocompromised patients receive postexposure prophylaxis with varicella zoster immune globulin if they present within 96 hours of exposure. Furthermore, susceptible patients should be vaccinated.

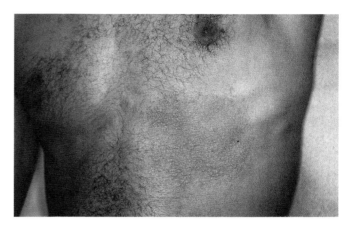

FIGURE 20.21 ■ HZV (Shingles). A painful eruption of many tiny vesicles on an erythematous base in this patient with HIV. (Photo contributor: Jeffery Gibson, MD.)

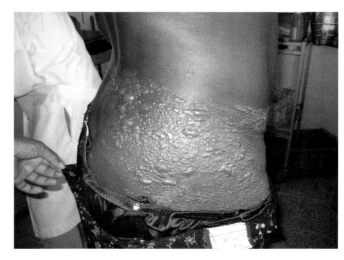

FIGURE 20.22 ■ HZV—Multiple Dermatomes. Severe painful shingles (vesicles and bullae) spanning multiple cutaneous dermatomes in this HIV patient. (Photo contributor: John Omara, MD.)

Pearls

1. Worsening cases of herpes zoster, complicated herpes zoster, or ophthalmic zoster all require intravenous acyclovir and admission.

2. Herpes zoster encephalitis can occur months after the cutaneous phase and can be difficult to diagnose. Common presenting symptoms include mental status changes, headache, fever, photophobia, and vomiting.

3. Ensure follow-up for patients diagnosed with shingles who are less than 50 years old, since they may require workup of a potential underlying immunodeficiency.

4. Proper exposure of the patient on physical examination is essential: examine the skin in patients complaining of chest pain, back pain, or extremity pain to avoid unnecessary work-ups or embarrassing misdiagnoses.

5. The presence of vesicles on the tip of the nose (Hutchinson sign) indicates involvement of the nasociliary branch of cranial nerve V and is associated with a higher risk of ocular involvement.

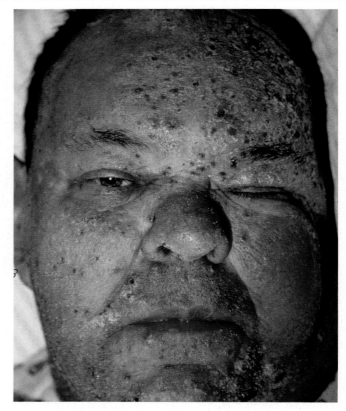

FIGURE 20.23 ▪ Disseminated Herpes Zoster Infection. Vesicles are seen over the entire face, representing disseminated HZV infection (multiple dermatomal distributions). (Photo contributor: the Department of Dermatology, National Naval Medical Center, Bethesda, MD.)

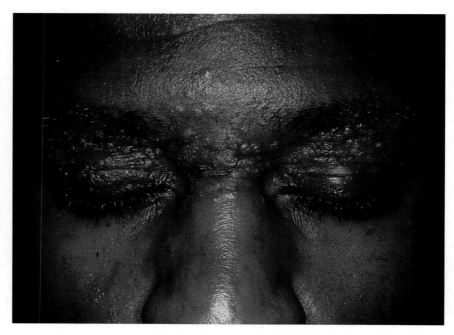

FIGURE 20.24 ▪ Ophthalmic Herpes Zoster. This patient has vesicles in the ophthalmic division of cranial nerve V bilaterally. (Photo contributor: Daniel L. Savitt, MD.)

Clinical Summary

Eosinophilic folliculitis, commonly seen in advanced HIV patients, is a pruritic skin eruption usually involving the face, neck, trunk, and extremities manifesting in the form of pustules and papules. The skin lesions usually start as small pustular groups that later coalesce to create irregular erosions and plaques with central hyperpigmentation. The associated pruritus is often so intense that the lesions become excoriated. Most patients with this condition will demonstrate CD4 cell counts of less than 250/µL. Approximately half of these patients will have moderate eosinophilia and moderate leukocytosis. The etiology of eosinophilic folliculitis is unknown, but is commonly thought of as an inflammatory process associated with immune dysfunction. It has become less common with the advent of highly active antiretroviral therapy.

Emergency Department Treatment and Disposition

The diagnosis requires dermatology consultation and referral for biopsy. Antihistamines, potent topical steroids, itraconazole, topical permethrin, retinoids, metronidazole, dapsone, and ultraviolet B phototherapy have all shown variable levels of efficacy.

Pearls

1. The severe pruritus associated with this condition helps distinguish it from bacterial folliculitis. Symptomatic treatment for pruritus is necessary, and the disease generally improves with improving HIV therapy.
2. Dermatological referral is warranted prior to initiating definitive therapy.
3. Patients with eosinophilic folliculitis may present with prurigo nodularis and lichen simplex chronicus as a result of severe itching and rubbing.

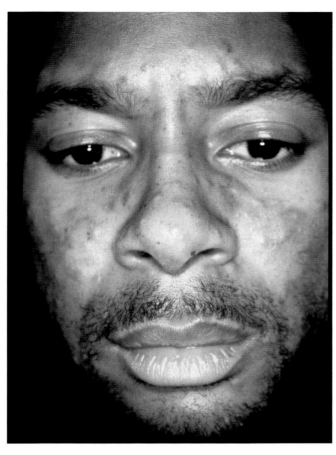

FIGURE 20.25 ■ Eosinophilic Folliculitis. The rash of eosinophilic folliculitis consists of small groups of pustules and vesicles, as seen on the face of this patient. (Photo contributor: the Department of Dermatology, National Naval Medical Center, Bethesda, MD.)

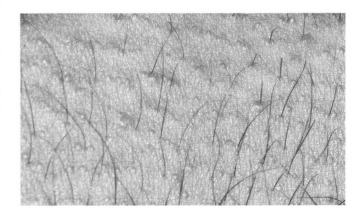

FIGURE 20.26 ■ Eosinophilic Folliculitis. A magnified view showing pustules at the base of each hair follicle. (Photo contributor: the Department of Dermatology, National Naval Medical Center, Bethesda, MD.)

Clinical Summary

As HIV infection progresses and the CD4 cell count declines, herpes simplex virus (HSV) infections become more frequent and severe, with delayed healing and prolonged shedding. There has recently been a dramatic increase in the incidence of genital HSV infections in both men and women, with both HSV-1 and HSV-2 accounting for infections. The lesions can be oral, labial, esophageal, genital, or rectal; lesions tend to be multiple, shallow, vesicular, and painful. Ulcerations are often associated with regional adenopathy. HSV esophagitis is often associated with oral or labial HSV. In contrast to cytomegalovirus (CMV) where there is a large solitary esophageal ulcer, multiple small ulcers characterize HSV esophagitis. Perirectal lesions are often beefy red and extremely tender, with a predilection for the gluteal cleft. Perirectal HSV may also be associated with proctitis and anal fissures.

Ocular HSV may be demonstrated by observing dendritic lesions after fluorescein staining. HSV is associated with a syndrome of acute retinal necrosis characterized by pain, keratitis, and iritis that may lead to retinal detachment. Recurrent herpetic whitlow in HIV patients can be severe, with extensive cutaneous erosions on the fingers. Dissemination can cause encephalitis, aseptic meningitis, transverse myelitis, pneumonitis, hepatitis, and colitis. The diagnosis is usually made clinically but can be confirmed a Tzanck test, biopsy, or culture.

Emergency Department Treatment and Disposition

Acyclovir (200 mg five times a day for 10 days) or famciclovir (500 mg tid for 7 days) are standard treatments. Valacyclovir should be used with caution in patients with HIV since it is associated with TTP. Ocular HSV requires prompt ophthalmology consultation. Severe, refractory, or disseminated HSV is an indication for admission and intravenous acyclovir. Intravenous acyclovir should be used with caution in dehydrated patients because it can crystallize in the renal tubules. For frequent recurrent oral or genital outbreaks, suppressive regimens (acyclovir 600 to 800 mg qid) are indicated.

Pearls

1. Anticipate disseminated disease in HIV patients; presentations of HSV may be atypical compared to HSV in immunocompetent individuals.
2. Suspect HSV in any HIV patient with a poorly healing, painful perirectal lesion.
3. Resistance to acyclovir and cross-resistance to ganciclovir are relatively common. Foscarnet may be considered as an alternative.
4. Genital infection in pregnancy is of particular concern due to the risk of transmission during delivery. If lesions are diagnosed in the pregnant female, close follow-up for treatment and definitive management during the pregnancy is mandatory.
5. Severe dysuria may accompany urogenital HSV lesions. Having the patient urinate sitting in a warm water bath sometimes helps to sooth the intense dysuria. Topical local anesthetics may be used to ease the pain of these mucosal lesions as well.

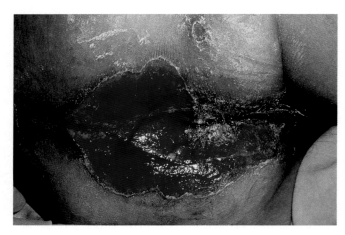

FIGURE 20.27 ■ Herpes Simplex Virus in an HIV Patient. Severe, recurrent perirectal HSV lesions in an HIV patient. (Photo contributor: Briana Hill, MD.)

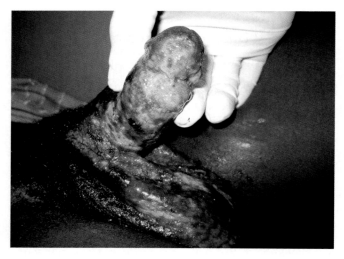

FIGURE 20.28 ■ Severe HSV on Genitalia. Severe ulcerative HSV lesions on the penis and scrotum of an HIV patient. (Photo contributor: John Omara, MD.)

Clinical Summary

Human scabies, caused by the *Sarcoptes scabiei* mite, is one of the most common contagious dermatoses. In HIV patients, this organism can cause "crusted scabies," also known as Norwegian scabies, which denotes an overwhelming scabies infestation. In typical scabies, the mites cause extremely pruritic burrows, vesicles, and papules in a characteristic distribution involving the finger webs, sides of the hands and feet, breasts, waist, and groin. Pruritus is most intense at night. In contrast, crusted scabies typically affects the hands and the feet with asymptomatic crusting. Norwegian scabies typically does not cause significant pruritus. Typical scabies involves approximately 15 mites per infected individual, whereas Norwegian scabies involves a hyperinfestation with thousands to millions of mites per individual. Scabies is spread by direct physical contact including sexual contact, and can occur in epidemic form. Transmission is common from mother to infant. Transmission through infected linens or clothing is common in cases of Norwegian scabies. Risk factors include poor hygiene, crowding, and exposure to pets.

Most often the diagnosis of scabies is made clinically, with evidence of burrows and severe pruritus in a characteristic distribution. Definitive diagnosis is made from examination of shavings from the lesions. Placing mineral oil over a suspected lesion and then shaving it with a number 15 blade can demonstrate the mites, which are usually 0.3 to 0.4 mm in length. Sometimes eggs, egg casings, or feces can be seen. Norwegian scabies is diagnosed similarly, with demonstration of the mites on a mineral oil or potassium hydroxide microscopic examination.

Emergency Department Treatment and Disposition

Topical Permethrin 5% cream has a low toxicity and is the treatment of choice for scabies. Patients are instructed to apply the cream from the neck down and leave it on for 8 to 14 hours before removal. One application is usually sufficient for treatment in nonimmunocompromised patients. The patient's clothes and bedding should be washed in hot water. Antihistamines should be prescribed to alleviate the pruritus. Often the pruritus persists after treatment as a hypersensitivity to the mites and their feces and eggs. Any complicating secondary skin infection should be treated with appropriate systemic antibiotics. Localized infections can be treated with topical steroids.

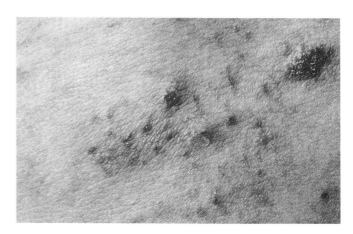

FIGURE 20.29 ■ Scabies. Typical scabies rash showing unroofed papules secondary to scratching. Several small burrows are also seen. (Photo contributor: George Turiansky, MD.)

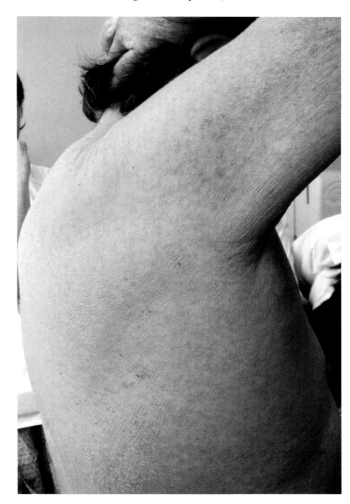

FIGURE 20.30 ■ Norwegian Scabies. Overwhelming scabies infestation causing "crusted scabies" in this patient with HIV. Hyperinfestations involve thousands to millions of mites. (Photo contributor: Francisco Bravo Puccio, MD, With Permission: The Gorgas Course in Clinical Tropical Medicine, Universidad Peruana Cayetano Heredia, Lima, Peru.)

For HIV patients with Norwegian scabies, permethrin should be applied to the face, scalp, behind the ears, and from the neck downward. Repeat treatments may be needed. For severe or refractory cases, oral ivermectin (200 mg/kg for one dose) can be tried with the exception of pregnant or lactating women.

Pearls

1. Often secondary staphylococcal infections complicate the diagnosis, including impetigo, ecthyma, paronychia and furunculosis.

2. Oral antibiotics are often indicated for Norwegian scabies because of skin breakdown.

3. Close contacts of infected patients should be treated simultaneously. Inform patients that although the scabicide will kill the mites, itching may last for weeks. Patients often seek repeat treatments and inappropriately receive additional scabicides, which can cause contact dermatitis.

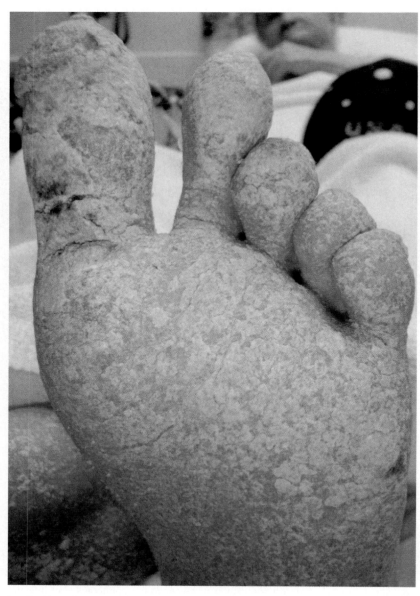

FIGURE 20.31 ■ Norwegian Scabies. Crusted lesions with hyperkeratotic scales on this patient's foot. Millions of mites were seen under microscopy in scrapings of the lesions. (Photo contributor: Larry Mellick, MD.)

Clinical Summary

Molluscum contagiosum is a poxvirus that causes flesh-colored, dome-shaped lesions on affected individuals. Usually molluscum contagiosum is an asymptomatic benign disease, but may become severe in HIV patients. Typical presentations consist of groups of 2 to 20 small, discrete, shiny lesions with central umbilication. Lesions can become generalized, as direct skin-to-skin transmission is common. Commonly infected regions include the crural folds, trunk, axilla, and genitals, with sparing of the palms and soles. The incubation period for the virus ranges from 2 weeks to 6 months.

Emergency Department Treatment and Disposition

If the diagnosis is suspected in the emergency department, the patient should be reassured and referred to a dermatologist. Usually self-limited with spontaneous remission, treatment outside of genital lesions is for cosmetic reasons only.

Pearl

1. Clinically, it may be difficult to distinguish between cutaneous *Cryptococcus* and molluscum contagiosum. Dermatology or infectious disease consultation and biopsy may be required.

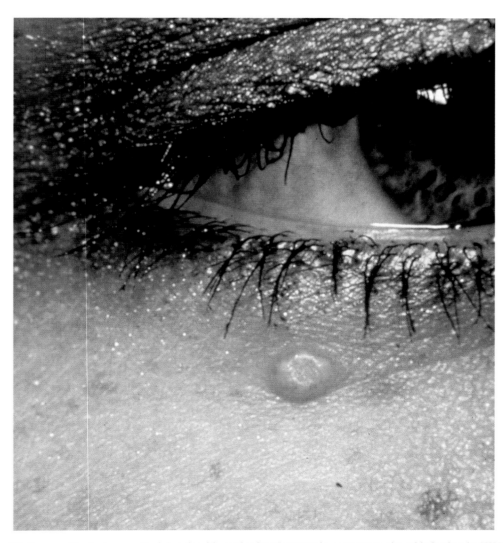

FIGURE 20.32 ■ Molluscum Contagiosum. Facial rash with ocular involvement is a common site of infection in HIV patients. Note the central umbilication. (Photo contributor: the Department of Dermatology, National Naval Medical Center, Bethesda, MD.)

Clinical Summary

Dermatophyte infections are common superficial fungal infections involving the scalp (tinea capitis), body (tinea corporis), feet (tinea pedis), crural fold (tinea cruris), and nails (onychomycosis). Infection is very common in healthy individuals, but can be varied and atypical in patients with HIV. HIV patients also can demonstrate a much more severe and extensive form of disease. Three different dermatophytes are the usual source of infection: epidermophyton, trichophyton, and microsporum.

Tinea capitis is seen as an enlarging scaling patch on the scalp that may progress to a kerion. The initial lesion can be overlooked until alopecia is present. Untreated permanent scarring can occur. Tinea pedis is the most common dermatophyte infection seen in practice. Usually self-limited, intermittent, recurrent, and intensely pruritic, these lesions can often be secondarily infected due to mechanical irritation. Tinea corporis is the most common fungal infection seen in HIV patients. Usually it begins as an intensely pruritic, oval scaling erythematous lesion that spreads centrifugally and can merge with other lesions. Tinea cruris is an infection involving the crural fold, much more common in men then women. It usually begins as a macular patch on the inner thigh, opposite the scrotal sac.

Emergency Department Treatment and Disposition

Tinea capitis responds to griseofulvin; however other oral agents that can be effective include terbinafine, itraconazole, or fluconazole. Treatment usually is carried out for at least 3 weeks, with topical treatments ineffective. Tinea pedis can usually be treated with a topical antifungal cream for 4 weeks. Often patients have tried outpatient, over-the-counter antifungal medications without success. Extensive treatment can be initiated with griseofulvin, terbinafine, or itraconazole orally. Tinea corporis often responds to daily application of topical antifungal medications, however systemic oral agents described above are also effective. Tinea cruris usually responds to topical antifungal medications.

Pearls

1. Confirming the diagnosis with a KOH preparation is important before initiating therapy, especially in diffuse disease. Often HIV patients suffer from a variety of skin infections that mimic dermatophyte lesions (eczema).
2. Athletes are especially at risk when close skin-to-skin contact occurs (wrestling, football). Oral treatment in these cases is preferred, with restriction in sports for 2 weeks or until lesions heal.

3. Some Dermatophyte infections fluoresce under the Wood lamp examination.

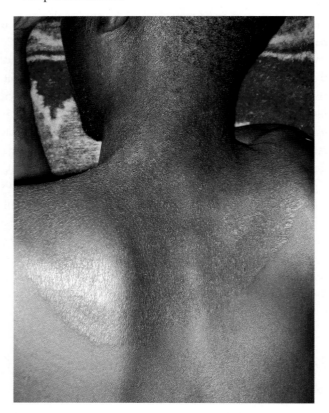

FIGURE 20.33 ■ Tinea Infection. Tinea infection involving the scalp, neck, and upper back of this HIV-infected patient. (Photo contributor: Seth W. Wright, MD.)

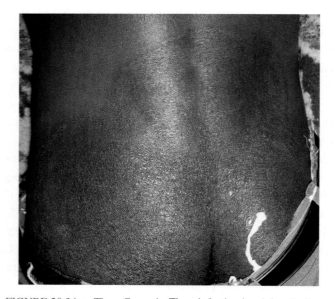

FIGURE 20.34 ■ Tinea Corporis. Tinea infection involving the lower back and buttocks of the patient in Fig. 20.33. (Photo contributor: Seth W. Wright, MD.)

Clinical Summary

Pneumocystis jirovecii (formerly *carinii*) pneumonia (PCP) is the most common opportunistic infection in HIV-infected patients. Clinical suspicion for PCP pneumonia in any HIV patient presenting with complaints of dyspnea and nonproductive cough should remain high. Presentations can be indolent, acute, or subacute, with associated symptoms including fever, fatigue, anorexia, weight loss, and chest pain. The CBC is usually normal except for lymphopenia, while serum LDH is often elevated. Arterial blood gases most often reveal a respiratory alkalosis, Po_2 of 70 mm Hg or less, and an increased A-a gradient of 35 mm Hg or more. Radiographic chest findings are variable with diffuse interstitial alveolar infiltrates being common. Patients who develop respiratory failure should be treated with mechanical ventilatory support. Patients who develop PCP pneumonia are at higher risk for pneumothorax, both spontaneously and associated with mechanical ventilation. There is evidence that PCP pneumonia is transmitted via person-to-person, thus respiratory isolation is warranted.

Emergency Department Treatment and Disposition

Management of patients with PCP pneumonia is complex and starts with meticulous supportive care. The initial treatment regimen is based on a number of factors, including prior PCP suppressive therapy, efficacy of treatment, patient tolerability to the treatment, severity of disease, toxicity of treatment, allergies, and drug–drug interactions. The timing of initiation of highly active antiretroviral therapy (HAART) in patients who are not already on these medications is controversial. Patients generally will improve after initiation of HAART therapy; however potential risks include immune reconstruction illness and drug–drug interactions. Trimethoprim-sulfamethoxazole, orally or intravenously, is generally the first-line standard treatment. Pentamidine, clindamycin-primaquine, trimetrexate-leucovorin, atovaquone, and trimethoprim-dapsone are also effective. Treatment with corticosteroids should be initiated if the Po_2 is less than 70 or the A-a gradient is greater than 35. Since patients will often worsen after 48 to 72 hours after diagnosis, hospitalization for moderate to severe illness is warranted. The CDC recommends prophylaxis against *P jirovecii* in patients with a history of PCP pneumonia, CD4 cell counts less than 200/μL, or a history of oropharyngeal candidiasis.

Pearls

1. Include PCP in the differential diagnosis of any HIV patient who presents with a persistent fever or respiratory complaint.
2. Patient with mild to moderate disease should have oxygen saturation measurements at rest and ambulation. If hypoxic or tachypneic, an ABG should be performed to determine the need for initiation of corticosteroid therapy.
3. Maintain a low threshold for admitting moderately ill patients, patients who require corticosteroid therapy, or patients who cannot readily obtain close outpatient follow-up.

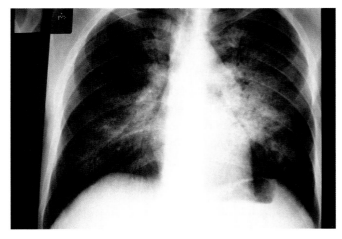

FIGURE 20.35 ■ *Pneumocystis jirovecii* Pneumonia (PCP). Chest radiograph showing diffuse interstitial alveolar infiltrates of PCP. (Photo contributor: Edward C. Oldfield III, MD.)

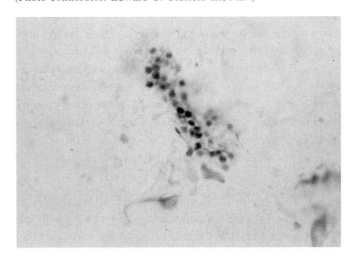

FIGURE 20.36 ■ PCP on Silver Stain. *Pneumocystis jirovecii* seen on methenamine-silver stain of a bronchoalveolar lavage sample from an HIV patient with PCP. (Photo contributor: Lawrence B. Stack, MD.)

Clinical Summary

Thrombocytopenia occurs in 40% to 70% of all HIV patients. It can occur independently at all stages of HIV infection and may be encountered as the initial presentation of disease. HIV-associated anemia and granulocytopenia can occur concomitantly as course of the HIV infection worsens, with thrombocytopenia seen in 30% of patients with CD4 counts less than 200/μL. HIV patients with thrombocytopenia often present to the emergency department with bleeding (especially from the oral mucosa), ecchymosis, and petechiae. Secondary causes of thrombocytopenia are generally seen as the result of opportunistic infections, malignancy, or medications.

Emergency Department Treatment and Disposition

The emergency physician's efforts are initially focused on stabilization of the patient with two large intravenous lines, type and cross-match, and crystalloid infusion if significant bleeding has occurred. Because of the complexity of the differential diagnosis and potentially complicated treatment of HIV thrombocytopenia, an infectious disease specialist should be consulted early. In most cases, HIV patients with platelet count greater than 50,000 can be managed conservatively with spontaneous remission of approximately 20%. Zidovudine can increase platelet counts up to two-fold in over 50% of patients. If the platelet count is less than 20,000, many infectious disease specialists recommend γ-globulin infusion and parenteral steroids. Other possible treatments include dapsone, danazol, interferon-α vincristine, anti-D immunoglobulin, splenic irradiation, and splenectomy. Even if the patient is to be managed conservatively, bone marrow analysis should be performed to rule out other causes of thrombocytopenia.

Pearls

1. Perform thorough skin and oral examinations in all patients with HIV looking for manifestations of thrombocytopenia.
2. Take a careful drug history and consider other infectious etiologies before assuming the thrombocytopenia is directly secondary to HIV infection.
3. Spontaneous bleeding is rare unless the platelet count is less than 10,000.

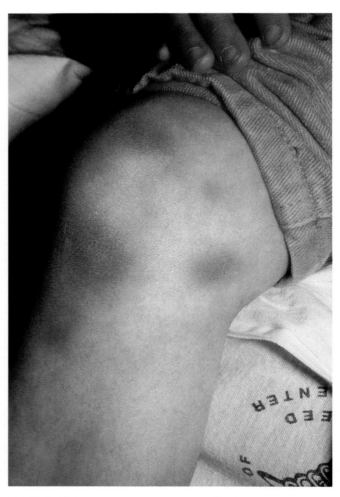

FIGURE 20.37 ■ Thrombocytopenia. Ecchymosis in an HIV patient with thrombocytopenia. (Photo contributor: Edward C. Oldfield III, MD.)

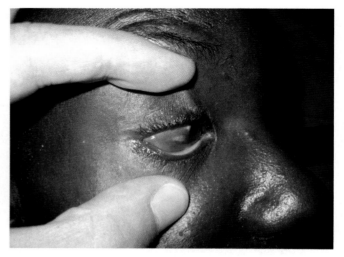

FIGURE 20.38 ■ HIV-Associated Thrombocytopenia. A large spontaneous subconjunctival hemorrhage is noted in this patient with HIV. (Photo contributor: John Omara, MD.)

Clinical Summary

HIV patients have a 5 to 20 times higher rate of drug reactions than non-HIV patients. Up to 5% of emergency department visits by HIV patients are due to complications of therapy. Many of these manifest dermatologically, in order of decreasing frequency: (1) exanthems, (2) urticaria/angioedema, (3) fixed drug reactions, (4) erythema multiforme, and (5) photosensitivity reactions. The most common medications associated with rashes are antivirals, antibiotics, and antifungals.

Emergency Department Treatment and Disposition

The emergency physician may need to consult an infectious disease specialist, a pharmacist, or a dermatologist to help clarify the existence of a drug reaction. Clues besides recent initiation of a new drug are eosinophilia greater than 1000 or elevated liver function tests. Individual treatment varies depending on the situation. The offending agent should be discontinued. Antihistamines and steroids are indicated in certain situations.

Pearls

1. Ask about alternative and nonprescription medicines.
2. Half of all HIV patients will react adversely to sulfa drugs.
3. Beware of serious drug reactions such as Stevens-Johnson syndrome and toxic epidermal necrolysis (TEN).

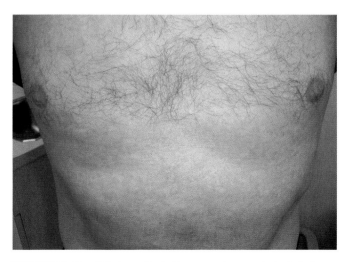

FIGURE 20.40 ■ Efavirenz Rash. Drug exanthem typical of efavirenz. (Photo contributor: Stephen Burdette, MD.)

FIGURE 20.41 ■ Efavirenz Rash. Close-up image of drug exanthem caused by efavirenz in an HIV patient. (Photo contributor: Stephen Burdette, MD).

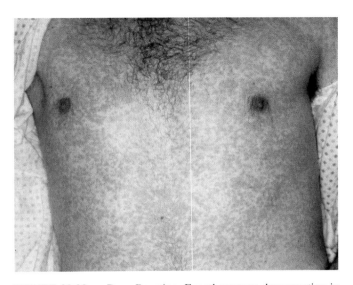

FIGURE 20.39 ■ Drug Reaction. Exanthematous drug reaction in an HIV patient. (Photo contributor: Kenneth Skahan, MD.)

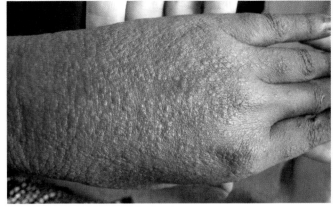

FIGURE 20.42 ■ Nevirapine Rash. Drug exanthema caused by Nevirapine in this HIV patient. (Photo contributor: Seth W. Wright, MD.)

Clinical Summary

Acute necrotizing ulcerative gingivitis (ANUG), also known as Vincent angina or trench mouth, is commonly seen in HIV patients. It is a distinct and rapidly progressive ulceration typically starting at the tip of the interdental papilla, spreading along the gingival margins, eventually destroying the periodontal tissue. The triad associated with ANUG is oral pain, halitosis, and ulcerations. Other signs and symptoms include "metallic taste," "wooden teeth" sensation, tooth mobility, fever, adenopathy, and malnutrition. The cause of this aggressive, destructive process in HIV patients is a polymicrobial infection by oral anaerobes (*Treponema, Selenomonas, Fusobacterium, Porphyromonas, Prevotella*). ANUG represents a spectrum of disease from mild ulcerations to severe cellulitis and spread of the infection to the soft tissues, cheeks, lips, and bones.

Emergency Department Treatment and Disposition

ANUG is most frequently seen in four population groups: (1) HIV patients, (2) malnourished children, (3) young adults who are under a great deal of stress, and (4) polysubstance abusers. The first steps for the emergency physician are to eliminate other potentially more serious life-threatening infections and to address hydration status. Treatment includes (1) eliminating contributing factors (stress, poor nutrition, poor sleep, alcohol, and tobacco use), (2) chlorhexidine rinses twice a day, (3) surgical debridement by an oral surgeon if needed, and (4) oral penicillin and metronidazole.

Pearls

1. Beware Ludwig angina (brawny submandibular induration and tongue elevation) associated with severe progression of ANUG as acute airway compromise is possible.
2. Noma (cancrum oris, gangrenous stomatitis), a rare disease of childhood associated with malnutrition, is characterized by an anaerobic destructive infectious process of the orofacial tissues that can clinically resemble ANUG.

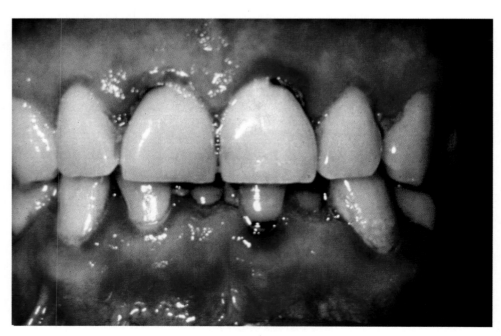

FIGURE 20.43 ■ Acute Necrotizing Ulcerative Gingivitis (ANUG). ANUG (Vincent angina or "trench mouth") caused by spirochetal and fusiform bacteria in an HIV patient. Note the punched-out ulcerations of the interdental papillae, which are pathognomonic. (Photo contributor: the Department of Dermatology, National Naval Medical Center, Bethesda, MD.)

Chapter 21

TROPICAL MEDICINE

Seth W. Wright
Meg Jack

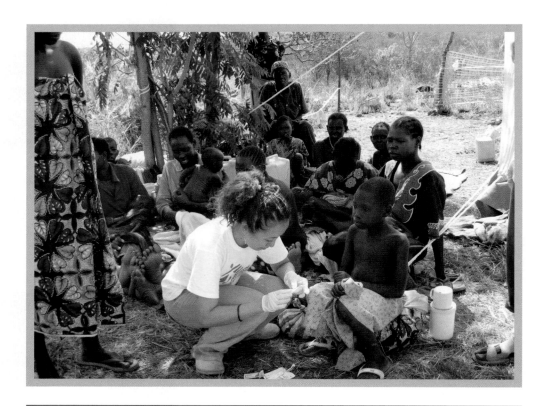

Clinical Summary

Free-living ameba, usually harmless residents of soil and water, can occasionally cause devastating illness in humans. There are three distinct human illnesses caused by these protozoa. Primary amebic meningoencephalitis (PAM) is a disease of previously healthy individuals and is caused by *Naegleria fowleri*. Granulomatous amebic encephalitis (GAE) is caused by *Acanthamoeba* species and *Balamuthia mandrillaris* and occurs in both healthy and immunocompromised persons. PAM and GAE are found worldwide but are more common in tropical regions. *Acanthamoeba* also causes chronic amebic keratitis, which is related to contact lens use and is thus a disease primarily of wealthier countries.

PAM is a devastating illness that is usually fatal and often occurs in children with a history of recent fresh-water exposure. The organism enters through the nose of the victim and penetrates the cribriform plate to the subarachnoid space and brain. Patients present with an acute illness that is indistinguishable from bacterial meningitis. Patients with GAE often present with an initial focus of infection in the skin or respiratory tract followed by neurologic changes reflective of extensive brain involvement. Amebic keratitis from *Acanthamoeba* has been increasingly recognized in recent years and is typically a result of contaminated contact lens saline solutions.

Emergency Department Treatment and Disposition

The mainstay of management is consideration of these uncommon diseases in emergency department patients. PAM is almost always fatal but one survivor was successfully treated with amphotericin B, miconazole, and rifampin. Isolated cutaneous disease from *Acanthamoeba* and *B mandrillaris* has been cured, but brain involvement is fatal and usually diagnosed at autopsy. Patients with suspected amebic keratitis should have immediate ophthalmologic referral.

Pearls

1. Lack of response to usual antimicrobials in a patient with severe meningitis symptoms should lead to the suspicion of PAM, particularly with recent fresh-water exposure.
2. It is thought that global warming might increase the rate of *N fowleri* infection as the organism thrives in water over 30°C.

3. Consider *Acanthamoeba* infection in all contact lens wearers with a corneal infection.
4. Early amebic keratitis can mimic the dendritic pattern of herpes simplex infection.

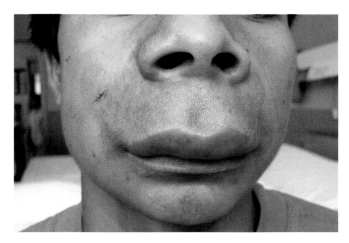

FIGURE 21.1 ■ Ameba. Twenty-one year old patient from South America with 1 year of symptoms from *Balamuthia mandrillaris*. The primary site often involves the mid-face and oral cavity. This patient did not have intracranial involvement. (Photo contributors: Seth W. Wright, MD and Universidad Peruana Cayetano Heredia, Lima, Peru.)

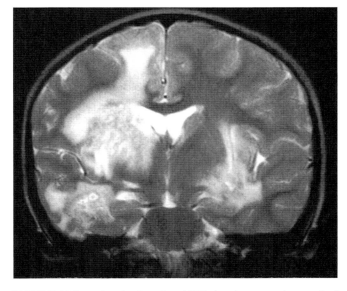

FIGURE 21.2 ■ Ameba Imaging. MRI showing extensive cerebral involvement in a fatal case of *Balamuthia mandrillaris*. (Photo contributors: Rob Greidanus, MD and Universidad Peruana Cayetano Heredia, Lima, Peru.)

Clinical Summary

Anemia in the tropics is a common consequence of various nutritional deficiencies, infections, parasites, genetic disorders, or chronic diseases. The prevalence and causes of anemia in tropical countries differs significantly from developed countries. Greater than 50% of young children and pregnant women in Africa and South Asia are anemic.

Deficiencies of iron, folic acid, and vitamin B_{12} from consumption of carbohydrate-rich staple diets and poor meat consumption are a common cause of anemia. Hookworm infection is a common cause of anemia, particularly in children and pregnant women. Malaria causes hemolysis and hypersplenism and should always be considered in anemic patients. Other parasitic illnesses causing anemia include visceral leishmaniasis (kala-azar) and African trypanosomiasis (sleeping sickness). Hemoglobinopathies, including sickle cell anemia and thalassemia, are common in Africa, the Middle East, and South Asia. Severe hemolytic anemia can result in patients with G6PD deficiency. Anemia of chronic disease, particularly from HIV/AIDS and tuberculosis, is common.

Emergency Department Treatment and Disposition

Treatment depends on the suspected cause(s) of the anemia. A low threshold for malaria treatment is important, particularly in children and pregnant women. Empiric treatment for hookworm is usually advisable. Iron and folate supplementation can lead to a dramatic increase in red cell counts in patients with nutritional deficiencies. Red blood cell transfusion is rarely needed in stable patients, even those with extremely low counts.

Pearls

1. Both sickle cell trait and G6PD deficiency may be protective against malaria and are common in tropical regions.
2. Administration of the antimalarial agent primaquine to patients with G6PD deficiency can lead to fatal hemolysis.
3. Thrombocytopenia in conjunction with anemia is highly suggestive of malaria in endemic areas.
4. Anemia in pregnancy should be screened for and aggressively treated as this improves both maternal and fetal outcomes.

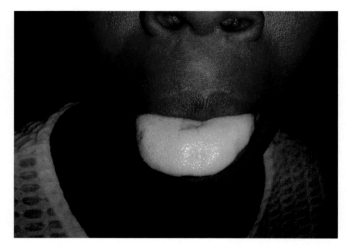

FIGURE 21.4 ■ Anemia. Pale tongue in a severely anemic Haitian woman. Pale mucus membranes, palms, and soles are often good indicators of anemia, particularly in dark skinned individuals. (Photo contributor: Andreas Fischer, RN.)

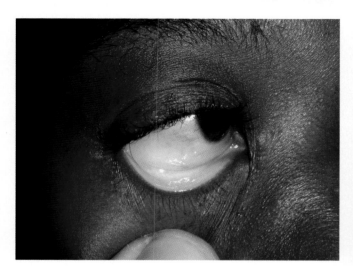

FIGURE 21.3 ■ Anemia. Conjunctival pallor in a Haitian woman with complaints of weakness (Hgb = 2.2). (Photo contributor: Andreas Fischer, RN.)

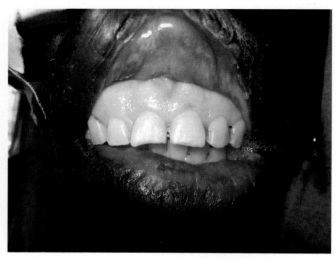

FIGURE 21.5 ■ Anemia in AIDS. Gums of Ugandan patient with end-stage AIDS and Hgb of 3.0. (Photo contributor: Seth W. Wright, MD.)

Clinical Summary

Cholera is a severe diarrheal disease caused by *Vibrio cholerae*, a gram-negative bacterium. It is spread via the fecal-oral route and is seen in areas of poor hygiene and overcrowding. Contamination of food and water are principle modes of infection. Endemic disease is present in many areas of the world with occasional epidemics. Incidence of disease decreases with age.

Cholera is characterized by massive, watery, gray, and painless diarrhea. The stool resembles "rice water" without blood or pus. Patients may have associated vomiting. Anuria, renal failure, hypotension, and circulatory collapse can occur within hours of diarrhea onset. Mortality rates as high as 20% to 50% among severe cases can be seen if adequate rehydration is not available. Death rates of less than 2% are seen with good case management.

Emergency Department Treatment and Disposition

The mainstay of treatment is adequate hydration. Oral rehydration solutions are adequate for mild and moderate dehydration. Patients with severe dehydration are treated with IV lactated Ringer solution and oral rehydration. Adult patients may require 10 to 15 L in the first 24 hours. Monitoring of electrolytes and renal function is ideal, but often not available in areas struck by cholera epidemics. Hypokalemia is common. Antibiotics are not required for recovery as the illness is self-limiting, but doxycycline may reduce the volume of diarrhea and shorten the duration of illness.

Pearls

1. Cholera is one of only three diseases, along with plague and yellow fever, that are internationally notifiable to the World Health Organization.
2. John Snow's removal of the Broad Street water pump handle during the 1854 cholera epidemic in London is considered to be the beginning of modern field epidemiology.
3. People with blood group O are nine times as likely to develop life-threatening symptoms.
4. Rapid cholera test kits are available and are essential for early confirmation of disease in the first suspected cases.

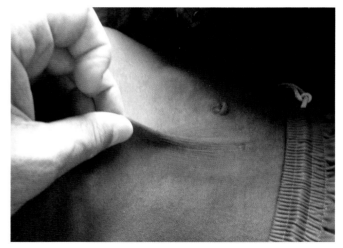

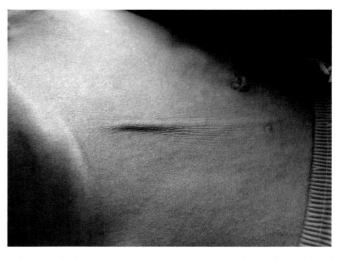

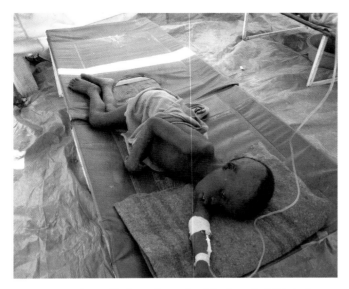

FIGURE 21.6 ■ Cholera. Severely dehydrated child during an outbreak in Uganda. Lethargy and sunken eyes are typical findings. IV fluids are typically reserved for severe cases. The child is on a typical cholera cot. (Photo contributor: Seth W. Wright, MD.)

FIGURES 21.7 ■ Dehydration in Cholera. "Tenting" of the skin of a dehydrated cholera patient. The presence of tenting implies moderate to severe dehydration. (Photo contributor: Seth W. Wright, MD.)

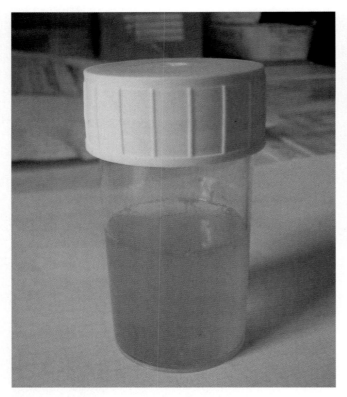

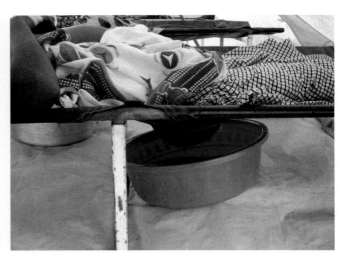

FIGURE 21.9 ■ Cholera Cot. Patient on cholera cot. Use of the cholera cot allows for monitoring of fluid output and allows for easier waste control in patients too weak to leave the bed. (Photo contributor: Seth W. Wright, MD.)

FIGURE 21.8 ■ Rice Water Stool. Typical "rice water" stool from cholera patient. Patients with cholera often lose a liter or more of watery stool an hour. (Photo contributor: Seth W. Wright, MD.)

Clinical Summary

Ascaris lumbricoides is the most common roundworm infection in humans endemic where sanitation is poor. Adult worms live in the small intestine and produce enormous numbers of eggs, which are excreted in the feces but are not immediately infectious as they require 3 to 8 weeks in soil to mature into an infective second-stage larval form. Ingested eggs hatch in the jejunum, and migrate through the intestinal wall into the bloodstream and are transported to the lungs. Larval worms burrow through the alveolar walls, pass through the trachea, and are swallowed back into the small intestine where they develop into adults.

Most infections are asymptomatic. Patients may present for care if they pass a worm in their stool. A heavy worm burden may lead to abdominal pain or intestinal obstruction. Failure to thrive and decreased cognitive development are seen in heavily infected children. Migrating worms may cause biliary obstruction, appendicitis, or liver abscesses.

Diagnosis is from identification of a passed worm or examination of stool for the eggs.

Emergency Department Treatment and Disposition

Outpatient treatment with mebendazole or albendazole is usually effective but only on the adult intestinal stage worm. Thus, it is recommended that a stool examination be done at 2 to 3 months and re-treatment initiated if positive for eggs.

Pearls

1. Marked peripheral eosinophilia can be seen during the migratory stage.
2. While in the lungs, migrating worms can cause a temporary eosinophilic pneumonitis, known as "Löffler's syndrome," which presents with asthma-like symptoms.
3. Vegetables grown in areas of poor hygiene should be thoroughly cooked or soaked in a solution of diluted iodine.
4. Infection is not spread directly from person to person as the eggs transmitted in stool need to mature in soil.

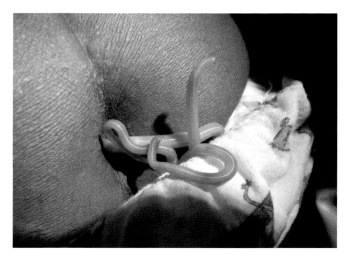

FIGURE 21.10 ■ Ascariasis. Worms spontaneously extruding from the anus of a boy with a high fever. Worms often migrate in patients with fever. (Photo contributor: Seth W. Wright, MD.)

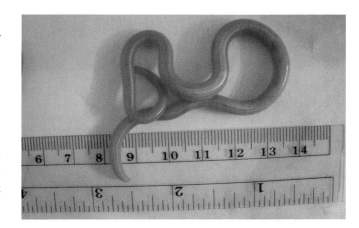

FIGURE 21.11 ■ Ascariasis. Adult ascaris worm after passage from the anus. (Photo contributor: Seth W. Wright, MD.)

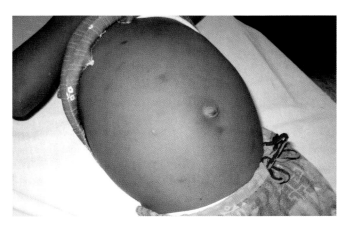

FIGURE 21.12 ■ Ascariasis. Distended abdomen of Haitian girl with a large ascaris worm burden. (Photo contributor: Seth W. Wright, MD.)

Clinical Summary

Cutaneous larva migrans (CLM), also known as "creeping eruption," is the most common dermatologic problem seen in travelers following a trip to the tropics. CLM is a parasitic infection that occurs worldwide but is most commonly seen in warm, tropical environments and is particularly common following beach vacations. While CLM also occurs in the United States, most commonly in the Southeast, it is now relatively uncommon due to shoe wearing habits and routine deworming of dogs and cats.

CLM is most commonly caused by dog and cat hookworms, *Ancylostoma caninum* and *A braziliense*, with humans being an accidental host. The infected animal passes eggs in its feces where they hatch, molt, and feed on bacteria in the soil. In the usual animal host, the larvae will penetrate the dermis and migrate through the lungs before reaching the intestines where they mature into adults. However, upon accidental contact with a human host, the larval worm penetrates the skin and attempts dermal migration. The worm remains under the skin since it lacks collagenase and cannot penetrate deeper layers. The larvae are unable to complete their life cycle, and, if left untreated, are trapped in the epidermis and will die in 2 to 8 weeks.

CLM is commonly seen on the lower extremities of travelers who walk barefoot on beaches with contaminated sandy soil. Symptoms are manifested by an erythematous tract with a distinctive serpiginous pattern. The tract is markedly pruritic and may feel like a thread on palpation.

Emergency Department Treatment and Disposition

Treatment consists of mebendazole, albendazole, or topical application of thiabendazole. Antipruritics may help symptoms.

Pearls

1. The lesions advance a few millimeters to several centimeters daily as the larva migrates.
2. Excoriation and secondary infections frequently occur. This can make the distinctive wandering rash more difficult to visualize.
3. Biopsy of the lesions is often not helpful for diagnosis since the organism lies 1 to 2 cm away from the leading edge of the eruption.

4. Gnathostomiasis, obtained after eating a larval worm in undercooked or raw fish, can cause a similar syndrome. The skin finding is often on the anterior abdominal wall and may be associated with significant peripheral eosinophilia.

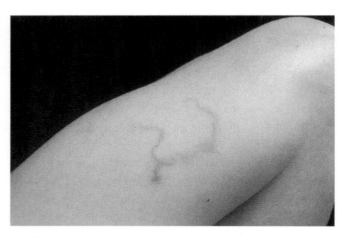

FIGURE 21.13 ■ Cutaneous Larva Migrans. A serpiginous, linear, raise, tunnel-like erythematous lesion outlining the path of migration in the larva. Upon palpation, it feels like a thread within the superficial layers of the skin. (Reproduced, with permission, from Wolff K, Johnson RA, Suurmond D. *Fitzpatrick's Color Atlas & Synopsis of Clinical Dermatology*. 5th ed. New York, McGraw-Hill, 2005; p 863.)

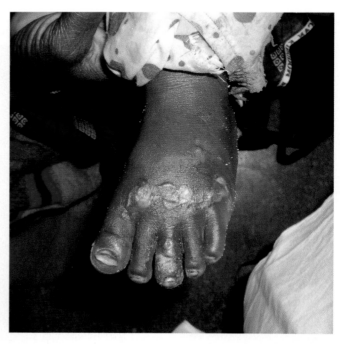

FIGURE 21.14 ■ Cutaneous Larva Migrans. CLM with secondary infection on the foot of a toddler from Zambia. (Photo contributor: Meg Jack, MD.)

Clinical Summary

Cysticercosis is caused by the dissemination of the larval form of the pork tapeworm *Taenia solium*. It affects 50 million people worldwide with increasing incidence in the United States, largely due to immigration and increased travel. Two distinct types of diseases exist, taeniasis (intestinal tapeworm) and cysticercosis, with occurrence depending on the stage the parasite was ingested. Taeniasis is acquired from ingesting cysts from infected, undercooked pork which develop into an adult tapeworm in the intestines. Eggs passed in the stool are highly infectious and may survive in the environment for months. People with an intestinal tapeworm can infect themselves with cysticercosis (anus-hand-mouth route) or it is attained from unhygienic food preparation. Once the eggs are ingested, they hatch, penetrate the bowel wall, and travel to the subcutaneous tissue, skeletal muscle, and brain though they may involve any organ. Symptoms are dependent on the area involved with significant morbidity associated with ocular, cardiac, and neurologic involvement. They will eventually die and leave calcified lesions.

Intestinal taeniasis is diagnosed through identification of the eggs through stool samples or by passage of an intact worm or worm segments. CT and MRI have facilitated recognition of neurocysticercosis with visualization of a contrast-enhancing ring lesion. Diagnosis may also be made by biopsy, serum, or CSF antibody testing. Neurocysticercosis should be strongly considered in endemic regions or in immigrants with new onset seizures. Symptoms generally occur when the cysts are dying due to swelling and inflammation.

Emergency Department Treatment and Disposition

Seizures are treated with standard medications. Calcified lesions do not require specific anticysticercal therapy. Viable cysts can be treated with albendazole or praziquantel, but should be done with expert consultation. Inpatient management is advisable if viable cysts are to be treated as inflammatory reactions may occur. Corticosteroids are recommended in this situation. Surgical intervention may be indicated for obstructing neurologic lesions or intraocular lesions.

Pearls

1. Infection is most common in rural, developing countries where pigs are allowed to roam freely with ingestion of infected human feces. This completes the cycle and propagates infection.

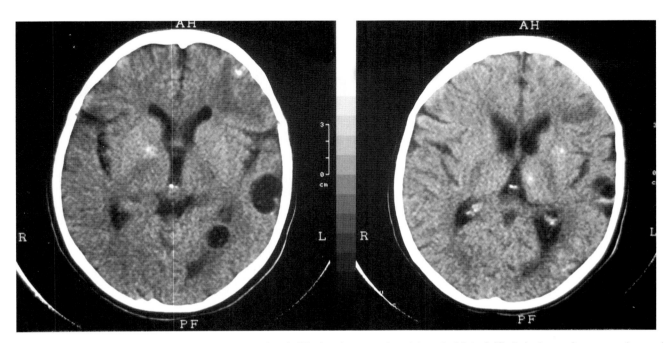

FIGURE 21.15 ■ Neurocysticercosis. Noncontrast head CT showing new (cystic) and old (calcified) lesions of neurocysticercosis. (Photo contributors: Seth W. Wright, MD and Universidad Peruana Cayetano Heredia, Lima, Peru.)

2. Cysticercosis and taeniasis are rare in Muslim countries where eating pork is forbidden; however, cysticercosis is still possible due to ingestion of infected food products.

3. The adult tapeworm can attain a length of 20 ft or more and can live up to 20 years in the intestine.

4. Most people with an intestinal pork tapeworm do not have cysticercosis.

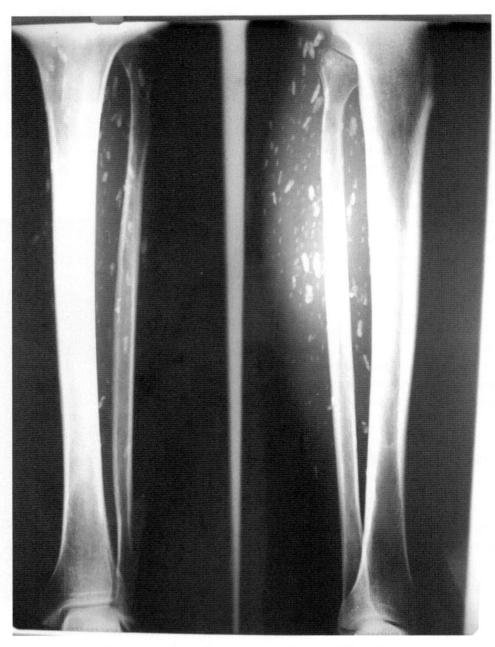

FIGURE 21.16 ■ Cysticercosis Cysts. Multiple calcified soft tissue cysts noted as an incidental finding on a lower leg radiograph in a patient with disseminated cysticercosis. (Photo contributors: Seth W. Wright, MD and Universidad Peruana Cayetano Heredia, Lima, Peru.)

Clinical Summary

Dengue fever, also known as "breakbone fever," is the most important mosquito-borne viral disease. Dengue is a rapidly emerging illness due to reintroduction of *Aedes* species mosquitoes into areas of previous eradication. It is now distributed throughout tropical and subtropical regions and widespread epidemics have occurred in the Caribbean and Southeast Asia, among other regions of the world. Dengue is one of the most common causes of fever in returned travelers.

The incubation period is usually 3 to 7 days with resolution of symptoms within 10 days. Clinical infection ranges from subclinical symptoms to a hemorrhagic state leading to shock. Most commonly, it is characterized by fever, severe myalgias, retro-orbital pain, and headache. The fever is often bimodal. A rash, seen in approximately 50% of cases, is usually maculopapular but may be mottled, flushed, or petechial. The disease can be graded from I to IV based upon the degree of thrombocytopenia, spontaneous bleeding, plasma leakage, and shock. These more severe forms constitute dengue, hemorrhagic fever, and dengue shock syndrome. There are four serotypes; exposure to one serotype provides lifelong immunity. Previous infection with one serotype may predispose an individual to a more severe infection with another serotype. Thus, the hemorrhagic fever is more common in indigenous individuals than the previously unexposed traveler.

The diagnosis is primarily clinical. The presence of thrombocytopenia, leukopenia, and hemoconcentration is suggestive and confirmatory tests with PCR or IgM antibodies via ELISA are available.

Emergency Department Treatment and Disposition

Supportive therapy is the only treatment available. Patients with mild illness are treated as outpatients. Admission of those with severe illness, hemorrhagic manifestations, shock, or an uncertain diagnosis is warranted.

Pearls

1. Consider dengue fever in recently returned travelers with fever, headache, and myalgias, particularly travelers to the Caribbean or Southeast Asia.

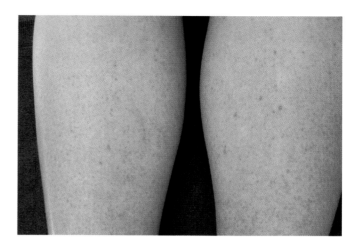

FIGURE 21.17 ■ Dengue Rash. Maculopapular rash from dengue on legs of an American medical worker during an outbreak in Guyana. (Photo contributor: Seth W. Wright, MD.)

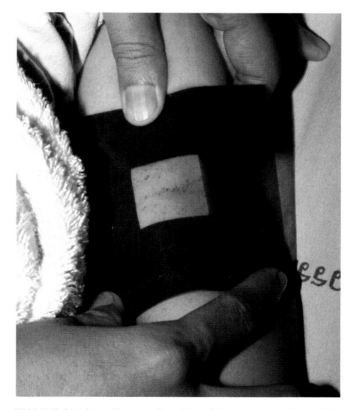

FIGURE 21.18 ■ Dengue Petechiae. Measurement of petechiae following a tourniquet test in a patient with dengue. Twenty or more petechiae in the template area are suggestive in the clinical diagnosis of dengue. (Photo contributor: WHO/TDR.)

2. The incubation period is usually rapid and patients will often have marked leukopenia, neutropenia, and thrombocytopenia.

3. The fever tends to be high and may suddenly resolve and then return; otherwise known as a "saddle back" fever pattern.

4. A positive "tourniquet test" to determine capillary fragility is highly suggestive of dengue. A blood pressure cuff is applied and inflated to a point between the systolic and diastolic blood pressures for 5 minutes. The test is positive if there are more than 20 petechiae per square inch.

5. Occasional cases of dengue occur in South Texas in people with no history of travel.

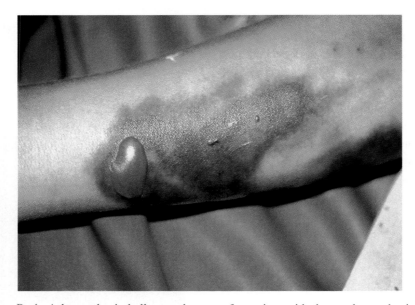

FIGURE 21.19 ■ Dengue Rash. A hemorrhagic bullae on the arm of a patient with dengue hemorrhagic fever. (Photo contributor: WHO/TDR.)

Clinical Summary

Elephantiasis affects more than 120 million people worldwide with over 40 million severely disfigured. It is not a specific disease but rather a syndrome caused by chronic obstruction of lymphatics. The most common cause is lymphatic filariasis which is caused by thread-like worms, *Wuchereria bancrofti, Brugia malayi, and B timori*. The infection is transmitted to humans by mosquitoes. Adult worms lodge in the lymphatics disrupting the fluid balance between tissues and blood vessels causing lymphedema of the extremities, breast, or genito-urinary system. The infection is generally acquired in child-hood, although clinical manifestations may take years to develop. Adult worms live for 4 to 6 years, producing millions of microfilariae that circulate in the blood and lymphatic system. Acute symptoms of lymphadenopathy and dermal inflammation may precede and later accompany chronic swelling. With persistent infection and inflammation, the skin develops a hyperkeratotic, pebbly appearance which may become ulcerated and darkened. Bacterial and fungal super-infections contribute to morbidity.

Mosquito nets and insect repellants are the main means of prevention of lymphatic filariasis. Parasites may be detected microscopically in the blood but the nocturnal periodicity makes identification challenging. Availability of the "card test" which identifies circulating antigens has overcome this problem and is available in some areas.

Emergency Department Treatment and Disposition

Treatment of lymphatic filariasis depends upon the presence or absence of other filarial organisms and includes various combinations of albendazole, ivermectin, and diethylcarbamazine (DEC). Cleansing of the affected areas and topical antibiotics aid in thwarting secondary disease. Local massage and elevation of the extremity improve lymphatic flow.

Pearls

1. Elephantiasis bears a heavy social burden due to physical limitations, disfigurement, sexual disability, and social stigmatization. Affected patients are frequently shunned by their families, unable to work and unwed.

2. Testicular hydrocele is the most common manifestation of chronic *W bancrofti* infection in males in endemic areas.

3. Tourists have a very low risk of transmission as multiple infective mosquito bites are required over months to years.

4. *W bancrofti* occasionally causes an acute asthma-like condition known as tropical pulmonary eosinophilia.

5. Podoconiosis is a noninfectious cause of elephantiasis that occurs in people who walk barefoot in areas with large amounts of volcanic ash. Kaposi sarcoma is another emerging cause of nonfilarial elephantiasis in sub-Saharan Africa.

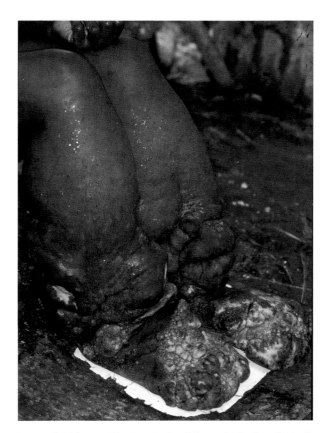

FIGURE 21.20 ■ Elephantiasis. Bilateral elephantiasis from lymphatic filariasis in an elderly Haitian man. (Photo contributor: WHO/TDR.)

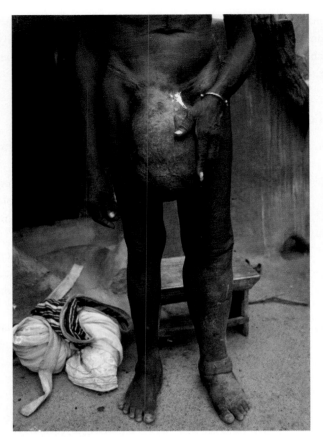

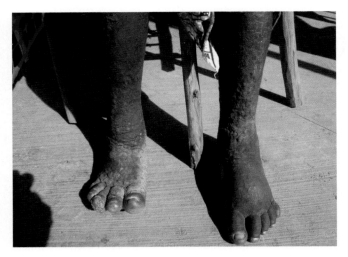

FIGURE 21.22 ▪ Elephantiasis. Nonfilarial elephantiasis due to extensive Kaposi sarcoma in a 26-year-old Ugandan woman with AIDS. (Photo contributor: Seth W. Wright, MD.)

FIGURE 21.21 ▪ Elephantiasis. A large hydrocele and unilateral elephantiasis from lymphatic filariasis in a man from Ghana. (Photo contributor: WHO/TDR.)

Clinical Summary

Meningococcal disease in developed countries usually consists of occasional sporadic cases and small outbreaks. In contrast, massive epidemics of serogroup A or C meningococcal meningitis occur in tropical countries, most notably in sub-Saharan Africa. These seasonal outbreaks tend to occur during the dry season along a wide swath of equatorial Africa known as the "meningitis belt."

The clinical presentation of epidemic meningitis is the same as that seen in developed countries. This typically consists of initial fever, headache, photophobia, and neck stiffness. Coma and death typically ensue if not treated. Diagnosis is with a spinal tap, although patients are often treated based on clinical grounds during a known outbreak. Mortality rates of less than 10% are obtainable. Large-scale vaccination programs are effective in decreasing spread of the disease within the affected areas and in adjacent population centers.

Emergency Department Treatment and Disposition

The mainstay of treatment is with antibiotics and supportive care. Penicillin and ampicillin are still the treatments of choice in many settings and are usually efficacious. Many countries and nongovernmental agencies are using single-dose oily chloramphenicol injections with success. Ceftriaxone is an excellent choice when available.

Pearls

1. Diarrhea can be an early finding in patients with meningococcal meningitis.
2. The use of single-dose oily chloramphenicol injections has allowed for easier management of large numbers of patients in limited-resource settings. A second dose is given in 24 hours if there has been no clinical improvement.
3. Massive outbreaks of meningitis have occurred during the Hajj, a pilgrimage to Mecca, in Saudi Arabia. They are the only country that requires proof of vaccination before entry.
4. An often-used critical threshold for the definition of an epidemic in Africa is 15 cases per 100,000 population per week. This would be equal to over 1400 cases per week in the Chicago metropolitan area.

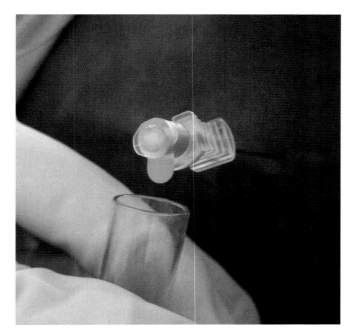 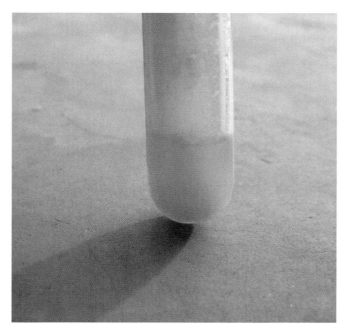

FIGURE 21.23 ■ Meningitis Spinal Fluid. CSF obtained from a 33-year-old Ugandan woman treated during an epidemic of serogroup A meningococcal meningitis. (Photo contributor: Seth W. Wright, MD.)

Clinical Summary

Endemic goiter is one of a spectrum of iodine deficiency disorders and is characterized by thyroid gland enlargement. This condition can occur in any location where environmental iodine is limited, but is rarely seen in developed countries as dietary iodine supplementation is routine. Dietary iodine deficiency is related to lack of environmental iodine and is often seen in mountainous areas away from the sea as iodine is leached from the soil by snow and rain. Iodine deficiency disorders are common in widespread areas of Africa, Asia, and South America.

Patients with inadequate iodine in their diet have decreased thyroid hormone production and increased pituitary thyroid-stimulating hormone (TSH) production. The thyroid is stimulated by the excessive TSH and becomes hyperplastic and enlarged. Patients are typically euthyroid.

Emergency Department Treatment and Disposition

Prevention with supplemental iodine, usually via salt, is the mainstay of goiter management at the community level. Individual patients with goiter can be treated with potassium iodide solution or Lugol's iodine with iodized salt as a permanent solution. Surgical treatment can be indicated for massive goiter, particularly in the setting of tracheal compression.

Pearls

1. Goiters in developed countries are most likely to be caused by defects in thyroid hormone production, resulting in an increase in TSH.
2. Iodine deficiency is the most common cause of preventable mental retardation (endemic cretinism) in the world.
3. Some dietary staple items, such as cabbage, cassava, lima beans, and sweet potatoes, have a goitrogenic factor which may be superimposed upon primary iodine deficiency.
4. Malignancy is not a common complication despite the massive size of many goiters.

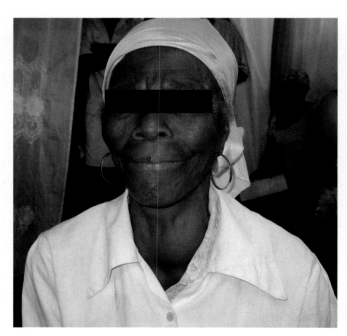

FIGURE 21.24 ■ Goiter. Easily visualized and palpable goiter in Haitian woman. (Photo contributor: Seth W. Wright, MD.)

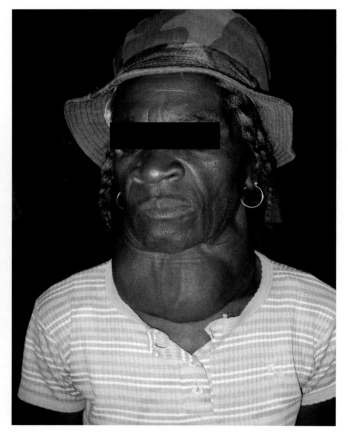

FIGURE 21.25 ■ Goiter. Patient from mountainous inland region of Haiti with massive goiter. This island nation has a high rate of goiter due to the complex interaction of poverty, political instability, deforestation, and erosion of soil. (Photo contributor: Ian D. Jones, MD.)

Clinical Summary

Leishmaniasis is a parasitic disease spectrum ranging from self-healing ulcers to disseminated cutaneous, mucocutaneous, and visceral forms. It is zoonotic and is spread to humans by the bite of a sand fly. The incubation period is 2 to 6 months, though it may range from days to years, with relapse possible.

The primary cutaneous lesion begins as an enlarging papule which develops a scaly appearance or more commonly an ulcerative lesion with indurated edges and a central crater. These lesions usually heal spontaneously in 6 to 12 months but may progress to other forms. Mucocutaneous involvement or "espundia" is often disfiguring. Initial symptoms of nasal congestion and epistaxis may progress to perforation of the nasal septum and collapse of the nasal bridge, causing a "tapir nose" deformity. Visceral involvement, known as "kala-azar," typically involves the spleen and liver and is generally fatal without treatment. It is associated with fever, anemia, cachexia, splenomegaly, and may progress to hemorrhagic symptoms and secondary infections.

The characteristic parasites can be identified from a smear or biopsy of the lesion identifying amastigotes (Leishman-Donovan bodies) of the parasite. Culture and PCR are also diagnostic options.

Emergency Department Treatment and Disposition

No specific emergency department treatment exists for leishmaniasis. Treatment of mucosal or cutaneous disease is with pentavalent antimony or amphotericin B after referral to an experienced clinician. Protective clothing, bed nets, and insect repellent are the most effective ways of avoiding transmission as the flies are usually active from dusk to dawn. Patients with suspected visceral leishmaniasis should be treated by a physician experienced in tropical medicine or infectious diseases as the treatment is difficult and often toxic.

Pearls

1. More than 90% of the world's cases of visceral leishmaniasis are in India, Bangladesh, Nepal, Sudan, and Brazil, while more than 90% of the world's cutaneous forms are located in Afghanistan, Algeria, Brazil, Iran, Iraq, Peru, Saudi Arabia, and Syria.
2. Leishmaniasis is common in the Middle East and many cases have been identified in troops deployed to that region.
3. Leishmaniasis should be considered in immigrants from Latin America, who present with a chronic skin lesion or mucosal lesions.
4. With visceral involvement, the primary cutaneous lesion will usually have resolved before clinical symptoms of kala-azar have developed.
5. After treatment of the visceral form, depigmented or nodular cutaneous lesions that are often confused with leprosy may occur.

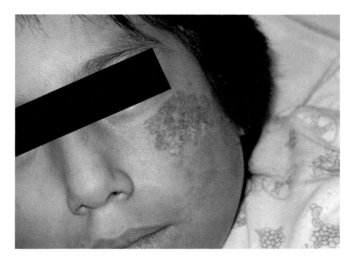

FIGURE 21.26 ■ Leishmaniasis. Cutaneous leishmaniasis in a girl from the highlands of Peru. Most leishmania lesions are on exposed areas of the body. (Photo contributors: Rob Greidanus, MD and Universidad Peruana Cayetano Heredia, Lima, Peru.)

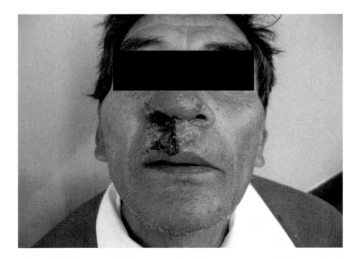

FIGURE 21.27 ■ Leishmaniasis. Mucocutaneous leishmaniasis (espundia) and "tapir-nose" deformity from *Leishmania brazilensis*. (Photo contributors: Rob Greidanus, MD and Universidad Peruana Cayetano Heredia, Lima, Peru.)

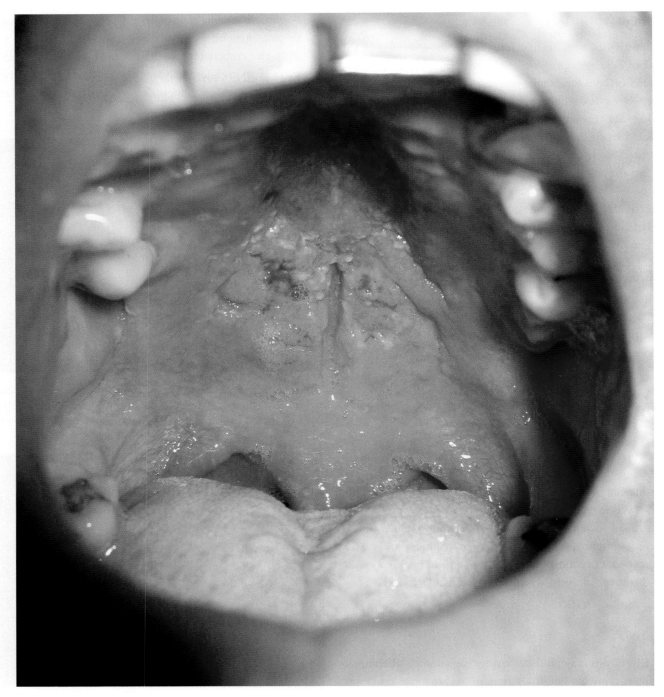

FIGURE 21.28 ■ Mucosal Leishmaniasis. Oral mucosal leishmaniasis caused by *L brazilensis*. Mucosal involvement can occur years after spontaneous resolution of a nontreated cutaneous lesion. (Photo contributors: Seth W. Wright, MD and Universidad Peruana Cayetano Heredia, Lima, Peru.)

Clinical Summary

Hydatid cysts are parasitic infections caused by the larval stage of *Echinococcus granulosis* tapeworms. The life-cycle is maintained between canines and various farm animals (usually sheep or cattle). Adult worms inhabit the small intestine of canines and eggs are passed in the stool. Farm animals become infected when they feed upon stool-contaminated material. The lifecycle is completed when dogs or other canines ingest the larval cysts that form in infected farm animals. Humans can be infected from ingestion of contaminated canine fecal material and are considered accidental hosts.

Hydatid cysts may affect any organ, but the liver is most commonly involved (>60% of cysts) followed by the lungs (20%). Diagnosis in uncertain cases may be aided by serologic testing. Changes in farming practices have led to a marked decline in hydatid cysts in most industrialized countries but they remain common in many developing areas. Most cases in the United States are in immigrants from highly endemic regions.

Emergency Department Treatment and Disposition

Hydatid cysts are often an incidental finding when x-rays, CT scans, or ultrasounds are done for other purposes. These patients can be referred for follow-up. Patients with symptomatic cysts may need admission and treatment. Depending on the size and location of the cyst, treatment may include percutaneous aspiration, surgical resection, or treatment solely with medication. Care must be taken with surgical intervention to avoid spillage of cysts, which may lead to anaphylaxis.

Pearls

1. Liver cysts may produce obstructive jaundice, abdominal pain, and cholangitis (triad of right upper quadrant adnominal pain, fever, and jaundice).
2. Cysts are slow growing with an estimated average cyst growth of 1-1.5 cm per year.

3. A chronic cough, pleuritic chest pain, hemoptysis, and dyspnea may be seen with lung involvement.
4. Though cerebral involvement is uncommon, it is seen more often in children. Symptoms may include headache, dizziness, focal neurologic deficits, or decreased level of consciousness.

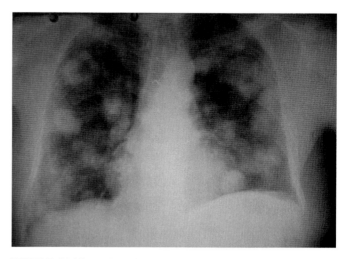

FIGURE 21.29 ■ Hydatid Cyst Radiograph. Chest x-ray showing multiple hydatid cysts. (Photo contributors: Rob Greidanus, MD and Universidad Peruana Cayetano Heredia, Lima, Peru.)

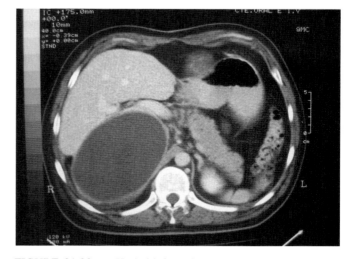

FIGURE 21.30 ■ Hydatid Cyst CT. Scan demonstrating large hydatid cyst in the liver. (Photo contributors: Seth W. Wright, MD and Universidad Peruana Cayetano Heredia, Lima, Peru.)

Clinical Summary

Mycobacteria other than tuberculosis and leprosy cause disorders primarily seen in tropical countries. These differ from *Mycobacterium tuberculosis* and *M leprae* as they are usually environmental saprophytes, not obligate human/animal pathogens. Human exposure may be via inhalation, contaminated water, or contamination of a preexisting wound.

Buruli ulcer is the most important disorder caused by infection with *M ulcerans*. It is a slow-growing ulcer with extensive necrosis and deep undermining of wound edges.

A variety of other cutaneous forms of mycobacterial diseases exist. Fish tank granuloma (from *M marinum*) is seen following handling of tropical fish tanks and occasionally in fishermen. Posttraumatic abscesses are caused by the rapidly growing mycobacteria, *M fortuitum* and *M chelonae*.

Disseminated disease from *M avium* complex is a late stage opportunistic infection in HIV/AIDS, occasionally seen in immunocompetent individuals.

Emergency Department Treatment and Disposition

These illnesses should be considered by the treating emergency physician when patients present with typical skin lesions and in severely immunocompromised AIDS patients. Buruli ulcer is typically treated with surgical excision as chemotherapy is usually ineffective. Other infections are treated with macrolide or other antibiotics.

Pearls

1. Buruli ulcer is the third most common mycobacterial disease worldwide, after tuberculosis and leprosy.

2. Consider *M marinum* infection on patients with a hand lesion following tropical fish tank manipulation.

3. Fast growing mycobacteria such as *M chelonae* cause "cold abscesses," often seen after nonsterile injections are given for cosmetic purposes. These may occur in mini-epidemics.

4. Some postulate that Crohn disease and sarcoidosis may be caused by yet unidentified mycobacteria.

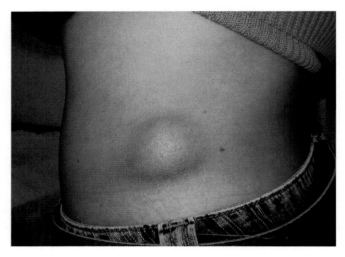

FIGURE 21.32 ■ Cold Abscess. A cold abscess following a cosmetic injection for weight loss. (Photo contributors: Seth W. Wright, MD and Universidad Peruana Cayetano Heredia, Lima, Peru.)

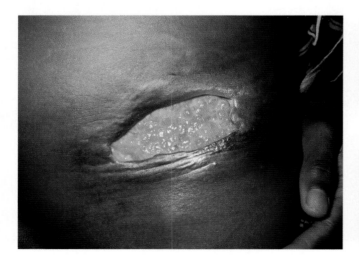

FIGURE 21.31 ■ Buruli Ulcer. Typical shallow base and deep undermining of the edges in a patient from Benin. (Photo contributor: World Health Organization.)

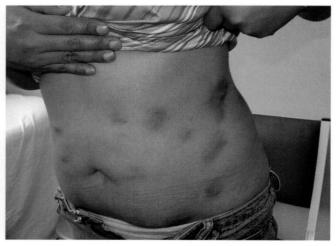

FIGURE 21.33 ■ Cold Abscesses. A patient with multiple recurrent cold abscesses from *M chelonae* following nonsterile weight loss injections in Peru. (Photo contributors: Rob Greidanus, MD and Universidad Peruana Cayetano Heredia, Lima, Peru.)

Clinical Summary

Leprosy, also known as "Hansen disease," is a chronic infectious disease caused by *Mycobacterium leprae*, an acid-fast rod-shaped bacillus. It primarily causes anesthetic skin lesions and peripheral nerve complications. Though the overall rate of infection is declining, it is still common in many parts of the world, including areas of South America, South Asia, and Africa. Severity of illness is proportional to the patient's ability to produce a cell-mediated response creating a range of symptoms from localized disease (tuberculoid leprosy) to disseminated disease (lepromatous leprosy), with many having borderline disease which falls between the two extremes.

Localized disease (paucibacillary) is limited to a single or few skin lesions. Lesions are typically sharply demarcated flat plaques with elevated margins which are hypopigmented and markedly anesthetic. This is often accompanied by marked peripheral nerve thickening. The most severe form (multibacillary) is lepromatous leprosy characterized by multiple small, erythematous, hyperpigmented macules, papules, or nodules. The peripheral nerves have less palpable findings, but more diffuse nerve involvement is seen in a stocking glove pattern. This results in loss of bone length and insensate extremities leading to repetitive trauma with ensuing infection and loss of digits. With diffuse infiltration of the face, the characteristic "leonine facies" is exhibited.

Diagnosis is primarily clinical along with staining of a slit skin smear or biopsy for acid-fast bacilli. PCR can aid in the diagnosis.

Emergency Department Treatment and Disposition

There is no specific emergency department therapy for leprosy. Patients with suspected leprosy should be referred to the national program (common in many endemic countries) or a clinician experienced with the management of this illness. Multidrug therapy is curative with varying combinations of dapsone, rifampin, and clofazimine. The class of disease dictates type and length of treatment.

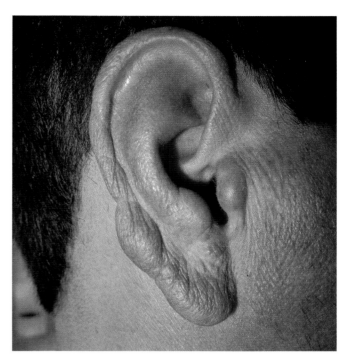

FIGURE 21.34 ■ Leprosy. Typical thickened skin on the external ear of a patient with lepromatous leprosy. (Photo contributors: Rob Greidanus, MD and Universidad Peruana Cayetano Heredia, Lima, Peru.)

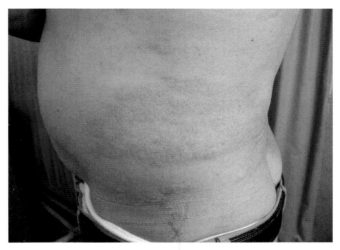

FIGURE 21.35 ■ Leprosy Skin Lesions. Anesthetic skin lesions in a Peruvian patient with borderline leprosy. Borderline disease is not as localized as tuberculoid leprosy and not as widespread as lepromatous disease. (Photo contributors: Rob Greidanus, MD and Universidad Peruana Cayetano Heredia, Lima, Peru.)

Pearls

1. About 100 cases of leprosy are reported each year in the United States.
2. The combination of skin lesions and neuropathy should suggest the diagnosis but neurological findings may be subtle leading to a delay in diagnosis.
3. Approximately 75% of people are able to mount a strong, cell-mediated immune response effectively eradicating the microbe.
4. Multidrug therapy has been made available by WHO free of charge to all patients worldwide since 1995, and provides a highly effective cure for all types of leprosy.
5. The mode of transmission is unknown, though bacilli are present in wounds and respiratory transmission is suspected. The fear of contagion and social rejection continues to cause distress despite studies revealing that it is not highly infectious and that treated individuals do not require isolation.

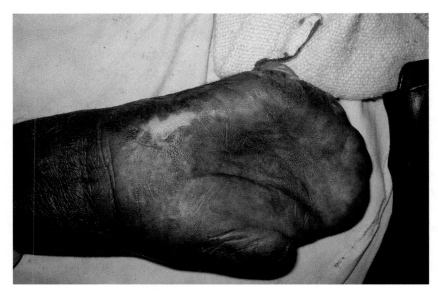

FIGURE 21.36 ■ Leprosy. Late-stage leprosy in a patient in Zambia with amputation of all hand digits. The palmer skin is relatively preserved while the skin on the wrist is thickened due to bacillary infiltration. (Photo contributor: Seth W. Wright, MD.)

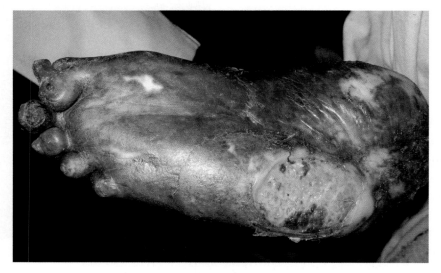

FIGURE 21.37 ■ Leprosy. Chronic foot changes of leprosy with ulceration and shortening of the toes. Extremity damage in leprosy results from loss of sensation, repeated trauma, neurotrophic atrophy, and direct bacillary deposition. (Photo contributor: Seth W. Wright, MD.)

Clinical Summary

Malaria is the most deadly vector-borne disease in the world, killing more than 1 million people annually. This parasitic disease is transmitted by the night-biting female *Anopheles* mosquito and is caused by four protozoa of the genus *Plasmodium* (*P falciparum, P malariae, P ovale, P vivax*) with *P falciparum* causing the most morbidity and mortality. It is most common in tropical areas, particularly sub-Saharan Africa and Southeast Asia, with specific species predominating in geographic areas.

The parasites undergo a hepatic cycle and then enter circulating red blood cells, feed on hemoglobin, and replicate inside the cell. Lysis of the cell releases toxic metabolic by-products and further parasites into the blood stream, causing cyclical clinical manifestations. Symptoms include fever, rigors, headache, myalgias, and malaise. *Plasmodium falciparum* infection can cause massive hemolysis due to overwhelming parasitemia. Parasitized erythrocytes lose flexibility leading to microcirculatory obstruction, hypoxia to vital organs, and splenomegaly. Symptoms from *P ovale* and *P vivax* may be delayed for many months due to hepatic dormancy.

Diagnosis is established by identification of the parasites on thick and thin smears. Rapid antigen kits are available in some regions. Bednets, insecticides, and protective clothing are effective adjuncts for prevention. Chemoprophylaxis with an appropriate agent is highly recommended for travelers to endemic regions.

Wright stain—thin smear for malaria

Uses: To evaluate for the presence of ring trophozoites.
Materials: Air-dried blood smear, Coplin jar of Wright stain, slide rack, pH 7.2 buffer, blotting paper.

Method

1. Place a drop of blood on the middle of a slide.
2. Hold another slide evenly on top of the slide at a 45-degree angle and drag the slide over the drop of blood to the opposite edge to spread the blood evenly.
3. Allow the blood to dry for 5 to 10 minutes.
4. Stain air-dried smears in a closed Coplin jar of Wright stain for 5 minutes.
5. Place the slide on a rack.
6. Rinse and treat with pH 7.2 buffer primed with 1 mL Wright stain per 400 mL for 3 minutes.
7. Rinse in pH 7.2 buffer for 20 seconds.
8. Blot dry and mount on microscope at ×100 (oil immersion).

Emergency Department Treatment and Disposition

Treatment depends upon geographic location of exposure, suspected species, and national policy in many endemic areas. Chloroquine is first-line therapy for the few remaining places without resistance. Quinidine is the usual treatment for severe malaria in the United States, while much of the world uses quinine or artemisinin-combination therapy. Artesunate is available from the CDC for residents of the United States. Evaluation of CDC or WHO guidelines by geographic region is highly recommended for both prophylaxis and treatment. Close attention to supportive therapy is mandatory. Patients in developing countries are often treated as outpatients. With rare exception, returning travelers with suspected malaria should be admitted for management and treatment. Admission is always warranted for patients with suspected or confirmed *P falciparum*, symptoms of cerebral malaria, life-threatening symptoms, children, pregnant women, or immunocompromised individuals.

Pearls

1. Malaria should be strongly considered in any patient exhibiting fever following recent travel to the tropics and is the single most common cause of fever in this population.

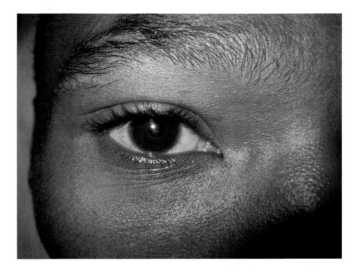

FIGURE 21.38 ■ Malaria Jaundice. Jaundice due to acute hemolysis in a Haitian teenager with documented *P falciparum* infection. (Photo contributor: Seth W. Wright, MD.)

2. The classic cyclical fevers do not always occur.
3. The average incubation period for *P falciparum* is about 13 days with a longer average period in the other species. Incubation periods for all species can be variable.
4. Parasitemia fluctuates over time with the highest incidence during episodes of fever. Failure to identify the parasites on initial smears is not an indication to withhold therapy when the diagnosis is likely.
5. Natives of highly endemic areas will often have partial immunity to malaria. This partial immunity is lost in pregnancy or lack of repeated exposure. Immigrants going back to their native country are at very high risk for severe infection due to loss of immunity.

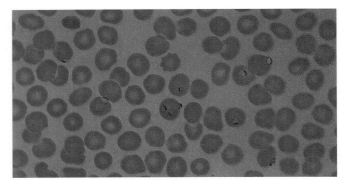

FIGURE 21.39 ■ *Plasmodium falciparum* Thin Film. Ring forms (trophozoites) of P falciparum are seen on the Wright stain thin film in a patient with intermittent fever who had recently traveled to Africa. (Photo contributor: James P. Elrod, MD, PhD.)

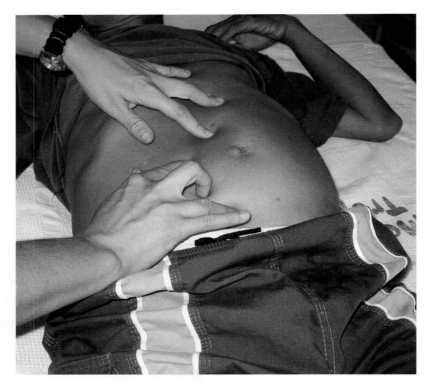

FIGURE 21.40 ■ Malaria. Massive splenomegaly in a patient with hyperreactive malarial splenomegaly. This condition can occur in patients with chronic infection but malaria smears are often negative. (Photo contributors: Seth W. Wright, MD and Universidad Peruana Cayetano Heredia, Lima, Peru.)

Clinical Summary

Mycetoma is a localized, chronic, granulomatous involvement of subcutaneous tissue with possible extension to underlying bone. Two classifications include eumycetoma, caused by filamentous fungi, and actinomycetoma, comprising of bacteria of actinomycetes species. The organism is inoculated into the subcutaneous tissue following minor trauma, most commonly involving the lower extremity and the hand, though it may arise anywhere on the body. Initially, a painless subcutaneous swelling is seen with induration, numerous suppurative nodules, and sinus tracts developing years later. Remote abscesses may be seen due to hematogenous extension though this is uncommon. Both types have similar clinical findings; however, eumycetoma causes more morbidity. Expulsion of grains containing aggregates of the organisms is common. Despite surgical excision of the affected area, it has a high recurrence rate with frequent need for amputation. Actinomycetoma occurs more frequently (60%) and has a much better outcome. Mycetomas are not contagious and are rarely fatal, but may cause significant disfigurement.

The presence of black grains is diagnostic of a fungal origin, while pale grains could be either fungal or from an actinomycetes species. Further identification of the causative organism may be done by means of various stains, culture, or by serology available in some centers.

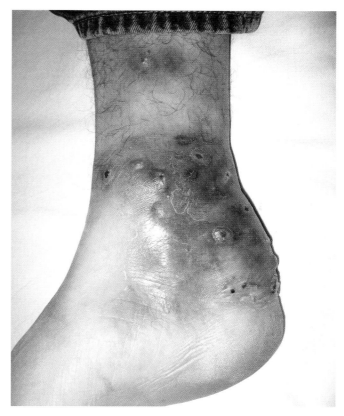

FIGURE 21.41 ■ Mycetoma. A eumycetoma with typical chronic sinus drainages in the foot and ankle of a 33-year-old agricultural worker in Peru. Treatment was with itraconazole. (Photo contributors: Rob Griedanus, MD and Universidad Peruana Cayetano Heredia, Lima, Peru.)

Emergency Department Treatment and Disposition

There is no specific emergency department management except referral. Surgical resection of large lesions may supplement treatment by reducing organism load. Eumycetoma is treated with 1 to 2 years of antifungal agents, while actinomycetoma responds to various combinations of trimethoprim-sulfamethoxazole, dapsone, streptomycin, and amikacin.

Pearls

1. It is possible to see this disease in the southern United States, but occurrence is rare. More commonly, it is seen in young male adults living in rural areas of Africa, Mexico, South America, or India who work as farmers or laborers. Walking or working barefoot is a risk factor for lower extremity disease.

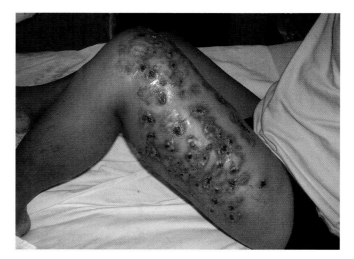

FIGURE 21.42 ■ Mycetoma. A large actinomycetoma of the upper leg with extensive active and healed sinus tracts. (Photo contributors: Stuart Skinner, MD and Universidad Peruana Cayetano Heredia, Lima, Peru.)

2. Patients may complain of a deep itching sensation rather than pain. If pain is present, it may indicate secondary infection or bone involvement.

3. Sweating of the affected area is commonly seen.

4. A similar condition, botryomycosis, is caused by a chronic *Staphylococcus* infection with sinus formation.

5. It was first described in the Madura district of India and is often referred to as "Madura foot."

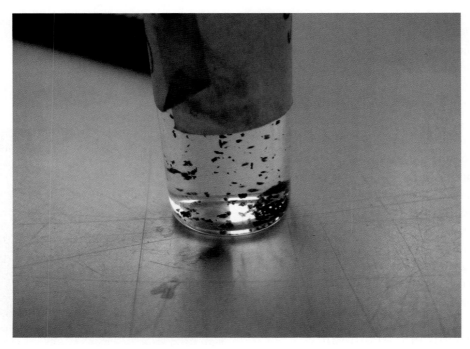

FIGURE 21.43 ■ Mycetoma Granules. Sinuses discharge characteristic dark granules (sclerotia) from a eumycetoma. The granules represent microcolonies of the organism. (Photo contributors: Seth W. Wright, MD and Universidad Peruana Cayetano Heredia, Lima, Peru.)

Clinical Summary

Myiasis is the invasion of living tissue of humans or animals by maggots, the larvae of flies. Infection is most commonly subcutaneous, but may be seen in wounds and body cavities. The human botfly (*Dermatobia hominis*) is a major cause of furuncular myiasis in the New World and uses mosquitoes to courier eggs to the host. A papule develops as the larvae feed followed by a pruritic furuncle. The larva may be observed surfacing through a central punctum. After maturation, it emerges and falls to the ground, where it pupates in the soil and evolves into an adult fly.

The Tumbu fly, found in Africa, also causes furuncular myiasis and is spread from eggs deposited in soil, sand, or clothes. Screw worm species are found in the Old and New Worlds. These worms are notorious for direct deposition of eggs after flying into the nasal cavity, leading to nasal cavity myiasis. Feeding maggots can cause extensive tissue damage. Wound myiasis, caused by numerous fly species, is seen in open sores and gangrenous tissues. Prevention of myiasis is through wearing protective clothing, utilizing insect repellant, and covering of wounds.

Emergency Department Treatment and Disposition

Causing the larva to surface facilitates removal in furuncular myiasis. This may be done with injection of lidocaine at the base of the lesion or through suffocation after application of occlusive substances such as Vaseline. Incisional extraction is challenging due to the larva's tapered shape and many rows of spines and hooks that it uses to grip the tissue. Wound myiasis is treated with thorough debridement of the wound. Secondary infection is the only indication for antibiotics but this is uncommon due to bacteriostatic activity in the gut of the larva. Leaving portions of the larvae after removal may incite an inflammatory reaction or bacterial infection.

Pearls

1. Screw worms are major problems for livestock. A sterile male release program has eliminated the screwworm from the United States.

2. Myiasis is self-limiting and usually not harmful but it does cause psychological distress to the host, especially when the larvae surface. Though rare, deaths from meningitis have occurred after tissue penetration from infection in the eye, nose, or ear canal.

3. Some feel that fly maggots are a useful method of wound debridement. Packets of fly maggots have been commercially developed for this purpose.

4. A widespread flea (*Tunga penetrans*) causes lesions known as tungiasis. The lesions are usually located on the foot or ankle.

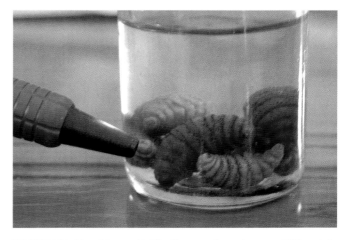

FIGURE 21.44 ■ Human Botfly. Preserved specimens of *D hominis*. (Photo contributors: Rob Greidanus, MD and Universidad Peruana Cayetano Heredia, Lima, Peru.)

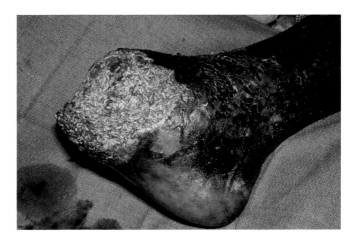

FIGURE 21.45 ■ Wound Myiasis. Wound myiasis in an elderly patient following dressing removal. (Photo contributor: the Department of Emergency Medicine, University of Cincinnati.)

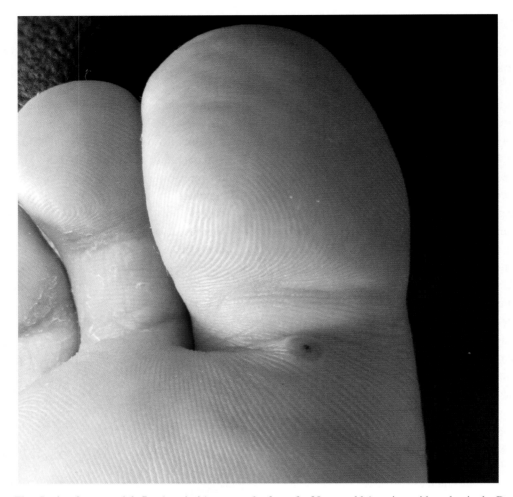

FIGURE 21.46 ■ Flea. Lesion from an adult flea (tungiasis) seen on the foot of a 30-year-old American aid worker in the Democratic Republic of Congo. Technically, this is not myiasis. (Photo contributor: Seth W. Wright, MD.)

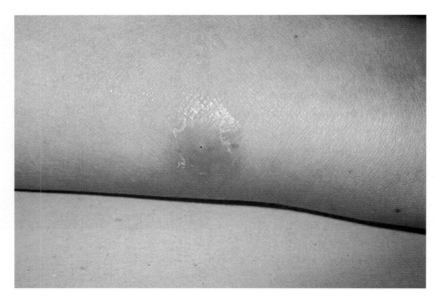

FIGURE 21.47 ■ Myiasis. Wound on the arm of a woman who had visited the Amazon jungle. A *D hominis* larva was extracted from the wound. (Photo contributors: Seth W. Wright, MD and Universidad Peruana Cayetano Heredia, Lima, Peru.)

Clinical Summary

Protein energy malnutrition (PEM) applies to a group of disorders including kwashiorkor and marasmus. These are characterized by an imbalance between the body's supply and demand of energy and nutrients. Kwashiorkor means "the sickness of weaning" as it is often seen following weaning after the birth of a sibling. Kwashiorkor usually occurs between the ages of 1 to 4 and when there is a deficiency of dietary protein in the presence of normal to high carbohydrate intake. The etiology is complex but there is decreased synthesis of proteins resulting in hypoalbuminemia. Kwashiorkor is an acute illness manifested by edema secondary to fluid and sodium retention. Patients have peripheral edema, moon facies, apathy, and a protuberant abdomen secondary to hepatomegaly. The skin can become hyperkeratotic and may split open in pressure-prone areas.

Marasmus is often seen under the age of 1 and is associated with inadequate intake of both protein and calories. This leads to the utilization of the body's own energy stores resulting in emaciation. These individuals do not have edema but rather a loss of subcutaneous fat, muscle wasting, and wrinkled loose skin. Marasmic-kwashiorkor refers to the combination of both forms simultaneously. Diagnostic laboratory studies are useful but often are not available. Patients with PEM may be left with permanent neurological and physical deficits due to lack of calories, vitamins, and essential amino acids.

Emergency Department Treatment and Disposition

These conditions are rarely seen or treated in developed countries, so acute treatment is often in clinics or hospitals with limited resources. These children often have an acute illness, such as measles, that should be treated as indicated. IV fluids are limited to those with shock as they are prone to congestive heart failure. WHO oral rehydration salt solution is usually used and is given at 5 mL/kg every 30 minutes orally or by NG tube for 2 hours and then 6 to 10 mL/h the next 6 hours. Low protein milk formula is then started with a goal of 100 kcal/kg/day. A normal diet is gradually started over a few weeks. Inpatient admission for evaluation, intervention, and arrangement of long-term care is advised when possible.

Pearls

1. Depigmentation of dark hair causes it to turn reddish and curly hair may become straight and brittle. Intermittent periods of proper nutrition may lead to alternating bands of light and dark hair known as "the flag sign."
2. Kwashiorkor is an acute illness, often of only several days duration. It is commonly precipitated by acute infections.
3. The mid upper arm circumference (MUAC) is often used for rapid assessment of nutritional status in developing countries.
4. Newer nutritional products, such as "Plumpy'nut," have been developed and allow for outpatient management of many malnourished children.
5. In developed countries, PEM is usually caused by abnormal metabolism, decreased absorption of nutrients from systemic diseases, or new dieting techniques.

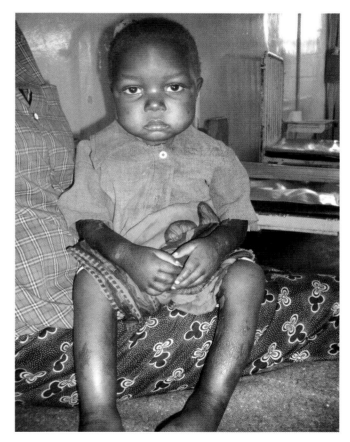

FIGURE 21.48 ■ Kwashiorkor. A Zambian child with typical light hair, moon facies, peripheral edema, and dry skin of kwashiorkor. (Photo contributor: Meg Jack, MD.)

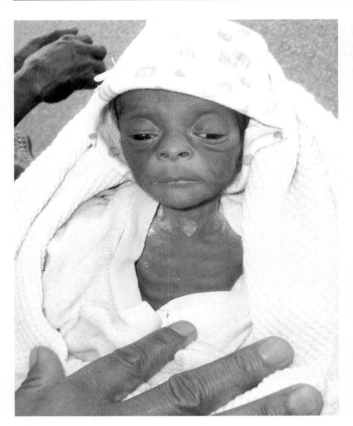

FIGURE 21.49 ■ Marasmus. An African infant with severe marasmus due to poor feeding following maternal death. The infant is severely underweight with loose skin and little subcutaneous fat. (Photo contributor: Meg Jack, MD.)

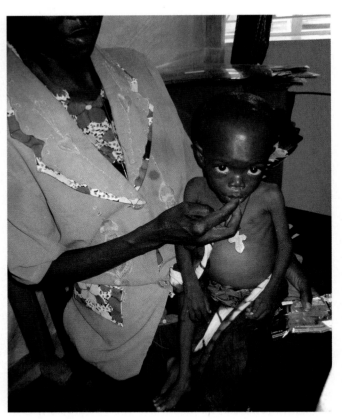

FIGURE 21.51 ■ Marasmus. An HIV-positive Ugandan girl recovering from marasmus. She is eating Plumpy'nut, a commonly used ready-to-use therapeutic food. (Photo contributor: Seth W. Wright, MD.)

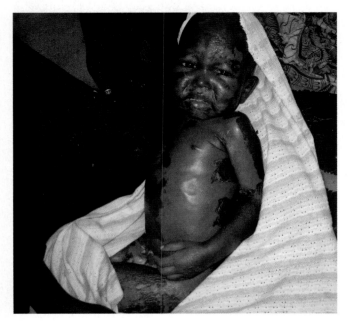

FIGURE 21.50 ■ Kwashiorkor. A Ugandan boy with acute kwashiorkor. The edema is typical of kwashiorkor. The rash is occasionally seen. The patient died several days after the photo was taken. (Photo contributor: Seth W. Wright, MD.)

Clinical Summary

Rabies is a viral zoonotic disease that humans typically acquire through the bite, less often through the lick or scratch, of an infected animal. Transmission via aerosolized virus has been documented in bat-infested caves and in laboratory workers. Human-to-human transmission has only been documented in transplant recipients. Infection can be prevented by pre-exposure or postexposure vaccination.

Rabies has the dubious distinction of having the highest case fatality rate of any infectious disease. Rabies is a severe progressive encephalitis and presents in one of two forms. Patients with the more common (80% of cases) "furious" form present with typical symptoms of agitation, laryngeal spasms, severe pain on swallowing, hydrophobia, confusion, agitation, and a host of other neurologic signs and symptoms. Patients with the paralytic form (20%) present with an ascending paralysis. Patient often have preceding paresthesias and pain at the site of the exposure. Autonomic instability is common in all patients prior to death. The diagnosis of rabies in developing countries is primarily clinical. Fluorescent antibody testing, biopsy, and PCR are done in areas where available.

Emergency Department Treatment and Disposition

Management of clinical rabies is traditionally supportive as the outcome has been uniformly fatal. Vaccination after development of clinical rabies is futile. Treatment in developing countries is usually limited to sedation with benzodiazepines and other comfort measures. Survival of one patient in Wisconsin has been reported using an induced coma (midazolam and ketamine) and antiviral agents (ribavirin and amantadine). This regimen is not practical in most developing countries where the majority of cases are located.

Pearls

1. The majority of rabies cases in the United States are caused by insect-eating bats, but most patients are unable to give a history of a bite.
2. Hawaii is the only US state to be considered rabies free.
3. The shortest incubation period is in those with extensive bites and in those with bite wounds to the face and scalp.

4. The less common paralytic form of rabies can present similar to Guillain-Barré syndrome.
5. Human-to-human transmission is extremely rare or non-existent. Nevertheless, postexposure prophylaxis of close contacts is recommended as virus is present in saliva.

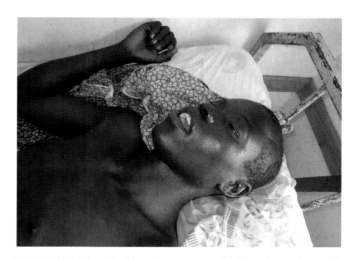

FIGURE 21.52 ■ Rabies. Twenty-year old Ugandan patient with furious rabies on the fourth day of clinical illness after a dog bite 2 months earlier. The neck is visibly swollen due to subcutaneous emphysema. The patient developed spontaneous pneumomediastinum due to forceful vomiting during a period of severe laryngeal spasms. (Photo contributor: Seth W. Wright, MD.)

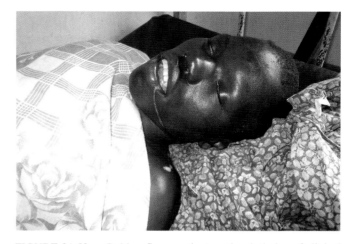

FIGURE 21.53 ■ Rabies. Same patient on the sixth day of clinical illness. The patient is now unable to swallow or control secretions due to laryngeal pain and spasms. (Photo contributor: Seth W. Wright, MD.)

Clinical Summary

Sporotrichosis is a subacute or chronic subcutaneous infection caused by the fungus *Sporothrix schenckii*. The illness is acquired from moss, decaying vegetation, hay, and soil and is usually seen in those whose vocation brings them into contact with the environment. The two primary manifestations involve the cutaneous and lymphocutaneous systems; however, osteoarticular, pulmonary, and disseminated forms (primarily in patients with AIDS) may be seen from direct inoculation or through hematologic seeding.

The extremities are most commonly involved with the initial lesion at the site of injury from a thorn, barb, pine needle, or wire. After approximately 1 to 10 weeks, a localized red, purple, or pink papule develops, often resembling an insect bite. The papule evolves into one or more nodules that form painless chronic ulcers with a nonpurulent, clear discharge. In the lymphocutaneous form, the nodules will progress proximally along lymphatic tracts and blood vessels. Many strains do not grow at temperatures above 35°C, decreasing their ability to spread and commonly resulting in a localized lesion. It is not communicable from person to person though it may be acquired through exposure to infected animals with cats being the most infectious.

Wearing gloves and long sleeves while working in the outdoors and avoidance of skin contact with sphagnum moss are the mainstays of prevention. Confirmatory diagnosis is made through serology or cell culture with identification of the cigar-shaped fungus.

Emergency Department Treatment and Disposition

Treatment with potassium iodide or itraconazole is effective with complete recovery in cutaneous and lymphocutaneous forms. Variable response to treatment is seen in patients with systemic involvement.

Pearls

1. This diagnosis should be considered when a cutaneous lesion is found on a patient involved with landscaping, rose gardening, Christmas tree farming, berry picking, baling of hay, and in veterinarians.

2. Lesions typically are noted on the distal upper extremity and the patient may have already failed multiple treatments with antibacterial agents.

3. While first described in the United States (southern and central United States), it is most common in Mexico, Central and South America, Japan, and Africa. In Peru, the incidence is approximately 1 in 1000 people.

4. Sporotrichosis is easily confused with leishmaniasis and the two illnesses coexist in many locations. Lymphatic spread is more characteristic of sporotrichosis but possible with either.

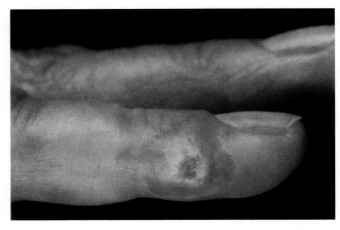

FIGURE 21.54 ■ Sporotrichosis. Typical finger lesion of sporotrichosis. (Reproduced, with permission, from Wolff K, Johnson RA, Suurmond D. *Fitzpatrick's Color Atlas & Synopsis of Clinical Dermatology*. 5th ed. New York: McGraw-Hill; 2005: p 739.)

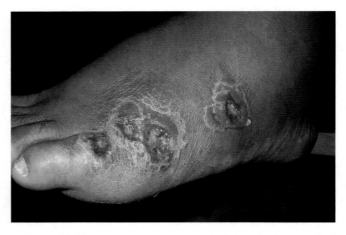

FIGURE 21.55 ■ Sporotrichosis. Typical lymphatic spread of sporotrichosis along the lateral aspect of the foot in a 30-year-old resident of the Peruvian Amazon. (Photo contributors: Seth W. Wright, MD and Universidad Peruana Cayetano Heredia, Lima, Peru.)

Clinical Summary

Tuberculosis (TB) is a chronic bacterial infection spread from human to human through respiratory droplets containing *Mycobacterium tuberculosis*, an acid-fast bacillus. Upon inhalation, the organisms are transported to regional lymph nodes where the immune system forms granulomas or "tubercles." Most people undergo complete healing following exposure with only a positive PPD. However, it may lie dormant as latent disease until the immune system is suppressed, leading to release of organisms. Tuberculosis occurs worldwide but is much more common in impoverished nations.

The organisms are dependent on high oxygen content and are typically found in the upper lobe or superior segment of the lower lobes of the lungs. Though it is primarily a respiratory illness, 15% of cases will exhibit extrapulmonary manifestations involving the adrenal glands, long bones, vertebrae, GI tract, GU tract, lymph nodes, meninges, pericardium, or peritoneum. Patients with HIV infection have a much higher prevalence of extrapulmonary disease. Common symptoms of active tuberculosis are fever, night sweats, malaise, weight loss, cough, hemoptysis, and pleuritic chest pain. Diagnosis is made by the PPD and chest x-ray but is confirmed through AFB smears and sputum culture. The mainstay of diagnosis in resource-limited countries is the AFB smear.

Emergency Department Treatment and Disposition

Typical first-line chemotherapy consists of isoniazid, rifampin, pyrazinamide, and ethambutol for 2 months followed by isoniazid and rifampin for 4 months. Patients in developed countries are usually admitted with respiratory isolation. Outpatient therapy is common in developing countries. After 2 weeks of treatment, the person usually is no longer contagious. Poor long-term adherence is a major contributing factor to the development of multi-drug-resistant strains. Directly observed therapy (DOT) where patients are observed taking the medication may be required to ensure compliance and is routine in most countries.

Pearls

1. One person infects 10 to 15 people per year with one cough generating approximately 3000 infective droplets. Any immunocompromised person with pulmonary symptoms should be placed in respiratory isolation until TB is excluded.

2. "Scrofula" refers to cervical lymph node involvement of TB, while vertebral involvement is called "Potts disease."

3. In highly endemic regions, the BCG (Bacille Calmette Guerin) vaccine is given to infants; however, it is not as effective in adults and may create a false-positive reaction with PPD placement.

4. For PPD tests, greater than 5 mm induration is positive in patients who have HIV, a suspicious chest x-ray, or an exposure. Greater than 10 mm is positive in IV drug users, high-prevalence groups (immigrants, long-term care facilities), children less than 4 year old, or in patients with medical conditions that increase progression of the disease (diabetes, cancer). Greater than 15 mm is positive in most others.

5. TB is the most important opportunistic infection in HIV patients in sub-Saharan Africa. The HIV epidemic has led to a massive increase in the incidence of TB in many countries.

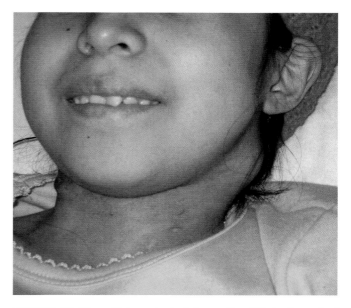

FIGURE 21.56 ■ Tuberculosis Adenopathy. Bilateral cervical adenopathy (scrofula) in a Peruvian child with documented TB. Cervical adenopathy in a child in highly endemic areas is strongly suggestive, and is the most common form, of extrapulmonary TB. (Photo contributors: Seth W. Wright, MD and Universidad Peruana Cayetano Heredia, Lima, Peru.)

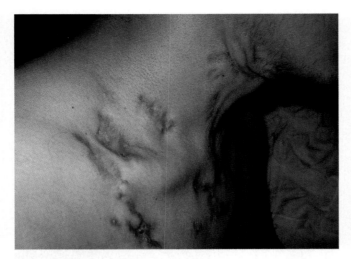

FIGURE 21.57 ■ Tuberculosis Scarring. Chronic discharging sinuses with extensive scar formation in a Peruvian man with extrapulmonary tuberculosis. (Photo contributors: Seth W. Wright, MD and Universidad Peruana Cayetano Heredia, Lima, Peru.)

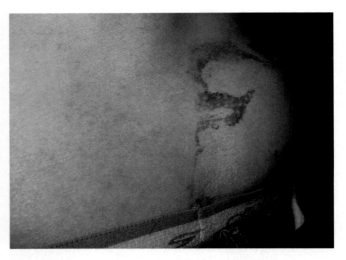

FIGURE 21.58 ■ Tuberculosis Cold Abscess. Cold abscess on the lower back of a patient with tuberculosis infection of the sacroiliac joint. (Photo contributors: Seth W. Wright, MD and Universidad Peruana Cayetano Heredia, Lima, Peru.)

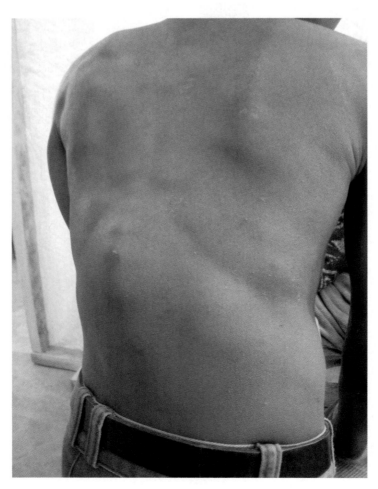

FIGURE 21.59 ■ Severe spinal deformity ("gibbus") in an 8-year-old Ugandan boy with Potts disease. (Photo contributor: Seth W. Wright, MD.)

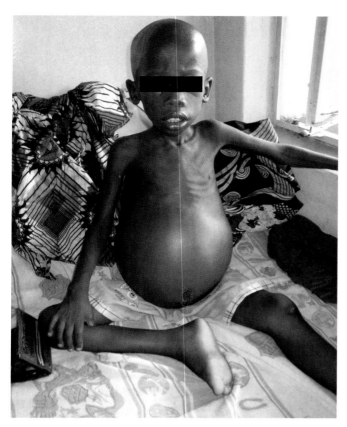

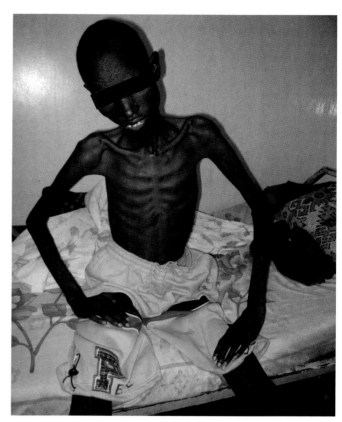

FIGURE 21.60 ▪ Abdominal Tuberculosis. Severe wasting and ascites in a Ugandan boy with abdominal tuberculosis. (Photo contributor: Seth W. Wright, MD.)

FIGURE 21.61 ▪ Pulmonary Tuberculosis. Severe wasting in a Sudanese soldier with smear positive pulmonary tuberculosis. His initial weight was 38 kg with a BMI of 11. His weight increased to 52 kg and BMI to 15 by the end of the 2-month intensive phase of treatment. (Photo contributor: Seth W. Wright, MD.)

Clinical Summary

Tetanus is an acute illness caused by *Clostridium tetani*. The infective spores are widely distributed in soil and are resistant to heat and disinfectants. Disease occurs when toxin forms after growth of the organism in wounds and is characterized by acute onset of skeletal muscle rigidity and convulsive spasm.

The toxin affects inhibitory GABA and glycine receptors, leading to unopposed contraction and spasm of skeletal muscle. Initial symptoms involve the facial musculature producing trismus (lockjaw) and risus sardonicus, otherwise known as the sneering grin. As larger muscle groups are involved, one may see opisthotonos, flexion and abduction of the arms, clenching of the fists against the thorax, and extension of the lower extremities. Other symptoms include laryngeal spasm resulting in asphyxia, seizures, hyperthermia, hypertension, diaphoresis, and tachycardia. Reflex spasms may be triggered by minimal external stimuli. Fractures, dislocations, and rhabdomyolysis may occur due to forceful sustained muscle contractions.

Emergency Department Treatment and Disposition

Diagnosis is primarily clinical. Treatment includes airway protection, metronidazole or penicillin, active immunization with tetanus vaccine, tetanus immune globulin, benzodiazepines, and supportive therapy. Wounds should be cleansed and debrided to eliminate further toxin production. Tetanus immune globulin facilitates removal of unbound tetanus toxin but does not affect toxin attached to nerve endings. Recovery of nerve function requires sprouting of new terminals and formation of new synapses which may take months to occur.

Pearls

1. There are three clinical forms of tetanus: local, cephalic, and generalized disease (most common).
2. Neonatal tetanus occurs in infants born without passive immunity 4 to 14 days after birth. Inoculation usually occurs through infection of the umbilical stump and is common in developing countries.
3. Tetanus may mimic an acute abdomen.
4. In developed countries, tetanus is primarily a disease of the elderly and inadequately vaccinated immigrants.
5. Tetanus disease does not infer immunity.

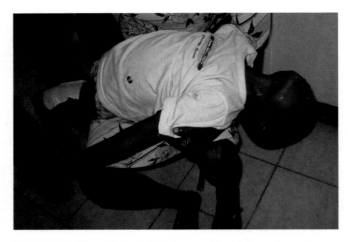

FIGURE 21.62 ■ Tetanus. Fatal generalized tetanus in an 8-year-old Haitian child resulting from an infected puncture wound on the left thigh. Severe opisthotonic posturing and rigid jaw clenching are evident. (Photo contributor: Seth W. Wright, MD.)

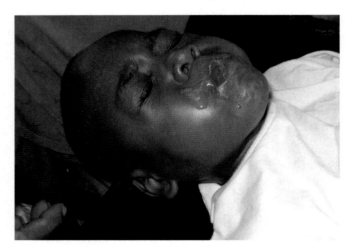

FIGURE 21.63 ■ Tetanus. Severe facial tetany. The distorted grin and raised eyebrows seen in tetanus is known as risus sardonicus. (Photo contributor: Seth W. Wright, MD.)

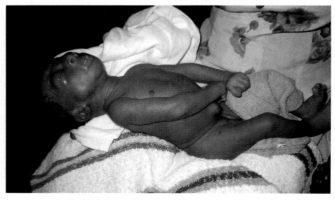

FIGURE 21.64 ■ Neonatal Tetanus. Neonatal tetanus in an 11-day-old infant. Ophthistonic posturing, muscular rigidity, and inability to swallow are seen. (Photo contributor: Seth W. Wright, MD.)

Clinical Summary

Trachoma is the leading cause of infectious blindness in the world. It is endemic in areas of Africa, Asia, Latin America, the Middle East, and aboriginal communities in Australia. Trachoma is a chronic follicular conjunctivitis caused by *Chlamydia trachomatis* and is prevalent in populations with limited access to adequate sanitation and clean water. It is spread from person to person through ocular and respiratory secretions with flies constituting a major means of transmission.

Although symptoms occur along a continuum, there are two distinct phases, the active phase and the scarring (cicatricial) phase. The active phase presents with mild itching, irritation, and discharge from the eye associated with inflammation of the conjunctivae, particularly the superior tarsal plate. With progression, symptoms include marked photophobia, blurred vision, and eye pain. The cicatricial phase occurs after repeated or severe infection with chronic inflammation causing the upper lid to shorten (entropion) with subsequent inversion of the eyelashes (trichiasis). Trichiasis causes painful corneal abrasions which over time leads to corneal edema, ulceration, scarring, opacities, and ultimately blindness. The lacrimal glands may be affected leading to dryness and increased eye irritation. Trachoma usually affects both eyes. Trachoma is a clinical diagnosis but may be confirmed by culture. Community-based efforts on education of hygiene and behavior modification can decrease the incidence in the community.

Emergency Department Treatment and Disposition

For acute and subacute infections, the most effective treatment is a single dose of azithromycin but may also be treated with tetracycline ophthalmic ointment. Eyelid surgery to correct trichiasis and entropion may prevent blindness.

Pearls

1. Trachoma was once endemic to North America and Europe, but has disappeared with improved sanitation and living conditions.

2. It is extremely contagious and may be spread through direct contact with eye, nose, or throat secretions of infected people.

3. Young children are particularly susceptible, but the disease progresses slowly and the more painful symptoms may not emerge until adulthood.

4. Adult women are at much greater risk due to their close contact with small children who are the main reservoir of infection.

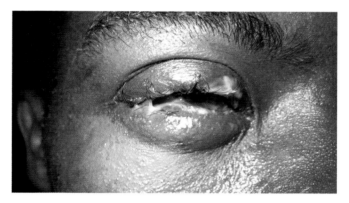

FIGURE 21.65 ■ Trachoma. Extensive inflammatory response with trichiasis in a Haitian patient. (Photo contributor: Seth W. Wright, MD.)

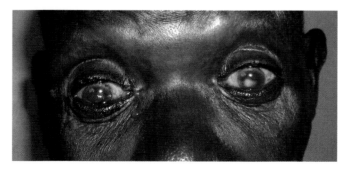

FIGURE 21.66 ■ Trachoma. Chronic corneal scarring with excessive tearing in an African patient. (Photo contributor: Meg Jack, MD.)

Clinical Summary

The epidemiology of snakebites in tropical regions differs considerably from that seen in more temperate climates. In general, the absolute number of venomous snakes is higher in the tropics and snakes are often located in areas of high population density. The prevalence of bites are also higher due to differences in agricultural and hunting practices, high rates of flooding, lack of adequate footwear in many locations, and housing that allows infiltration of snakes into living areas.

The annual mortality of snakebite in India possibly exceeds 20,000 and has been stated to be the fifth most common cause of death in Burma (Myanmar). In some native populations in South America up to 2% to 20% of adult deaths are from snakebite. Snakebite is a significant cause of mortality and morbidity in tropical countries and a major occupational hazard. Places where snakebites are common are often in remote locations and medical care may not be immediately available.

Signs and symptoms will depend upon the type of envenomation and the amount of toxin injected. Local pain and swelling is common. Bruising, swelling, and blistering are seen with many snakebites. Clotting disturbances and frank hemorrhage are seen with many viper bites while shock can occur from bleeding, vasodilatation, vascular leak, or myocardial depression. Elapid bites and sea snake bites are notable for neurotoxicity.

Emergency Department Treatment and Disposition

Patients should be reassured and kept as immobile as possible. Any involved extremity should be splinted. Tourniquets are usually discouraged but may be useful in some neurotoxic snakebites. Many modalities such as suction, incision, pumping apparatus, cryotherapy, and electrical shocks have been advocated but are of no proven benefit and may be harmful. Specific antivenin is used as indicated but is often not available or prohibitively expensive.

Pearls

1. Venomous snakes can be found at altitudes as high as 4000 m in equatorial tropical regions.
2. Neurotoxicity is seen in bites of elapids such as kraits, coral snakes, mambas, and cobras, but is not a feature of the African spitting cobra. The most common cause of death in neurotoxic envenomation is respiratory paralysis.
3. Ptosis is often an early sign of neurotoxicity.
4. Snake venom ophthalmia is the syndrome caused by the spitting cobras. Severe pain, swelling, and corneal ulceration are seen and blindness can ensue as a secondary complication.
5. A simple bedside 20-minute blood clotting test can be used to determine the presence of significant coagulopathy in areas without laboratory coagulation capability.

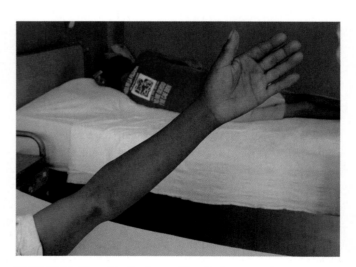

FIGURE 21.67 ■ Fer-De-Lance Bite. Patient was bit on the index finger by *Bothrops atrox*, also known as the common lancehead or sometimes fer-de-lance, while clearing brush in rural Peru. This pit viper causes more deaths than any other New World snake. (Photo contributors: Seth W. Wright, MD and Universidad Peruana Cayetano Heredia, Lima, Peru.)

Clinical Summary

Traditional and complementary medical practices are common in all areas of the world. While frequently used in developed countries, these practices are even more prevalent in the tropics and among indigenous populations. The World Health Organization has estimated that as many as 80% of people in some countries rely upon traditional medical practices. Traditional medicine is common due to varied religious, spiritual, and cultural traditions and strongly held beliefs. Poverty, lack of education, decreased access to standard medical therapy, and mistrust of Western concepts of medicine all play a role in the prominent nature of traditional medicine in many countries.

Traditional medicine practices are as varied as the societies of the world. Local practices for acute and chronic illnesses might include prayer, meditation, diets, fasting, massage, exercise, herbal remedies, acupuncture, skin scraping, and scarification. The concepts underlying these practices are also varied. Underlying principles of traditional therapies in some societies are related to the balance or homeostasis between negative (bad, dark, devil, etc) and positive (good, light, angels, etc) forces. Ayurvedic medicine is practiced throughout South Asia and roughly translates to "knowledge of life." This common practice seeks to promote spiritual harmony based upon the theory that health exists when there is a balance between three fundamental bodily humors. Other concepts such as witchcraft or the "evil eye" are prominent in dozens of countries. The evil, or covetous, eye may be felt to be the cause of a curse, misfortune, or disease and various amulets, decorations, or procedures may be used to ward off the unwanted effects.

Pearls

1. More than 70% of Americans using traditional therapies will not inform their physician of their use.
2. The majority of pediatric fevers from malaria are treated with herbal medicines at home in many African countries.
3. Coin rubbing (cao gio) is a common treatment for minor illnesses in Southeast Asia and is commonly seen in immigrants to the United States. This should not be mistaken for child abuse.
4. Many common medications, including several important antimalarial agents, are derived from traditional herbal remedies.
5. Ayurvedic and Unani systems have a recognized place in national health programs in India and have hundreds of thousands of registered practitioners.

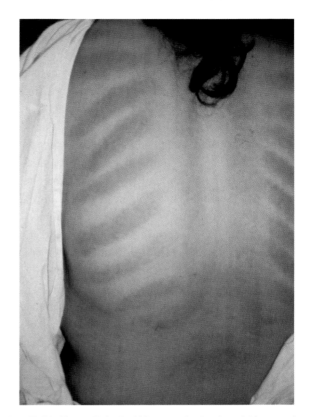

FIGURE 21.68 ■ Coin Rubbing. Typical coin-rubbing marks on the back of a Southeast Asian immigrant with a minor illness. (Photo contributor: Seth W. Wright, MD.)

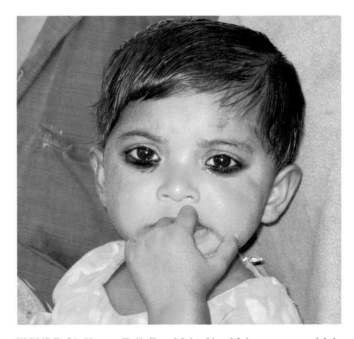

FIGURE 21.69 ■ Evil Eye Make-Up. Make-up on a girl in Bangladesh used to ward off the "evil eye," a sickness transmitted by someone who is envious, jealous, or covetous. (Photo contributor: Seth W. Wright, MD.)

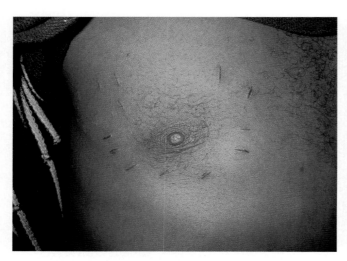

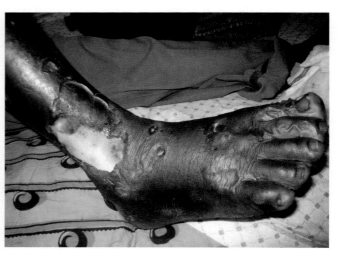

FIGURE 21.70 ■ Traditional Healing Practice. Razor marks placed by a traditional healer in a Zambian patient with fever and cough. A chest x-ray showed an infiltrate corresponding to the razor marks. (Photo contributor: Seth W. Wright, MD.)

FIGURE 21.71 ■ Traditional Healing Practice. Necrotizing fasciitis of the leg and foot as a complication of a Ugandan traditional healing practice. A traditional healer had made small ankle razor wounds for treatment of pedal edema. (Photo contributor: Seth W. Wright, MD.)

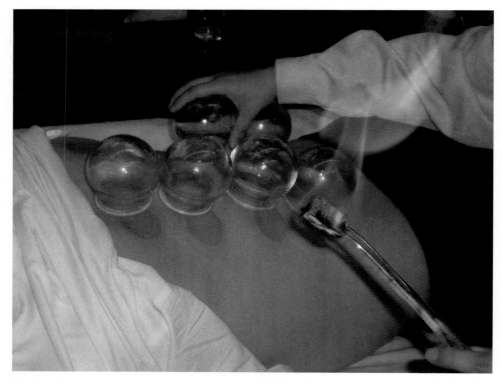

FIGURE 21.72 ■ Fire Cupping. Fire cupping is used in traditional Chinese medicine for a variety of ailments including musculoskeletal pain and various respiratory, digestive, and gynecologic diseases. The distinctive temporary cupping marks develop as a result of the vacuum that forms within the cups as the heated air cools. (Photo contributor: Allison Bollinger, MD.)

Chapter 22

AIRWAY PROCEDURES

Steven J. White
Richard M. Levitan
Lawrence B. Stack

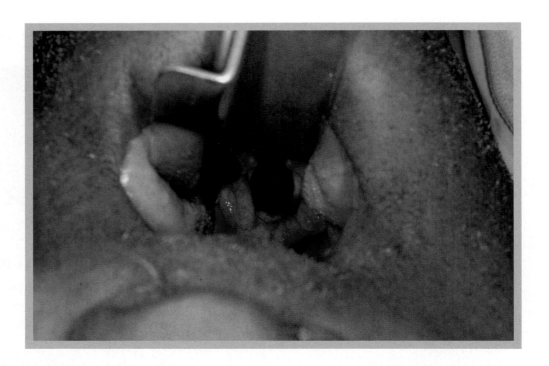

MAXIM: *Patients will not die if they are not intubated; they will die if their lungs are not ventilated and their blood is not oxygenated.*

Summary

The goal for airway management in any patient must be to maintain adequate ventilation and oxygenation. This does not necessarily mean intubation. Correct bag-valve-mask (BVM) ventilation/oxygenation technique is an underrated skill that will buy you time in the patient with a difficult airway. Proper steps for optimal two-person BVM ventilation include:

1. Positioning—ear to sternal notch alignment (when clinical scenario permits). Neck slightly flexed, head slightly extended.

2. Jaw thrust—displace mandible anteriorly with pressure from long, ring and small fingers on mandible, not soft tissues.

3. Mask compression—thumb and index fingers should apply firm pressure to face and nasal bridge.

4. Oral/nasal airways—may help maintain airway patency during BVM ventilation.

5. Use 7mg/kg tidal volume, over 1 to 2 seconds at 12 breaths/min.

Pearls

1. Be an expert at BMV ventilation.

2. Ear to sternal notch positioning is most beneficial in obese patients and those with obstructive sleep apnea.

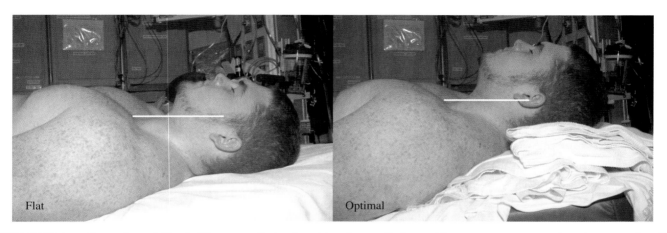

Flat

Optimal

FIGURE 22.1 ■ Ear to Sternal Notch Alignment. Optimal position for ventilation and laryngoscopy occurs when the external auditory canal and the sternal notch are aligned in the horizontal plane. This position optimizes airway patency and ventilation mechanics. (Photo contributor: Lawrence B. Stack, MD.)

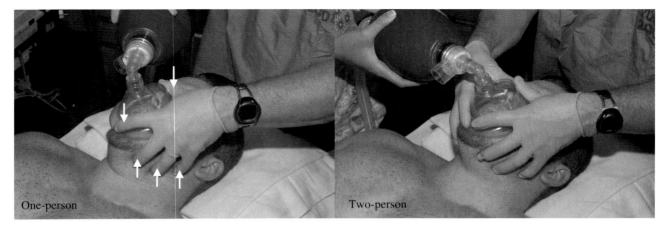

One-person

Two-person

FIGURE 22.2 ■ Bag-Valve-Mask Ventilation. Correct positioning and forces during bag-valve-mask ventilation are demonstrated for the one- and two-person techniques. Upward force on the mandible, not soft tissue, is key to effective jaw-thrust technique. (Photo Contributor: Lawrence B. Stack, MD.)

3. Keeping dentures in place facilitates BVM while removing them facilitates orotracheal intubation.

4. Mid-face and mandibular disfiguration from whatever cause will interfere with optimal BVM ventilation.

5. Consider LMA, Combitube, Air-Q if unable to intubate or obtain adequate seal for BVM ventilation.

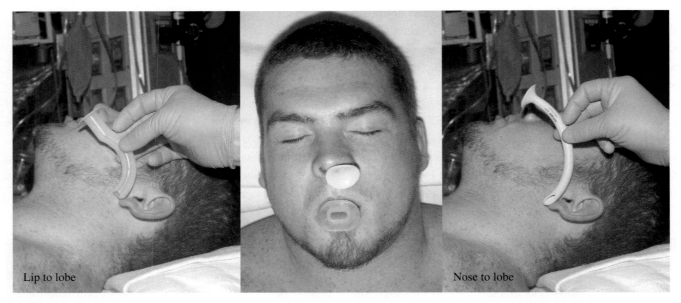

Lip to lobe

Nose to lobe

FIGURE 22.3 ■ Nasal and Oral Airways. Appropriate sized and placed nasal and oral airways maximize upper airway patency during bag-valve-mask ventilation. (Photo contributor: Lawrence B. Stack, MD.)

MAXIM: *Patients with airway problems should be positioned for their comfort, not ours.*

Summary

If physically able and mentation is normal, a patient with airway difficulty will assume a position which optimizes their airway patency and gas exchange, usually sitting up and leaning forward. Such patients include those with incomplete airway obstruction, flash pulmonary edema, and massive airway bleeding from oropharyngeal trauma. Unfortunately, during preparation for intubation, such patients often are placed supine prematurely, increasing the patient's respiratory distress and anxiety, increasing the likelihood of spontaneous emesis and aspiration, and decreasing his ability to handle oropharyngeal bleeding or secretions. In these clinical situations, we should rethink the desire to immediately place a patient supine for endotracheal intubation. Intubation can be accomplished with the patient sitting up, by either:

1. Altering the intubation technique
2. Altering the intubator position relative to the patient

Pearls

1. Keep patients in optimal position for spontaneous ventilation until they are sedated just prior to intubation, then, place them supine.
2. Consider intubating a patient sitting upright if you feel the supine position will compromise their ability to be ventilated.
3. Titrating ketamine in small doses (10 mg every 1-2 minutes) may facilitate intubation in a patient who is awake and sitting upright.

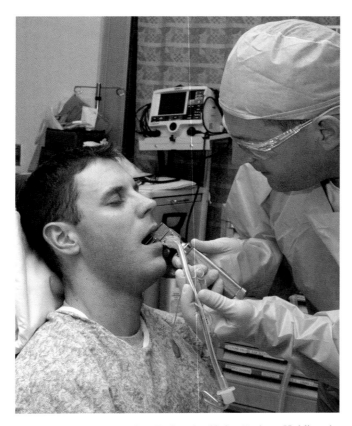

FIGURE 22.4 ■ Intubation Facing the Sitting Patient. Holding the laryngoscope in the right hand and displacing the mandible forward and passage of the tube with the left hand is an alternative position to supine intubation. (Photo contributor: Lawrence B. Stack, MD.)

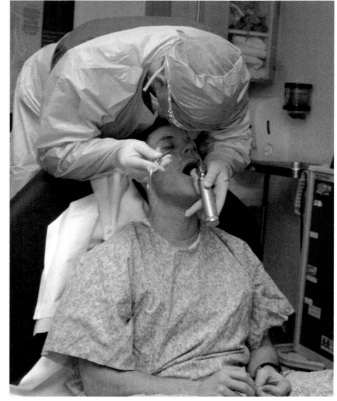

FIGURE 22.5 ■ Intubation above the Sitting Patient. Standing above a patient and intubating in the conventional manner is an alternative airway management position in a patient who may be difficult to ventilate in the supine position. An assistant may be necessary to hold the patient upright if sedated and/or paralyzed. (Photo contributor: Lawrence B. Stack, MD.)

MAXIM: *Endotracheal intubation is not always the best initial intervention for airway problems.*

Summary

Some patients in respiratory distress may benefit from other interventions, short of intubation. Patients with flash pulmonary edema may have dramatic improvement with intravenous nitroglycerin, intravenous furosemide, and BiPAP (Bi-Level Positive Airway Pressure) ventilation. Patients with airway narrowing (edema, neoplasm, stricture, foreign body) can have significant decreased work of breathing by decreasing airway resistance to inspired gas using administration of helium-oxygen (HELIOX) mixture. HELIOX, usually as a 78:22 helium: oxygen mixture, is much less dense than either air or 100% oxygen by virtue of helium replacing nitrogen or oxygen, respectively. This lowers resistance to laminar flow by as much as 25% to 20% and the effects are immediate.

Pearl

1. Alternative ventilatory adjuncts include HELIOX, CPAP, BiPAP, and Vapotherm. These adjuncts may prevent the need for intubation in selected patients.

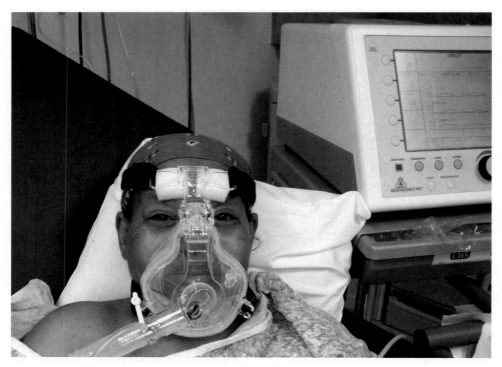

FIGURE 22.6 ■ Bi-Level Positive Airway Pressure. This patient with COPD rapidly improved with the application of BiPAP. (Photo contributor: Steven J. White, MD.)

MAXIM: *The most important initial airway intervention may be to ask for help.*

Summary

Clinical scenarios where asking for help include:

1. The patient with possible laryngeal injury/tracheal disruption, for whom a nonendoscopic intubation attempt can result in tracheal disruption and fatally lost airway

2. The patient who has recently undergone neck surgery, who has pending loss of airway from an expanding hematoma; definitive and life-saving intervention in this case is to open up the recent incision and evacuate the hematoma

3. The patient with suspected epiglottitis, where an immediate operative tracheostomy or cricothyroidotomy may be required if intubation fails due to epiglottic edema

Pearls

1. Emergency physicians are airway experts, but know your limitations.

2. Do not let your ego get in the way of proper patient airway management and care.

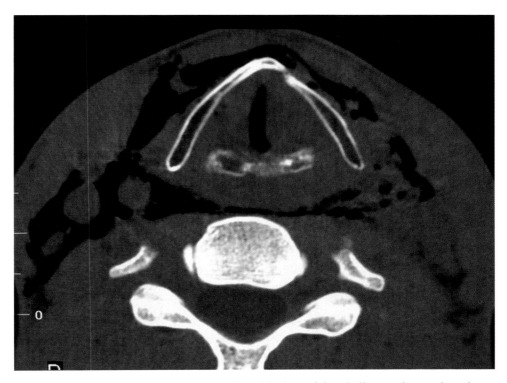

FIGURE 22.7 ■ Laryngeal Fracture. This 17-year-old male was kicked in the neck by a bull at a rodeo causing a laryngeal fracture. (Photo contributor: Rudy Kink, MD.)

MAXIM: *Think before you paralyze.*

Summary

Before committing to rapid-sequence induction (RSI) for direct laryngoscopy, consider the following:

1. Are any planned medications contraindicated?
2. Can rescue ventilation be achieved?
3. Is direct laryngoscopy possible?
4. What are my secondary and tertiary backup plans in the event of primary plan failure?
5. Are my equipment and personnel ready for RSI?

Pearls

1. A good backup plan to direct laryngoscopy should have at least one alternative intubation technique, one alternative ventilation technique, and one surgical airway technique.
2. Prepared equipment, correct patient position, proper drug dosing, having a backup plan, effective communication, and good technique will promote first-pass intubation.

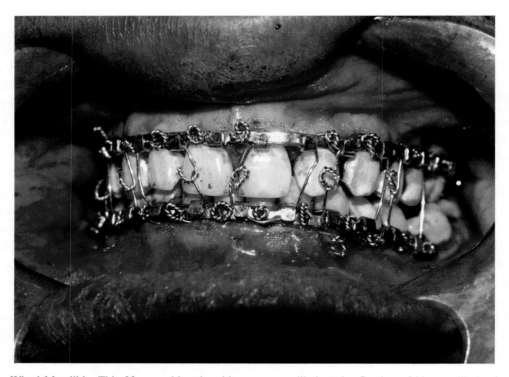

FIGURE 22.8 ■ Wired Mandible. This 33-year-old male with recent mandibular wire fixation of his mandibular fracture. A nasal or neck approach would be the only options for an emergency airway in this patient if no wire cutters were available. (Photo contributor: David Effron, MD.)

Patient Preparation

The optimal position to maximize laryngoscopic visualization of the larynx is:

1. The head extended
2. The neck flexed
3. The base of the ear aligned with the sternal notch (see Fig. 22.1)
4. The facial plane horizontal, parallel to the ceiling

This position most closely replicates in a supine posture that which the patient would assume sitting up. For very large individuals or those with significant morbid obesity, this may require creation of a textile ramp of blankets, sheets, or towels to raise the head and shoulders to proper elevation and alignment.

Technique

Optimal Epiglottoscopy

The key to using the laryngoscope to optimally visualize the glottic opening is to first visualize and control the epiglottis, a relatively fixed anterior structure. Pulmonary secretions, blood, and/or vomitus that pools in the posterior pharynx may obscure the posterior laryngeal structures, dependent with gravity. The epiglottis itself may be camouflaged in this pool of goo. One should carefully insert the laryngoscope blade with a goal of adequately visualizing *and controlling* the epiglottis. Failure to do so risks inserting the laryngoscope blade too deeply, and often results in displacing the larynx anteriorly to expose the esophagus, which, as a consequence of anterior-ward tension on the laryngoscope blade, may then look like a glottic opening begging for a tube. By carefully controlling the epiglottis, the intubating clinician will be able to locate important airway landmarks. Be careful to displace the tongue to the left side as you insert the blade. If the bulk of the tongue wraps around the blade, it can both impair your view and impede insertion of the endotracheal (ET) tube.

Progressive visualization of laryngeal structures is predictable:

1. Uvula and posterior pharynx
2. Epiglottis
3. Posterior arytenoids cartilages and interarytenoid notch
4. Glottic opening
5. Vocal cords
6. Esophagus

Bimanual Laryngoscopy

Even with well-performed laryngoscopy, adequate visualization of the laryngeal structures may be difficult. Bimanual laryngoscopy (external laryngeal manipulation by the operator), where the laryngoscopist performs laryngoscopy while simultaneously manipulating the external larynx facilitates optimal visualization. This eliminates any delay or miscommunication between an assistant and laryngoscopist. Once optimal position is found, an assistant can maintain that position. Alternatively, an assistant's hand, placed on the laryngeal structures, guided by the laryngoscopist's hand can maintain optimal position after the laryngoscopist removes his hand from the assistant's hand.

Optimizing Biomechanics

Holding the laryngoscope handle and blade where the proximal end of the blade is in the palm of the hand creates a natural extension of the forearm and provides fine control of the blade tip. Effort mechanics are more efficient with this grip. Placing the elbow close to the body requires less effort and more mechanical control than if the elbow abducted from the body.

Lip Commissure Retraction

The lip commissure is the junction of the upper and lower lips. Lateral retraction of the patient's right lip commissure by an assistant facilitates visualization of oral structures and insertion of the ET tube into the oral cavity. Retraction of the lip commissure aids in keeping the ET tube from blocking the view of the glottic opening during advancement of the ET tube. Using the retracted lip commissure as a fulcrum or "toggle," gives optimal control of the ET tube tip, especially when the stylet is in the "straight to cuff" shape. Retraction may also facilitate intubation by allowing clockwise rotation of the tube if the ET tube tip becomes hung up on the proximal tracheal cartilages.

Stylet Shape

A stylet should be used with all oral intubations in which a laryngoscope is employed. The laryngoscopist will typically fashion an inexpensive stylet, essentially a malleable wire, into a shape of their preference, to permit control of the distal ET tube tip. One should take care not to place too much bend or curvature to the stylet, because such a configuration can actually impair the glottic view and control of the ET tube tip. Optimal stylet configuration has been described as "straight to the cuff" and then a gentle anterior bend of 30 degrees.

Even with a correct bend on the stylet, it may be difficult to advance the styletted ET tube into the trachea. The tip of the left-sided beveled tube can impact and catch on the anterior tracheal cartilages, preventing advancement. This can often be remedied with a generous clockwise or rightward rotation of tube and stylet, which acts to rotate the bevel anteriorly and depress the ET tube tip.

Pearls

1. The key to first-pass intubation success is identification and control of the epiglottis during direct laryngoscopy.
2. The glottic opening lies between the epiglottis and inter-arytenoid notch. Identification and passing the tube between these structures will improve first-pass success.
3. While most intubations are performed without difficulty, if a difficult airway is anticipated and there is time to prepare, optimize the patient's ear-to sternal notch position.

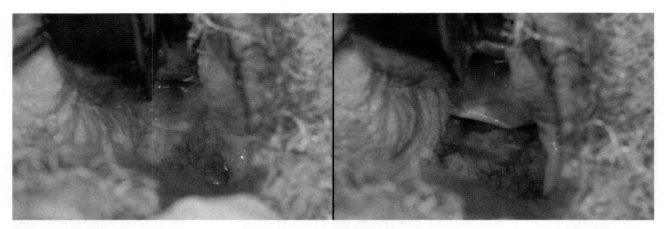

FIGURE 22.9 ■ Epiglottic Camouflage. Vomitus, blood, and pulmonary secretions may pool in the posterior pharynx and obscure the gravity-dependent epiglottis. Elevating anterior laryngeal structures will expose the epiglottis. (Photo contributor: Lawrence B. Stack, MD.)

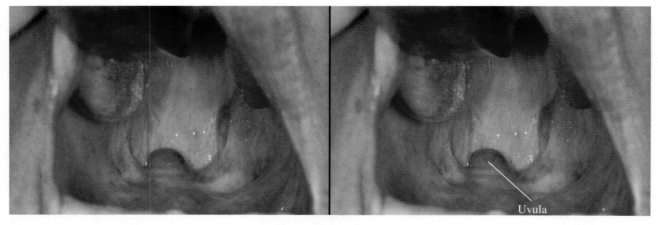

FIGURE 22.10A ■ Progressive Visualization—Uvula. The uvula and posterior pharynx are the first structures visualized during correct laryngoscopic technique. (Photo contributor: Lawrence B. Stack, MD.)

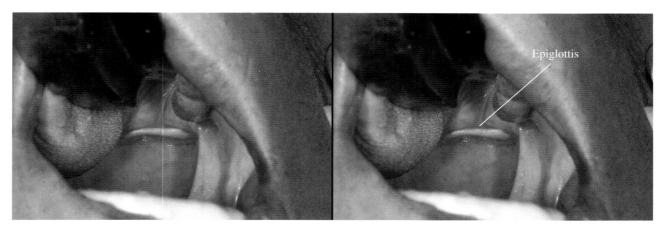

FIGURE 22.10B ■ Progressive Visualization—Epiglottis. The key to first-pass intubation is finding and identifying the epiglottis laryngoscopy. Following epiglottis will take one to the glottic opening. (Photo contributor: Lawrence B. Stack, MD.)

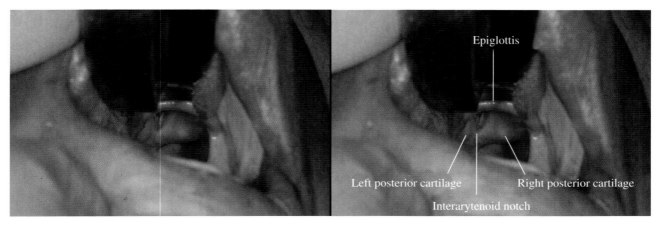

FIGURE 22.10C ■ Progressive Visualization—Interarytenoid Notch. The interarytenoid notch is a vertical cleft between the posterior cartilages. Above the notch lies the glottic opening. Below the notch is the esophagus. (Photo contributor: Lawrence B. Stack, MD.)

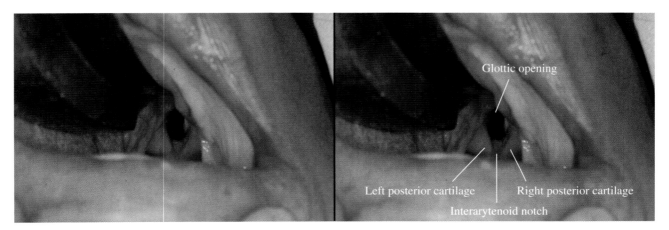

FIGURE 22.10D ■ Progressive Visualization—Glottic Opening. The posterior glottic opening is seen before the vocal cords are visualized. (Photo contributor: Lawrence B. Stack, MD.)

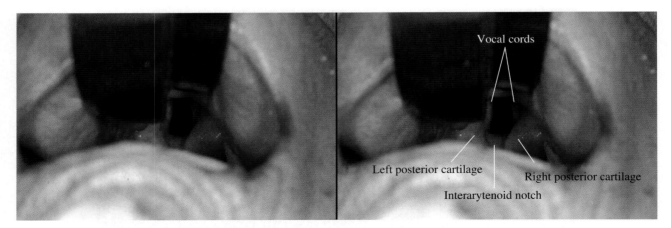

FIGURE 22.10E ■ Progressive Visualization during Laryngoscopy—Vocal Cords. The vocal cords have a distinct white appearance. (Photo contributor: Lawrence B. Stack, MD.)

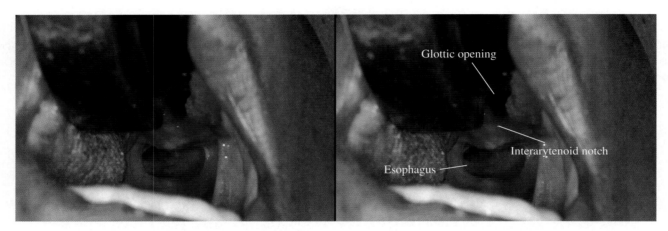

FIGURE 22.10F ■ Progressive Visualization during Laryngoscopy—Esophagus. The esophagus lies directly below the interarytenoid notch. (Photo contributor: Lawrence B. Stack, MD.)

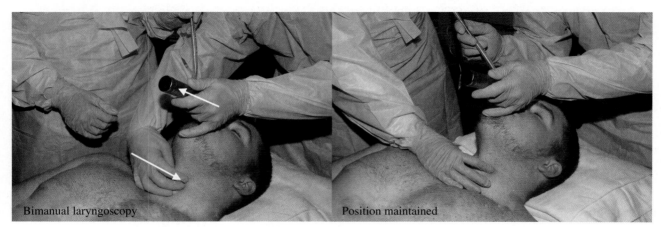

FIGURE 22.11 ■ Bimanual Laryngoscopy. Laryngoscopist uses right hand to manipulate laryngeal structures for optimal visualization during laryngoscopy. Once optimal position is identified, an assistant maintains it during intubation. (Photo contributor: Lawrence B. Stack, MD.)

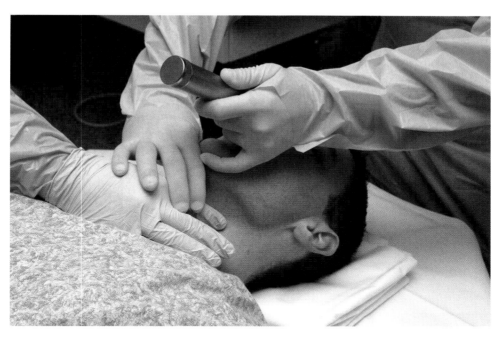

FIGURE 22.12 ▪ Bimanual Laryngoscopy. An alternative technique is to have the laryngoscopist place their hand on top of the assistant's hand which is on the laryngeal structures. When optimal visualization of laryngeal structures is made, the laryngoscopist removes their hand while the assistant maintains appropriate positioning. (Photo contributor: Lawrence B. Stack, MD.)

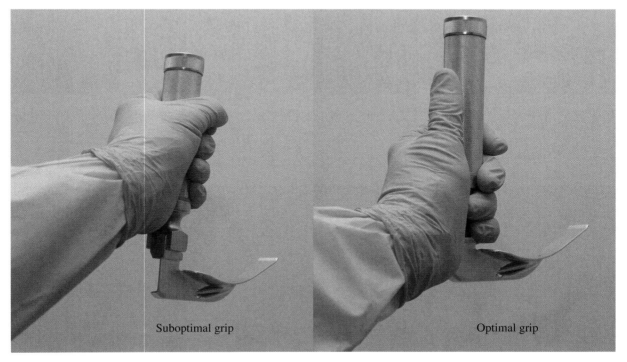

FIGURE 22.13 ▪ Laryngoscope Grip. The laryngoscope should be gripped as low as possible and the thumb extended. This makes a natural extension of the forearm. (Photo contributor: Lawrence B. Stack, MD.)

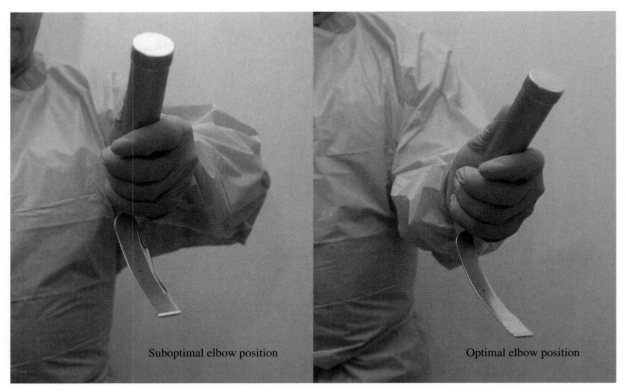

Suboptimal elbow position

Optimal elbow position

FIGURE 22.14 ▪ Laryngoscope Biomechanics. Keeping the elbow close to the body requires less effort and more control during laryngoscopy. (Photo contributor: Lawrence B. Stack, MD.)

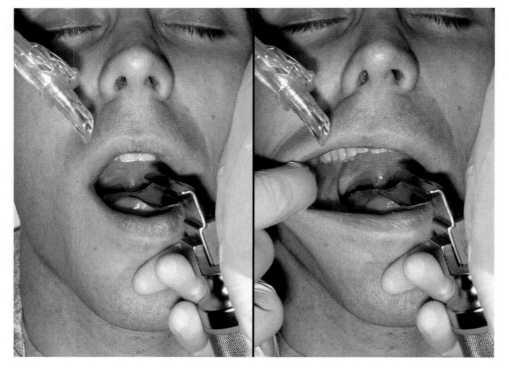

FIGURE 22.15 ▪ Lip Retraction. An assistant performs this maneuver as the laryngoscopist introduces the tube into the oral cavity while maintaining visualization of critical structures. (Photo contributor: Lawrence B. Stack, MD.)

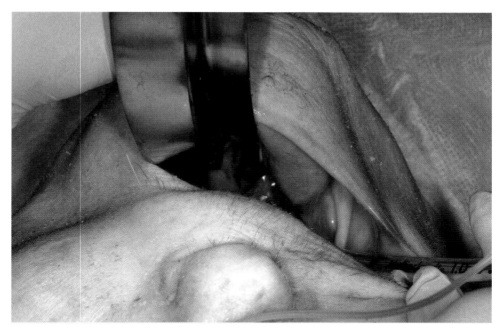

FIGURE 22.16 ■ Toggling of the ET Tube. Use the retracted lip commissure as a fulcrum allows fine control of the ET tube tip during intubation. (Photo contributor: Lawrence B. Stack, MD.)

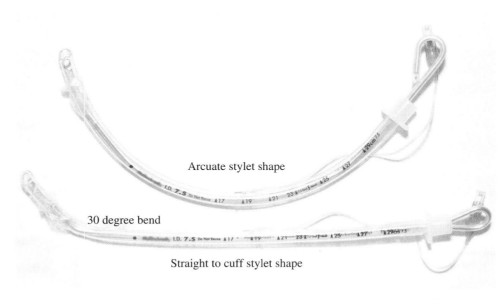

FIGURE 22.17 ■ Stylet Shape. Straight to cuff with a 30 degree bend is the optimal stylet shape as this offers the most ET tube tip control and view of the glottic opening. (Photo contributor: Lawrence B. Stack, MD.)

Equipment

The Eschmann stylet, also known as a "gum elastic bougie" or simply "bougie," is a 60-cm long, flexible introducer, which is designed to assist intubation of the anterior larynx, especially those with an "epiglottis-only" view. The tip of the Eschmann stylet has an anterior fixed flexion with an angle of 40 degrees to facilitate entering an anterior glottic opening.

Technique

Using a laryngoscope, one obtains the best view possible of the glottic opening. In the case of limited glottic view, the Eschmann stylet is inserted such that the tip is introduced just under the epiglottis and probes for the glottic opening. The intubator should feel a tactile "pop" as the bougie enters the trachea and he may also have a tactile sensation of "speed bumps" as the bougie is advanced and tracks across the tracheal cartilaginous rings. However, the more sensitive indicator of tracheal bougie position is the resistance encountered as the tip abuts against the carina, at approximately 27 to 30 cm. Should the bougie be inserted into the esophagus, no such endpoint is encountered.

While continuing to hold anterior traction with the laryngoscope, the laryngoscopist should direct an assistant to thread the endotracheal tube over the Eschmann stylet again while maintaining anterior traction; the intubator should then advance the ET tube over the Eschmann stylet to the appropriate insertion depth. Resistance to tube advancement may indicate "arytenoid arrest" and can be remedied by rotating the tube counterclockwise 90 degrees followed by attempts to advance the ET tube tip past the arytenoid cartilages.

A one-handed technique can be employed in which the ET tube is preloaded onto the bougie, which is then curled in the right hand with approximately 20 cm of bougie protruding through the distal end. The laryngoscopist performs laryngoscopy as before, maintains anterior traction on the mandible, and inserts the bougie through the glottic opening as above. He then uncoils the ET tube/bougie and advances the pair until resistance of the carina is met, confirming intratracheal position. The ET tube is then advanced to the proper depth and the bougie is removed.

Use of the Eschmann stylet does not have to be limited to the anticipated difficult airway. In fact, to gain proficiency, we recommend that practitioners use it as their routine stylet, as it has come to be used in the UK. The practitioner will then be better prepared for the unanticipated anterior larynx/limited view airway.

Pearls

1. The bougie is an excellent adjunct in the limited view or "epiglottis view" airway.
2. The bougie is best deployed as a two-person technique.
3. Stall of ET tube advancement when using the bougie is most frequently due to catching the bevel on the right arytenoid cartilage and can be relieved by rotating the tube counterclockwise.

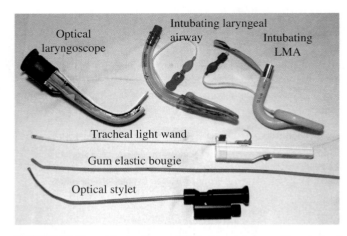

FIGURE 22.18 ■ Alternatives to Direct Laryngoscopy. If optimized direct laryngoscopy does not allow for visualization of the glottis, alternative methods should be considered. (Photo contributor: Lawrence B. Stack, MD.)

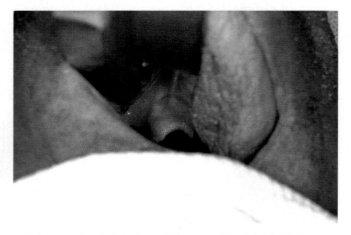

FIGURE 22.19 ■ Epiglottis-Only View. In this view, despite optimal laryngoscopy, the epiglottis may be all that is seen. The bougie may be a reasonable alternative in this situation. (Photo contributor: Lawrence B. Stack, MD.)

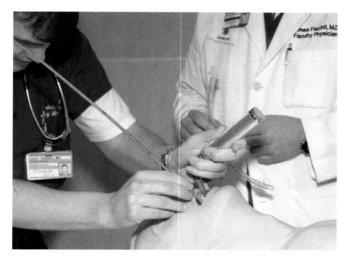

FIGURE 22.20 ■ Passing the Bougie. The two-person technique for using the bougie. Standard DL is preformed and the bougie is used like a stylet, but hugging the underside of the epiglottis. (Photo contributor: Lawrence B. Stack, MD.)

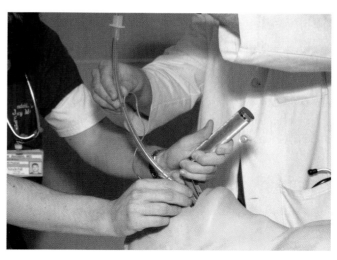

FIGURE 22.22 ■ Tube over the Bougie. An assistant places the bougie over the tube while direct laryngoscopy is maintained. (Photo contributor: Lawrence B. Stack, MD.)

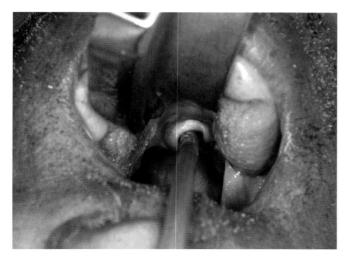

FIGURE 22.21 ■ Bougie under the Epiglottis. Here the bougie is hugging the underside of the epiglottis. Tracheal rings can be felt by "tactile speed bumps" confirming correct placement. (Photo contributor: Lawrence B. Stack, MD.)

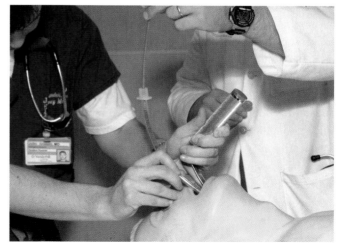

FIGURE 22.23 ■ Tube Advancement Stall. Stalling of tube advancement while using the bougie is most likely due to catching the right arytenoids cartilage with the bevel of the ET tube. (Photo contributor: Lawrence B. Stack, MD.)

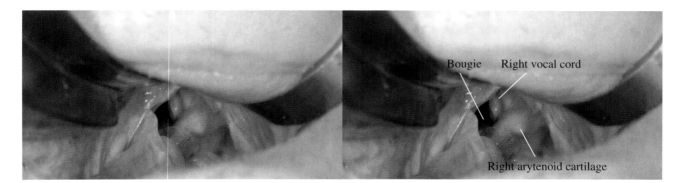

FIGURE 22.24 ■ Arytenoid "Arrest." The right arytenoid cartilage is caught between the bougie and the bevel of the ET tube, stalling advancement of the tube. Counterclockwise rotation of the tube will release the tube and allow it to advance. (Photo contributor: Lawrence B. Stack, MD.)

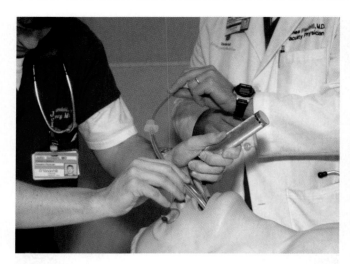

FIGURE 22.25 ▪ Arytenoid "Escape." Turning the tube counter-clockwise, as shown here, will release the bevel of the ET tube from the arytenoid cartilage and allow the tube to advance. (Photo contributor: Lawrence B. Stack, MD.)

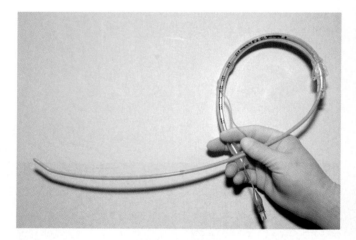

FIGURE 22.26 ▪ One-Handed Bougie Configuration. Holding the bougie in this manner will allow one person to pass the bougie. (Photo contributor: Lawrence B. Stack, MD.)

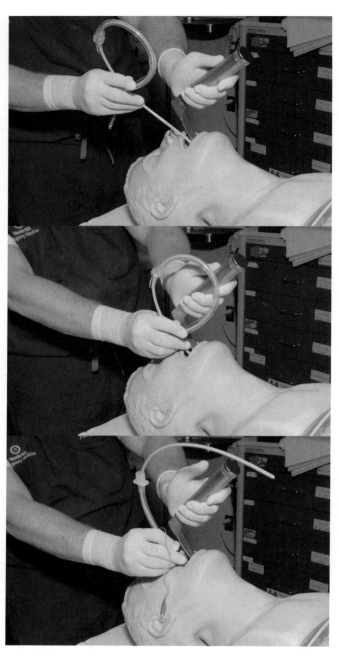

FIGURE 22.27 ▪ One-Handed Bougie Technique. Passing the bougie using the one-handed technique. See text for details. (Photo contributor: Lawrence B. Stack, MD.)

Equipment

Optical stylets consist of fiberoptic bundles (image and light-conducting) within a malleable metal conduit, attached to a handle/power source. Two common optical stylets in use are the Levitan and the Shikani models. The Levitan stylet is shorter and easier to wield but requires that the ET tube be precut to 28 cm in length, a design compromise to accommodate tubes of different sizes. An optical stylet can greatly facilitate intubation of the anterior larynx. Since one cannot always predict the difficult anterior airway, we believe that it is sensible to use one of these stylets for each standard laryngoscopic intubation.

Technique

Optical stylets can be used in two ways: (1) with ET tube loaded, the optical stylet can be used much like a conventional stylet, in concert with a laryngoscope. In the event of epiglottis-only view with the laryngoscope, the styletted ET tube is advanced under the epiglottis, the glottic opening visualized, and the tube/stylet is advanced into the trachea. Position is readily confirmed by visualization of anterior tracheal rings, (2) the optical stylet and ET tube can be inserted without use of a laryngoscope, by elevating the mandible using the left hand, and guiding the stylet around the curvature of the tongue.

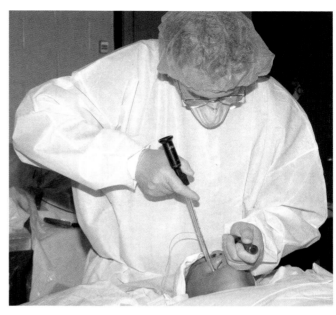

FIGURE 22.29 ■ Optical Stylet as Stylet. The optical stylet used as a conventional stylet during laryngoscopy. If the view is "epiglottis only," the device can be used to view laryngeal structures. (Photo contributor: Lawrence B. Stack, MD.)

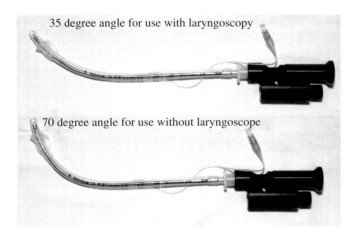

35 degree angle for use with laryngoscopy

70 degree angle for use without laryngoscope

FIGURE 22.28 ■ Optical Stylet. The Levitan optical stylet with varying angles depending if a laryngoscope is used. (Photo contributor: Lawrence B. Stack, MD.)

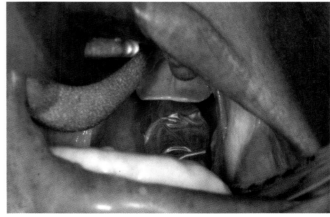

FIGURE 22.30 ■ Epiglottis-Only View. This demonstrates the "epiglottis-only" view and correct positioning of the optical stylet for viewing the laryngeal structures. Note the tip of the optical stylet is toggled just under the epiglottis. (Photo contributor: Lawrence B. Stack, MD.)

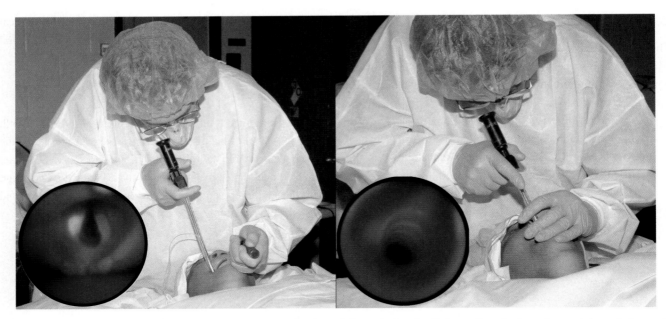

FIGURE 22.31 ■ Optical Stylet with Laryngoscopy. Note the view of the optical stylet (left panel) and when advanced through the cords (right panel). (Photo contributor: Lawrence B. Stack, MD.)

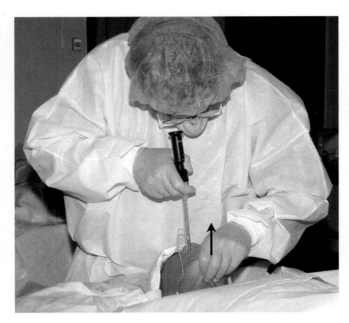

FIGURE 22.32 ■ Optical Stylet Used Alone. The optical stylet used without laryngoscopy. Note the left hand elevates the mandible. The stylet is then guided around the curvature of the tongue for laryngeal structure viewing. (Photo contributor: Lawrence B. Stack, MD.)

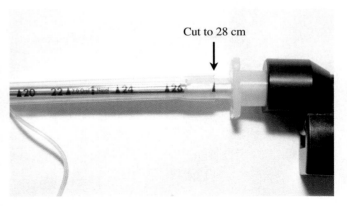

FIGURE 22.33 ■ Levitan Optical Stylet. The Levitan optical stylet requires that ET tubes be cut to 28 cm before use. (Photo contributor: Lawrence B. Stack, MD.)

Equipment

The optical laryngoscope is a relatively inexpensive device, which holds promise for the out-of-hospital environment. It consists of a curved tubular handle/blade that connects a viewing eyepiece to an illuminated prism at the tip of the device, which permits visualization of the anterior larynx. The device has clips that hold an ET tube in place in a side channel in such a way that the ET tube can be visualized as it is slid along the channel into the trachea. Although the optical laryngoscope does not incorporate high-quality optics (device is intended for single use), it does provide a panoramic view of the larynx. The optical laryngoscope provides an economical option for EMS and air medical crews, in addition to hospital crash carts and emergency department airway kits.

Technique

The device with ET tube attached is inserted into the mouth down the center of the tongue, neck-head neutral, advancing the device blade tip into the vallecula. The endotracheal tube is then inserted under direct visualization. If the ET tube does not align with the glottic opening, the device is slightly withdrawn and twisted slightly until the tube can be passed into the trachea.

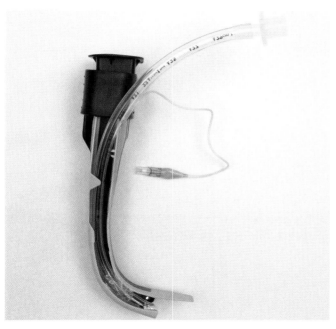

FIGURE 22.34 ■ Optical Laryngoscope. The optical laryngoscope, loaded with an ET tube. (Photo contributor: Lawrence B. Stack, MD.)

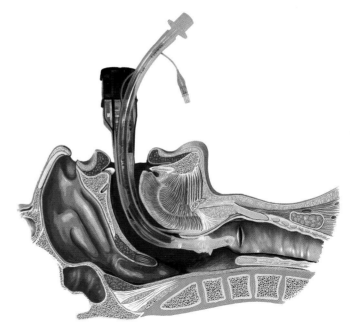

FIGURE 22.35 ■ Optical Laryngoscope in the Vallecula. Anatomical drawing demonstrating the proper placement of the tip in the vallecula. (Photo contributor: Prodol, Inc.)

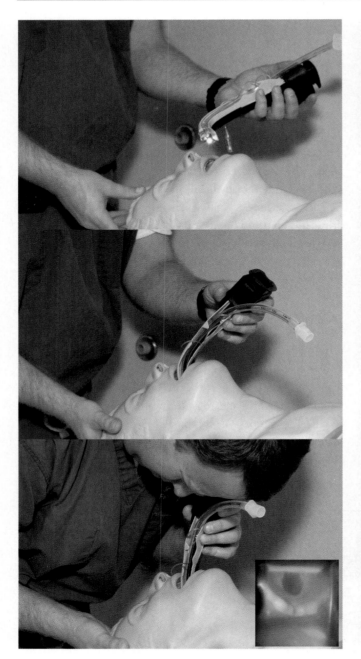

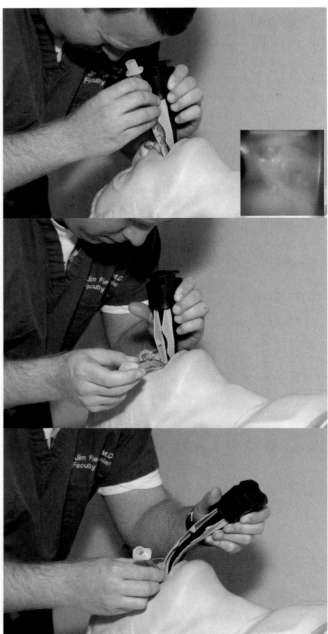

FIGURE 22.36 ■ Optical Laryngoscope Insertion. Progressive steps demonstrating insertion. Note visualization of laryngeal structures when the optical laryngoscope is in the correct position. (Photo contributor: Lawrence B. Stack, MD.)

FIGURE 22.37 ■ Optical Laryngoscope Tube Passage and Removal. Progressive steps demonstrating passage of the ET tube and removal of the optical laryngoscope by peeling the tube away from the device. (Photo contributor: Lawrence B. Stack, MD.)

Equipment

The tracheal light wand is a device which consists essentially of a bright light bulb on the end of a wire. The best tracheal light wand incorporates (a) a very bright distal light encased in a tube-like flaccid stylet, (b) a removable stiffening wire to provide rigidity and allow the stylet to conform to the required bending angle, (c) a handle which comprises a water-proof battery housing, on-off magnetic reed switch, and a track which provides for easy length adjustment of the stylet for different size endotracheal (ET) tubes. There is cam-like locking device to firmly secure the tube to the stylet. The stylet is marked in centimeter markings to align with those on the endotracheal tube, ensuring that the distal bulb is always at the proper position at the tip of the ET.

Technique

The intubation technique relies on the unique appearance and location of the transilluminated glow of the skin overlying the anterior neck to provide feedback to the intubator about the ET tube tip position and the subsequent stylet movements needed for tracheal placement and advancement. For intubation, the stylet is bent at the distal 5 cm, conveniently labeled with "BEND HERE." The bend angle is critical and depends upon the head and neck position of the patient. For a patient who is in a neutral head/neck position, such as a patient in a halo device, the stylet should be configured to about an 80 degree acute angle. If the patient is hyperflexed, a more acute angle is required, approximately 60 degrees. Finally, for patients who are hyperextended, an obtuse angle of 110 or 120 degrees would be appropriate.

The technique can be performed with the intubator facing the patient, or with the intubator at the head of the bed behind the patient. The light wand should be held in the dominant hand with a pencil grip at the ET tube hub/handle junction. With his nondominant hand, the intubator should grasp the tongue with gauze, gently distracting forward. This acts to bring the epiglottis anteriorly. The light wand/ET tube is introduced into the center of the mouth and advanced to the hypopharynx while maintaining anterior pressure, holding the elbow high and the arm abducted, to keep the stylet bulb anterior. Advancement stops when the intubator recognizes an orange glow on the anterior neck tissues or when tube advancement meets resistance. The appearance and position of this glow determines the next maneuver.

If transillumination positional feedback indicates that the tube tip is in one of the pyriform fossae, the stylet/ET tube is withdrawn slightly and rotated toward the midline and reinserted. This process is continued repeatedly in an iterative manner until the correct midline glow indicating tracheal position is encountered. At that point, the stiffening wire is

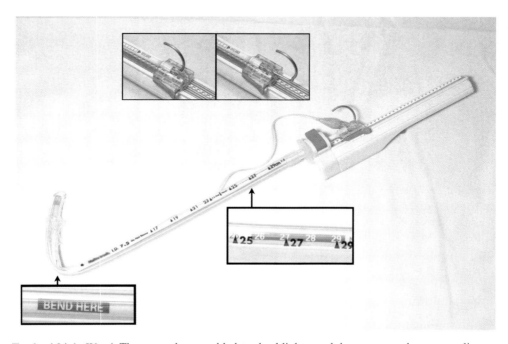

FIGURE 22.38 ■ Tracheal Light Wand. The correctly assembled tracheal light wand demonstrates the correct alignment of the centimeter markings (insert) on the tube, the correct location of the bend (insert), and the correct engagement of the wire portion of the stylet (insert). (Photo contributor: Lawrence B. Stack, MD.)

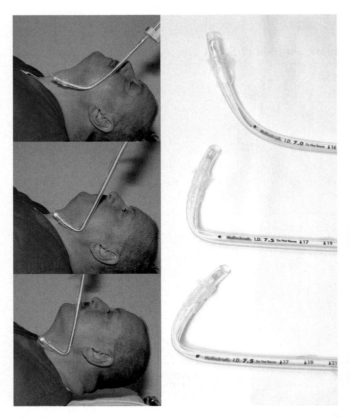

FIGURE 22.39 ■ Tracheal Light Wand Bend Angle. The head/neck position and suggested corresponding bend angle. (Photo contributor: Lawrence B. Stack, MD.)

withdrawn several centimeters, resulting in a caudad displacement of the glow as the intratracheal stylet "relaxes." The tube and stylet is then advanced until the glow just disappears below the sternal notch. The tube is now confirmed to be intratracheal and the tube tip is confirmed to be reliably in the mid-trachea, with no need for confirmatory chest radiograph.

Failure to modify the position of the transilluminated glow usually indicates that the stiffening wire has displaced from the locking notch that keeps the wire from rotating in place.

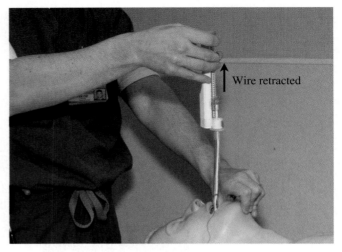

FIGURE 22.41 ■ Tracheal Light Wand Technique. Once the tracheal position is encountered, the stiffening wire is retracted several centimeters before advancing ET tube into the trachea. (Photo contributor: Lawrence B. Stack, MD.)

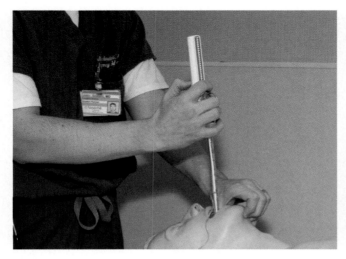

FIGURE 22.40 ■ Tracheal Light Wand Positioning. The correct position is demonstrated here. The device is placed in the center of the mouth while the left hand is lifting the tongue anteriorly. (Photo contributor: Lawrence B. Stack, MD.)

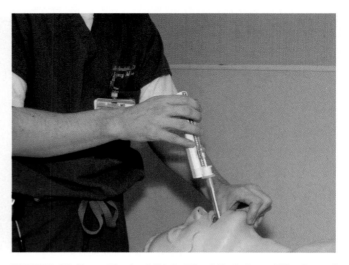

FIGURE 22.42 ■ Tracheal Light Wand Technique. ET tube and stylet are advanced until the light glow just disappears below the sternal notch. (Photo contributor: Lawrence B. Stack, MD.)

TABLE 22.1 ■ TRACHEAL LIGHT WAND MANEUVER DECISIONS			
Glow Appearance	**Position of Glow**	**Anatomic Position of Stylet Tip**	**Next Maneuver**
Bright orange, well localized	High neck/submental	Vallecula	Remove stylet, decrease acuity of bend angle
Dull orange glow	Right/left of neck midline	Right/left pyriform fossa	Partially withdraw stylet, rotate slightly to midline, re-advance, keeping tip anterior
No glow or very dim	If present, thin line at lateral neck, may be bilateral	Esophagus	Remove stylet, increase acuity of bend angle
Bright midline glow	Thyroid prominence	Glottic opening	Withdraw stiffening wire by 3 cm, advance stylet/ET tube until glow just disappears beyond sternal notch

(Photo contributor: Lawrence B. Stack, MD.)

Equipment

The Glidescope is a video laryngoscope composed of an integrated blade/handle which houses a blade tip-mounted camera and light source, connected by cable to a video LCD display. The Glidescope affords an excellent view of the laryngeal structures with little anteriorly directed force. Use of proprietary stylet, conformed to angle of Glidescope blade is recommended. A more portable version, suitable for out-of-hospital use, is marketed as the Glidescope Ranger.

Technique

The blade is inserted into the mouth, along the center of the tongue and advanced to visualize the epiglottis and laryngeal structures. Little to no anterior force is required, and, in contrast to standard laryngoscope, levering the blade is recommended to enhance the view.

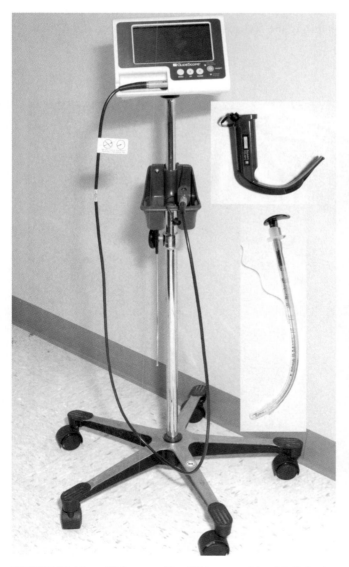

FIGURE 22.43 ■ Glidescope. The Glidescope video LDC display on a stand with blade (inset) and proprietary stylet (inset). (Photo contributor: Lawrence B. Stack, MD.)

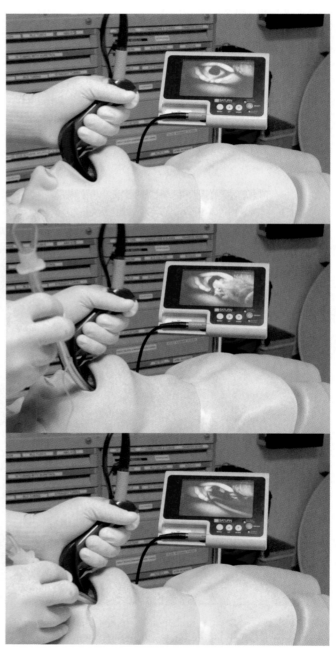

FIGURE 22.44 ■ Glidescope in Use. The Glidescope in action demonstrating progressive images of passage of an ET tube. (Photo contributor: Lawrence B. Stack, MD.)

Digital intubation relies on tactile definition of intubation landmarks, primarily the epiglottis but often the posterior cartilages and inter-arytenoid notch.

Technique

Digital intubation technique is performed with the intubator facing the patient from the side. With the gloved nondominant hand, the intubator should insert the index and third fingers into the patient's mouth. He should next "walk" the fingers down the tongue to progressively displace the tongue anteriorly as the fingers are advanced to the epiglottis. The epiglottis will have a feel similar to the earlobe. As the third finger encounters the epiglottis, the finger traps and holds the epiglottis anteriorly. The endotracheal tube, with stylet configured to an open "C," is introduced by the dominant hand into the corner of the mouth and advanced to the palmer side of the intraoral index finger. The intraoral index finger is then used to guide the ET tube tip to the third finger, where the ET tube is slipped between the epiglottis and third finger. The third finger is used to keep the ET tube anterior against the laryngeal surface of the epiglottis while the ET tube is advanced by the dominant hand and assisted by the intraoral index finger. It is often possible to palpate the arytenoid cartilages/inter-arytenoid notch, in which case one need only ensure that the ET tube tip remains anterior to those cartilages and is prevented from drifting posteriorly to the esophageal inlet. The posterior cartilages project cephalad, feeling like snake fangs. Correct ET tube position can be confirmed by palpating the arytenoid cartilages posterior to the ET tube.

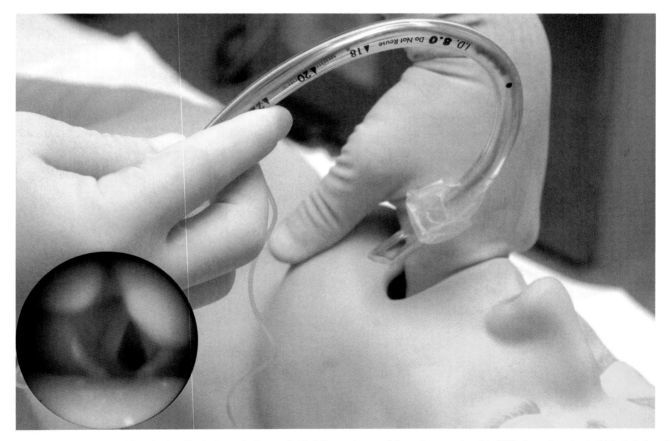

FIGURE 22.45 ■ Digital Intubation Technique. Index and third finger inserted into the mouth with "C"-shaped stylet held in left hand. Third finger holds epiglottis anteriorly (insert). (Photo contributor: Lawrence B. Stack, MD.)

The laryngeal mask airway (LMA) was originally designed to facilitate ventilation during anesthesia for short operating room procedures. It has been shown to provide improved ventilation in cardiac arrest and failed airway cases and has a shallow learning curve, promoting its use by relative novices.

Equipment

The LMA consists of a short-curved tube connected to a small mask with inflatable cuff. The shape promotes blind insertion with an endpoint detected as resistance, as the leading edge of the cuff just enters and obstructs and the esophageal inlet. The inflated cuff then seals around the laryngeal inlet. The distal "mask" incorporates a small grate to prevent prolapse of the epiglottis within the mask. The LMA has several configurations including a disposable model, the LMA "Unique" and a model that facilitates blind oral intubation, the intubating LMA, or I-LMA. LMAs are available in three adult sizes, #3 (30-50 kg), #4 (50-70 kg), and #5 (>70 kg). They are also available in pediatric sizes from size 0 to 2.5 for infants through toddlers.

Technique

The LMA is inserted into the mouth and held against the hard palate while being advanced into the hypopharynx. The LMA is advanced until resistance is met, and the cuff is then inflated with 20 to 40 mL of air to affect a seal. The mask should be lubricated prior to insertion.

Because the LMA aligns with the glottic opening, it is possible to intubate the trachea through the LMA with minimal interruption of ventilation. The distal grate prevents anything larger than a 6.0 ID ET tube through a #3 and #4, and a 7.0 ID ET tube through a #5. In addition to passing a small ET tube directly, it is also possible to pass a flexible fiberoptic scope or a rigid fiberoptic scope (Levitan or Shikani) through the LMA under direct visualization. One must be sure to have an endotracheal tube, sized to pass through the LMA, loaded onto the stylet prior to passage. It is recommended to rotate the ET tube counterclockwise 90 degrees to orient the bevel posteriorly, rotating clockwise as the tube is passed into the glottis.

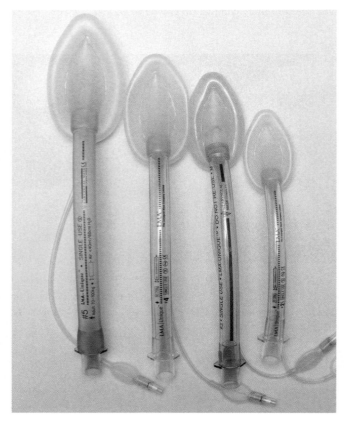

FIGURE 22.46 ■ LMA Unique. Adult sizes 3, 4, and 5 and pediatric size 2.5 are seen here. (Photo contributor: Lawrence B. Stack, MD.)

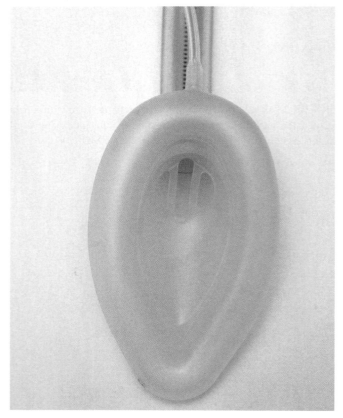

FIGURE 22.47 ■ LMA Unique. The laryngeal surface of the LMA Unique with inflated cuff. Note the "grate" which prevents epiglottic prolapse into the mask. (Photo contributor: Lawrence B. Stack, MD.)

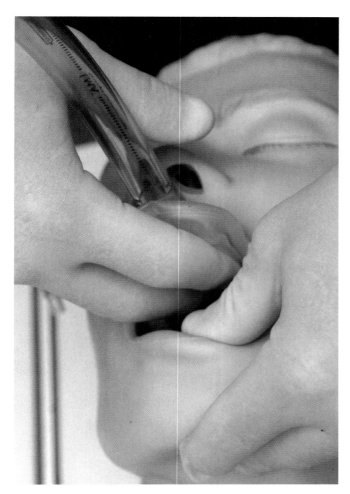

FIGURE 22.48 ■ LMA Insertion. LMA with deflated cuff is held against the hard palate during insertion by the index and third fingers. (Photo contributor: Lawrence B. Stack, MD.)

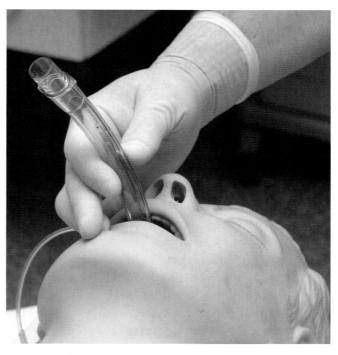

FIGURE 22.49 ■ Correct LMA Placement. The LMA is correctly seated when resistance is met. Slight adjustments may be needed once seated. (Photo contributor: Lawrence B. Stack, MD.)

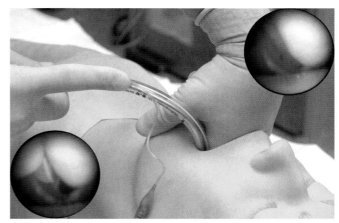

FIGURE 22.50 ■ Digital Intubation-ET Tube Passage. Intraoral index finger guides ET tube to third finger (insert) which directs the tube into the glottic opening (insert). (Photo contributor: Lawrence B. Stack, MD.)

Equipment

The intubating laryngeal mask airway (iLMA) is a modification of the original LMA and incorporates a larger metal-reinforced tube lumen with integrated metal handle and a more acute bend to facilitate insertion. Instead of the distal grate, there is a bar that elevates the epiglottis as the ET tube exits the iLMA. The manufacturer supplies a special silicone ET tube that exits the iLMA at a shallower angle, facilitating glottic passage. A well-lubricated standard ET tube can be used but must be inserted with the curve oriented opposite to the curve of the LMA, a maneuver that allows the ET tube to exit at the proper angle.

Technique

The iLMA is inserted well lubricated with cuff deflated, using the handle to keep the iLMA against the palate during insertion to prevent downfolding of the epiglottis. Once inserted, the cuff is inflated and the iLMA position is adjusted to optimize ventilation. Use of quantitative capnography, with waveform, can help to optimize the position prior to intubation.

Once the lubricated tube is passed into the trachea and the correct position is confirmed, the mask can be withdrawn by using a "tube stabilizer," either that supplied by the manufacturer or another commercially available stabilizer.

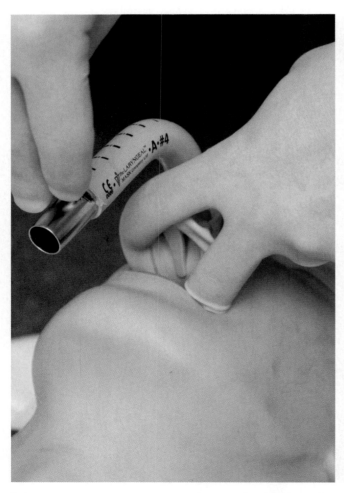

FIGURE 22.51 ■ I-LMA Insertion. I-LMA with deflated cuff is held against the hard palate during insertion by the index and third fingers. (Photo contributor: Lawrence B. Stack, MD.)

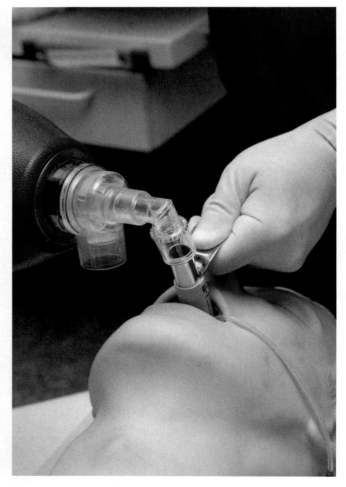

FIGURE 22.52 ■ Correct I-LMA Placement. The I-LMA is correctly seated when resistance is met. Slight adjustments may be needed once seated. Confirmation is best made with capnography. (Photo contributor: Lawrence B. Stack, MD.)

Equipment

The reusable intubating laryngeal airway (ILA) is similar in concept to the classic LMA but has structural features that provide easier and more stable insertion with less likelihood of tube kink. In addition, it has a unique "keyhole" like airway outlet which helps to direct an endotracheal (ET) tube to the midline at the proper glottic entry angle. Because it has a larger lumen, the ILA can accommodate standard ET tube up to 8.5 mm ID. The ILA comes in five sizes—1.0 (<5 kg), 1.5 (10-20 kg), 2.4 (20-50 kg), 3.5 (50-70 kg), and 4.5 (70-100 kg), accommodating maximum ET tube sizes of 4.5, 5.5, 6.5, 7.5, and 8.5 respectively.

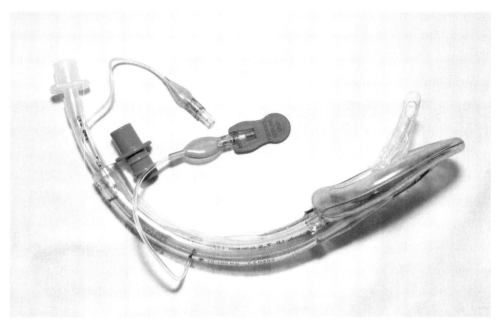

FIGURE 22.53 ■ Intubating Laryngeal Airway. Intubating laryngeal airway demonstrating an ET tube through the device lumen. (Photo contributor: Lawrence B. Stack, MD.)

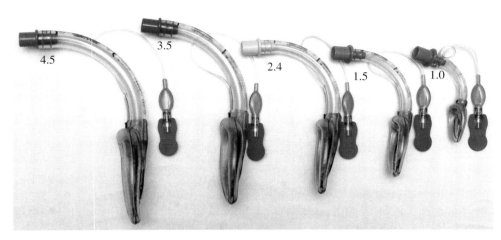

FIGURE 22.54 ■ Intubating Laryngeal Airway Sizes. Intubating laryngeal airway in five different sizes. (Photo contributor: Lawrence B. Stack, MD.)

Technique

The mandible is displaced anteriorly with a jaw lift maneuver, bringing the tongue and epiglottis forward, the ILA is then inserted into the mouth, advancing with a downward and inward force to follow the curve of the oropharynx/hypopharynx. The insertion endpoint is firm resistance to further insertion. The cuff is then inflated with approximately 20 mL of air or until the pilot balloon is firm. Ventilation can proceed by attaching a ventilating bag to the proximal port.

Intubation can be accomplished through the ILA in a well-sedated/chemically paralyzed patient after first removing the proximal 15-mm adaptor port. A well-lubricated standard endotracheal (ET) tube can then be inserted through the ILA. This procedure can also be aided by using a light wand or optical stylet through the ET tube to facilitate optimal alignment for intubation.

Once the ET tube is inserted, the ILA can be easily removed by inserting the disposable tube stabilizer/stylet.

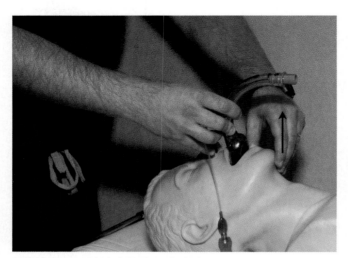

FIGURE 22.55 ■ Intubating Laryngeal Airway Insertion. The ILA is inserted by displacing the tongue and jaw anteriorly. The ILA is advanced down the curvature of the oropharynx and hypopharynx. (Photo contributor: Lawrence B. Stack, MD.)

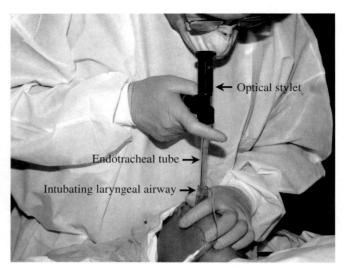

FIGURE 22.57 ■ Optical Stylet Facilitation of ET tube Placement. An optical stylet is placed through the ET tube that is within the lumen of the Air-Q. (Photo contributor: Lawrence B. Stack, MD.)

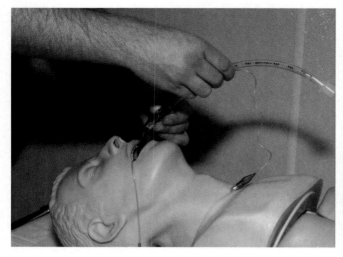

FIGURE 22.56 ■ ET tube Insertion through ILA. ET tube is advanced through the ILA. (Photo contributor: Lawrence B. Stack, MD.)

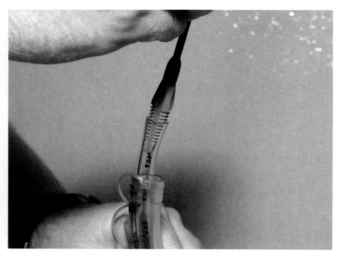

FIGURE 22.58 ■ Intubating Laryngeal Airway Removal. Removal of the ILA while keeping the ET tube in place is accomplished by using the disposable tube stabilizer (blue). (Photo contributor: Lawrence B. Stack, MD.)

The Combitube is dual-lumen, double-cuff tubular device which is designed to be inserted blindly, to enter either the esophagus (most likely) or trachea. It can be an airway of last resort in management of the failed airway and is within the skill set of advanced life support and, in some jurisdictions, basic life support EMS providers.

Equipment

The Combitube comes in two sizes: 37F for patients of height from 4 to 6'6" and 41F for patients taller than 6'6".

Technique

Combitube insertion is straightforward, but should be reserved for those patients who have no active gag, and are unresponsive or chemically sedated. Placement is facilitated by distracting the mandible anteriorly and can be accomplished most easily by using a laryngoscope in the usual manner. However, Combitube insertion is commonly done using manual displacement. As the mandible is displaced anteriorly, the Combitube, well-lubricated with water-soluble lubricant, is inserted into the mouth and advanced until the double line of the proximal tube is located at the level of the alveolar ridge. At this point, the pharyngeal cuff, with blue pilot balloon and injection port well-marked "#1," is inflated with 85 mL of air (100 mL for 41F), followed by inflation of the distal cuff (presumed esophageal) through the "#2" port colored white using 5 to 10 mL air. Ventilation is then first attempted through the #1 blue lumen, which has a blind distal end; air flow exits the #1 lumen through a series of holes and is prevented from entering the esophagus by the distal balloon which seals the proximal esophagus and from regressing through the mouth by the pharyngeal balloon which seals the hypopharynx, leaving the only course for airflow to be into the trachea to the lungs. Even though preferential esophageal intubation occurs overwhelmingly, blind tracheal placement is also possible, in which case ventilation of lumen #2—"white" will replicate endotracheal tube ventilation. In that case, the pharyngeal lumen can be deflated. One should determine the correct lumen for ventilation by the adjunctive use of capnometry, attaching the capnometer sequentially to the #1 and #2 lumens. One should be able to detect a distinct difference in capnometer reading/appearance. Choosing the wrong lumen to ventilate has the same end-effect as inadvertent esophageal intubation and the same meticulous care that is exercised in determining endotracheal tube

location should be extended to confirm the ventilating lumen of the Combitube. In the event that neither lumen provides sufficient ventilation and there is no air egress from the mouth, the pharyngeal balloon may have caused the epiglottis to fold over the tracheal inlet. This can be remedied by deflating both cuffs and pulling the Combitube back about 3 cm. Both cuffs should be reinflated and the ventilation sequence repeated.

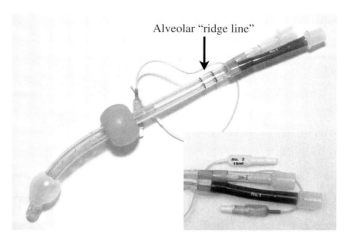

Alveolar "ridge line"

FIGURE 22.59 ■ Combitube. The 37 F Combitube for patients up to 6 ft 6 in. in height. (Photo contributor: Lawrence B. Stack, MD.)

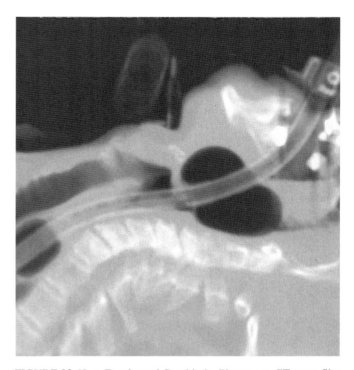

FIGURE 22.60 ■ Esophageal Combitube Placement. CT scout film demonstrating esophageal placement of the Combitube. (Photo contributor: Steven J. White, MD.)

If there appears to be an air leak from the mouth, additional air can be added to the pharyngeal balloon inflation port.

Intubation around the Combitube will require deflation of the pharyngeal cuff. Prior to Combitube removal and cuff deflation, a nasogastric suction tube should be passed into the esophagus for decompression and evacuation of stomach contents. Under direct visualization with laryngoscope or with use of optical stylet, Glidescope or flexible fiberoptic endoscopy, the clinician should direct deflation of the pharyngeal cuff only,

until the airway landmarks can be visualized. Intubation can then be performed; in the event of laryngoscopy failure, the pharyngeal cuff should be reinflated to permit resumption of ventilation and consideration of additional measures.

Pearl

1. Prolonged or over-inflation of the pharyngeal cuff can cause massive glossal edema from impaired venous return.

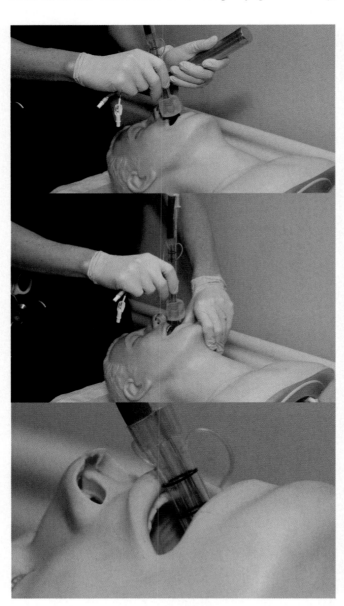

FIGURE 22.61 ■ Combitube Insertion Techniques. Laryngoscope-assisted combitube insertion and manual-distraction combitube insertion techniques. Double line at the alveolar ridge confirms proper depth. (Photo contributor: Lawrence B. Stack, MD.)

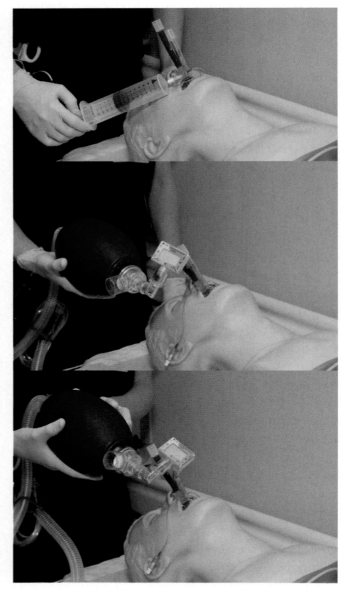

FIGURE 22.62 ■ Esophageal Combitube Placement. Once inserted to proper depth, balloons are filled. 85 mL in balloon #1 and 10 mL in balloon #2. End tidal CO_2 detector color change on lumen #1 confirms esophageal placement of the Combitube. (Photo contributor: Lawrence B. Stack, MD.)

Patient Preparation

The nares should be inspected for patency and the side deemed most hospitable to tube passage should be anesthetized and vasoconstricted. Additionally, it is helpful to confirm nasal patency by inserting a well-lubricated nasal trumpet. Lidocaine jelly can be used as the lubricant to provide additional topical anesthesia. We favor the use of disposable atomizers to instill 2 mL of a mixture of tetracaine 1% phenylephrine 0.5%, which yields excellent mucosal anesthesia and vasoconstriction. Favorable intubation conditions can be achieved in about 5 minutes.

In preparation for nasal intubation, the ET tube can be conformed into a circle by inserting the tip into the 15-mm proximal adaptor, and soaked in warm water to soften the tube for nasal passage. Success can also be enhanced by the use of a special endotracheal tube, called an Endotrol control tip endotracheal tube. This tube incorporates a length of nylon fishing line within a channel in the anterior wall of the ET tube. Pulling on the proximal loop "trigger" causes anterior deflection of the tube tip.

Technique

Once the selected naris is suitably anesthetized, the intubator faces the patient, who can be sitting up or supine, and inserts the tube into the naris, parallel to the nasal floor/perpendicular to the facial plane (not along the nasal axis). To minimize trauma to the nasal turbinates, the bevel of the tube should face the turbinates. This implies that if the left naris is being intubated, the tube can be inserted along the normal curve of the nose-nasopharynx; however, if the right naris is being intubated, the tube should be inserted with the curve of the tube in a cephalad direction. This should be done until the tube is advanced to the nasopharynx, at which point the tube is rotated to the correct anatomic configuration. As the tube is slowly advanced to the hypopharynx, the intubator listens closely for transmitted breath sounds, rotating the tube right or left to maintain maximal transmission. It takes a more-severe-than-expected rotation externally to generate a small rotation of the supraglottic tube tip. The tube is then rapidly advanced unless resistance is encountered, as would be expected with pyriform sinus tube tip position. Correct intratracheal placement should elicit cough, a reflex deep inspiration, and a loss of phonation. The intubator may also be sprayed with coughed secretions. If breath sound transmission decreases with advancement, the tube is withdrawn and re-advanced, preferably with more ante-

rior displacement of the tip if the Endotrol tube is used. If such a tube is not available, anterior displacement can be produced by partially inflating the endotracheal tube cuff.

The audible feedback to determine tube tip position can be enhanced by the attachment of the Beck Airway Airflow Monitor (BAAM), which creates an amplified sound with air movement, much like the sound of a tea kettle. Alternatively, one can remove the diaphragm/bell from a stethoscope and insert the distal end of the stethoscope tubing into the proximal end of the endotracheal tube. In addition to amplifying transmitted sounds, this trick also can spare the intubator from a sputum ear wash. Positional feedback can also be enhanced by use of a quantitative waveform capnometer/capnograph.

Pearls

1. Blind nasotracheal intubation offers a viable option in the event that oral intubation is rendered impossible in the short term, such as a patient who has a wired jaw or large subglossal hematoma.
2. The blind nasotracheal intubation technique requires maintenance of spontaneous respirations because the intubator relies on audible variation in transmitted breath sounds via the endotracheal tube.
3. The TrachLight light wand can be used for blind NT intubation, with the stiffening wire removed. Tube tip position is determined identically to that with orotracheal transillumination, with identical repositioning maneuvers, except that rotational maneuvers are likely to be more extreme as noted above.

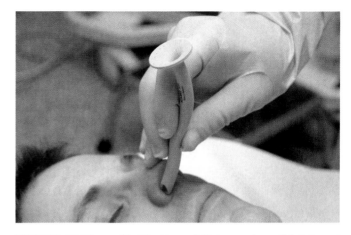

FIGURE 22.63 ■ Verification of Patency. A well-lubricated nasopharyngeal airway will verify patency of the nasal passage prior to NTT insertion. (Photo contributor: Lawrence B. Stack, MD.)

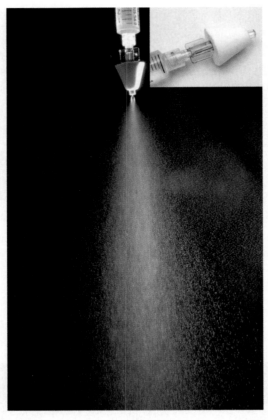

FIGURE 22.64 ■ Atomizer. A disposable atomizer used to deploy topical vasoconstrictors and analgesics prior to NTT insertion. (Photo contributor: Lawrence B. Stack, MD.)

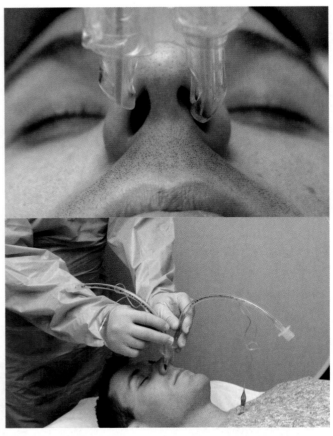

FIGURE 22.66 ■ Bevel Placement for NT Intubation. When inserted into the nose, the bevel of the tube should face the turbinates to minimize the trauma to these structures. (Photo contributor: Lawrence B. Stack, MD.)

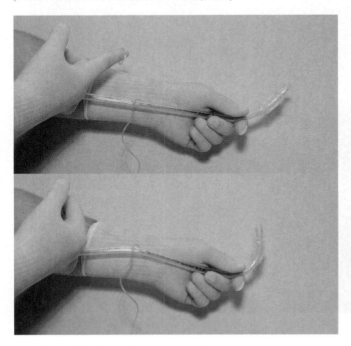

FIGURE 22.65 ■ Endotrol ET tube. Demonstration of the ET tube tip control using the Endotrol trigger. (Photo contributor: Lawrence B. Stack, MD.)

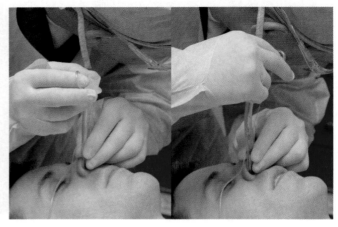

FIGURE 22.67 ■ Maneuvering for Maximized Breath Sounds. Once the ET tube is in close proximity of the glottic opening, the intubator must rotate the tube left or right till maximum air movement is heard, then advance the tube. (Photo contributor: Lawrence B. Stack, MD.)

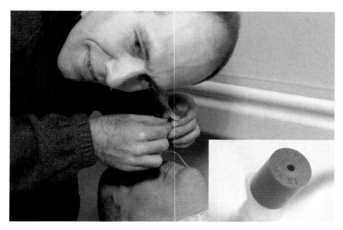

FIGURE 22.68 ■ Beck Airway Airflow Monitor (BAAM). The BAAM makes an amplified sound to help identify location of maximized air movement. (Photo contributor: Lawrence B. Stack, MD.)

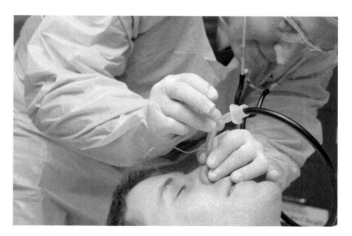

FIGURE 22.69 ■ Stethoscope Airflow Monitor. Removing the diaphragm/bell from a stethoscope and placing it in the end of the ET tube will enhance identify the location of maximum air movement. (Photo contributor: Lawrence B. Stack, MD.)

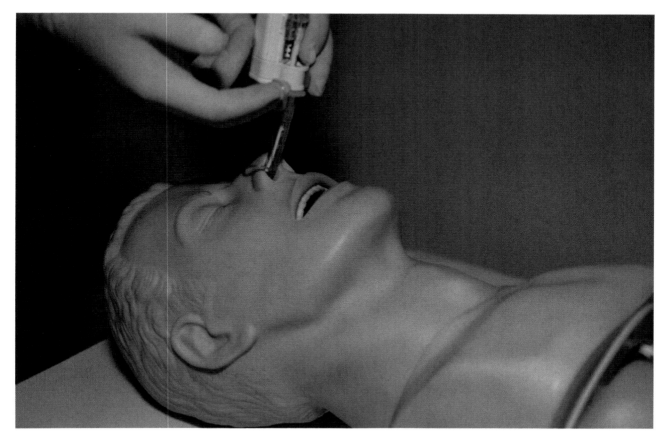

FIGURE 22.70 ■ Tracheal Light Wand Augmentation of NT Intubation. Remove the stiffening wire, and place the stylet into the ET tube and use conventional landmarks to guide maneuvering decisions for proper tube placement. (Photo contributor: Lawrence B. Stack, MD.)

There are two methods of nasal flexible fiberoptic technique: (1) scope first and (2) tube first.

Patient Preparation

For both methods, the nose is prepared as described above under blind nasotracheal intubation.

Technique

Scope First

The largest possible endotracheal tube, preferably 7.0 mm ID, is inserted over the endoscope to the most proximal position of the endoscope. The fiberoptic endoscope is then inserted through the selected naris. Under direct visual guidance, the endoscope is advanced along the floor of the nose, navigating under the inferior turbinate. The endoscope tip is manipulated by a combination of trigger deflection (up/down) and scope rotation (left/right) to keep the lumen in the center of the optical field. As the tube is advanced to the posterior nasopharynx, the scope tip is deflected downward to reveal the epiglottis and laryngeal inlet. The scope is advanced further, with the operator maneuvering the scope tip to keep the glottic opening in the center of the optical field. With the endoscope tip just above the cords, 2 mL of 1% lidocaine should be injected through the injection port of the fiberscope to provide vocal cord anesthesia prior to tube passage. The endoscope advancement continues until the endoscope tip is approximately 3 to 5 cm above the carina. The tube is then gently advanced over the fiberoptic sheath into the naris

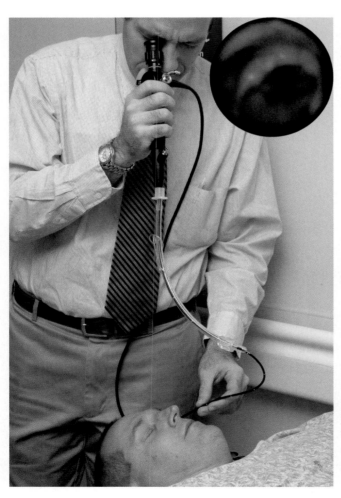

FIGURE 22.71 ■ Scope-First Method. The ET tube is placed at the proximal extreme. The endoscope is then guided to the glottic opening and the tube is then advanced over the endoscope. (Photo contributor: Lawrence B. Stack, MD.)

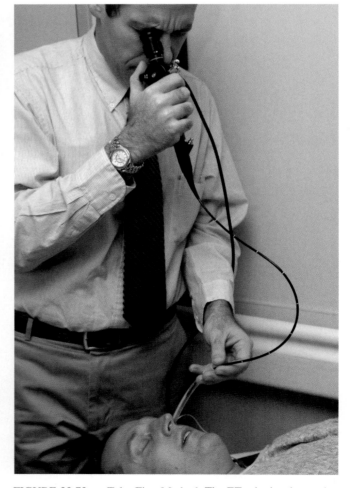

FIGURE 22.72 ■ Tube-First Method. The ET tube is advanced to the hypopharynx. The endoscope is then advanced through the tube and maneuvered to the glottic opening. The tube is then advanced over the endoscope. (Photo contributor: Lawrence B. Stack, MD.)

and to the trachea. If resistance is encountered at 14 to 16 cm, the tube may be impacting upon the right arytenoid. As discussed previously, this can be corrected by a severe counterclockwise rotation. The tube tip should be verified to be the correct distance from the carina.

If during endoscope navigation through the nose, the view becomes blurry because of adherent secretions, the tip can be cleared by gently deflecting the tip into "pink" mucosa. If one becomes lost or disoriented during scope advancement or if there is no obvious lumen through which to advance, the endoscope should be withdrawn slightly and the tip maneuvered to provide a recognizable view. The endoscope should not be advanced if a lumen is not readily apparent.

Tube-first

To avoid some of the technique difficulty inherent with nasal navigation, the endotracheal tube can be passed through the naris and advanced into the hypopharynx first, before scope insertion. The endoscopist then inserts the intubating fiberscope through the endotracheal tube, advances it to and through the glottic opening to the appropriate distance above the carina. Tube advancement proceeds as described above. The tube-first method may also facilitate endoscopic intubation in the event of epistaxis.

Transtracheal jet ventilation (TJV), also know as percutaneous translaryngeal jet ventilation and needle cricothyrotomy, is an easily performed rescue technique which secures a temporary access for ventilation in the event of failed intubation attempts. It should be viewed as a temporizing measure, but one which can afford hours of sufficient ventilation and oxygenation to provide a significant time window for other airway access. Transcricoid needle aspiration was once a mainstay of medical care to obtain sterile pulmonary cultures; it has been demonstrated to be a safe method of access with minimal complications, primarily bleeding.

The primary misconception about TJV is that it is only good for oxygenation not ventilation. With proper equipment and ventilating pressure head, it is possible to supply the same minute volume as achieved with bag ventilation. Minute volume (tidal volume $\times$ respiratory rate) is the primary determinant of P_{CO_2}.

Equipment

Proper equipment for TJV includes: (1) 18G or larger catheter or needle, to which a syringe can be attached. Cook catheter manufactures a specific TJV catheter, which has a wire-reinforced wall to resist bending and kinking, (2) high-pressure tubing with in-line flow valve, optional (but recommended) pressure gauge, (3) quick connect to wall oxygen outlet, (4) DIHSS connection to accessory port of oxygen tank regulator, and (5) pressurized oxygen source at 50 PSI. This is the pressure which is supplied by wall outlets in hospitals as well as from oxygen tank regulators before the oxygen flow meter (requires an accessory port on the regulator).

Technique

The technique is as follows:
1. Identify the thyroid cartilage and the cricothyroid membrane directly caudally.
2. Prepare the neck with suitable antiseptic; anesthetize the skin overlying the cricothyroid membrane with 1% lidocaine.
3. Isolate the trachea between the thumb and third finger of the sterilely gloved nondominant hand, using the index finger to palpate the cricothyroid membrane landmark. With a syringe attached, preferably containing sterile water or remaining lidocaine, insert the catheter through the cricothyroid membrane at a 30-degree angle to the horizontal, aiming toward the feet. Once through the skin,

begin aspirating as the catheter is advanced. Air and bubbles entering the syringe confirm entry into the trachea.
4. Carefully slide the catheter off the needle and into the trachea.
5. *Crucial step:* Reattach syringe and reconfirm tracheal position.
6. Attach high-pressure manual jet ventilator to catheter.
7. Begin ventilation at approximate ratio of 1 second insufflation to 5 seconds of exhalation; watch carefully that the chest falls after ventilation, signifying sufficient expiration.
8. Continue to manually secure the catheter at all times until more definitive airway control has been secured.

Pearls

1. During TJV, if the patient has an oxygen requirement, it will be necessary to apply a non-rebreather oxygen face mask so that the gas that is entrained by the Bernoulli effect is enriched with oxygen.
2. During DJV, the clinician must take great care to ensure that (a) the catheter is truly within and stays within the trachea and (b) that the chest falls after each rise with insufflation.
3. Transtracheal jet ventilation can be used in the patient with airway obstruction as long as it is primarily inspiratory obstruction and not complete inspiratory and expiratory. Exhalation for this technique must occur through whatever glottic and pharyngeal lumen is present.
4. If one predicts a high likelihood of difficult airway, one can choose to prophylactally insert a transtracheal catheter under more controlled circumstances than a crashing patient with failed airway. This may buy time for additional airway maneuvers in the event that the primary and secondary airway plans do in fact fail.

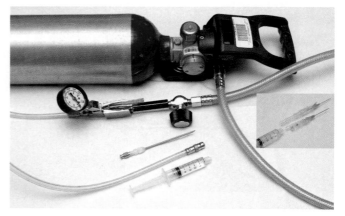

FIGURE 22.73 ■ Transtracheal Jet Ventilation Equipment. See text for details. (Photo contributor: Lawrence B. Stack, MD.)

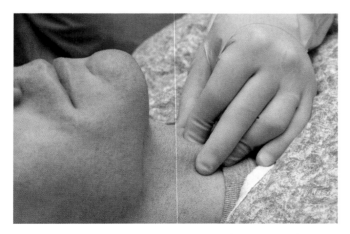

FIGURE 22.74 ■ Identify Landmarks. Identify thyroid cartilage and cricothyroid membrane. (Photo contributor: Lawrence B. Stack, MD.)

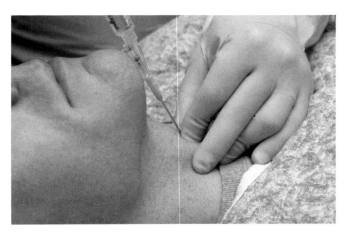

FIGURE 22.75 ■ Enter Cricothyroid Membrane. Once through the skin, begin aspirating, looking for air. (Photo contributor: Lawrence B. Stack, MD.)

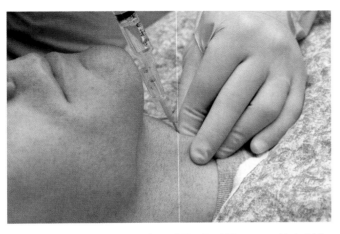

FIGURE 22.76 ■ Confirmation of Tracheal Entrance. Air bubbles seen during aspiration confirm entrance into the trachea. (Photo contributor: Lawrence B. Stack, MD.)

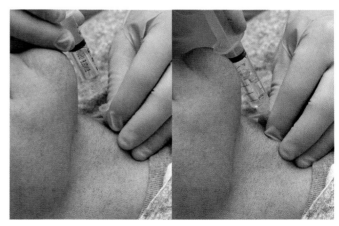

FIGURE 22.77 ■ Reconfirm Tracheal Position. Reattach syringe and aspirate to reconfirm tracheal placement before insufflating oxygen. (Photo contributor: Lawrence B. Stack, MD.)

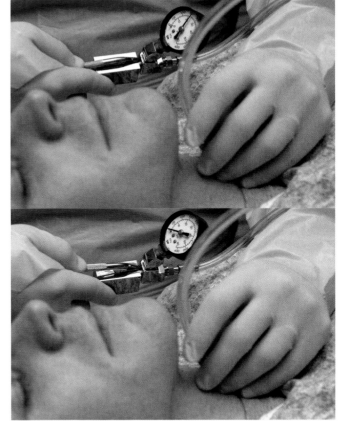

FIGURE 22.78 ■ Insufflation 1 Second—Exhalation 5 Seconds. Maintain control of the needle and pressure tubing at all times. (Photo contributor: Lawrence B. Stack, MD.)

Equipment

The Melker kit includes all the equipment necessary: catheter, thin-walled needle, Seldinger wire, cuffed tracheostomy tube 5.0 mm ID, and tapered introducer.

Technique

1. Identify the thyroid cartilage and the cricothyroid membrane directly caudally.
2. Prepare the neck with suitable antiseptic; anesthetize the skin overlying the cricothyroid membrane with 1% lidocaine.
3. Isolate the trachea between the thumb and third finger of the sterilely gloved nondominant hand, using the index finger to palpate the cricothyroid membrane landmark. With a syringe attached, preferably containing sterile water or remaining lidocaine, insert the catheter through the cricothyroid membrane at a 30 degree angle to the horizontal, aiming toward the feet. Once through the skin, begin aspirating as the catheter is advanced. Air and bubbles entering the syringe confirm entry into the trachea.
4. Carefully slide the catheter off of the needle and into the trachea.
5. Reattach syringe and reconfirm tracheal position.
6. Thread Seldinger wire through catheter into trachea; lack of resistance to wire passage confirms correct position.
7. Remove catheter and with the included scalpel, make a small incision at the wire-skin entry site.
8. Insert tracheostomy tube with dilator/introducer over wire into trachea. Expect significant resistance. Inability to pass dilator may indicate an inadequate skin incision.
9. Withdraw dilator/introducer and wire as one unit, inflate cuff, and initiate ventilation.
10. Secure tracheostomy tube with tracheostomy ties.

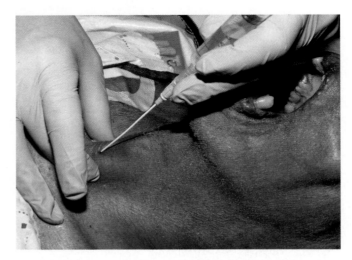

FIGURE 22.80 ■ Identify Landmarks. Palpate thyroid cartilage and cricothyroid cartilage caudally. Angle needle 30 degrees caudad to enter the trachea. (Photo contributor: Lawrence B. Stack, MD.)

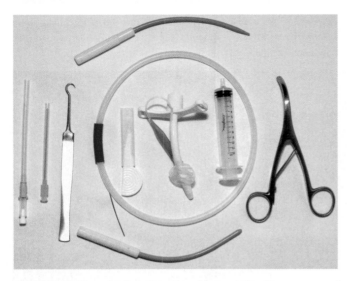

FIGURE 22.79 ■ Melker Cricothyroidotomy Kit. Components of the kit produced by Cook Inc. (Photo contributor: Lawrence B. Stack, MD.)

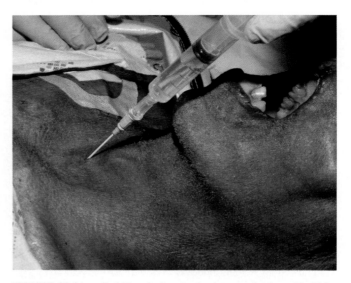

FIGURE 22.81 ■ Bubbles during Aspiration. Aspiration of bubbles during needle advancement confirms tracheal placement. (Photo contributor: Lawrence B. Stack, MD.)

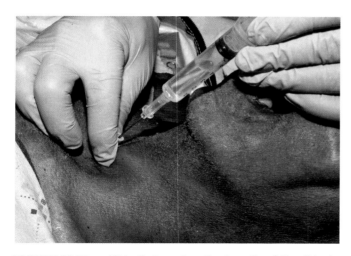

FIGURE 22.82 ■ ■ Slide Catheter into Trachea. Carefully slide the catheter off the needle into the trachea. (Photo contributor: Lawrence B. Stack, MD.)

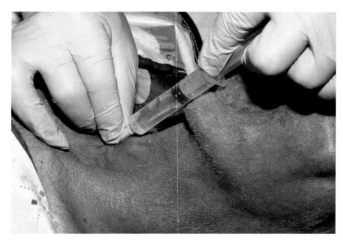

FIGURE 22.83 ■ ■ Confirm Tracheal Placement. Again, aspirate bubbles from the catheter to confirm tracheal placement. (Photo contributor: Lawrence B. Stack, MD.)

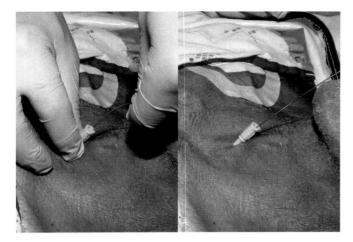

FIGURE 22.84 ■ ■ Thread Wire. Lack of resistance during threading of Seldinger wire confirms tracheal placement. (Photo contributor: Lawrence B. Stack, MD.)

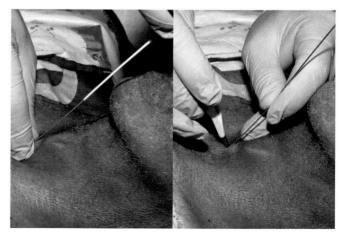

FIGURE 22.85 ■ ■ Incision at Wire Entry Site. Remove catheter and make incision at the wire entry site. (Photo contributor: Lawrence B. Stack, MD.)

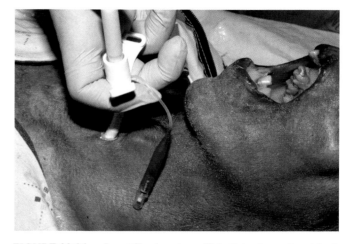

FIGURE 22.86 ■ ■ Insert Tracheostomy Tube/Introducer. Insert both devices over the wire and into the trachea. (Photo contributor: Lawrence B. Stack, MD.)

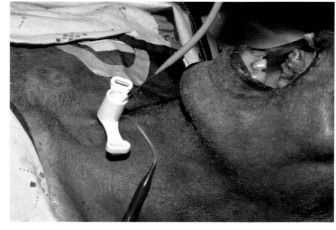

FIGURE 22.87 ■ ■ Remove Wire and Introducer. Remove these devices together as a single unit. (Photo contributor: Lawrence B. Stack, MD.)

Technique

1. Identify the thyroid cartilage and the cricothyroid membrane directly caudally.
2. Cleanse skin surface with appropriate antibacterial medication.
3. Anesthetize skin surface with 1% lidocaine.
4. While stabilizing the trachea with the gloved nondominant hand, make a vertical incision through the skin overlying the cricothyroid membrane.
5. Dissect the tissues over the cricothyroid membrane in a horizontal direction, until the cricothyroid membrane is exposed.
6. Incise the cricothyroid membrane horizontally and insert a tracheal hook to stabilize and control the trachea.
7. If a tracheal dilator is available, insert it into the trachea to dilate and control the trachea to facilitate tube insertion.
8. Insert a cuffed tracheostomy tube, or a 6.0 ID endotracheal tube.
9. Inflate cuff and initiate ventilation.

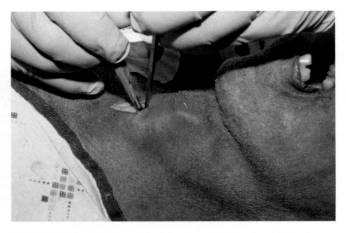

FIGURE 22.89 ■ Horizontal Incision through Cricothyroid Membrane. Insert a tracheal hook through the incision to gain proximal control of the trachea. (Photo contributor: Lawrence B. Stack, MD.)

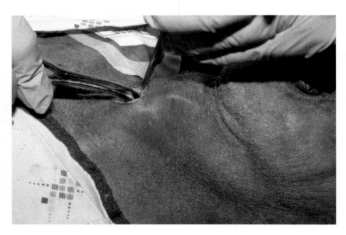

FIGURE 22.90 ■ Insert Tracheal Dilator. Then rotate dilator cephalad. (Photo contributor: Lawrence B. Stack, MD.)

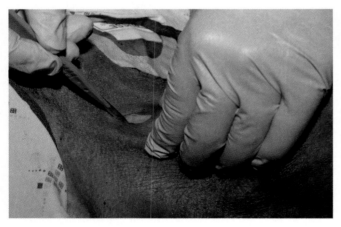

FIGURE 22.88 ■ Incision over Cricothyroid Membrane. Stabilize the proximal trachea; make a vertical incision over the cricothyroid membrane. (Photo contributor: Lawrence B. Stack, MD.)

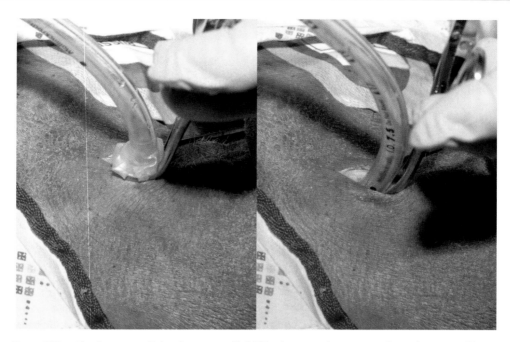

FIGURE 22.91 ■ Insert ET or Tracheostomy Tube. Insert a cuffed ET tube or tracheostomy tube and remove dilator. (Photo contributor: Lawrence B. Stack, MD.)

Chapter 23

ECG ABNORMALITIES

James V. Ritchie
Michael L. Juliano
R. Jason Thurman

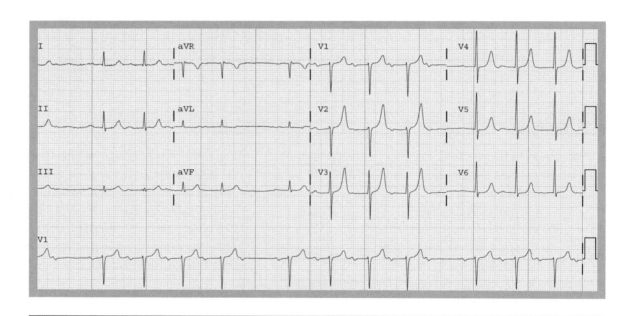

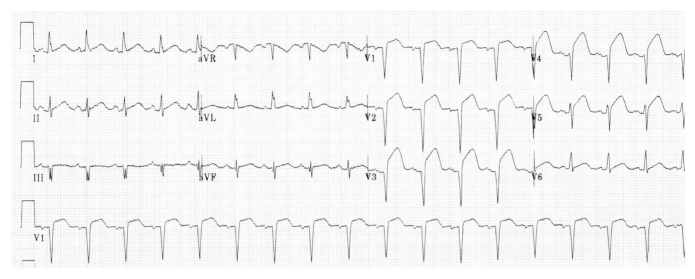

FIGURE 23.1A ■ Acute Anteroseptal Myocardial Infarction. (ECG contributor: James V. Ritchie, MD.)

ECG Findings

- ST segment elevation in the anterior precordial leads.
- Commonly-used terminology for injury location:
  - V3-V4: Anterior injury.
  - V_1-V_4: Anteroseptal injury.
  - V_3-V_6: Anterolateral injury. Leads I and aVL may also be involved, especially if the circumflex artery is affected (high lateral injury).
- Reciprocal ST segment depressions are often present in the inferior leads (II, III, aVF).

Pearls

1. The left anterior descending artery supplies blood to the anterior and lateral left ventricle and ventricular septum.
2. Normal R-wave progression (increasing upward amplitude with R wave > S wave at V_3 or V_4) may be interrupted.
3. The development of pathologic Q waves in any of the V leads other than V_1 strongly suggests that the injury has progressed to an infarction, as seen in this example.

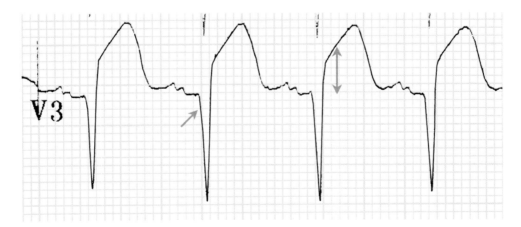

FIGURE 23.1B ■ Pathologic ST-segment elevation beyond 1 mm (double arrow) with pathologic Q waves (arrow) in lead V_3. The ST segment demonstrates a convex upward, or "tombstone" morphology.

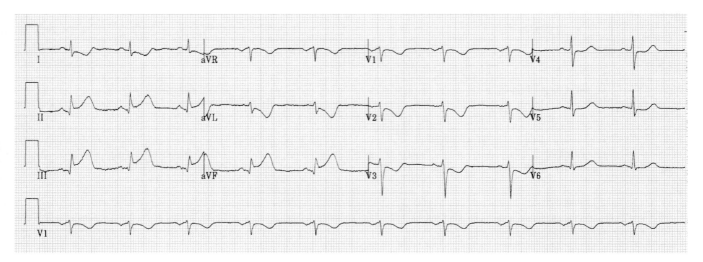

FIGURE 23.2A ■ Acute Inferior-Posterior Myocardial Infarction. (ECG contributor: James V. Ritchie, MD.)

ECG Findings

- ST segment elevation in inferior leads (II, III, aVF)
- Reciprocal ST segment depressions in the anterior leads (V_1-V_3) and possibly high lateral leads (I, aVL)

Pearls

1. The right coronary artery supplies blood to the right ventricle, the SA node, the inferior portions of the left ventricle, and usually to the posterior portion of the left ventricle and the AV node.
2. Infarctions involving the SA node may produce sinus dysrhythmias including tachycardias, bradycardias, and sinus arrest.
3. Infarctions involving the AV node may produce AV blocks.
4. In the presence of acute inferior injury, especially if the ST segment elevation in III is higher than in II, a right-sided ECG should be obtained to look for right ventricular involvement. The administration of nitroglycerin in the presence of acute right ventricular infarction can precipitate profound hypotension, as these patients are preload dependent.
5. Since the right coronary artery so often supplies the posterior left ventricle, look carefully for evidence of a posterior infarction (as present in the example) and consider obtaining an ECG with posterior leads.

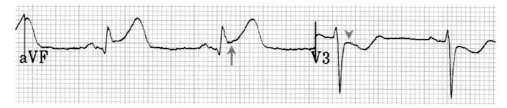

FIGURE 23.2B ■ ST-segment elevation is present in the inferior leads (II, III, aVF) (arrow), with reciprocal ST depression in the anterior leads (V_2-V_4) (arrowhead) and high lateral leads (I, aVL).

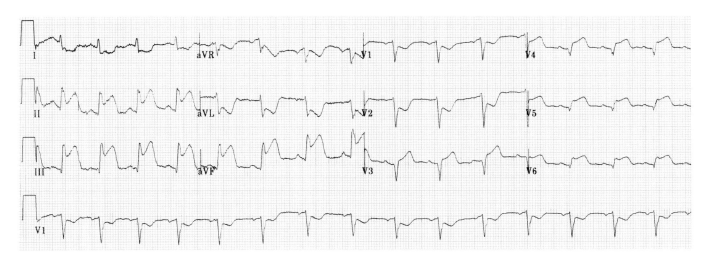

FIGURE 23.3A ■ Right Ventricular Myocardial Infarction. **This ECG was obtained with right-sided lead placement. (ECG contributor: Thomas Bottoni, MD.)**

ECG Findings

- ST elevation in right-sided V leads (V_4R, V_5R)
- ST elevation greater in lead III than lead II suggests RV MI
- ST elevation in the normally-obtained V_1 also strongly suggests RV MI
- Often associated with inferior MI and/or posterior MI

Pearls

1. The smaller muscle mass of the right ventricle produces a less intense injury pattern that is overwhelmed by the left ventricle in the normally obtained ECG. Placement of right-sided V leads, with V_1-V_6 in mirror-image locations on the right side of the chest, is important in detecting right ventricular injury.

2. The heart with an injured right ventricle is very preload-dependent. Beware of lowering preload with nitrates in any patient with suspected RV MI as severe hypotension may occur. Treat hypotension with volume.

3. Obtain a right-sided ECG in any patient with inferior or posterior MI, and in any patient with a significant hypotensive response to nitrates.

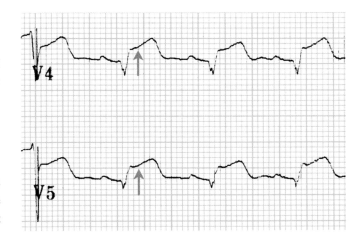

FIGURE 23.3B ■ ST elevation in V_4R and V_5R (arrows), with the V_4 and V_5 leads placed in their mirror-image locations on the right side of the chest. Any ST elevation seen in the right-sided precordial leads is significant.

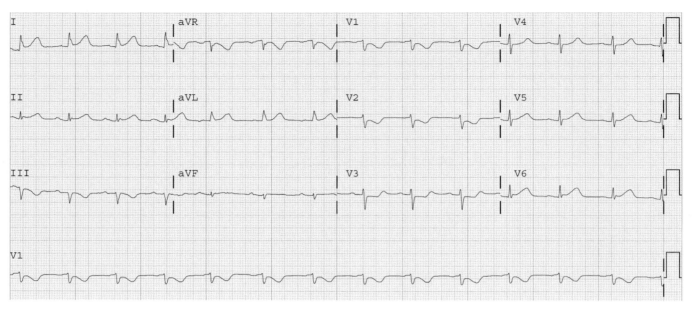

FIGURE 23.4A ▪ Acute Posterior-Lateral Myocardial Infarction. (ECG contributor: Ian D. Jones, MD.)

ECG Findings

- With acute injury pattern—ST segment depression in lead V_1 and/or V_2 with acute injury pattern.
- With infarction pattern—Small S wave and large R wave greater than 4 ms duration in lead V_1 or V_2 with infarction.
- With infarction pattern—R-wave/S-wave ratio greater than 1 in lead V_1 or V_2 with infarction.

Pearls

1. The posterior portion of the left ventricle has no EKG electrodes directly overlying it and is the last portion of ventricle to depolarize. It receives its blood supply from either the right coronary artery (in 85% of individuals) or the circumflex artery (in 15% of individuals).
2. V_1 and V_2 are primarily affected as the most anterior leads and indirectly assess the posterior left ventricle, though in an "inverted" orientation. Instead of observing downgoing Q waves and ST elevation large upgoing R waves and ST depression are seen. By holding the EKG up to a backlight upside down and horizontally flipped, the more classic injury pattern can be observed by looking *through* the EKG paper (see Fig. 23.4C).
3. Posterior involvement may be confirmed with posterior leads. V_8 is located at inferior tip of left scapula; V_9 is positioned between V_8 and the spine at the same level.
4. Frequently inferior MI is also present with posterior MI, since the right coronary artery serves both areas. In the above example, there is subtle ST elevation in the lateral leads, indicating posterior-lateral injury.

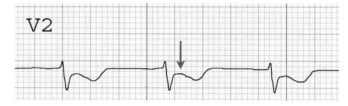

FIGURE 23.4B ▪ This tracing demonstrates injury in the posterior LV, manifesting as acute ST depression in V_2 (arrow).

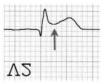

FIGURE 23.4C ▪ By inverting and rotating the EKG, the "classic" ST-elevation injury pattern is easily seen (arrow).

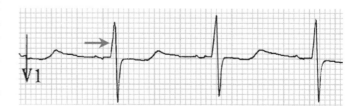

FIGURE 23.4D ▪ The ST depression is subtle and downsloping. However, the R-wave amplitude approximates that of the S wave and the R wave duration is significant (>4 ms). This is actually an "inverted Q wave" from this patient's posterior infarction that has evolved since the initial tracing.

737

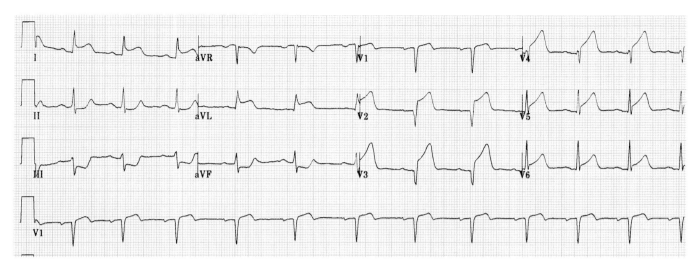

FIGURE 23.5A ■ Left Main Coronary Artery Lesion (widowmaker). (ECG contributor: James V. Ritchie, MD.)

ECG Findings

- ST segment elevation in the precordial leads (V_2-V_6) and high lateral leads (I, aVL)
- Reciprocal ST segment depressions in the inferior leads (II, III, aVF)

Pearls

1. The left main coronary artery branches into the left anterior descending artery and the circumflex artery. It supplies blood to the ventricular septum and the anterior and lateral aspects of the left ventricle, usually sparing the posterior and inferior portion, which is most often served by the right coronary artery.

2. Normal R-wave progression (increasing R wave amplitude across the precordial leads) may be interrupted.

3. Risk of cardiogenic shock is high since so much of the left ventricle is served by the left main coronary artery.

4. A left main coronary thrombosis is also known as the "widowmaker lesion."

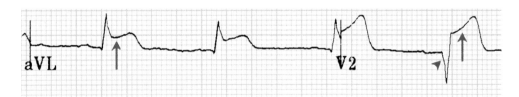

FIGURE 23.5B ■ Significant ST elevation is present in the precordial leads (V_2-V_6) and high lateral leads (I and aVL) (arrows). In this example, significant Q waves have appeared, signaling infarction (arrowhead).

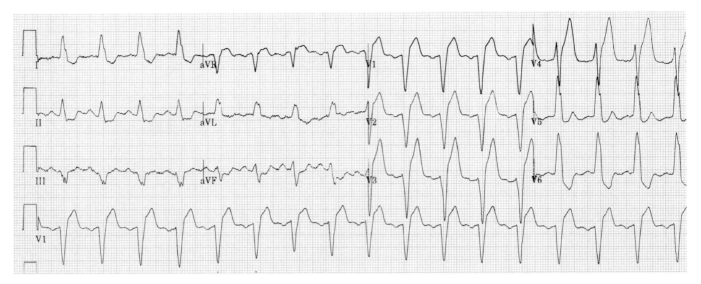

FIGURE 23.6A ■ Acute Myocardial Infarction by Sgarbossa Criteria in the setting of underlying LBBB. (ECG contributor: James V. Ritchie, MD.)

ECG Findings

- ST elevation greater than or equal to 1 mm concordant with QRS deflection (score = 5)
- ST depression greater than or equal to 1 mm in leads V_1, V_2, V_3 concordant with QRS deflection (score = 3)
- ST elevation greater than or equal to 5 mm discordant with QRS deflection (score = 2)

Pearls

1. These scored criteria may be used to diagnose acute myocardial infarction in the setting of a LBBB. However, most myocardial ischemia in the setting of LBBB does not produce these changes. An absence of these findings should not be used as evidence against acute coronary syndrome.
2. Score of greater than or equal to three gives a specificity for myocardial infarction of 90%.
3. The first and third criteria listed above may also be used in ECGs with wide QRS complexes resulting from a pacemaker or idioventricular rhythm.

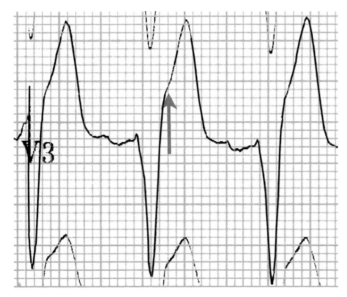

FIGURE 23.6B ■ The ST elevation is greater than 5 mm discordant from the primary QRS deflection (arrow).

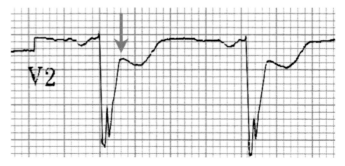

FIGURE 23.6C ■ The ST depression is greater than 1 mm concordant to the primary QRS deflection (arrow).

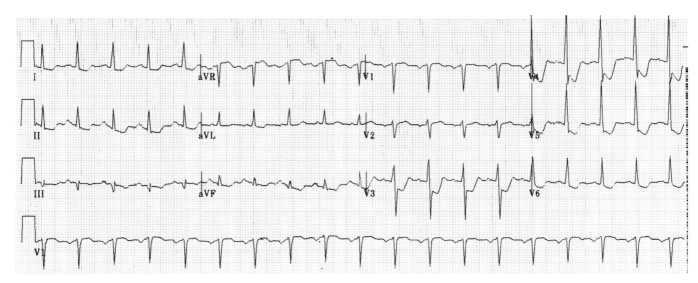

FIGURE 23.7A ■ Subendocardial Ischemia. (ECG contributor: James V. Ritchie, MD.)

ECG Findings

- ST segment depression greater than or equal to 1 mm in anatomically adjoining leads
- ST segments may be horizontal or downsloping with acute ischemia

Pearls

1. Some ST depression in the lateral precordial leads (V_4-V_6) is common at higher heart rates, and is commonly seen during exercise treadmill tests, but such depression should not be downsloping unless ischemia is also present.

2. ST elevation in other leads suggests that the depression may represent reciprocal changes from acute injury rather than subendocardial ischemia.

3. Downsloping ST depression may also be seen in left ventricular hypertrophy, but this depression should not be dynamic, and should be stable with serial ECGs. ST depression from ischemia will be dynamic, changing with time on serial ECGs. Remember the axiom, "One ECG begets another!"

4. Isolated ST depression in leads V_1 and V_2 may represent posterior ischemia.

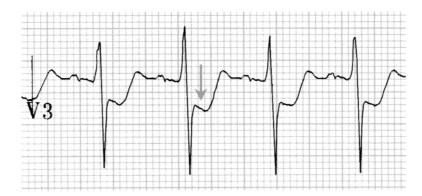

FIGURE 23.7B ■ Downsloping ST segments depressed greater than 1 mm (arrow). These changes were dynamic over time. The patient sustained a nontransmural myocardial infarction.

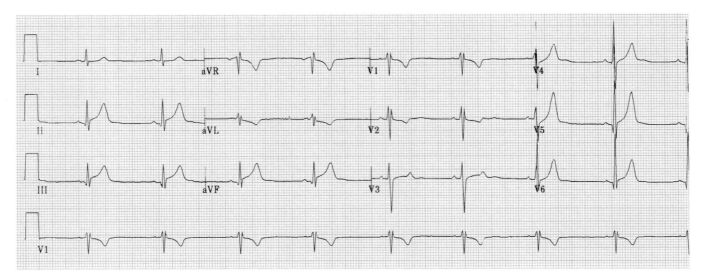

FIGURE 23.8A ■ Hyperacute T Waves. T waves in a patient with acute myocardial ischemia. (ECG contributor: James V. Ritchie, MD.)

ECG Findings

- T wave amplitude/QRS amplitude greater than 75%
- T waves greater than 5 mV in the limb leads
- T waves greater than 10 mV in the precordial leads
- T waves have asymmetric appearance

Pearls

1. Hyperacute T waves occur very early (within minutes) during myocardial injury and are transient.
2. The term "hyperacute T waves" is reserved for the early stages of myocardial infarction. "Prominent T waves" can also be seen with left ventricular hypertrophy, early repolarization, or with hyperkalemia.
3. Serial ECGs are useful in distinguishing transient hyperacute T waves from other causes of tall, peaked T waves. Once again, one ECG begets another.

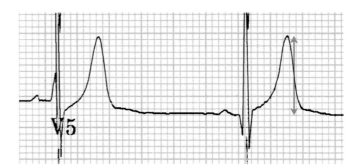

FIGURE 23.8B ■ T-wave height is greater than 10 mm in V_5 (double arrow) and is asymmetric. This height was transient and was significantly diminished in a tracing obtained 15 minutes later. Note also in the 12-lead ECG example above the presence of inferior ST elevation.

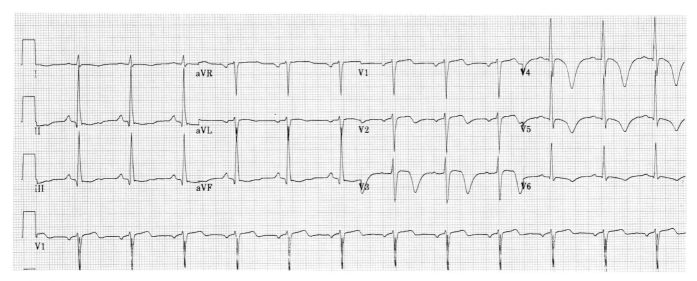

FIGURE 23.9A ■ Wellens Waves. Wellens Waves are present and are indicative of a high-grade LAD lesion. (ECG contributor: James V. Ritchie, MD.)

ECG Findings (Two Classic Types)

- Biphasic T waves in anterior and/or lateral leads
- Deeply inverted, symmetrical T waves in the same leads

Pearls

1. These characteristic patterns of T wave changes are closely associated with critical left anterior descending artery stenosis.

2. The changes are classically apparent on ECG *after* resolution of chest pain.

3. These changes are transient, and often are not associated with cardiac enzyme elevations.

4. Wellens waves are not associated with changes in R-wave progression.

5. Serial electrocardiograms may assist in differentiating Wellens Waves from stable, nonspecific findings.

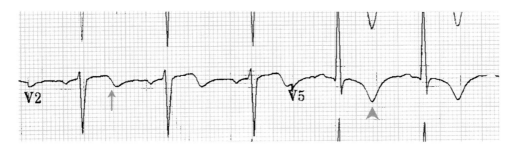

FIGURE 23.9B ■ Biphasic T waves with the later segment inverted, as in V_2 above (arrow), or deep symmetric inverted T waves, as in V_5 above (arrowhead). These findings in the precordial leads, in the setting of suspected ACS, strongly suggest an underlying high-grade LAD lesion.

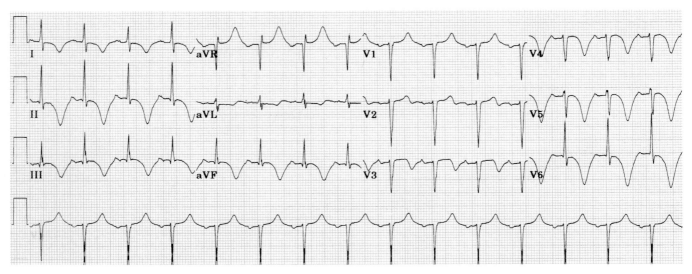

FIGURE 23.10A ■ Cerebral T Waves. This ECG was obtained on a patient with a severe acute hemorrhagic CVA. (ECG contributor: James V. Ritchie, MD.)

ECG Findings

- Inverted, wide T waves are most notable in precordial leads (can be seen in any lead).
- QT interval prolongation.

Pearls

1. These are associated with acute cerebral disease, most notably an ischemic cerebrovascular event or subarachnoid hemorrhage.

2. They may be accompanied by ST segment changes, U-waves, and/or any rhythm abnormality.

3. Differential diagnosis includes extensive myocardial ischemia.

4. Strongly suspect an intracranial etiology in a patient with altered mental status and these electrocardiographic findings.

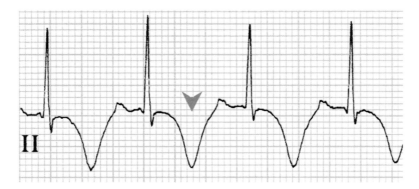

FIGURE 23.10B ■ Deep, symmetrical, inverted T waves (arrowhead) with a prolonged QT interval.

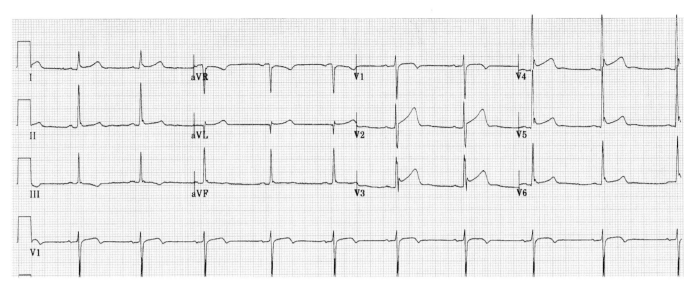

FIGURE 23.11A ■ Early Repolarization. (ECG contributor: James V. Ritchie, MD.)

ECG Findings

- ST elevation, usually in the anterior leads.
- J-point elevation, but usually less than one-third the total height of the T wave.
- ST segment is "concave upward," or "holds water," or "is smiling at you."
- J-point notch strongly suggests early repolarization, but is not always present.

Pearls

1. This is a normal variant and is especially common in young healthy males, but also may be present in other groups. However, the presence of any clinical suspicion for ongoing myocardial ischemia should prompt further investigation and must override the finding of apparent early repolarization on ECG.
2. Q waves and reciprocal ST-segment depression in other leads should *not* accompany early repolarization. If present, they strongly suggest ischemia as the cause for the ST elevation.

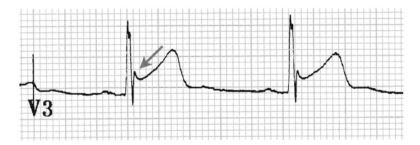

FIGURE 23.11B ■ ST elevation in precordial leads, with a concave-upward ST segment and a J-point notch (arrow).

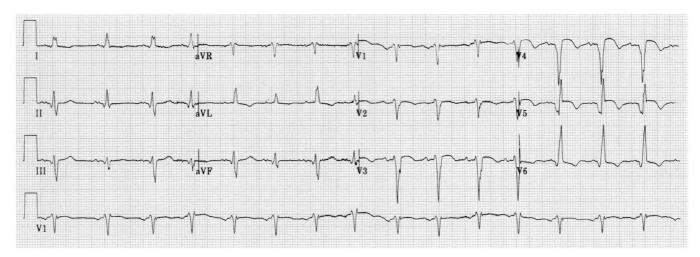

FIGURE 23.12A ■ Left Ventricular Aneurysm. This ECG was obtained on an asymptomatic patient with history of MI 2 years prior. (ECG contributor: James V. Ritchie, MD.)

ECG Findings

- ST elevation in anterior contiguous leads
- Deep pathologic Q waves in anterior leads

Pearls

1. ST segment elevation which occurs in the setting of a myocardial infarction should resolve within days under normal circumstances.
2. Persistent ST-segment elevation occurring for weeks or longer after a myocardial infarction is suspicious for ventricular aneurysm.
3. Ventricular aneurysms may follow a large myocardial infarction in the anterior portion of the heart.
4. The aneurysm consists of scarred myocardium, which does not contract but bulges outward during systole.
5. Potential complications from ventricular aneurysm include congestive heart failure, myocardial rupture, arrhythmias, and thrombus formation.
6. Suspect an LV aneurysm when these findings appear in the ECG of a patient who does not demonstrate symptoms suggesting ACS. However, one should also be vigilant for the presence of "silent" ACS.

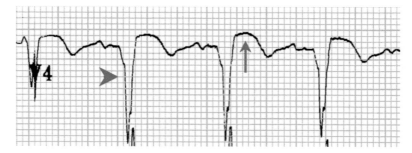

FIGURE 23.12B ■ Persistent ST elevations (arrow) and deep, pathologic Q waves (arrowhead) in an asymptomatic patient with a history of anterior myocardial infarction 2 years earlier.

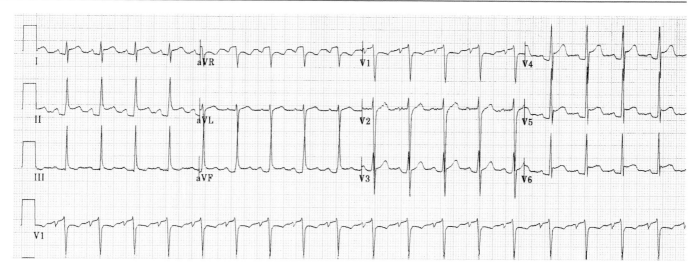

FIGURE 23.13A ■ Acute Pericarditis. (ECG contributor: James V. Ritchie, MD.)

ECG Findings

- Diffuse ST elevation in noncontiguous leads
- PR depression
- T wave flattening or inversion

Pearls

1. Pericarditis may produce inflammation of the epicardium. This is most often demonstrated on the ECG as a widespread injury pattern.

2. Pericarditis does *not* produce abnormal Q waves. The presence of abnormal Q waves must prompt consideration of acute or old coronary syndrome, including Dressler syndrome or postinfarct pericarditis.

3. Pericarditis may be focal, resulting in regional rather than diffuse EKG changes.

4. Benign early repolarization and myocarditis may also appear as ST elevation in many noncontiguous leads.

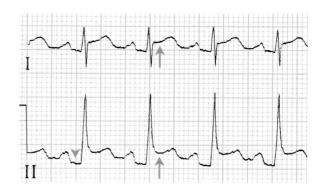

FIGURE 23.13B ■ ST elevation in noncontiguous leads I and II (arrows) with PR depression (arrowhead). No pathologic Q waves or reciprocal changes are present.

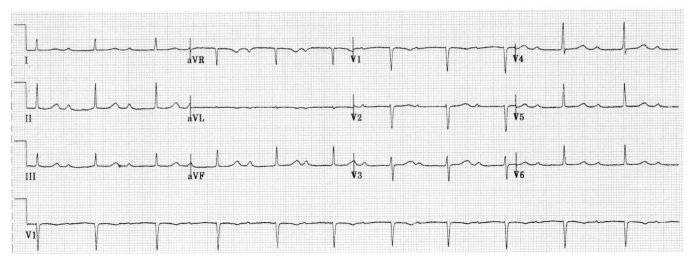

FIGURE 23.14A ■ First-Degree AV Block. (ECG contributor: James V. Ritchie, MD.)

ECG Findings

- A PR interval greater than 200 ms (normal 120-200 ms) with no significant variation in PR intervals between beats.
- Each P wave is followed by a QRS complex.

Pearls

1. This type of heart block usually does not affect heart function and can be considered non-pathologic (especially in athletes or patients with higher vagal tone).
2. First-degree block may also be due to heart disease (myocarditis, rheumatic fever) or drugs (digoxin, amiodarone, β-blockers, calcium channel blockers).

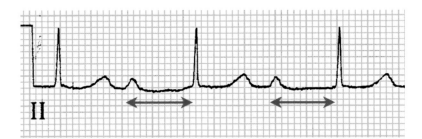

FIGURE 23.14B ■ The PR interval is fixed (double arrows) and is longer than 0.2 seconds, or five small blocks.

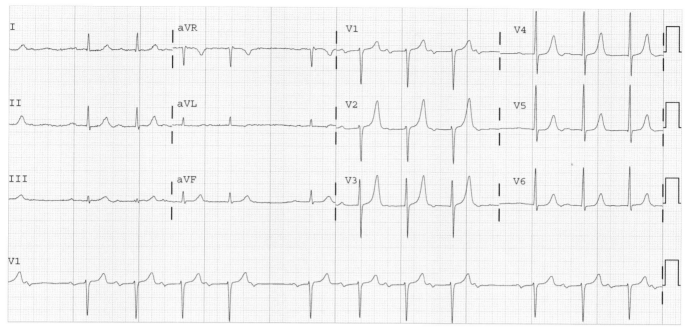

FIGURE 23.15A ▪ Second-Degree AV Block (Mobitz I, Wenckebach). (ECG contributor: James Paul Brewer, MD.)

ECG Findings

- Progressive PR-interval prolongation throughout the cardiac cycle until a P wave occurs without a QRS complex ("dropped" beat).
- After the dropped QRS complex, the cycle continues again with the PR interval of the first beat in the cycle always shorter than the PR interval of the last beat in the previous cycle.
- P wave may be hidden by the preceding T wave.

Pearls

1. The number of P-QRS complexes prior to the "dropped" beat may vary.

2. A clue to the diagnosis of Mobitz type I heart block can be found in the appearance of grouped QRS complexes
3. This type of block is normally asymptomatic, and may be seen in athletes.
4. These patients have low risk of progression to complete heart block, and usually do not require a pacemaker. However, Mobitz type I heart block may be caused by inferior myocardial infarction or drugs (digoxin, amiodarone, β-blockers, calcium channel blockers).

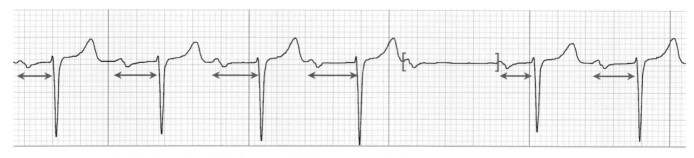

FIGURE 23.15B ▪ The PR interval gradually increases (double arrows) until a P wave is not followed by a QRS and a beat is "dropped" (brackets). The process then recurs. P waves occur at regular intervals, though they may be hidden by T waves.

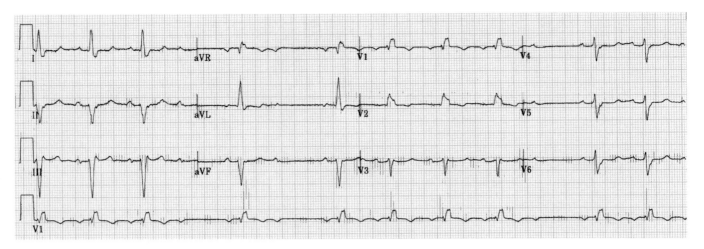

FIGURE 23.16A ▪ Type II Second-Degree AV Block (Mobitz II). (ECG contributor: Michael L. Juliano, MD.)

ECG Findings

- The PR interval remains constant and does not increase (as seen with Mobitz type I) with each cardiac cycle prior to the "dropped" QRS complex.
- P-P interval is constant, and R-R interval is constant until the dropped beat.
- R-R interval encompassing the "dropped" QRS should be roughly equal to two P-P intervals.

Pearls

1. This type of heart block is associated with disease of the conduction system distal to the AV node. A pacemaker is usually indicated.
2. Mobitz type II block can accompany myocardial infarction and has a high chance of progression to a complete heart block.

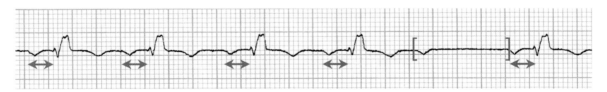

FIGURE 23.16B ▪ The PR interval is constant (double arrows) until the dropped beat (brackets).

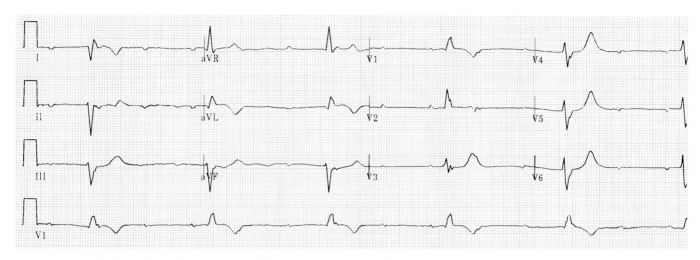

FIGURE 23.17A ■ Third-Degree AV Block (Complete Heart Block). (ECG contributor: James V. Ritchie, MD.)

ECG Findings

- Atrial and ventricular electrical activities are entirely disassociated.
- The P-P and R-R intervals remain constant.
- P waves may be hidden in the QRS complex or may distort the shape of the T wave.
- The atrial rate is usually faster than the ventricular rate.

Pearls

1. Third-degree block is also called complete heart block because no impulses are conducted from the atria to the ventricles.

2. Ventricular rate and QRS morphology depend upon the location of the escape pacemaker.

3. AV node escape rate is typically 40 to 60 bpm, with a narrow QRS complex.

4. Ventricular escape rate is usually 20 to 40 bpm, with a widened QRS complex.

5. Complete heart block may be caused by myocardial infarction, conduction system disease, or drugs such as digoxin.

6. Complete heart block may dramatically decrease cardiac output. Rescue cardiac pacing is often required.

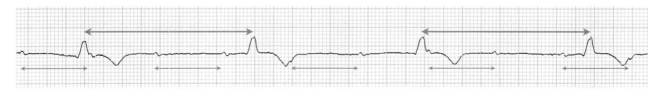

FIGURE 23.17B ■ The P-P interval is uniform (lower double arrows) and the R-R interval is uniform (upper double arrows), but the P waves and QRS complexes are disassociated.

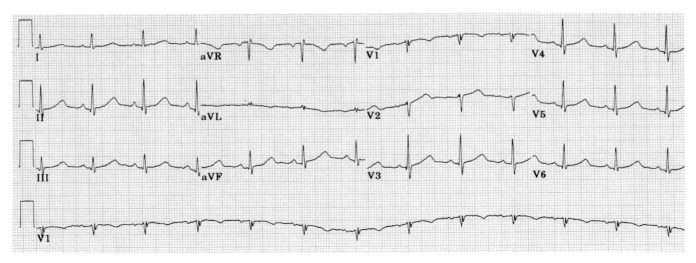

FIGURE 23.18A ■ Prolonged QT Interval. (ECG contributor: James V. Ritchie, MD.)

ECG Findings

- Normal QTc interval is less than 440 ms.
- QTc interval greater than 440 ms is considered prolonged.
- QTc interval greater than 500 ms is considered moderately prolonged.
- QTc interval greater than 550 ms is markedly prolonged.

Pearls

1. The QT interval is measured form the beginning of the QRS complex to the termination of the T wave (or U wave if present) and should be measured in the EKG lead with the longest appearing QT interval that has a distinct T wave with a clear termination point.

2. The QT interval will increase with bradycardia and decrease with tachycardia, thus it is important to use the corrected QT interval ($QTc = QT/\sqrt{R\text{-}R}$ interval) for heart rates other than 60 (in which the QTc = QT).

3. Prolonged QT intervals may be congenital. The vast majority are acquired, usually due to medications or electrolyte abnormalities (hypokalemia, hypomagnesemia, hypocalcemia, and hyperphosphatemia).

4. Numerous medications may prolong the QT interval in therapeutic or toxic doses.

5. Prolongation of the QT interval predisposes to Torsades de pointes.

6. Look carefully for prolonged QT intervals in patients who present with syncope.

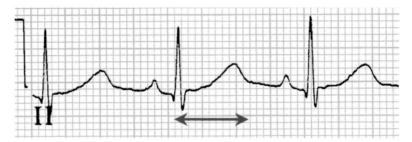

FIGURE 23.18B ■ QT Interval Prolongation. QT of 440 ms, QT$_c$ of 498 (double arrow). Note the QT Interval is measured from the beginning of the QRS complex to the termination point of the T wave.

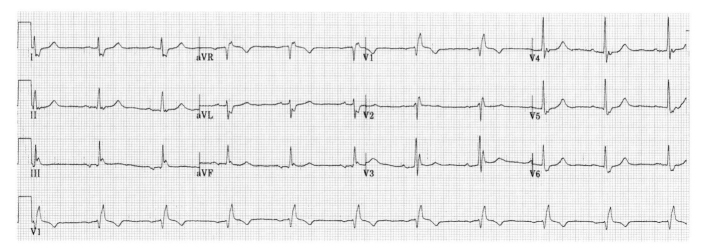

FIGURE 23.19A ■ Right Bundle Branch Block. (ECG contributor: James V. Ritchie, MD.)

ECG Findings

- Wide QRS complex, at least 120 ms (three small blocks).
- QRS complex has sR' or rsR' in leads V_1 and V_2.
- Slurred S wave V_6 and I.

Pearls

1. The signal exiting the AV node is carried rapidly to the LV through the intact left bundle, but is delayed into the right ventricle, where depolarization must propagate cell-to-cell. Since the RV myocardial mass is much smaller than that of the LV, this delay in depolarization is best seen in the leads overlying the right ventricle, leads V_1 and V_2.

2. Acute right heart strain, as may occur with pulmonary embolism, may result in new onset RBBB.

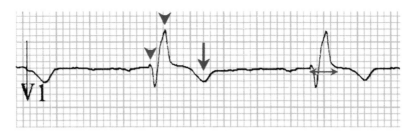

FIGURE 23.19B ■ rsR' pattern in V_1 (arrowheads), with T wave downgoing (arrow). QRS duration greater than 120 ms (double arrow).

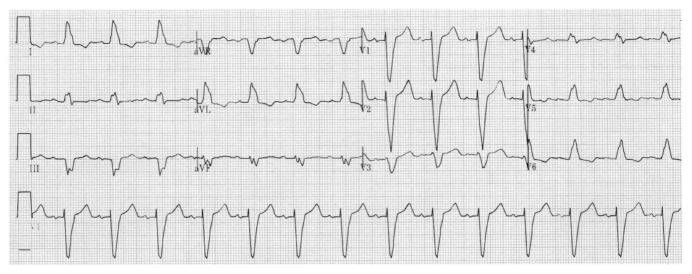

FIGURE 23.20A ■ Left Bundle Branch Block. (ECG contributor: James V. Ritchie, MD.)

ECG Findings

- Wide QRS complex, at least 120 ms (three small blocks).
- T wave appears on the opposite side of the baseline from the QRS complex.
- The QRS precordial axis is normal or deviated to the left.
- QRS complex deflection is predominately downward in lead V_1 and upward in lead V_6.

Pearls

1. The signal exiting the AV node does not proceed through the left ventricular conduction system. It must propagate more slowly cell-to-cell through the myocardium, starting in the septum. Therefore, the QRS is wider and the bulk of the depolarization signal is deflected toward the far lateral aspect of the heart.

2. Acute myocardial infarction may produce a new onset LBBB on ECG. Therefore, patients with new onset LBBB with a clinical presentation consistent with acute coronary syndrome should be treated as having an acute ST segment Elevation Myocardial Infarction (STEMI).

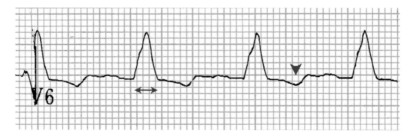

FIGURE 23.20B ■ The QRS is wider than 120 ms (double arrow). The T wave deflection is in the opposite direction from the QRS deflection (arrowhead).

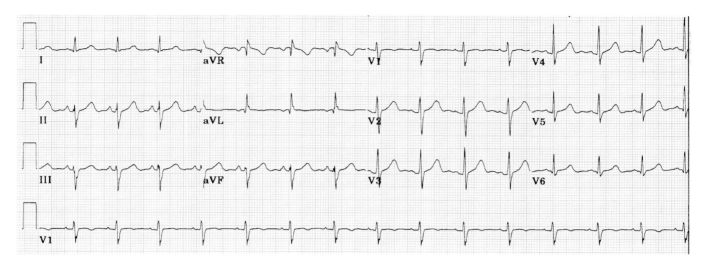

FIGURE 23.21A ▪ Left Anterior Fascicular Block. (ECG contributor: James V. Ritchie, MD.)

ECG Findings

- QRS complex widening, usually 90 to 120 ms
- Left axis deviation beyond minus 45 degrees with no other cause (such as inferior myocardial infarction)
- Small R wave and large S wave in the inferior leads
- Slurred S wave in V_5 and V_6

Pearls

1. The signal exiting the AV node is carried rapidly to the inferior aspect of the LV and all of the RV through the intact left posterior fascicle and right bundle, where quick depolarization occurs. However, conduction to the high lateral and upper portions of the left ventricle is slower and must proceed cell-to-cell due to the blocked left anterior fascicle. Therefore, the latter portion of the QRS depolarizes toward the upper lateral myocardium, manifested as strong left-axis deviation.

2. Left anterior fascicular block is the most common intraventricular conduction disturbance associated with acute anterior myocardial infarction, with the left anterior descending artery usually involved.

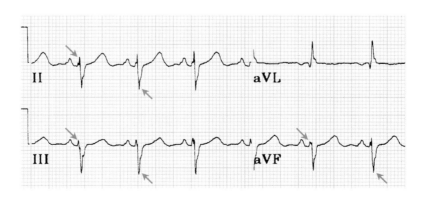

FIGURE 23.21B ▪ Small R waves, large S waves in all inferior leads (arrows), with QRS axis deviated left beyond minus 45 degrees.

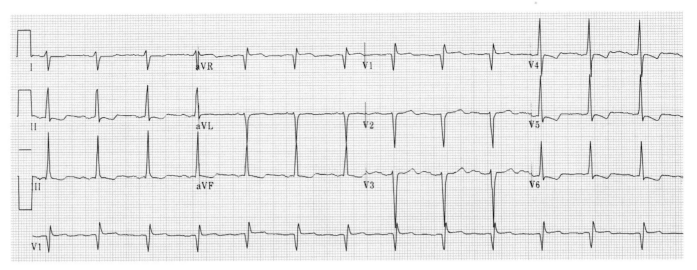

FIGURE 23.22A ■ Left Posterior Fascicular Block. (ECG contributor: James V. Ritchie, MD.)

ECG Findings

- QRS complex widening to 90 to 120 ms.
- Right axis deviation must be beyond 100 degrees and must have no other cause (such as lateral myocardial infarction).
- Small R wave and large S wave in the high lateral leads, I and aVL.
- Slurred S wave in V_5 and V_6.
- This example also contains unrelated ST changes.

Pearls

1. The signal exiting the AV node is carried rapidly to the upper aspect of the LV and all of the RV through the intact left anterior fascicle and right bundle, where depolarization is rapid. However, conduction to the inferior portion of the left ventricle is slower and must proceed cell-to-cell due to the blocked left posterior fascicle. Therefore, the latter portion of the QRS depolarizes toward the inferior myocardium, manifesting as strong right axis deviation.

2. Left posterior fascicular block may be associated with acute inferior myocardial infarction as well as with multiple cardiomyopathic conditions.

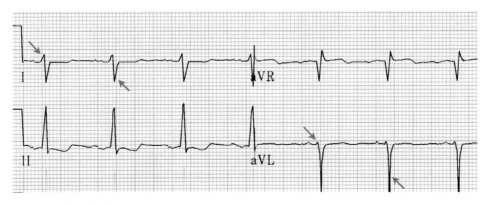

FIGURE 23.22B ■ Small R waves and large S waves in leads I and aVL (arrows).

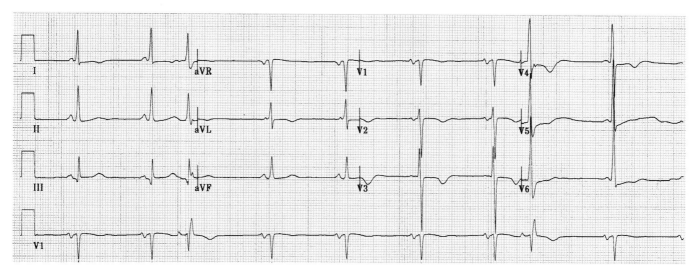

FIGURE 23.23A ■ Ashman Phenomenon. (ECG contributor: James V. Ritchie, MD.)

ECG Findings

- Aberrant ventricular conduction, usually with right bundle branch block pattern.
- Altered durations of the refractory period of the bundle branch or ventricular tissue are present, commonly due to atrial fibrillation, atrial ectopy, and atrial tachycardia

Pearls

1. After depolarization, tissue repolarizes during its refractory period. Refractory period changes with the preceding cardiac cycle, with longer R-R intervals producing longer refractory periods and shorter R-R intervals producing shorter refractory periods.
2. A longer R-R interval lengthens the following refractory period. When an early or premature (ectopic) depolarization

reaches the ventricular conduction system before it has completely repolarized, aberrant conduction may occur and be manifest on the ECG with a bundle-branch block pattern.

3. Ashman phenomenon most commonly appears with a right bundle branch block pattern, since the right bundle has a longer refractory period than the left bundle.
4. Ashman phenomenon is often seen in atrial fibrillation, when a long R-R interval is followed by a much shorter R-R interval.
5. In the setting of a premature atrial beat (as seen in this example), the earlier in the cycle the PAC occurs and the longer the preceding R-R interval is, the more likely aberrant conduction of the beat will occur.

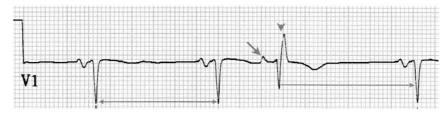

FIGURE 23.23B ■ After a relatively long R-R interval (double arrow), a PAC (diagonal arrow) is followed by an aberrantly conducted QRS with RBBB morphology (arrowhead). After a short pause (single arrow), the next beat is conducted normally as it has occurred outside of the refractory period set by the previous beat.

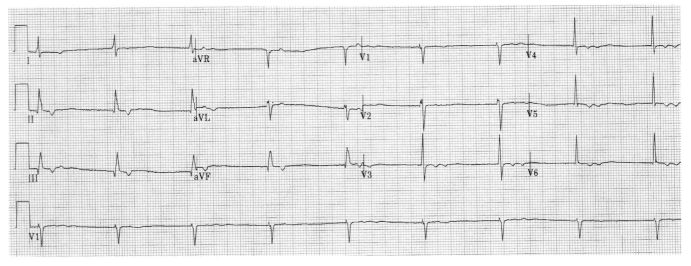

FIGURE 23.24A ■ Junctional Rhythm with Retrograde P Waves. (ECG contributor: James V. Ritchie, MD.)

ECG Findings

- The QRS complex is narrow, with a rate typically between 40 and 60 beats per minute.
- P waves are absent, retrograde, very slow, or unrelated to the QRS complex.

Pearls

1. When the atria fail to initiate a cardiac rhythm, or when no pacing signal reaches the lower AV node, the AV node or His bundle usually picks up the pacemaking responsibility.

2. P waves may be conducted retrograde and buried in the T wave as seen in this example. In the case of a complete AV block, the P waves have no relation to the QRS complex.

3. If a bundle branch block is also present, the QRS may be wide, and may be difficult to discern from a primary ventricular rhythm.

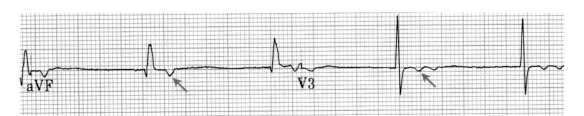

FIGURE 23.24B ■ The QRS is narrow. P waves are not present before the QRS. In this example, the signal which originated in the His bundle is conducted retrograde through the AV node into the atria, and retrograde P waves are apparent in the ST segment (arrows).

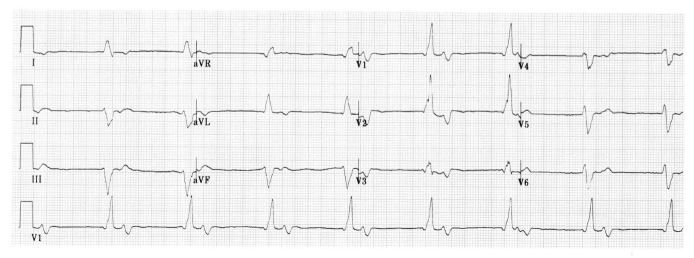

FIGURE 23.25A ▪ Ventricular Rhythm with Retrograde P Waves. (ECG contributor James V. Ritchie, MD.)

ECG Findings

- The QRS complex is wider than 120 ms, with a rate typically between 20 and 40 beats per minute.
- The T wave is discordant relative to the QRS.

Pearls

1. When the atria and the AV node fail to initiate a cardiac rhythm, or when no pacing signal reaches the ventricle, the ventricular tissue usually picks up the pacemaking responsibility.

2. P waves may also be conducted retrograde and buried in the T wave as seen in this example. In the case of a complete AV block, the P waves have no relation to the QRS complex.

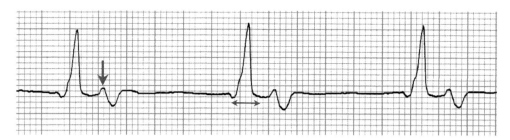

FIGURE 23.25B ▪ Wide-complex (double arrow) regular QRS at a rate of approximately 50 bpm. Retrograde P waves are seen in this example (arrow).

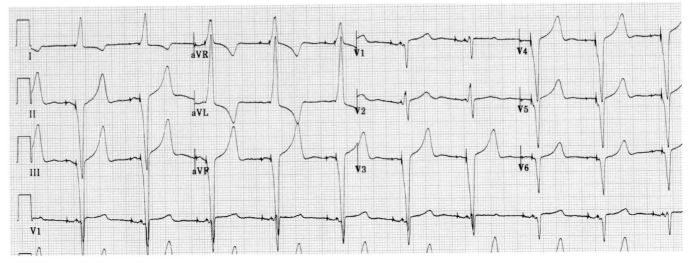

FIGURE 23.26A ■ Dual Chamber Pacemaker, Paced Rhythm. (ECG contributor: James V. Ritchie, MD.)

ECG Findings

- Very narrow signal of no discernable width, immediately followed by a P wave (if an atrial lead) or a QRS complex (if a ventricular lead). The narrow pacer "spike" amplitude varies, and can be larger than the QRS or may be indiscernible.

- A QRS complex initiated by a pacer spike will be wide, with morphology similar to a PVC or idioventricular rhythm. The axis is unlike typical bundle branch blocks, because the signal usually originates low in the right ventricle.

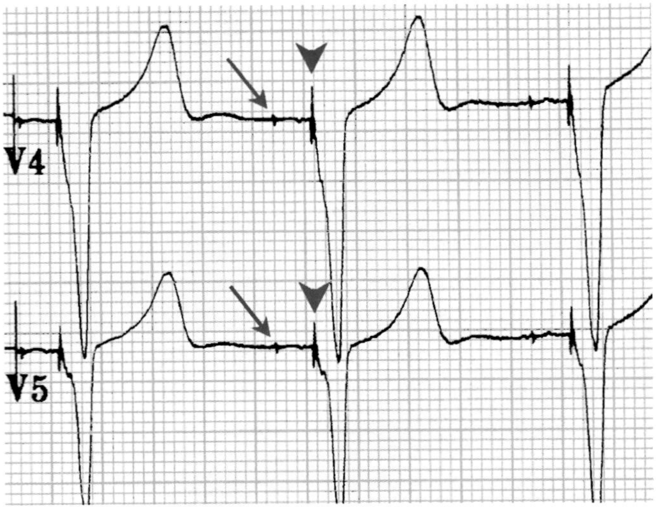

Pearls

1. Pacemakers are designated by the "five letter" system. In this system, the letter "A" denotes atrium, "V" denotes ventricle, "D" denotes dual (both chambers), and "O" denotes neither. The first three letters are the most commonly used:
   A. First letter—designates chamber(s) paced
   B. Second letter—designates chamber(s) sensed
   C. Third letter—designates pacemaker response to sensed electrical activity: T: triggered—fires even when beat sensed, I: inhibitory—holds when beat sensed, D: dual—atrial triggered and ventricle inhibited
   D. Fourth letter—extra options: P: programmable, M: multiprogrammable, C: communicating, R: rate adaptation, O: none

FIGURE 23.26B ■ Tiny pacer spikes (arrows) precede the P waves, and somewhat larger pacer spikes precede the QRS complexes (arrowheads). The QRS complexes are wide, with discordant T waves.

   E. Fifth letter—cardioverting options: P: pacing, S: shocking, D: dual (P+S), O: none
2. The two most common pacemaker malfunctions are failure to pace and failure to sense.
3. Some ECG machines perceive small pacer spikes as artifact and do not reproduce them on the printed tracing.

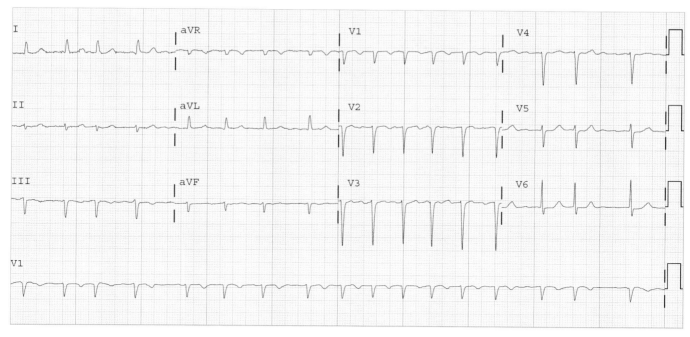

FIGURE 23.27A ▪ Atrial Fibrillation. (ECG contributor: R. Jason Thurman, MD.)

ECG Findings

- Electrical activity in the atria is chaotic. The ECG baseline, representing the ongoing chaotic atrial activity, is unorganized. The resulting "rumbling" baseline may have large or indiscernibly small amplitude.
- The AV node has a refractory period, and therefore does not conduct every signal it receives from the atria.
- Since the signals are received unpredictably, the AV node signals are sent to the ventricles in an "irregularly irregular" pattern creating varying R-R intervals.

Pearls

1. Most "irregularly irregular" rhythms are due to atrial fibrillation, but other rhythms may produce similar findings. These include multifocal atrial tachycardia, atrial flutter with variable AV block, and frequent PJCs.
2. Therapy is geared toward keeping the ventricular response at an appropriate rate.
3. Synchronized cardioversion may be indicated if a patient is unstable, but the risk of clot embolization must be carefully considered when planning nonemergent electrical cardioversion of atrial fibrillation.

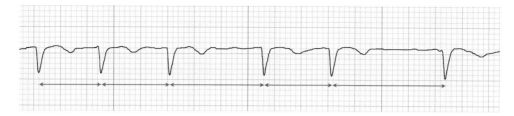

FIGURE 23.27B ▪ R-to-R interval varies in an "irregularly irregular" pattern (double arrows). The baseline "rumble," representing "F waves," may be very fine or even indiscernible.

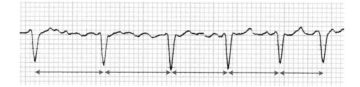

FIGURE 23.27C ▪ The baseline "rumble" may be very coarse resembling atrial flutter waves.

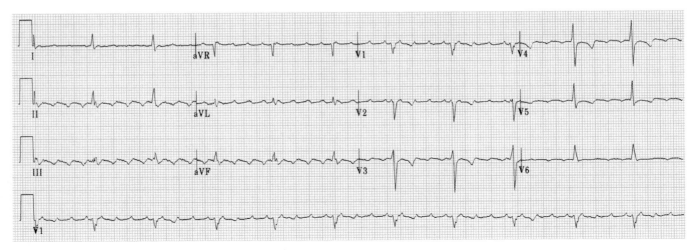

FIGURE 23.28A ■ Atrial Flutter. (ECG contributor: James V. Ritchie, MD.)

ECG Findings

- Electrical activity in the atria is ongoing and regular, self-propagating in a roughly circular movement.
- Flutter waves appear in a rapid sine wave or "sawtooth" pattern, usually in the inferior leads.
- Atrial activity in lead V_1 often appears as rapid P waves at a rate approximating 300 bpm.

Pearls

1. The AV node's refractory period prevents 1:1 conduction to the ventricles. Usually, conduction is blocked at a ratio of 1:2 to 1:4. The QRS complexes should appear with regular periodicity. However, AV conduction may be variable from beat-to-beat creating irregular R-to-R intervals.

2. A conduction ratio of 2:1 is usually difficult to discern, because the two flutter peaks between QRS complexes may look like normal P and T waves. A ventricular rate of 140 to 160 beats per minute should prompt consideration of the possibility of atrial flutter with 2:1 block.

3. Conditions that cause rapid repetitive tremors (such as Parkinson disease, rigors, shivering, or hepatic tremor) may mimic flutter waves on EKG (known as pseudoflutter).

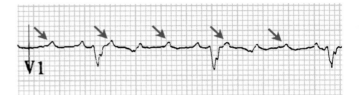

FIGURE 23.28B ■ Atrial flutter with 4:1 block. The flutter waves (arrows marking every other flutter wave) may be mistaken for P and T waves.

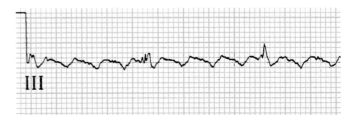

FIGURE 23.28C ■ The "sawtooth" pattern is most apparent in the inferior leads.

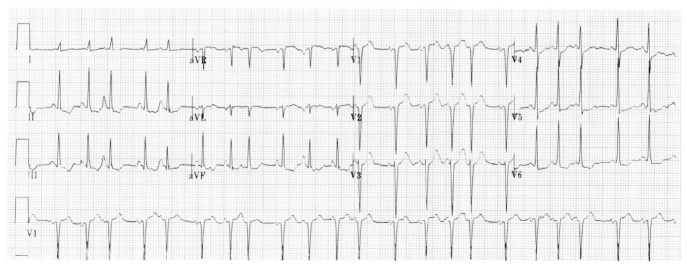

FIGURE 23.29A ■ Multifocal Atrial Tachycardia. (ECG contributor: James V. Ritchie, MD.)

ECG Findings

- Multiple P-wave morphologies with heart rate greater than 100 bpm
- A chaotic R-R interval
- Varying PR intervals

Pearls

1. Multiple atrial foci are capable of acting as pacemakers. When irritated by stretching, medications, or certain acute medical conditions, these foci compete in pacing the atria.

2. The different atrial foci produce P waves of different morphologies.

3. Since the atrial foci vary in distance to the AV node, PR intervals vary.

4. Multifocal atrial tachycardia (MAT) usually results from exacerbation of another condition which produces distention or irritation of the atria. The most common cause of MAT is COPD exacerbation. Treatment of the arrhythmia is by treating the underlying condition.

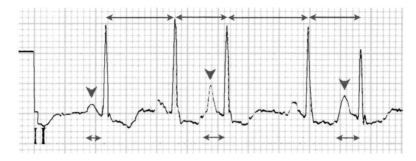

FIGURE 23.29B ■ Multiple P morphologies (arrowheads), varying PR intervals (lower double arrows), and varying R-R intervals (upper double arrows) with heart rate greater than 100 bpm.

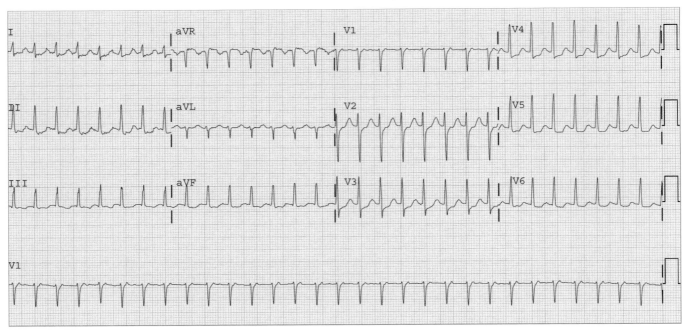

FIGURE 23.30A ■ Supraventricular Tachycardia (AVNRT). (ECG contributor: R. Jason Thurman, MD.)

ECG Findings

- Tachycardia, rate usually greater than 140 bpm
- Narrow QRS complex
- Absent, retrograde, or unusual P waves

Pearls

1. SVT occurs when the sinoatrial node rhythm is superseded by a faster rhythm, usually originating in the AV node.
2. Three common types are:
   A. Atrial tachycardia—originates from an ectopic focus in the atrium. P waves may have an unusual morphology or may be hidden by the preceding T wave.
   B. Atrioventricular nodal reentrant tachycardia (AVNRT) occurs when an electrical impulse continues around the AV node in a circular pattern causing rapid depolarizations of the ventricles. Since the AV node is the origin of the atrial depolarization, the P-wave deflection should be inverted if seen (eg, downgoing in II, III, aVF).
   C. Atrioventricular reentrant tachycardia (AVRT) as seen with bypass tracts outside of the AV node (WPW). Instead of intranodal reentrant activity as seen with AVNRT, an accessory tract provides the reentrant pathway to propagate the tachycardia.
3. Normal deflections seen in the ST-segments are relatively wide based. When you see "tight little turns" in the ST segment, you should strongly consider the presence of retrograde P waves.

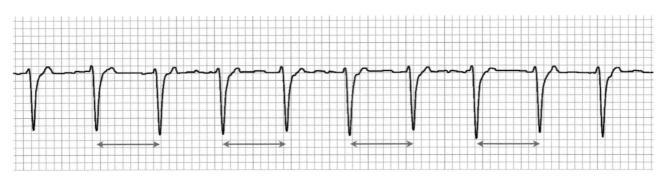

FIGURE 23.30B ■ A narrow-complex tachycardia, with no clear P waves preceding the QRS. R-R intervals are regular (double arrows), differentiating this from fine atrial fibrillation. This rhythm converted to a normal sinus rhythm after the administration of IV adenosine.

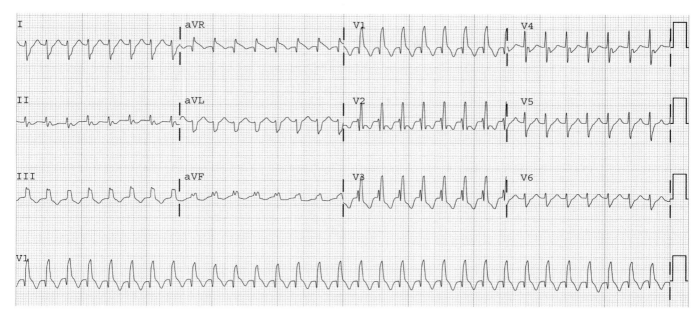

FIGURE 23.31A ■ Supraventricular Tachycardia with Aberrant Conduction, Underlying RBBB. (ECG contributor: Walter Clair, MD.)

ECG Findings

- Tachycardia (usually >120 bpm) with a wide QRS complex
- No "capture" or "fusion" beats or AV dissociation as seen with ventricular tachycardia
- QRS morphology consistent with one of the bundle branch block patterns

Pearls

1. When a person with a chronic wide-complex (aberrant) bundle branch block (BBB) enters a supraventricular tachycardia, the ECG will display a wide-complex tachycardia.

2. The rapid rate of a SVT may "outrun" the ventricular conducting system's ability to repolarize quickly, producing a rate-related bundle branch block. The signal then must propagate cell-to-cell, producing a wide-complex tachycardia. A typical bundle-branch pattern usually results.

3. An irregularly irregular or chaotic R-R interval, even if subtle, strongly suggests atrial fibrillation or flutter as the culprit SVT. In contrast, the R-R interval of ventricular tachycardia is almost never chaotic.

4. Ventricular rates of 140 to 160 should prompt consideration of atrial flutter with a 2:1 block.

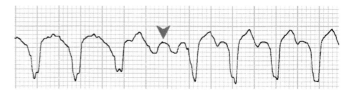

FIGURE 23.31C ■ Wide-complex tachycardia at approximately 150 bpm. The R-R interval is regular, except for one pause, when characteristic atrial flutter waves are apparent (arrowhead).

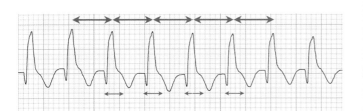

FIGURE 23.31B ■ Wide-complex tachycardia with a rate of 188 bpm. This patient has sudden onset of SVT with a known underlying RBBB. QRS complexes are wide (lower double arrows) and R-R intervals are regular (upper double arrows).

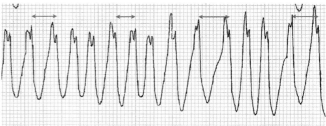

FIGURE 23.31D ■ Irregularity in the R-R interval, as seen most easily in the baseline (double arrows), strongly suggests the presence of rapidly conducted atrial fibrillation with aberrancy.

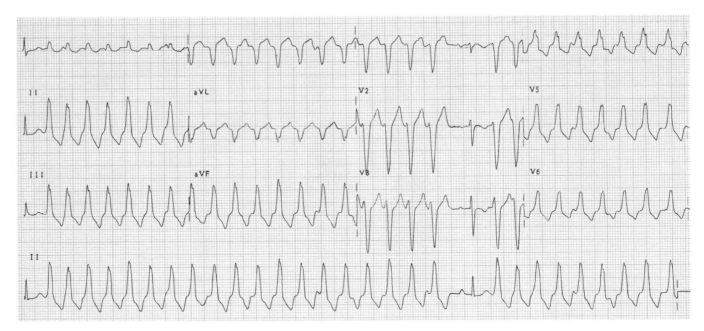

FIGURE 23.32A ■ Ventricular Tachycardia with Capture Beat. (ECG contributor: James V. Ritchie, MD.)

ECG Findings

- Tachycardia (usually >120 bpm) with a wide QRS complex.
- AV dissociation is present; P waves may appear periodically in the T wave or baseline.
- "Capture" beats may occur if atrial depolarization occurs prior to the intrinsic firing of the ventricle.
- "Fusion" beats may occur if atrial depolarization passes through the AV node at the same time as the intrinsic ventricle depolarization, producing a QRS that appears to be different or narrower than the other VT QRS complexes.

Pearls

Findings suggestive of VT versus aberrant SVT or antidromic WPW:

1. Apparent AV dissociation, capture, or fusion beats
2. An unusual QRS axis, between 180 to 270 degrees
3. Precordial concordance, in which QRS complexes in the precordium are all upgoing or all downgoing
4. A completely upgoing QRS in V_1
5. Predominately downgoing QRS in V_4, V_5, and V_6

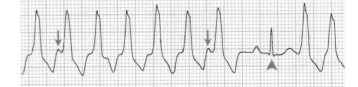

FIGURE 23.32B ■ A wide-complex tachycardia. AV dissociation is apparent, as P waves occasionally appear superimposed in the ST segment or just prior to the QRS (arrows). A capture beat occurs following a lapse in the VT (arrowhead).

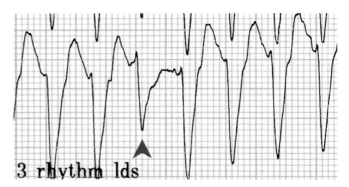

FIGURE 23.32C ■ Another example of ventricular tachycardia, featuring a fusion beat (arrowhead). (ECG contributor: Marc Mickiewicz, MD.)

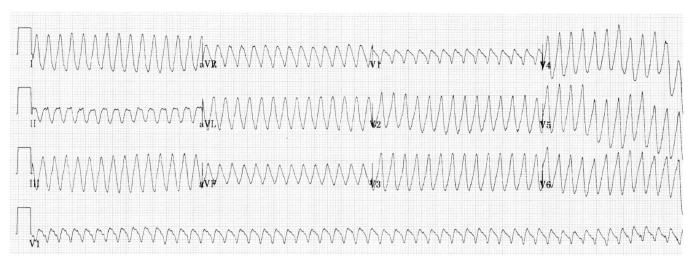

FIGURE 23.33A ■ Ventricular Flutter. (ECG contributor: James V. Ritchie, MD.)

ECG Findings

- Tachycardia with a wide monomorphic QRS complex
- Ventricular rate may be very rapid (300 bpm)
- Sine wave appearance with regular large oscillations

Pearls

1. Imagine an atrial flutter sawtooth with much larger amplitude.
2. When you see a very rapid wide-complex tachycardia (>240 bpm), consider ventricular flutter or WPW with atrial fibrillation or flutter.
3. WPW with atrial flutter may be indistinguishable from ventricular flutter.
4. Ventricular flutter is treated as ventricular tachycardia.
5. Ventricular flutter usually leads to ventricular fibrillation if not promptly corrected with antiarrhythmic medications or electrical cardioversion.
6. Patients with such a rapid rate are almost always unstable. Emergent cardioversion is indicated. If the patient appears to be stable enough for chemical cardioversion, choose a medication which is safe to use with WPW, such as procainamide or amiodarone.

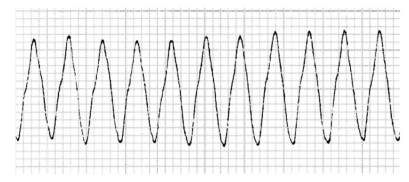

FIGURE 23.33B ■ Very rapid, regular, wide-complex tachycardia with sine-wave appearance. The rate in this example is 330 bpm. Differential diagnosis includes WPW with atrial flutter.

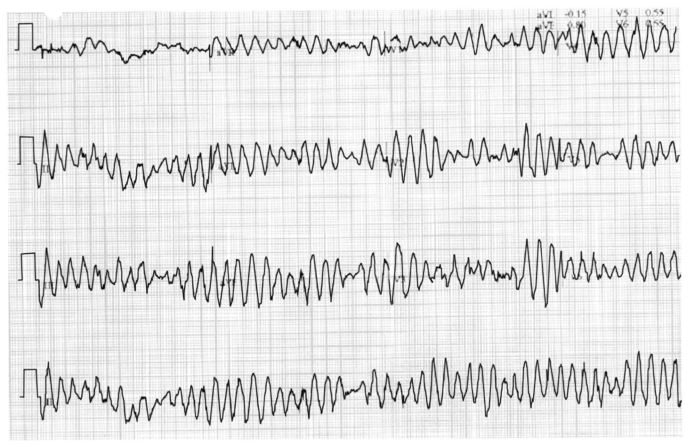

FIGURE 23.34A ■ Torsades de Pointes. (ECG contributor: James V. Ritchie, MD.)

ECG Findings

- Wide-complex tachycardia with QRS polymorphism.
- QRS morphology changes gradually throughout the tracing, appearing to rotate around the baseline to the opposite direction.

Pearls

1. The cyclic rotation of the QRS complex gives rise to the term Torsades de pointes (French meaning "twisting of the points").

2. Common precipitating factors are etiologies which prolong the QT interval such as: medications, electrolyte abnormalities (hypocalcemia, hypomagnesemia, hypokalemia), and hereditary disorders.

3. Torsades can also occur in the setting of myocardial ischemia without prolongation of the QT interval.

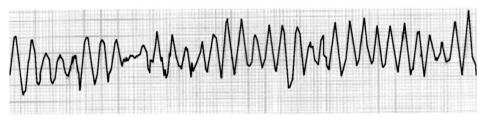

FIGURE 23.34B ■ Very rapid wide-complex tachycardia with sine-wave appearance and fluctuations in the amplitude of the QRS complexes consistent with Torsades de pointes.

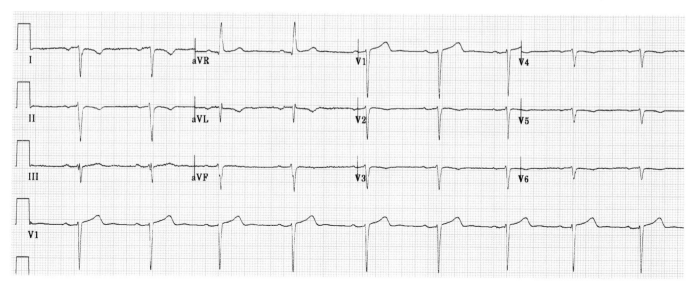

FIGURE 23.35A ■ Dextrocardia. (ECG contributor: James V. Ritchie, MD.)

ECG Findings

- P, QRS, and T are downgoing in lead I, a mirror image of normal.
- QRS deflections in V_4 to V_6 are small and downgoing.

Pearls

1. The orientation of the heart in the chest cavity is reversed with the predominant electrical activity moving left to right (as opposed to right to left).

2. Normally placed precordial leads in a patient with dextrocardia are actually placed over the thinner right ventricle instead of the left ventricle.

3. Reversing all EKG leads should produce an essentially normal EKG.

4. A "reversed" lead I with normal-appearing V leads strongly suggests accidental limb lead reversal.

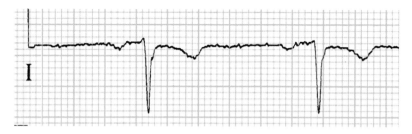

FIGURE 23.35B ■ The P wave, QRS, and T wave are downgoing in lead I. Differential diagnosis includes limb lead reversal and dextrocardia. The 12-lead ECG above represents Dextrocardia as evidenced in the abnormal precordial leads.

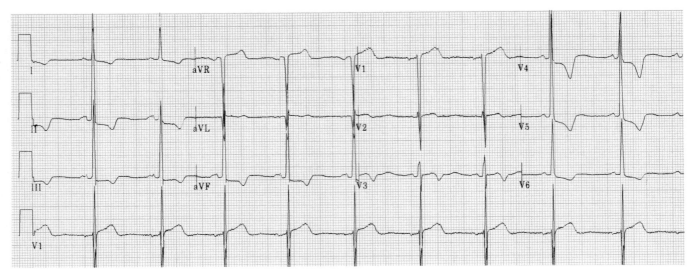

FIGURE 23.36A ■ Left Ventricular Hypertrophy with Strain Pattern. (ECG contributor: James V. Ritchie, MD.)

ECG Findings

- Large S waves in anterior precordial leads
- Large R waves in lateral precordial leads
- R wave in aVL + S wave in V_3 greater than 28 mm in males, greater than 20 mm in females
- S wave in V_1 + R wave in V_5 or V_6 greater than 35 mm if age over 40, greater than 40 mm if age 30 to 40, greater than 60 mm if age 16 to 30
- R wave in aVL greater than 11 mm
- T waves deflected opposite to QRS complex (strain pattern)

Pearls

1. The muscular left ventricle normally dominates the QRS morphology.

2. LVH can produce related changes such as left atrial abnormality. It may also produce ST-T wave changes, particularly in opposite deflections of the T wave with respect to the main deflection of the QRS complex. These ST deflections, often referred to as "LVH with strain," may be confused with ischemia.

3. LVH is often a sign of disease states such as systemic hypertension or aortic stenosis.

4. LVH may manifest on the ECG in many different ways. Several different systems for diagnosing LVH by ECG have been promoted. No one system is adequately sensitive *and* specific enough to warrant exclusion of all others.

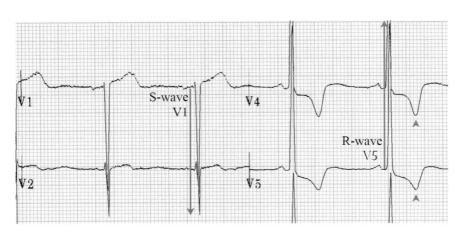

FIGURE 23.36B ■ The QRS deflections are very large. The R wave in V_5 plus the S wave in V_1 total approximately 75 mm (arrows). ST downsloping to inverted T waves in V_4 and V_5 (arrowheads) may also be seen, a finding often referred to as "LVH with strain."

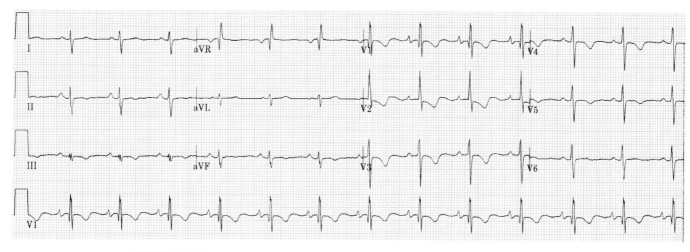

FIGURE 23.37A ■ Right Ventricular Hypertrophy. (ECG contributor: James V. Ritchie, MD.)

ECG Findings

- S wave amplitude increases in lateral leads (V_5, V_6, I, aVL).
- R wave amplitude increases in aVR, V_1, V_2, and may exceed the S-wave amplitude (especially in lead V_1).
- Right axis deviation (> +90 degrees).
- T wave inversions in relation to QRS complex.

Pearls

1. Hypertrophy of the right ventricle causes characteristic EKG changes as the predominant electrical signal of the left ventricle is overcome.
2. As right ventricular hypertrophy (RVH) persists, right atrial enlargement (RAE) may occur as seen in the example (P wave amplitude in V_1 >1.5 mm).
3. Congenital heart disease, pulmonic or mitral stenosis, and pulmonary hypertension are common causes of RVH.

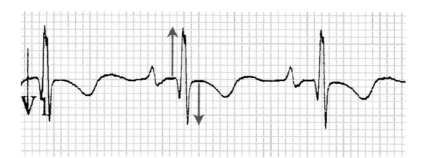

FIGURE 23.37B ■ The R wave amplitude exceeds the S wave amplitude (arrows) in lead V_1. In addition, the P wave upward deflection exceeds 1.5 mm, indicating concomitant right atrial enlargement.

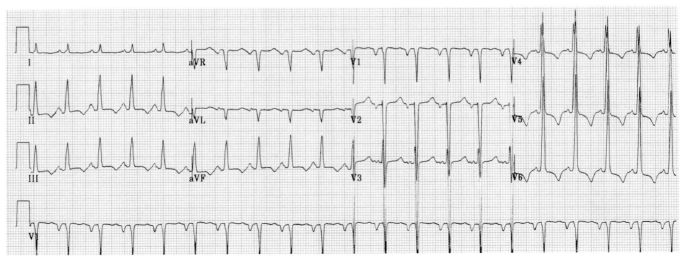

FIGURE 23.38A ■ Left Atrial Hypertrophy with LVH Present. (ECG contributor: James V. Ritchie, MD.)

ECG Findings

- Increased duration (width) of the P wave without affecting its upward amplitude (as commonly seen with right atrial abnormalities)
- Negative P wave deflection in lead V_1, with width and depth greater than 0.04 seconds (one small box)
- Wide P wave in lead II
- Notched P wave in II, III, or aVF with duration greater than or equal to 0.12 seconds (also known as P-mitrale)

Pearls

1. Normal P wave morphology has an amplitude of less than 2.5 mV (2.5 vertical boxes) and a duration (width) of less than 120 ms (3 small boxes).

2. The left atrium depolarizes after the right atrium and therefore has the most effect on the second portion of the P wave.

3. Causes of left atrial abnormality or P-mitrale include: valvular heart disease (mitral and aortic), CAD, cardiomyopathy, hypertension, and left ventricular hypertrophy.

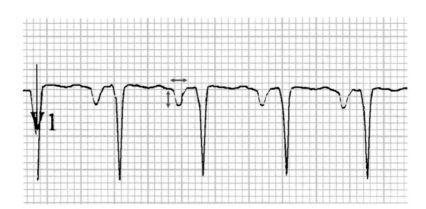

FIGURE 23.38B ■ The P wave in V_1 is downgoing. The downgoing segment is wider and deeper than one small block (double arrows).

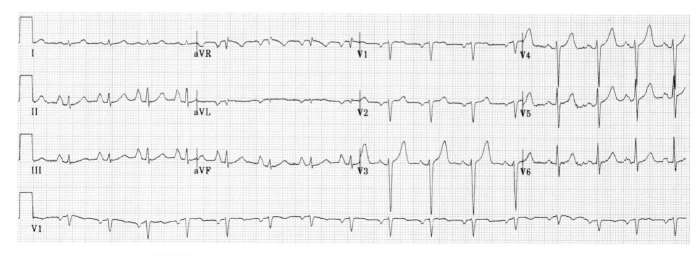

FIGURE 23.39A ■ Right Atrial Hypertrophy. (ECG contributor: James V. Ritchie, MD.)

ECG Findings

- Increased amplitude of P wave without affecting duration (as commonly seen with left atrial abnormalities)
- Peaked P waves (>2.5 mm) in leads II, III, aVF (also known as P pulmonale)
- P waves upward deflection greater than 1.5 mm in lead V_1 or V_2

Pearls

1. Normal P wave morphology has amplitude of less than 2.5 mV (2.5 small vertical boxes) and duration (width) of less than 120 ms (3 small boxes).

2. The right atrium depolarizes before the left atrium and therefore has the most effect on the first portion of the P wave.

3. RAE is often associated with right ventricular hypertrophy, COPD, some congenital heart diseases, pulmonary hypertension, and may be seen transiently in pulmonary embolus.

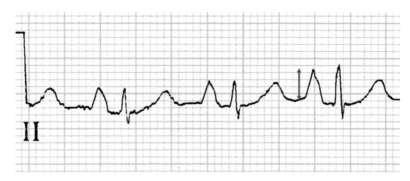

FIGURE 23.39B ■ The P wave in lead II (an inferior lead) is greater than 2.5 mm in amplitude (double arrow).

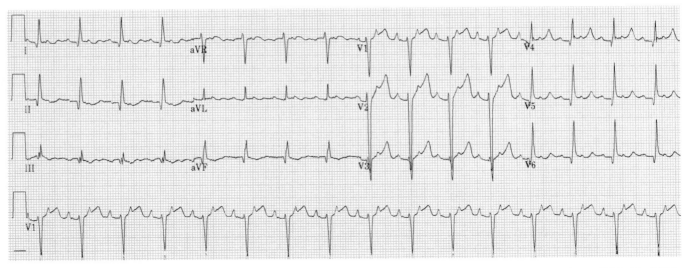

FIGURE 23.40A ■ Hypertrophic Cardiomyopathy with underlying Atrial Flutter with 2:1 Block. (ECG contributor: James V. Ritchie, MD.)

ECG Findings

- High-voltage QRS suggesting left ventricular hypertrophy
- Left atrial abnormality
- Prominent Q waves, especially in the lateral precordial leads
- Deep S waves in anterior precordial leads
- Poor R wave progression across precordium
- Lateral T wave inversions

Pearls

1. The ventricular myocardium hypertrophies abnormally, either concentrically or focally. Left ventricle outflow obstruction from the hypertrophy may lead to LVH without dilation.

2. HCM is also known as idiopathic hypertrophic subaortic stenosis (IHSS), hypertrophic obstructive cardiomyopathy (HOCM), and muscular subaortic stenosis (MSS).

3. ECG changes are variable and usually do not include all listed above.

4. Always consider this condition in young athletes with syncope or unusual dyspnea.

5. HCM is associated with a systolic ejection murmur that diminishes with increases in preload (having the patient squat) and augments with decreases in preload (Valsalva maneuver).

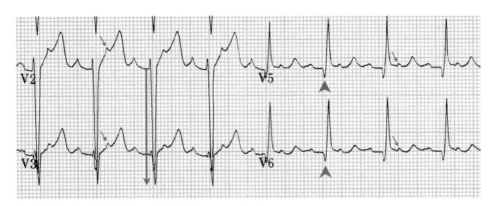

FIGURE 23.40B ■ Deep S-wave voltage (28 mm S in V_2, large arrow), and narrow Q waves in V_5 and V_6 (arrowheads). This patient also has atrial flutter with 2:1 block. The additional P waves appear in the ST segments (small arrows).

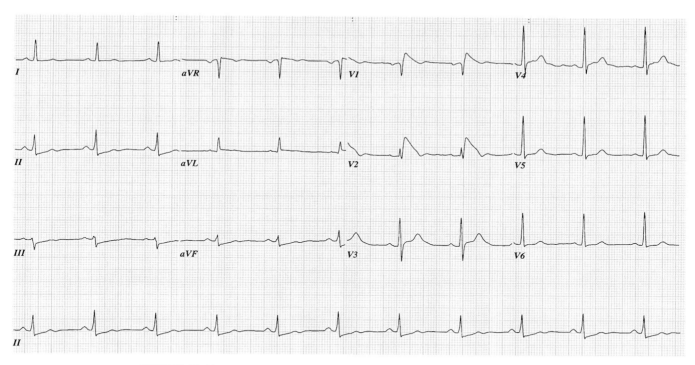

FIGURE 23.41A ■ Brugada Syndrome. (ECG contributor: Michael L. Juliano, MD.)

ECG Findings

- Incomplete or complete RBBB pattern in leads V_1, V_2, and sometimes V_3.
- ST elevation of at least 1 mV in leads V_1, V_2, and sometimes V_3 followed by T inversion (convex pattern) or upright T (concave, or "saddle back" pattern).

Pearls

1. This syndrome was first described in individuals who experienced sudden cardiac death with structurally normal hearts, but congenitally abnormal ion channels in myocyte cell membranes have been associated with the disease.
2. Concern for spontaneous ventricular dysrhythmia is high.
3. Consultation with a cardiologist is recommended for electrophysiological testing and intracardiac defibrillator placement.

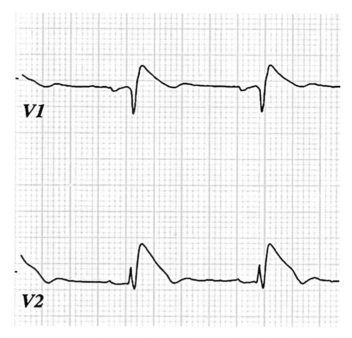

FIGURE 23.41B ■ RBBB pattern with ST elevation (type 1 Brugada syndrome).

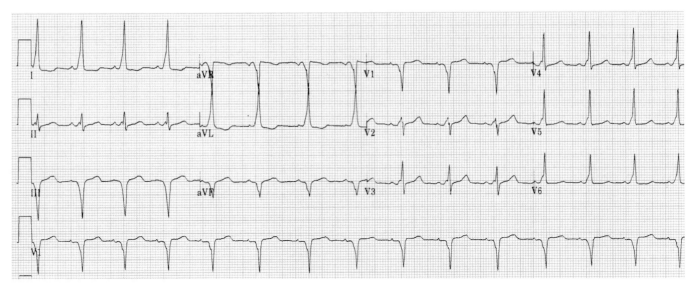

FIGURE 23.42A ■ Wolff-Parkinson-White Syndrome. (ECG contributor: James V. Ritchie, MD.)

ECG Findings

- Normal P waves
- Shortened PR interval
- Prolonged QRS interval
- Delta waves (slurring of the initial upstroke of R wave)

Pearls

1. Accessory tracts from the atria to the ventricles lead to depolarization of ventricles without using the AV node as the primary connecting route.
2. Tachycardia associated with WPW may be mistaken for ventricular tachycardia. Suspect WPW if the QRS complex is wide and tachycardia is extreme (ventricular rate >240).
3. Do not treat this tachycardia with AV nodal blocking agents (calcium channel blockers, β-blockers, digoxin). This may lead to unopposed ventricular stimulation through the accessory tract and may worsen the tachycardia.
4. Procainamide, amiodarone, and cardioversion are accepted methods for conversion of a tachycardia associated with WPW.
5. Depolarization via the accessory pathway may produce "pseudo-Q waves" as shown in leads III and aVF in this example.

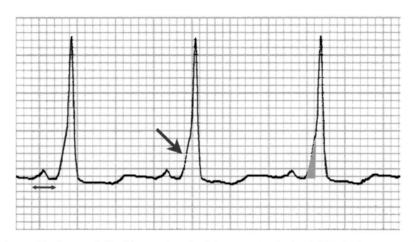

FIGURE 23.42B ■ The PR interval is shortened (double arrow) and a delta wave (upsloping initial QRS segment) is seen (arrow, shaded area).

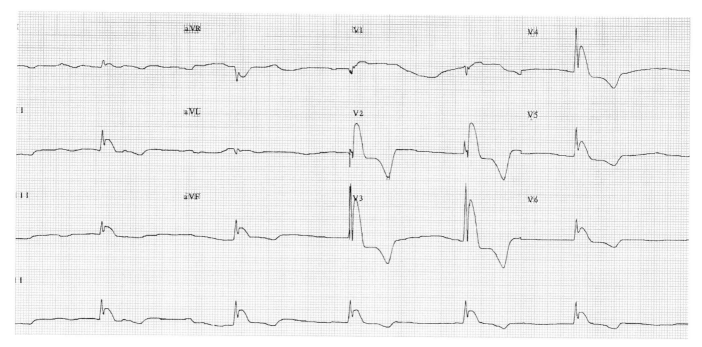

FIGURE 23.43A ■ Hypothermia with Osborne Waves ("J" Waves) Present. (ECG contributor: Michael L. Juliano, MD.)

ECG Findings

- Sinus bradycardia or atrial fibrillation with slow ventricular response.
- PR, QRS, and QT intervals are typically prolonged.
- Osborne or "J" wave (a positive deflection of the terminal portion of the QRS complex). The J wave may be subtle or large and "humped."

Pearls

1. The hypothermic patient's rhythm slows, proceeding from sinus bradycardia to atrial fibrillation with slow response and may proceed to other arrhythmias including ventricular fibrillation and asystole.
2. The amplitude of the "J" wave corresponds to the degree of hypothermia.
3. Myocardial damage and EKG changes associated with hypothermia are not necessarily due to low temperature. They may be indirectly caused by systemic circulatory issues such as hypoperfusion.
4. Defibrillation and many medications may be ineffective in the hypothermic patient. Rapid rewarming is indicated as an initial and critical resuscitative measure.

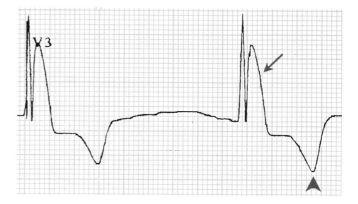

FIGURE 23.43B ■ A large Osborn wave (J wave) (arrow) follows the QRS, and is distinct from the T wave (arrowhead).

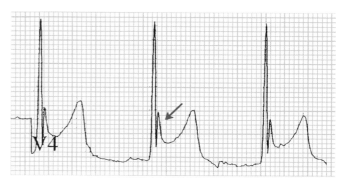

FIGURE 23.43C ■ This is a more typical appearance of a J wave (arrow).

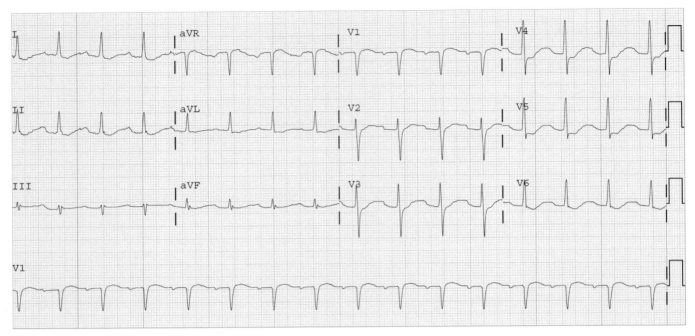

FIGURE 23.44A ■ Hypokalemia (ECG contributor: R. Jason Thurman, MD.)

ECG Findings

- Flattened or inverted T waves
- Prominent U waves
- ST segment depression
- Conduction disturbances

Pearls

1. Hypokalemia can produce varied ECG changes associated with the repolarization phase of the cardiac cycle.

2. Unlike hyperkalemia, in hypokalemia there is no direct correlation with the potassium level and the severity of ECG changes. However, more ECG changes may become apparent as the potassium level falls.

3. Suspect hypomagnesemia if the ECG does not normalize after potassium replacement.

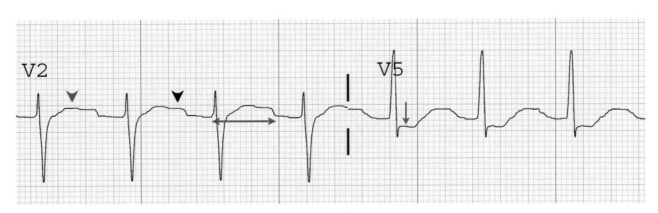

FIGURE 23.44B ■ This EKG demonstrates multiple findings consistent with hypokalemia: flattened T waves (blue arrowhead), U waves (black arrowhead), prolonged QT (QU) intervals (double arrow), and ST-segment depression (arrow). This patient's potassium level was 1.9.

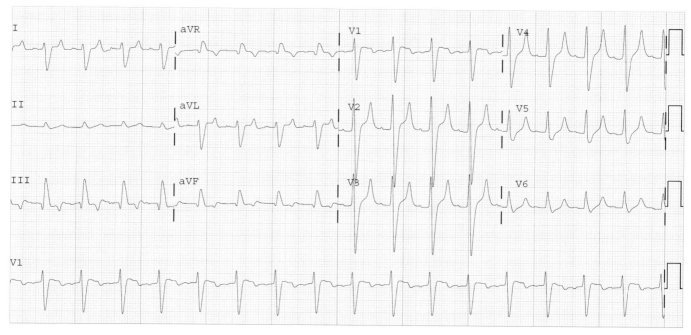

FIGURE 23.45A ■ Hyperkalemia (K 7.1). (ECG contributor: R. Jason Thurman, MD.)

ECG Findings

Findings are variable but tend to correlate with increasing serum potassium levels following the order below:

- Peaked T waves, tented with a narrow base (may be >10 mm high in precordial leads and/or >6 mm in limb leads)
- QT interval shortening

- QRS complex widening
- PR interval prolongation
- Decreased P wave amplitude
- As potassium levels approach and exceed 8.0 mEQ/L:
  - Indiscernible P waves
  - Sine wave appearance of QRS-T complex
  - Left or right bundle branch pattern
  - Ventricular tachycardia, fibrillation, or asystole

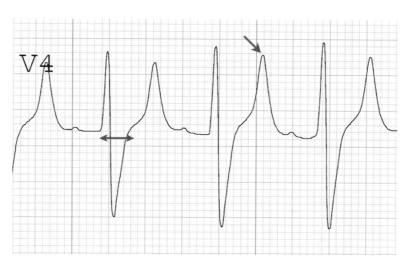

FIGURE 23.45B ■ Peaked T waves (arrow), widened QRS (double arrow), and subtle flattening of the P waves are seen in this patient with a serum K of 7.1.

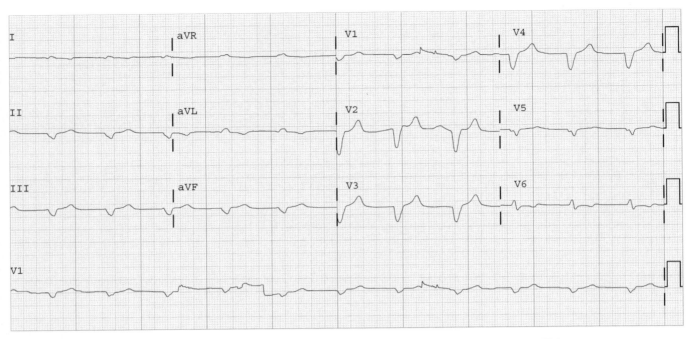

FIGURE 23.46A ■ Severe Hyperkalemia (K 8.5). (ECG contributor: Ben Heavrin, MD.)

Pearls

1. As the QRS complex widens, it appears more "blunted" than expected when compared with a left bundle branch block.

2. Acute treatment for hyperkalemia includes insulin and glucose, sodium bicarbonate, and β-agonists in an attempt to drive potassium into the cell. Intravenous calcium may be used to stabilize the myocardium but has no effect on serum potassium levels. These are temporizing measures which must be followed by definitive treatment of the underlying problem, which may include the need for dialysis.

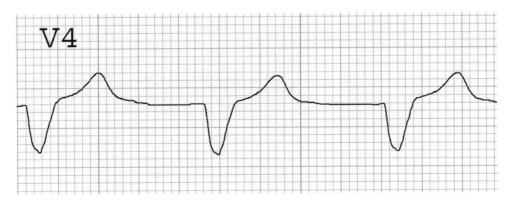

FIGURE 23.46B ■ Wide, blunted QRS with near sine-wave appearance. No P waves visible. Serum K was 8.5 in this patient. These abnormalities resolved with rapid treatment.

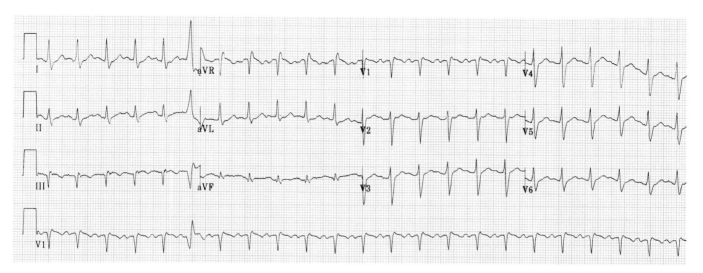

FIGURE 23.47A ■ Sinus Tachycardia and S1Q3T3 pattern in a patient with acute pulmonary embolism. (ECG contributor: James V. Ritchie, MD.)

ECG Findings

- Sinus tachycardia, nonspecific ST-T changes
- Precordial T wave inversions
- Prominent S wave in lead I, Q wave in lead III, and inverted T wave in III (S1/Q3/T3)
- Incomplete or complete RBBB, P pulmonale (lead II)
- May see right axis deviation

Pearls

1. No EKG pattern is diagnostic for pulmonary embolism. Small-to-moderate emboli may not affect the EKG.
2. With large emboli, increased resistance to pulmonary arterial flow produces right ventricle overload and dilation.
3. Increased right atrial pressures may produce "P pulmonale," (tall P waves >2.5 mm in lead II) or atrial dysrhythmias.

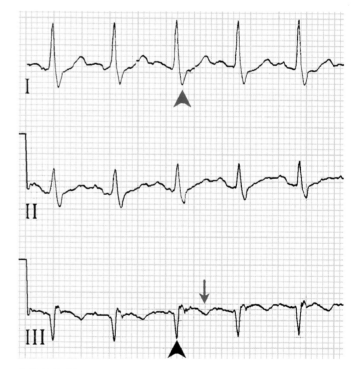

FIGURE 23.47B ■ S wave is apparent in lead I (blue arrowhead), Q wave in lead III (black arrowhead), and inverted T wave in lead III (blue arrow).

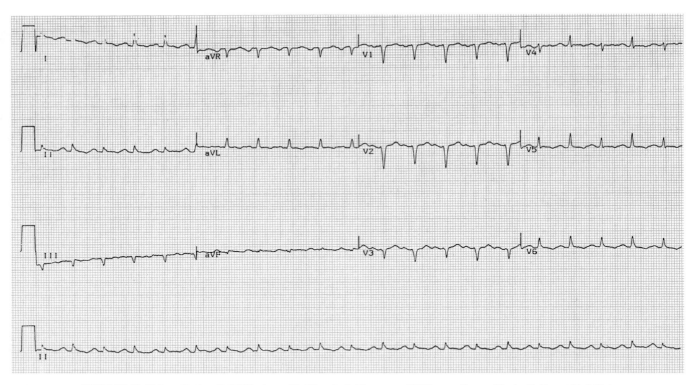

FIGURE 23.48A ■ Pericardial Effusion with Electrical Alternans. (ECG contributor: Kevin E. Zawacki, MD.)

ECG Findings

- Sinus tachycardia
- Low voltage of QRS complex (QRS averaging <5 mm height in limb leads, or <10 mm height in precordial leads)
- Electrical alternans (beat-to-beat change in electrical axis and/or amplitude of the QRS complex)

Pearls

1. A physiologically significant pericardial effusion compresses the heart, and affects the ability of the heart to fill properly. This typically results in a reflex sinus tachycardia to maintain cardiac output.

2. Pericardial effusion may be caused by pericarditis, malignancy, uremia, trauma, iatrogenic injury (CVL placement), aortic dissection with retrograde involvement of the pericardium, and free wall rupture after a myocardial infarction.

3. Initial treatment of physiologically significant pericardial effusion is with intravenous fluid bolus to increase preload. Pericardiocentesis should be reserved for hemodynamically threatening effusions due to a high associated morbidity. Surgical pericardial window may be necessary, especially in malignant effusions.

4. Electrical alternans is an uncommon finding. Pericardial effusion should be suspected in the setting of a sinus tachycardia and low voltage.

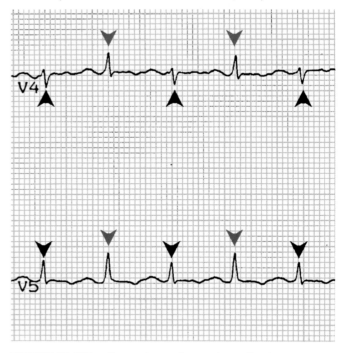

FIGURE 23.48B ■ Low voltage, sinus tachycardia, electrical alternans (arrowheads) demonstrate beat-to-beat alternating QRS electrical axis and/or amplitude. Electrical alternans is often best seen in the anterior precordial leads V_3 and V_4.

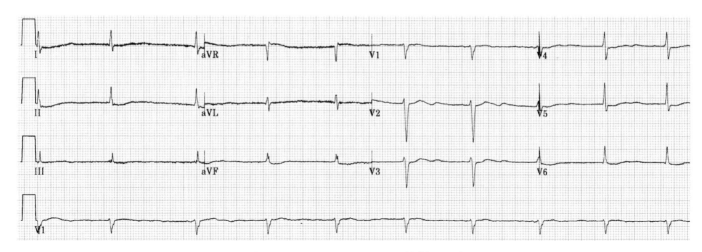

FIGURE 23.49A ■ Digoxin Effect with Evidence of Toxicity. (ECG contributor: James V. Ritchie, MD.)

ECG Findings

- ST segment shortening and depression leading to a "scooped" appearance
- QT interval shortening
- PR interval prolongation
- Decreased T wave amplitude
- Premature ventricular complexes are the most common dysrhythmia
- Bradydysrhythmias, various heart blocks, especially with findings consistent with increased automaticity (atrial tachycardia with block, atrial fibrillation with slow ventricular response, accelerated junctional rhythms)
- Bidirectional ventricular tachythms may rarely be seen (see Figure 17.67).

Pearls

1. ECG changes associated with digoxin can be seen from therapeutic or toxic levels.
2. ST segment changes may be exaggerated by myocardial disease or tachycardia.
3. An acute overdose of a digoxin is usually associated with hyperkalemia which may increase the height of the T wave.
4. Avoid calcium for treatment of hyperkalemia in the setting of digoxin toxicity as this may potentiate some adverse effects of digoxin.
5. A digoxin overdose can lead to almost any dysrhythmia, but it commonly blocks the transmission of impulses through the AV node leading to bradycardic rhythms and accelerated escape rhythms.

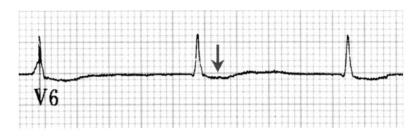

FIGURE 23.49B ■ The "sagging" appearance of the ST segment (arrow) is characteristic of digoxin therapy, and is not a sign of toxicity. However, this patient also has a sign of chronic digoxin toxicity. Atrial fibrillation is present, but the R-to-R interval has become regular. Digoxin toxicity has produced a total AV block but has also excited the AV node, producing a relatively accelerated junctional escape rate.

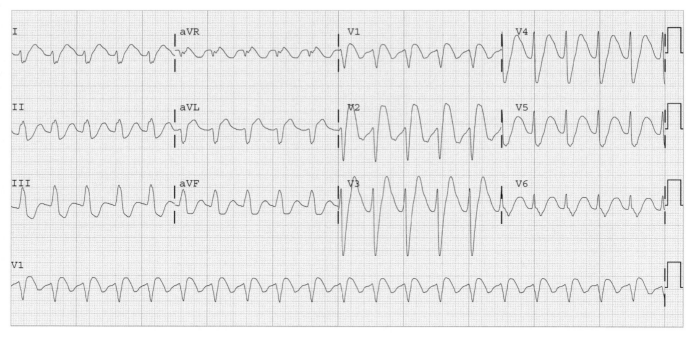

FIGURE 23.50A ■ Tricyclic Antidepressant Toxicity. (ECG contributor: Saralyn R. Williams, MD.)

ECG Findings

- Tachycardia
- QRS complex widening
- QT prolongation
- Prominent terminal R wave in aVR or V_1
- Prominent S in Lead I

Pearls

1. TCAs produce their effects by several mechanisms. Anticholinergic effects may induce tachycardia and sodium channel blockage may lead to QRS widening.

2. The QRS widening seen in a TCA overdose has a non-specific pattern and is typically unlike any bundle branch block morphology.

3. ECG effects are rate dependent and become more pronounced with tachycardia and acidosis.

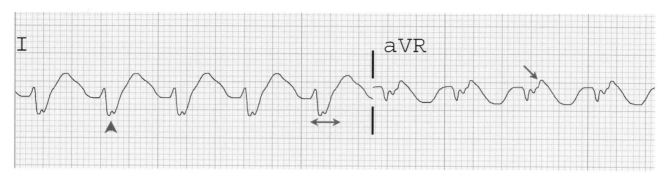

FIGURE 23.50B ■ Prominent S wave in lead I (arrowhead) with prominent terminal R wave in aVR (arrow). The QRS complex is wide (double arrow), the QT interval is prolonged, and the patient is tachycardic.

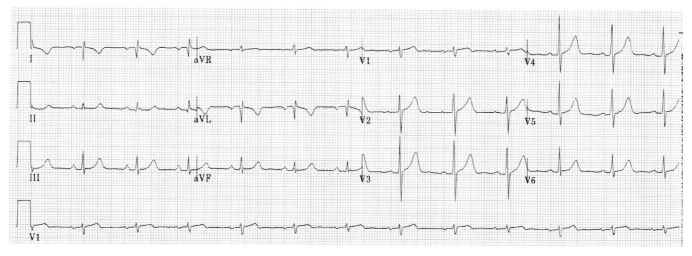

FIGURE 23.51A ■ Limb Lead Reversal. (ECG contributor: Michael L. Juliano, MD.)

ECG Findings (dependent on which leads are reversed)

- Reversal of the left arm (LA) and right arm (RA), most common
  - P, QRS, and T predominantly downgoing in lead I
  - P, QRS, T upgoing in lead aVR
  - Precordial leads unaffected
- Reversal of the leg leads (left leg [LL] and right leg [RL])
  - Does not commonly produce EKG changes because RL is used as a grounding electrode
- Reversal of LA-LL
  - Transposition of leads I and II and leads aVF and aVL with reversal of lead III
- Reversal of RA-RL
  - Transposition of aVR and aVL and inversion of lead II

- Incorrect precordial lead placement
  - Isolated reversal of the usual R-wave progression from V_1-V_6

Pearls

1. If the ECG seems to have an unusual axis or appearance, especially when compared with a prior ECG on the same patient, consider a lead misplacement and repeat the tracing, confirming correct lead positions.

2. A "reversed" lead I with normal-appearing V leads strongly suggests accidental limb lead reversal as opposed to dextrocardia. Dextrocardia features a "reversed" lead I while QRS deflections in V_4 to V_6 appear small and downgoing

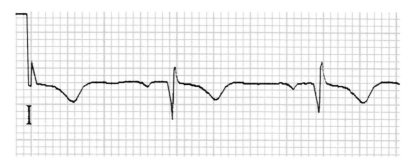

FIGURE 23.51B ■ The P wave, QRS, and T wave are inverted in lead I in this EKG. Normal-appearing V leads in the 12-lead ECG above suggest limb lead reversal rather than dextrocardia. The arm leads were indeed reversed, and correction produced a normal-appearing tracing.

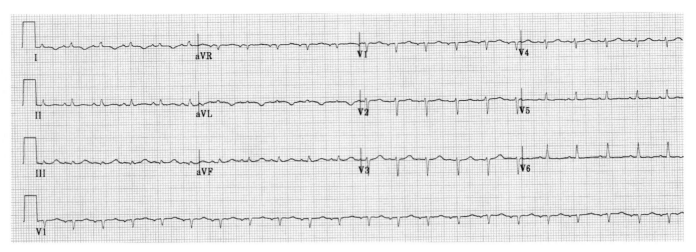

FIGURE 23.52A ■ Low-Voltage EKG. (ECG contributor: James V. Ritchie, MD.)

ECG Finding

- QRS amplitude of less than or equal to 5 mV in all limb leads or a sum of all limb lead QRS amplitude less than or equal to 30 mV and/or QRS amplitude less than or equal to 10 mV in all precordial leads

Pearls

1. Differential diagnosis includes: Normal variant, low standardization of the ECG machine, pericardial or pleural effusion, obesity/anasarca, COPD/emphysema, cardiac infiltrate (tumor, amyloid), myocardial infarction, myocarditis, cardiomyopathy, adrenal insufficiency, or hypothyroidism
2. Always check the calibration markings at the left of the ECG to check for low standardization of the ECG machine as an etiology for the observed tracing.

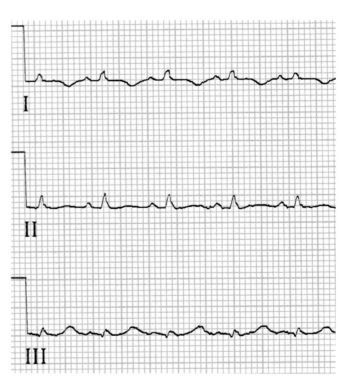

FIGURE 23.52B ■ QRS height is less than 5 mm in limb leads in this normally calibrated tracing.

Chapter 24

EMERGENCY ULTRASOUND

Paul R. Sierzenski
Jason Gukhool
Stephen J. Leech

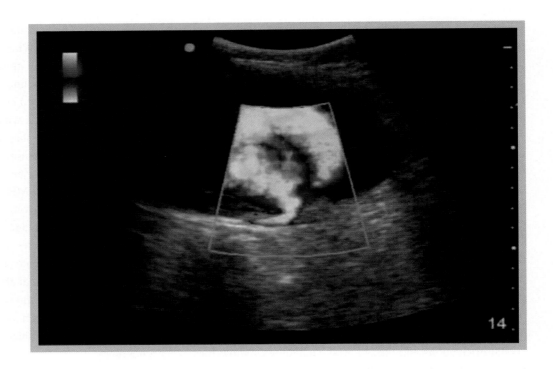

Emergency medicine ultrasound has the basic goal of improving patient care. This chapter strives to provide a "visual blueprint" for the reader who uses emergency medicine ultrasonography in his or her practice. It is intended to serve as a practical imaging reference when an emergency screening ultrasound examination (EUS) is being performed and assumes a basic knowledge and experience base in ultrasound examinations. For practitioners without this prerequisite body of knowledge, it may provide useful information about the scope of the EUS examination.

Success in performing an EUS is dependent on the physician's goal-directed approach to each examination. This demands that the physician uses ultrasound to identify, confirm, or exclude specific sonographic findings that are consistent with specific disease states or life-threatening conditions.

Basic ultrasound information—including transducer recommendations, scanning protocols, anatomic schematics, and ultrasound images—are presented throughout the chapter. Applicable protocols are patterned after imaging guidelines of the American Institute of Ultrasound in Medicine as well as the authors' collective experiences. The issues of the efficacy, accuracy, and/or sensitivity of this modality are not debated. Once again, this chapter is not presented as a primary instructional tool, but rather as a rapid visual review for the physician trained in EUS applications.

Transducers

Sonography is performed using transducers of varying frequencies and configurations (Fig. 24.1). Lower or higher frequencies are selected for more or less depth of penetration. Many manufacturers produce multifrequency transducers available with small or large footprints. Different crystal orientations and phased array technologies allow for purpose built probes that emphasize detail (linear) or maximize the viewing area (curved). The various transducers recommended for use in the EUS include:

- *Microconvex*: This transducer has the advantage of a tight curvature and small footprint that allows for easy access between ribs and for subxiphoid imaging. This is an excellent transducer for the E-FAST, especially for the beginner who may have difficulty scanning or interpreting images with rib shadowing present. This probe is also helpful in the thin patients with a high-positioned gallbladder requiring intercostal windows for optimal imaging. These transducers are generally more expensive than the standard curve-linear transducer.

- *Convex Array*: Considered a standard abdominal transducer, it provides wide near and far fields of view (ideal in evaluating the aorta in long axis). The large footprint of this type of transducer may make subxiphoid cardiac imaging difficult, as will the noted presence of "rib shadowing" which is inevitable with this transducer in scanning the right/left upper quadrants in the coronal plane. This is the transducer of choice for abdominal imaging and is used by many vascular laboratories in evaluating the abdominal aorta.

- *Phased Array*: This transducer is the transducer of choice for cardiac ultrasound. Whereas a typical probe's imaging sector is determined by physical orientation of its crystals, phased array technology allows for electronic steering of the ultrasound beam. This results in a narrow, near field of view and a wide, far-field sector similar to curved probe that is pie shaped in appearance. This allows for the phased array to use a small, flat footprint that is easy to move between ribs. These transducers are available in the 1.0- to 5.0-MHz ranges and will yield less resolution than the curved array transducers of higher frequencies. The advantage of this transducer is that the small footprint facilitates scanning through intercostal spaces for cardiac, thoracic, or upper abdominal imaging. The disadvantage is that the image quality is slightly less than that of geometrically steered (linear and curved array) transducers of the same frequency. This is not the preferred transducer for transabdominal pelvic sonography.

- *Linear*: This transducer is frequently used for imaging superficial (eg, intraocular) structures and for vascular ultrasound. It is commonly found in frequencies from 5.0 to 13.0 MHz and ranges from 25 to 38 mm in width. It can be helpful in abdominal imaging of the very thin patient or the patient with an extremely superficial gallbladder.

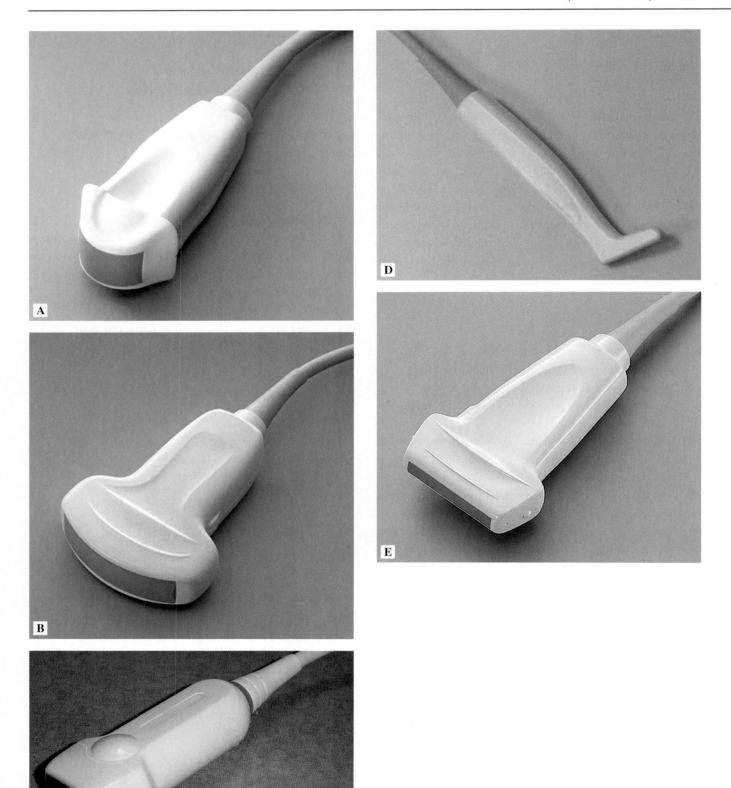

FIGURE 24.1 ■ Transducers. Transducers recommended for use in the emergency ultrasound (EUS). A. Microconvex. B. Convex array. C. Phased array. D. "Hockey puck" linear. E. Linear (A, B, and E Photo contributor: SonoSite, Inc; C and D, Photo contributor: Paul R. Sierzenski, MD, RDMS.)

Clinical Summary

The Extended Focused Assessment with Sonography for Trauma (E-FAST) is an organized series of sonographic windows or views that attempts to identify the presence or absence of fluid or air in anatomic potential spaces (eg, pericardium, pleural space or Morison pouch) or anatomically dependent areas (eg, pelvis, posteroinferior thorax, and splenorenal recess). The goal of this cardiac and thoracoabdominal survey is to identify or exclude immediate or potential life threats in the trauma or critically ill patient. Though initially intended for the evaluation of the traumatized patient, the E-FAST examination and its components are also extremely valuable in the evaluation of several emergent complaints and clinical conditions.

Indications

- Blunt abdominal trauma
- Penetrating thoracic/abdominal trauma
- Unexplained hypotension (trauma and nontrauma)
- Evaluation of the pregnant trauma patient
- Acute dyspnea with suspected pleural/pericardial effusion or tamponade

The FAST examination uses four primary sonographic windows to evaluate the patient. It is recommended that these windows are scanned in sequence, but isolated views may be obtained when indicated (eg, suspected pleural effusions in the dyspneic patient). The E-FAST examination incorporates imaging of both thoraces to identify pneumothoraces (Fig. 24.2). Finally, it is important to note that these are not "single" views, but a series of images in each plane as the transducer is moved to scan "through" the window of interest, much as a CAT scan obtains a series of images, so should an appropriately performed E-FAST.

Required Views for the E-FAST Examination

1. Subxiphoid-cardiac window (subcostal view)
2. Right upper quadrant (Morison pouch)
3. Left upper quadrant (splenorenal view)
4. Suprapubic window (pelvic view)
5. Right thorax
6. Left thorax

The technique and common findings for each of these views are presented in the next six topics.

Equipment: Recommended Transducers for the FAST Examination

- Microconvex
- Convex array
- Phased array

Most abdominal sonography is performed using transducers of 3.5 to 5.0 MHz. The FAST examination is an echocardiographic and thoracoabdominal examination. Ideally this is done using a single transducer that can image all three of these areas, but may result in some sonographic compromise or require the use of multiple probes.

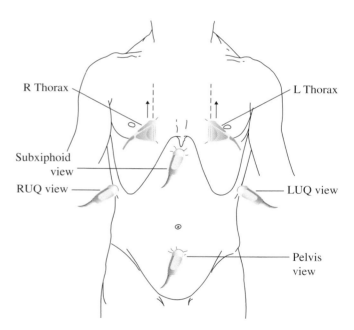

FIGURE 24.2 ■ E-FAST Trauma Series. Ultrasound transducer positions for rapidly detecting pericardial fluid, hemoperitoneum, or pneumothorax.

Patient Preparation

- The patient is supine, and the examination is generally performed from the right side of the patient.

Technique

- Direct the transducer indicator to the patient's right (in abdominal or general preset).
- The transducer is directed under the xiphoid process toward the left shoulder in a horizontal plane (Fig. 24.3).
- Pivot, sweep, and tilt the transducer to view of all four cardiac chambers.
- Identify the liver (if in view), heart, four cardiac chambers, and surrounding pericardium (Fig. 24.4).

Abnormal Findings

- Hemopericardium (pericardial effusion): Anechoic (black) region noted between the bright pericardium and the walls of the heart (occasionally internal echoes representing fibrin, clot, or cardiac tissue may be present) (Fig. 24.5).
- Pericardial clot: Small pericardial clots can be confused with a "fat pad," while large pericardial clots can be confused with liver tissue (Figs. 24.6, 24.7).
- Asystole: No cardiac activity present.
- Hyperdynamic cardiac activity: Extensive cardiac contraction with near-total or complete collapse of the cardiac chambers, often associated with tachycardia and hypovolemia.

Pearls

1. When the view is obscured by gas, slide the transducer slightly to the patient's right subcostal region, and use the liver as an echogenic window.
2. If unable to view the heart in the true subxiphoid or subcostal window, move to a parasternal long axis view (see "Cardiac Ultrasound [ECHO]," below).
3. A frequent mistake in imaging is to direct the transducer posterior toward the spine rather than cephalad toward the shoulder. You will often require less than a 30-degree angle between the transducer and the skin to view the heart.

4. Start imaging with the depth/scale setting at its maximum (eg, 24-35 cm). This should allow you to image the anterior and posterior pericardium in your initial view. Gradually decrease the depth/scale (eg, 14-18 cm) to fill the entire sector image with the heart as you continue to optimize your image.
5. Hypotensive patients with pericardial fluid/tamponade such as with right ventricular collapse warrant emergent pericardiocentesis (see Fig. 24.33).

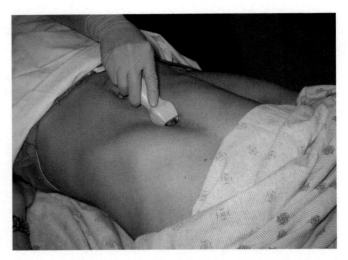

FIGURE 24.3 ■ Subxiphoid-Cardiac. The transducer is directed under the xiphoid process toward the left shoulder in a horizontal plane. (Photo contributor: Stephen J. Leech, MD, RDMS.)

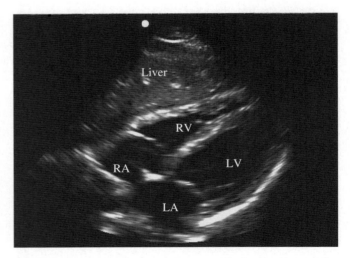

FIGURE 24.4 ■ Subxiphoid-Cardiac. The heart, four cardiac chambers, and surrounding pericardium are seen in this view. (Photo contributor: Stephen J. Leech, MD, RDMS.)

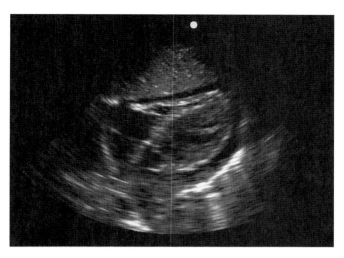
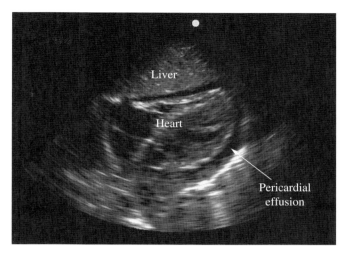

FIGURE 24.5 ■ Hemopericardium. The dark black, anechoic region between the bright pericardium and the walls of the heart represents a pericardial effusion. (Photo contributor: Stephen J. Leech, MD, RDMS.)

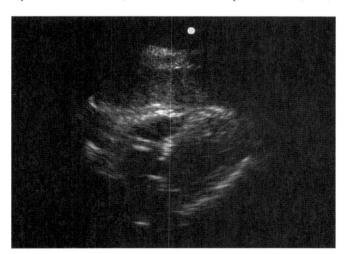
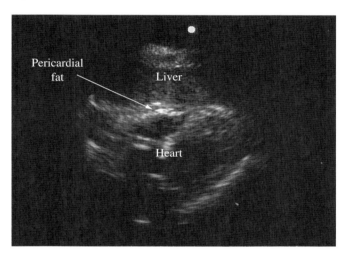

FIGURE 24.6 ■ Fat Pad. A subcostal cardiac view shows a separation between the right ventricle and the pericardium. This space is the result of an epicardial "fat pad" and is not a pericardial effusion. (Photo contributor: Stephen J. Leech, MD, RDMS.)

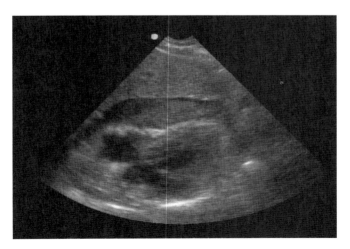
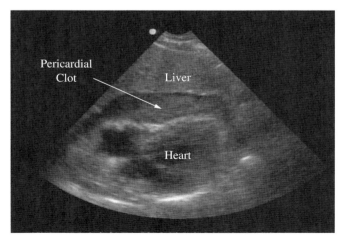

FIGURE 24.7 ■ Pericardial Clot. An echogenic mass that is isoechoic with the liver is seen within the anechoic hemopericardium. This represents pericardial clot in this patient. (Photo contributor: Paul R. Sierzenski, MD, RDMS.)

Patient Preparation

- The patient is supine.

Technique

- The transducer indicator is aimed toward the axilla/head.
- The transducer is oriented as a coronal section through the body in the midaxillary line, extending from the 9th through 12th ribs. Start between the 11th and 12th ribs initially, then move cephalad or caudal, anterior or posterior, to complete the evaluation (Fig. 24.8).
- Identify the interface of the liver and right kidney. This region is the potential space known as Morison pouch. Normally, these organs' surrounding tissues are in direct contact with one another or separated by adipose tissue of heterogeneous echoes (Fig. 24.9).
- Evaluate the right diaphragmatic recess and the subdiaphragmatic recess.

Abnormal Findings

- Hemoperitoneum: Anechoic (black) region between the liver and right kidney or in the subdiaphragmatic recess (Fig. 24.10).
- Right hemothorax: Anechoic (black) region above the level of the diaphragm.

- Solid organ injury: Solid organ injury such as hepatic and renal lacerations as well as organ rupture have been described but are not the goal of this examination and are beyond the scope of this chapter.
- Hydronephrosis: Dilatation of the renal sinus with black, anechoic fluid within the bright renal sinus (see "Renal Ultrasound").

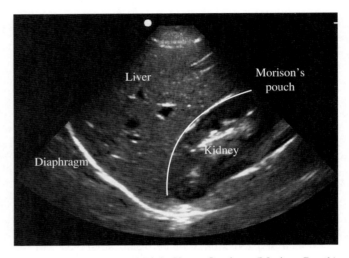

FIGURE 24.9 ■ Normal Right Upper Quadrant (Morison Pouch). At the liver and right kidney interface is the potential space known as "Morison pouch." Normally the surrounding tissues of these organs are in direct contact with one another. (Photo contributor: Stephen J. Leech, MD, RDMS)

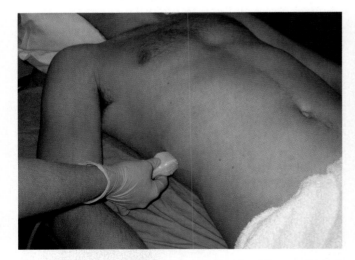

FIGURE 24.8 ■ Right Upper Quadrant Position. The transducer is directed as a coronal section through the body in the midaxillary line extending from the 9th through the 12th ribs. (Photo contributor: Stephen J. Leech, MD, RDMS.)

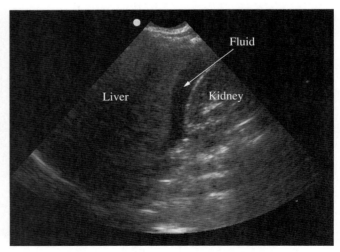

FIGURE 24.10 ■ Hemoperitoneum (Morison Pouch). The dark black, anechoic region between the liver and kidney or in the subdiaphragmatic recess represents fluid in Morison pouch. (Photo contributor: Stephen J. Leech, MD, RDMS.)

Patient Preparation

- The patient is supine.

Technique

- The transducer indicator is directed toward the axilla.
- The transducer is oriented as a coronal section through the body in the midaxillary to posterior axillary line extending from the 9th through 12th ribs. Start between the 11th and 12th ribs initially, then move cephalad or caudal, anterior or posterior, to complete the evaluation (Fig. 24.11).
- Identify the interface of the spleen and left kidney. This region is a physiologic potential space referred to as the splenorenal recess. Normally, the surrounding tissues of these organs are in direct contact with one another (Fig. 24.12).
- Evaluate the left diaphragmatic recess and the left subdiaphragmatic recess.

Abnormal Findings

- Hemoperitoneum: Anechoic (black) region between the spleen and left kidney or between the spleen and the diaphragm (Fig. 24.13).
- Hemothorax: Anechoic (black) region above the level of the diaphragm (Fig. 24.14).
- Solid organ injury: Solid organ injury such as splenic and renal lacerations as well as organ rupture have been described but are not the goal of this examination and are beyond the scope of this chapter.
- Hydronephrosis: Dilatation of the renal sinus with black, anechoic fluid within the bright renal sinus (see "Renal Ultrasound").

Pearls for RUQ and LUQ Views

1. The diaphragmatic recess includes a *superior region,* which is the inferior border of the right thorax, and an *inferior region (subdiaphragmatic recess),* which is the superior border of the abdomen. Fluid in the diaphragmatic recess can represent a hemothorax when located superior/cephalad to the diaphragm or a hemoperitoneum or subphrenic hematoma (inferior to the diaphragm) in the setting of trauma.
2. Identify the kidneys from the superior to the inferior poles in the coronal plane. It may seem easier at first to perform a short axis view; however, the sonographer

risks missing early a small fluid collection if only a middle renal transverse section is imaged.

3. If you are uncertain whether a finding is real or artifact, evaluate it in a second plane. Turn the transducer 90 degrees from your initial transducer position to see if the finding is still noted on the image. If the entire image is unchanged, it is less likely to be an artifact.
4. The liver is affixed to the diaphragm via the coronary ligament but the spleen lacks a similar attachment. Dependent fluid collects in the left subdiaphragmatic area more often than the right and this space should be evaluated sonographically during the examination.

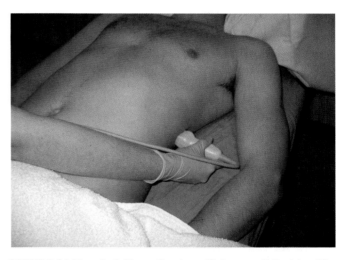

FIGURE 24.11 ■ Left Upper Quadrant (Splenorenal) Position. The transducer is directed as a coronal section through the body in the midaxillary line extending from the 9th through the 12th ribs. (Photo contributor: Stephen J. Leech, MD, RDMS.)

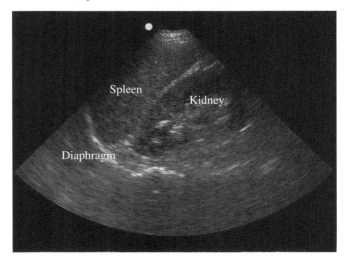

FIGURE 24.12 ■ Left Upper Quadrant (Splenorenal). The spleen and left kidney interface is a physiologic potential space (splenorenal recess). (Photo contributor: Stephen J. Leech, MD, RDMS.)

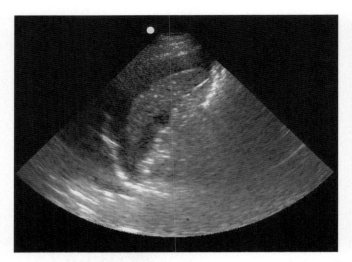
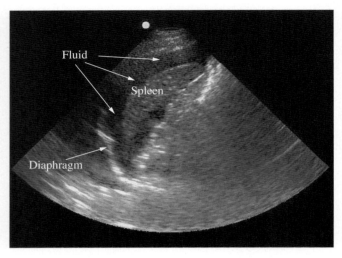

FIGURE 24.13 ■ Hemoperitoneum (Splenorenal Pouch). The anechoic area above the spleen and left kidney or between the spleen and the diaphragm represents fluid in the potential space. This image represents fluid above the spleen but below the level of the diaphragm. (Photo contributor: Stephen J. Leech, MD, RDMS.)

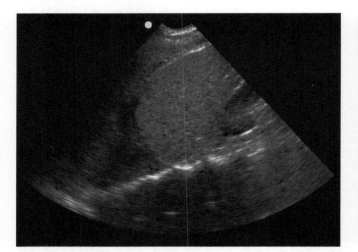
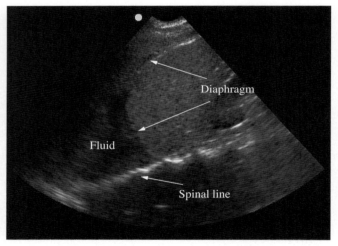

FIGURE 24.14 ■ Right Hemothorax. Fluid is identified in the chest as an anechoic "wedge," with the loss of the mirroring artifact and visualization of the "spinal line" beyond the costophrenic angle. This represents a hemothorax. (Photo contributor: Stephen J. Leech, MD, RDMS.)

Patient Preparation

- The patient is supine.

Technique

Sagittal View (Longitudinal)

- The transducer indicator is oriented toward the patient's head.
- The transducer is placed just above the symphysis pubis and is directed into the pelvis (Fig. 24.15).
- Identify the bladder (triangular in this view when fully distended), uterus (pear-shaped if present), and rectum (Fig. 24.16).

Technique: Transverse View

- The transducer indicator is oriented toward the patient's right.
- The transducer is placed about 1 to 2 cm above the symphysis pubis, with the beam angled caudally into the pelvis (Fig. 24.17).
- Identify the bladder (rectangular in this view when fully distended), uterus (oval hyperechoic structure if present), and rectum (Fig. 24.18).

Abnormal Findings

- Hemoperitoneum: Anechoic (black) regions between the bladder and uterus or the uterus and rectum or as loops of bowel floating lateral to the bladder in the transverse view and lateral or superior to the bladder in the sagittal view (Fig. 24.19).

Pearls

1. It is important to remember that the bladder is within the pelvis; therefore the transducer must be directed inferiorly into the pelvis to image the bladder and its neighboring structures.
2. When in the sagittal plane, rotate the transducer 90 degrees counterclockwise directing the transducer indicator toward the patient's right to obtain a transverse view.

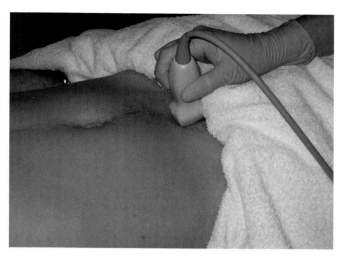

FIGURE 24.15 ■ Suprapubic Sagittal Position. The transducer is directed with the transducer indicator oriented toward the patient's head and placed just superior to the symphysis pubis. (Photo contributor: Stephen J. Leech, MD, RDMS.)

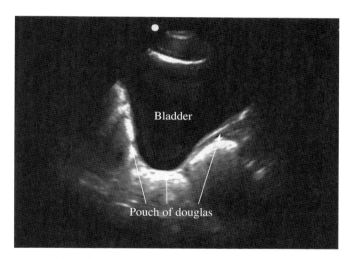

FIGURE 24.16 ■ Suprapubic Sagittal. In this view, when fully distended, the bladder is triangular in shape. If present, the uterus is pear-shape. Fluid may collect in the vesicouterine (V) (potential space seen between the bladder and uterus in this view) and/or rectouterine (D) (pouch of Douglas) (space seen posterior to the border of the uterus and rectum) pouches. (Photo contributor: Stephen J. Leech, MD, RDMS.)

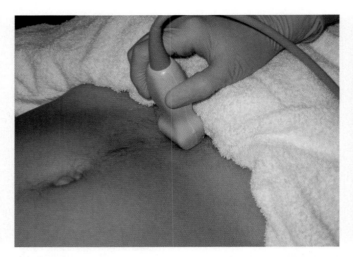

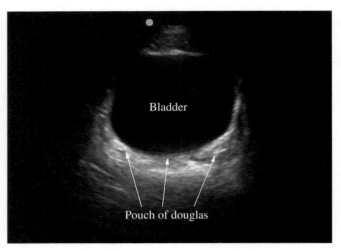

FIGURE 24.17 ■ Suprapubic Transverse Position. The transducer indicator is oriented toward the patient's right and the beam angled caudally into the pelvis. (Photo contributor: Stephen J. Leech, MD, RDMS.)

FIGURE 24.18 ■ Suprapubic Transverse. In this view, the bladder assumes a rectangular shape when fully distended. If present, the uterus is an oval hyperechoic structure. (Photo contributor: Stephen J. Leech, MD, RDMS.)

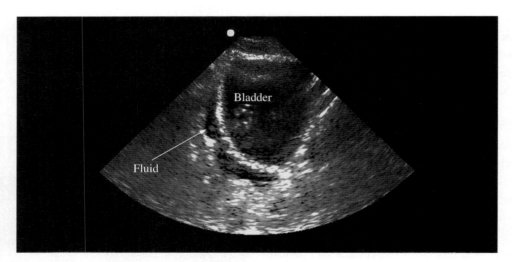

FIGURE 24.19 ■ Hemoperitoneum. Hemoperitoneum can be seen as dark black, anechoic regions between the bladder and uterus, as well as the uterus and rectum or as loops of bowel floating lateral to the bladder in the transverse view and lateral or posterior to the bladder in the sagittal view. (Photo contributor: Stephen J. Leech, MD, RDMS.)

Patient Preparation

- The patient is supine.
- Note: Evaluation for thoracic fluid is best performed as an extension of the RUQ and LUQ views by sliding the transducer up into the chest in a coronal plane.

Technique

- A high-frequency linear transducer is preferred.
- The transducer indicator is oriented toward the patient's head (Fig. 24.20).

Suspected Pleural Fluid (Hemothorax)

- The transducer is slid or placed in the fifth or sixth interspace in the midaxillary line.
- Identify the hyperechoic rib shadows and deeper linear echogenic structure that is the pleura.
- The depth should be adjusted so that the pleural line is positioned in the middle or upper half of the screen.
- In the fully inflated healthy lung, air prevents direct visualization of structures deep to the pleura. If fluid is present, it is identified as an anechoic (black) area that may contain heterogeneous echoes.
- The presence of pleural fluid may allow direct visualization of the lung or posterior structures (spine).

Suspected Pneumothorax

- The transducer is placed at the second or third interspace in the mid-clavicular line.
- Identify the hyperechoic rib shadows and deeper linear echogenic structure that is the pleura.
- The depth should be adjusted so that the pleural line is positioned in the middle or upper half of the screen.
- Pleural sliding—the motion of the visceral and parietal pleura sliding back and forth during normal respiration is readily seen on ultrasound. Using power Doppler, or M-mode over the pleural interface may highlight this motion.
- There are several key artifacts that are used to establish the *absence* of pneumothorax.
  - "Power slide": Power Doppler allows for the subtle movement of the pleura to be accentuated as a color flash. The presence of this is termed the "power slide" (Fig. 24.21).
  - The "seashore sign": It is described as "waves on the beach" and is noted with M-mode when no pneumothorax is present (Fig. 24.22A). (A "stratosphere sign" is seen when a pneumothorax is present, the result of the M-mode reflecting only a reverberation artifact [Fig. 24.22B]).
  - "Comet tail": When the two pleural surfaces are in direct contact with each other, they create a reverberation artifact that can be identified in the far field, resembling a "comet tail."

Abnormal Findings

- Hemothorax: Anechoic (black) regions between the pleural line and other structures. Heterogeneous echoes may be present due to clotted blood or other material.
- Pneumothorax: Careful identification of the absence of findings consistent with normal structures is crucial. Estimation of the pneumothorax size is possible by using transducer positions in which the pneumothorax is identified to gauge the size.

Pearl

1. The finding of a "lung point" is 100% diagnostic of a pneumothorax (Fig. 24.23).

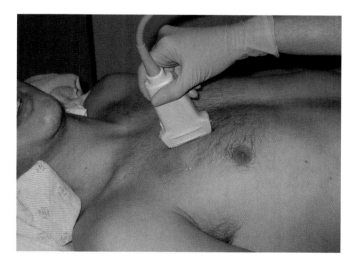

FIGURE 24.20 ■ Anterior Thorax Position. Here a linear transducer is placed in a midclavicular line at the 2nd to 3rd intercostal space, in a sagittal plane to evaluate for a pneumothorax. (Photo contributor: Stephen J. Leech, MD, RDMS.)

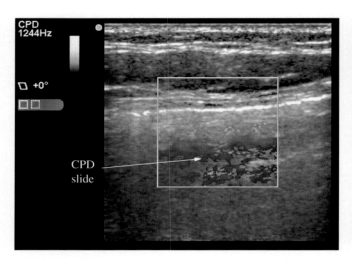

FIGURE 24.21 ▪ Power Slide Power Doppler. Imaging is used in the anterior thorax ultrasound to enhance the pleural sliding that confirms the absence of a pneumothorax. This nondirectional Doppler technique results in a Doppler "flash" when lung is imaged moving within the "Doppler box." It would not be present if a pneumothorax existed. A false-positive result can occur if the probe is moved. (Photo contributor: Stephen J. Leech, MD, RDMS.)

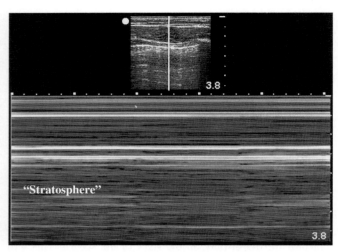

FIGURE 24.22B ▪ Stratosphere Sign (Pneumothorax). The "stratosphere sign" describes the M-mode appearance on thoracic ultrasound when pneumothorax is present. The near-field image resembles fairly equidistant lines, much like a series of plane condensation trails in the sky. (Photo contributor: Stephen J. Leech, MD, RDMS.)

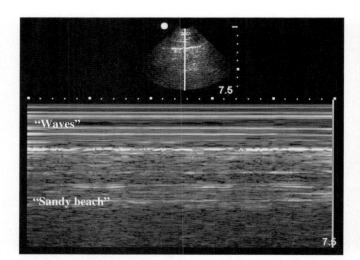

FIGURE 24.22A ▪ Seashore Sign. The "seashore sign" describes the M-mode appearance on thoracic ultrasound when there is no pneumothorax. The near-field image resembles waves on a beach, and the far-field image resembles a sandy beach. (Photo contributor: Stephen J. Leech, MD, RDMS.)

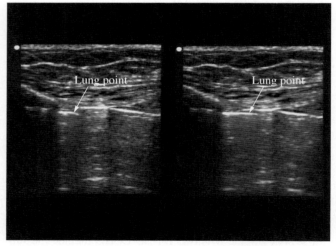

FIGURE 24.23 ▪ Lung Point. The "lung point" describes the location where the pneumothorax ends and begins. At this point the sliding "leading edge" of the lung is termed the lung point. It is seen in the series of images to move from the right to the left of the image as the patient exhales. (Photo contributor: Paul R. Sierzenski, MD, RDMS.)

Clinical Summary

Two-dimensional echocardiography (2D ECHO) can yield significant diagnostic information for the patient presenting with cardiac arrest, shock, shortness of breath, and a host of other complaints or physical findings. Although the physician can easily become intimidated by all the diagnostic possibilities that can be identified or potentially missed in performing echocardiography, one can, with experience, incorporate ED ECHO into the diagnostic armamentarium safely without becoming overextended.

It is important to note that by convention, unlike abdominal sonography, cardiac ultrasound is viewed with the transducer indicator for the display on the right of the screen. This will require the indicator on the transducer to be direct toward the patient's left in an anatomically transverse view. Longitudinal or sagittal views will still be obtained with the indicator directed cephalad. This may be disorienting for many who have not performed echocardiography before. Most ultrasound systems include cardiac presets that automatically reverse the indicator orientation to the right of the display screen. The following section describes a sonographic approach for a conventionally oriented image using standard cardiac windows.

Indications

- Cardiac arrest, PEA
- Penetrating thoracic/abdominal trauma
- Unexplained hypotension or shock
- Dyspnea
- Chest pain
- Acute myocardial infarction
- Suspected aortic dissection

Specific pathologic states investigated with ED ECHO include asystole, cardiac activity, pericardial effusion, and aortic root dilatation/dissection.

The sonographic windows for ED ECHO include the subxiphoid view presented within the trauma/FAST examination.

The ED ECHO utilizes cardiac windows that are familiar to cardiologists and sonographers alike. The four ED ECHO windows will allow the emergency physician to evaluate asystole, pericardial effusions, and the aortic root.

Required Views for Emergency Department

1. Subxiphoid (subcostal) (see "FAST Examination," above)
2. Parasternal long-axis view (PSLAx)
3. Parasternal short-axis view (PSSAx)
4. Apical four-chamber view (A4C)
5. Subxiphoid long-axis view (IVC)

The technique and common findings for each of these views are presented in the next five topics.

Equipment: Recommended Transducers for ECHO

- Phased array
- Microconvex

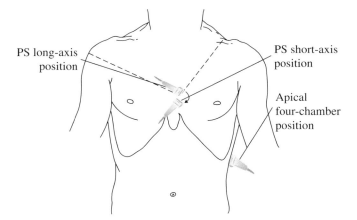

FIGURE 24.24 ■ Cardiac Ultrasound. Transducer positions for parasternal long axis, parasternal short axis, and apical four-chamber view to evaluate asystole, pericardial effusions, and the aortic root.

Patient Preparation

- The patient is supine.

Technique

- The transducer indicator should be directed toward the left in a cardiac preset.
- The transducer is placed inferior to the xiphoid process and directed cephalad toward the left shoulder in a horizontal plane (see Fig. 24.3).
- Pivot, sweep, and tilt the transducer to view all four cardiac chambers.
- Identify the heart, four cardiac chambers, and surrounding pericardium (see Fig. 24.4).

Abnormal Findings

- Hemopericardium (pericardial effusion): Anechoic (black) region noted between the bright pericardium and the walls of the heart (occasionally internal echoes representing fibrin, clot, or cardiac tissue may be present) (see Fig. 24.5).
- Asystole: No cardiac activity present.
- Hyperdynamic cardiac activity: Extensive cardiac contraction with near-total or complete collapse of the cardiac chambers, often associated with tachycardia.

Pearls

1. When the view is obscured by gas, slide the transducer slightly to the patient's right subcostal region, and use the liver as an echogenic window.
2. If unable to view the heart in the true subxiphoid or subcostal window, move to a parasternal long axis view (see "Cardiac Ultrasound [ECHO]," below).
3. A frequent mistake in imaging is to direct the transducer posterior toward the spine rather than cephalad toward the shoulder. You will often require less than a 30-degree angle between the transducer and the skin to view the heart.
4. Start imaging with the depth/scale setting at its maximum (eg, 24-35 cm). This should allow you to image the anterior and posterior pericardium in your initial view.

Gradually decrease the depth/scale (eg, 14-18 cm) to fill the entire sector image with the heart as you continue to optimize your image.

5. Hypotensive patients with pericardial fluid/tamponade such as with right ventricular collapse warrant emergent pericardiocentesis (see Fig. 24.33).

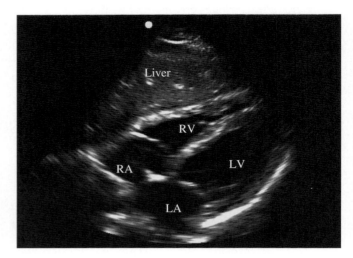

FIGURE 24.25 ■ Subxiphoid-Cardiac. The transducer is directed under the xiphoid process toward the left shoulder in a horizontal plane. (Photo contributor: Stephen J. Leech, MD, RDMS.)

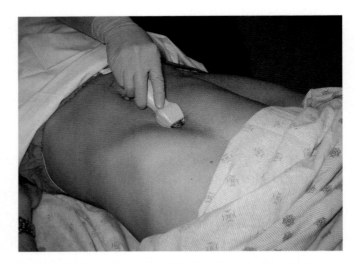

FIGURE 24.26 ■ Subxiphoid-Cardiac. The heart, four cardiac chambers, and surrounding pericardium are seen in this view. (Photo contributor: Stephen J. Leech, MD, RDMS.)

Patient Preparation

- The patient is supine or in the left lateral decubitus (LLD) position with the left arm extended above the head for easier transducer access.

Technique

- The transducer indicator directed at the right clavicle or shoulder.
- The transducer is placed in the fourth or fifth left parasternal intercostal space and the beam is directed posteriorly (Fig. 24.27).
- Identify the right ventricle, left atrium, left ventricle, aortic valve, aortic root, aortic outflow tract, and surrounding pericardium (Fig. 24.28).

Abnormal Findings

- Hemopericardium: Anechoic (black) region noted between the hyperechoic (bright) pericardium and the walls of the heart (see Fig. 24.5).
- Aortic root dilatation: An aortic root measurement greater than 3.8 to 4.0 cm is abnormal and indicates aneurismal dilatation that may suggest aortic dissection in the appropriate clinical setting. Further evaluation is recommended.
- Dilated descending aorta: The transverse descending thoracic aorta can be seen in the far field in this view posterior to the left atrium. A descending thoracic aorta greater than 4.0 cm is abnormal and indicates aneurismal dilatation that may suggest aortic dissection in the appropriate clinical setting. Further evaluation is recommended.

Pearls

1. A true parasternal long-axis view (a sagittal image through the heart) will visualize the aortic root within the image. If the aortic root is not present, you are likely in an oblique plane and will need to angle the transducer to optimize the image.
2. It is critical to make deliberate, slow, small adjustments of the transducer in imaging the heart, since even small movements at the skin surface can translate into large changes in beam angle at just 5 to 10 cm deep from the surface.
3. Normal spontaneous respiration is usually fine for cardiac imaging. Patients who are tachypneic can be very challenging, and verbally coaching the patient's breathing

patterns is best. If you note a great deal of artifact due to lung interposition, place the patient in the left lateral decubitus position; have him or her inhale and slowly exhale while you scan. When you have an acceptable window, ask the patient to stop exhaling and hold his or her breath while you capture your images.

4. Remember that the parasternal long axis is approximated by a line running from the right acromioclavicular joint and the left antecubital fossa (when the arm is lying by the patient's side).

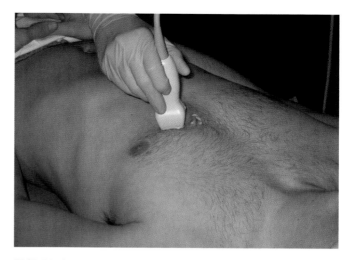

FIGURE 24.27 ■ Parasternal Long-Axis Position. The transducer is placed in the fourth or fifth left parasternal intercostal space with the transducer indicator oriented toward the right clavicle or shoulder. (Photo contributor: Stephen J. Leech, MD, RDMS.)

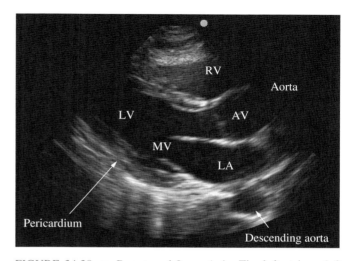

FIGURE 24.28 ■ Parasternal Long-Axis. The left atrium, left ventricle, aortic valve, aortic root, aortic outflow tract, and surrounding pericardium can be visualized. (Photo contributor: Stephen J. Leech, MD, RDMS.)

Patient Preparation

- The patient is supine or in the left lateral decubitus position.

Technique

- From the parasternal long-axis position, rotate the transducer 90 degrees clockwise (to the patient's left) or place the transducer in the fourth or fifth left parasternal intercostal space in a line connecting the left clavicle/shoulder and the right hip (Fig. 24.29).
- Identify the left ventricle (circular), right ventricle (crescent-shaped), and surrounding pericardium (Fig. 24.30).

Abnormal Findings

- Hemopericardium: Anechoic (black) region noted between the bright pericardium and the walls of the heart (Fig. 24.5).
- Dilated right ventricle: The right ventricle is normally a crescent-shaped structure. A rounded, dilated structure suggests elevated right-sided pressures, as seen with pulmonary emboli and severe pulmonary hypertension.

Pearl

1. The standard parasternal short-axis view is obtained with the image plane at the level of the papillary muscles. Visualization of the papillary muscles should ensure a true transverse section through the left ventricle and provides a prime location for the evaluation of left ventricular contraction and motion.

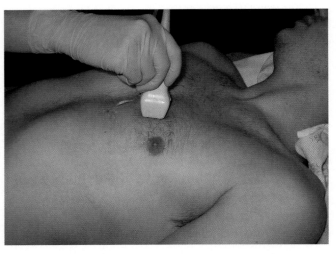

FIGURE 24.29 ■ Parasternal Short-Axis Position. From the parasternal long-axis position, rotate the transducer 90 degrees clockwise (to the patient's left) or place the transducer in the forth or fifth left parasternal intercostal space in a line connecting the left clavicle/shoulder and the right hip. (Photo contributor: Stephen J. Leech, MD, RDMS.)

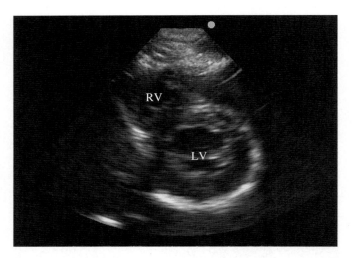

FIGURE 24.30 ■ Parasternal Short-Axis. The left ventricle (circular), right ventricle (crescent-shaped), aortic valve, and surrounding pericardium can be identified. (Photo contributor: Paul R. Sierzenski, MD, RDMS.)

Patient Preparation

- The patient is supine or in the left lateral decubitus position.

Technique

- The transducer indicator is directed toward the left axilla or directly posterior to the patient.
- The transducer is placed over the cardiac apex or the point of maximal intensity (PMI) with the beam directed toward the right clavicle/shoulder in a plane coronal to the heart (Fig. 24.31).
- Identify the left ventricle, right ventricle, left atrium, right atrium, and surrounding pericardium (Fig. 24.32).

Abnormal Findings

- Hemopericardium: Anechoic (black) region noted between the hyperechoic pericardium and the walls of the heart (see Figs. 24.5, 24.33).
- Dilated right atria/ventricle: If the right atria/ventricle are rounded or appear rigid and poorly contracting, this may suggest elevated right-sided pressures as seen with pulmonary emboli and severe pulmonary hypertension (Figs. 24.34, 24.35).

Pearls

1. See "Scan Pearls for the FAST Examination, Subxiphoid-Cardiac," item 4, above.
2. It is critical to realize the variance in the resting position of the heart. There can be significant differences in acoustic windows from patient to patient with the four-chamber apical view.

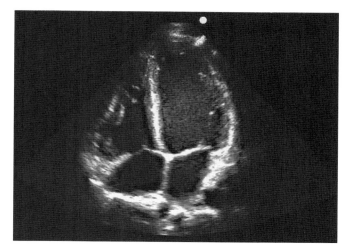

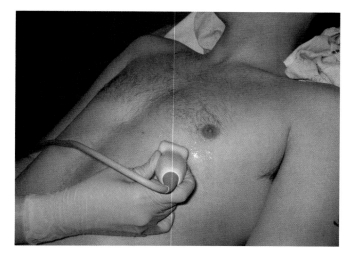

FIGURE 24.31 ■ Apical Four-Chamber Position. The transducer is placed over the cardiac apex or the point of maximal intensity, with the beam directed toward the right clavicle/shoulder in a plane coronal to the heart. The transducer indicator is directed toward the left axilla. (Photo contributor: Stephen J. Leech, MD, RDMS.)

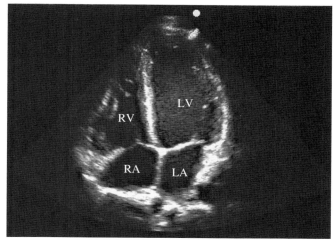

FIGURE 24.32 ■ Apical Four-Chamber. The right ventricle (RV), left ventricle (LV), right atrium (RA), left atrium (LA), and surrounding pericardium are visualized in this view. (Photo contributor: Stephen J. Leech, MD, RDMS.)

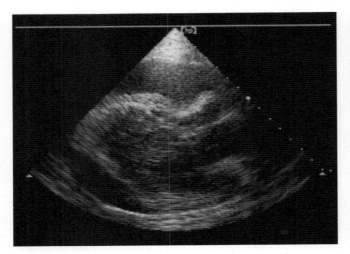

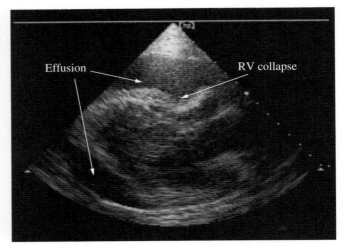

FIGURE 24.33 ▪ Hemopericardium with RV Collapse. Parasternal long axis view shows a circumferential hemopericardium with deep collapse of the right-ventricle-free wall. (Photo contributor: Paul R. Sierzenski, MD, RDMS.)

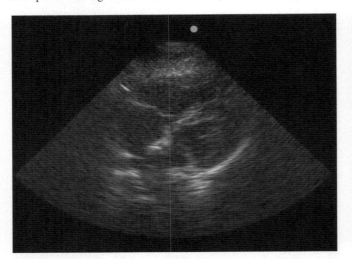

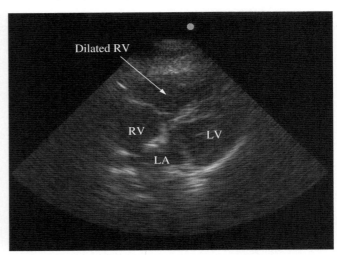

FIGURE 24.34 ▪ Dilated Right Ventricle. A significantly dilated right ventricle is noted in this patient with a massive pulmonary embolus as seen in this subcostal view. (Photo contributor: Stephen J. Leech, MD, RDMS.)

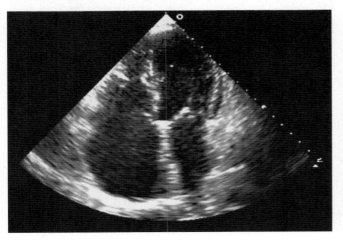

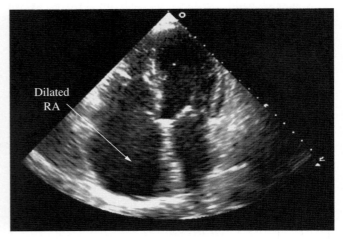

FIGURE 24.35 ▪ Dilated Right Atrium. The right atrium is dilated and the largest chamber seen in this apical four-chamber view of a patient with a history of severe tricuspid regurgitation. (Photo contributor: Ellen Sierzenski, RDCS.)

Patient Preparation

- The patient is supine.

Technique

- The transducer indicator is directed toward the patient's head.
- The transducer is placed subxiphoid and tilted over to the patients right to identify the inferior vena cava (IVC) as it enters the right atrium (Fig. 24.36).
- Identify the liver IVC, right atrium, and right hepatic vein (Fig. 24.37).
- Measure the IVC 2 to 3 cm distal to the entry point to the RV. Measure the IVC through the respiratory cycle at end inspiration and expiration (Fig. 24.38).

Abnormal Findings

- IVC Measurements: The general size of the IVC

IVC Size	IVC Change w/resp	Estimated CVP
<1.5	Total Collapse	0-5 mm Hg (Fig. 24.36)
1.5-2.5	>50% Collapse	5-10 mm Hg
1.5-2.5	<50% Collapse	11-15 mm Hg
>2.5	<50% Collapse	16-20 mm Hg
>2.5	No Change	>20 mm Hg (Fig. 24.39)

Pearls

1. Consider using M-mode through the IVC to aid in measurement for patients with high respiratory rates.
2. Some patients require a low anterior intercostal view to image the IVC as it enters the right atrium.

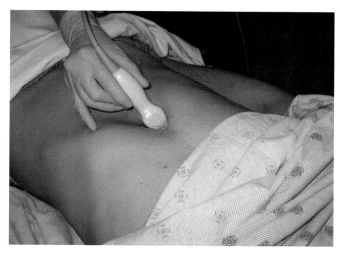

FIGURE 24.36 ■ Subxiphoid Long-Axis (IVC) Position. The transducer is placed in a subcostal position with the indicator to the patients head for a sagittal, long axis view. It is slid or angled to the right to identify the inferior vena cava (IVC) as it enters the right atrium. (Photo contributor:: Stephen J. Leech, MD, RDMS.)

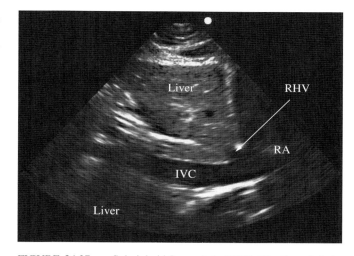

FIGURE 24.37 ■ Subxiphoid Long-Axis (IVC). The liver, inferior vena cava (IVC), diaphragm, right atrium (RA), and right hepatic vein (RHV) is noted. (Photo contributor: Stephen J. Leech, MD, RDMS.)

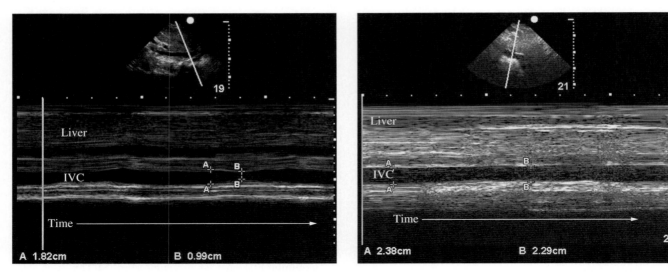

FIGURE 24.38 ■ Respiratory Cycle: Normovolemic IVC. (Left) Measurement of the IVC during the respiratory cycle using M-mode. (Right) Respiratory Cycle: Hypervolemic IVC. Note the plethoric, distended IVC with no change during respiratory cycle (M-mode). (Photo contributor: Stephen J. Leech, MD, RDMS.)

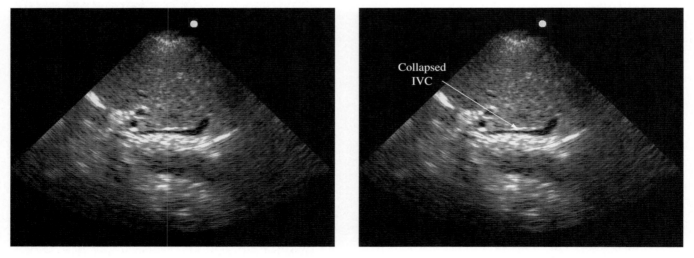

FIGURE 24.39 ■ IVC Collapse (Hypovolemia). Total collapse of the IVC in a hypovolemic patient. (Photo contributor: Stephen J. Leech, MD, RDMS.)

Clinical Summary

Ultrasound of the gallbladder can be among the most rewarding EUSs to perform. Patients can receive a rapid focused ultrasound to determine if gallstones or gallbladder pathology is the etiology of their presenting symptoms. Careful positioning of the patient is important with gallbladder and biliary ultrasound to minimize bowel gas, accentuate possible pathology, and verify suspected findings. This can be a technically difficult ultrasound to perform.

Indications

- Right-upper-quadrant pain
- Jaundice/icterus
- Epigastric pain

It is important to recognize the limited nature of gallbladder ultrasounds performed by emergency physicians. Thorough evaluation of the biliary tract is a routine component of a comprehensive abdominal ultrasound but can be technically difficult, especially in the patient with acute pain. For this reason, measurement of the hepatic and common bile ducts is not included as an initial key component to the basic gallbladder EUS. Techniques for measurement of the common bile duct are reviewed below; these should be performed by an emergency physician experienced in abdominal ultrasound. Although the sonographic identification of gallstones may seem straightforward, the sonographic findings for cholecystitis can frequently be subtle.

Required Views for Emergency Department Gallbladder Ultrasound

1. Sagittal view
2. Transverse view

The technique and common findings for each of these views are presented in the next two topics.

Equipment: Recommended Transducers for Gallbladder Ultrasound

- Convex array
- Microconvex
- Phased array

Most abdominal sonography is performed using transducer frequencies of 3.5 to 5.0 MHz. In rare instances, lower or higher frequencies are needed for more or less depth of penetration, decreasing and increasing resolution respectively.

Patient Preparation

- The patient is supine or in the left lateral decubitus position.

Techniques

Gallbladder Ultrasound Window 1: Sagittal View

- Initially, the transducer is placed in the subxiphoid region with the indicator directed toward the patient's head in a sagittal view and swept below the right costal margin to approximately the midclavicular line (Fig. 24.40).
- Identify the liver, portal vein, common bile duct, hepatic artery, gallbladder, and main lobar fissure (spanning these two structures). Measure the thickness of the common bile duct when visible (Fig. 24.41).
- Scan through the gallbladder completely from the medial to lateral borders of the gallbladder.

Gallbladder Ultrasound Window 2: Transverse View

- After identifying the gallbladder in the sagittal position, rotate the transducer 90 degrees counterclockwise (to the patient's right) (Fig. 24.42).
- Identify the liver, gallbladder, inferior vena cava, right kidney (if visualized), and common bile duct (if visualized) (Figs. 24.43-24.45).

Abnormal Findings

- Gallstones: Bright oval to round hyperechoic structure(s) within the gallbladder, often with a posterior shadowing (Figs. 24.46, 24.47).
- Pericholecystic fluid: An anechoic stripe that borders the outer gallbladder wall, visible in two views. This fluid is often, but not necessarily, circumferential (Fig. 24.48).
- Thickened gallbladder wall: A gallbladder wall that measures 4 mm or more is considered abnormal.
- Sonographic Murphy sign: The transducer is placed directly over the gallbladder and the patient is asked to inspire. If the patient experiences pain, it is considered a positive examination.
- Dilated common bile duct (CBD): A CBD with an internal diameter greater than 4.0 mm is dilated; however, documented measurements up to 8.0 mm can be normal in the elderly. One rule of thumb is that 4 mm up to age 40 and thereafter an increase of 1 mm per decade represents the normal range.

Pearls

1. Other positions—including prone, right lateral decubitus, semierect, and standing—may be helpful in scanning the gallbladder and are patient specific.

2. It is frequently necessary to have the patient take a deep breath and hold it to allow the gallbladder to descend into sonographic view.

3. Measure the anterior wall when evaluating wall thickness. The thickness of the posterior wall is often affected by "posterior enhancement"; therefore it may falsely appear thickened.

4. The duodenum is located medially to the gallbladder. It may be interpreted as a gallstone even by proficient sonographers if care is not taken to evaluate the gallbladder completely and to observe for peristalsis on areas suspected to be bowel.

5. If you suspect gallstones but do not visualize "shadowing," confirm that your focal point is at the area of interest and try changing the transducer frequency if possible (eg, increase from 3.5 to 5.0 MHz).

6. If pericholecystic fluid is suspected but difficult to determine, it may be helpful to increase the frequency or convert to a linear transducer.

7. The CBD lies just anterior to the portal vein, a structure with markedly hyperechoic walls compared to the hepatic veins. It may be more easily seen by positioning the patient in the left lateral decubitus position.

8. Most ultrasound systems provide a cinematic loop, or "cineloop," that will allow the sonographer to recall on average 20 to 40 images that occurred before the image was frozen. Scrolling through these images is helpful in identifying the cleanest and sharpest image of the CBD to measure.

9. The gallbladder tends to migrate inferiorly in elderly patients, so that it may lie significantly below the costal margin.

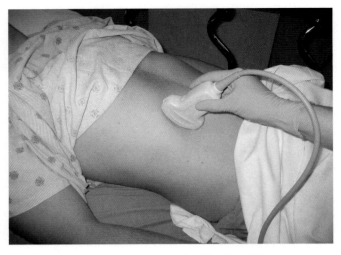

FIGURE 24.40 ▪ Gallbladder: Sagittal Position. The transducer is initially placed in the subxiphoid region with the orientation indicator directed toward the patient's head and moved along the right costal margin approximately to the midclavicular line. (Photo contributor: Stephen J. Leech, MD, RDMS.)

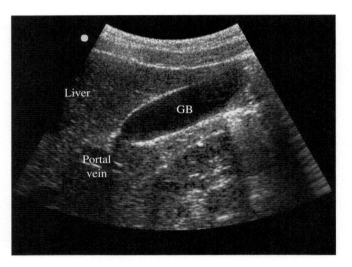

FIGURE 24.41 ▪ Gallbladder: Sagittal. Various structures can be seen in this sagittal view. The gallbladder and portal vein are within the liver. Moving the patient to the left lateral decubitus position may improve this view. (Photo contributor: Stephen J. Leech, MD, RDMS.)

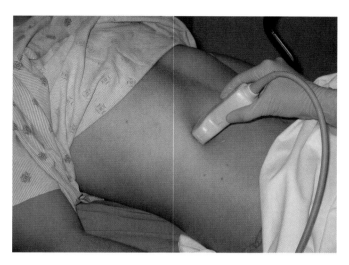

FIGURE 24.42 ■ Gallbladder: Transverse Position. The transducer is rotated 90 degrees counterclockwise from the sagittal position and moved along the right costal margin. (Photo contributor: Stephen J. Leech, MD, RDMS.)

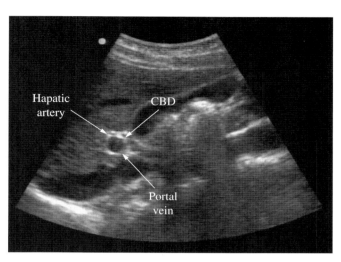

FIGURE 24.44 ■ Gallbladder: Portal Triad. The portal vein, common bile duct, and hepatic artery are readily seen in this transverse view. Although not apparent in the drawing, these structures are within the liver. Color-flow Doppler can facilitate identification of these structures. (Photo contributor: Paul R. Sierzenski, MD, RDMS.)

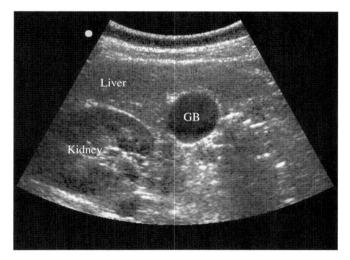

FIGURE 24.43 ■ Gallbladder: Transverse. Various structures can be seen in this transverse view. (Photo contributor: Stephen J. Leech, MD, RDMS.)

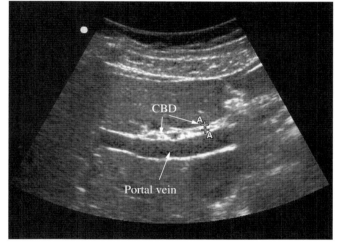

FIGURE 24.45 ■ Gallbladder: Common Bile Duct (CBD). The CBD is seen in this transverse view of the patient in Fig. 24.42. Once it is identified, its thickness should be measured. (Photo contributor: Stephen J. Leech, MD, RDMS.)

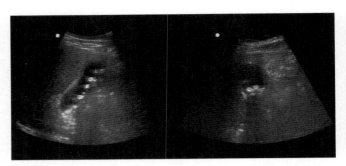
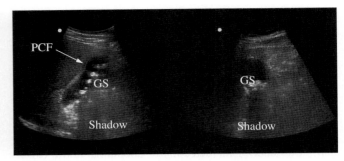

FIGURE 24.46 ▪ Gallbladder: Gallstone. The bright oval-to-round hyperechoic structures within the gallbladder with a posterior shadow are the classic gallstone presentation seen on ultrasound in sagittal and transverse views. A small amount of pericholecystic fluid is seen near the fundus in the sagittal view. (Photo contributor: Stephen J. Leech, MD, RDMS.)

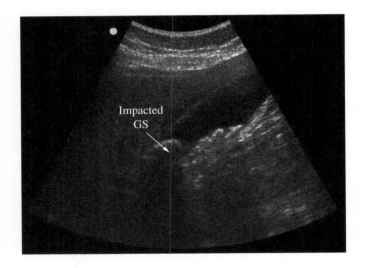

FIGURE 24.47 ▪ Gallbladder: Impacted Gallstone. A bright, hyperechoic structure is lodged at the neck of the gallbladder. Repositioning the patient reveals no movement of the stone verifying that it is impacted. (Photo contributor: Stephen J. Leech, MD, RDMS.)

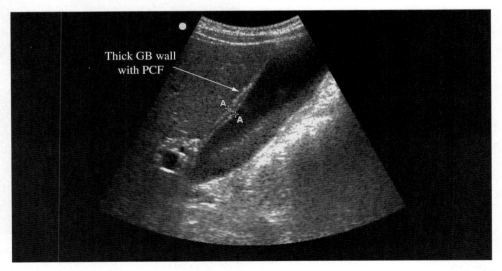

FIGURE 24.48 ▪ Gallbladder: Pericholecystic Fluid. A circumferential anechoic stripe that borders the outer gallbladder wall is consistent with pericholecystic fluid (PCF). A small gallstone with posterior shadowing and small amount of PCF is also seen. (Photo contributor: Stephen J. Leech, MD, RDMS.)

Clinical Summary

Emergency ultrasound of the abdominal aorta is used to diagnose or exclude an abdominal aortic aneurysm (AAA). As the general population ages, the frequency of AAA increases, and the use of ultrasound of the abdominal aorta in the ED for patients with abdominal, back, or flank pain should also increase. Though the sensitivity of transabdominal ultrasound for the detection of abdominal aortic dissection is limited, the presence of an intra-aortic flap is diagnostic for aortic dissection. Recognition of this finding is essential for emergency physicians.

Indications

- Abdominal, back, or flank pain
- Pulsatile abdominal mass
- Hypotensive patient with abdominal pain or distension
  Early diagnosis of AAA can improve patient survival. When a patient is unstable, there is no bedside test superior to an EUS of the aorta to diagnose an AAA. Since aortic aneurysms occur as both fusiform (most common) and saccular types, it is essential that the EUS of the aorta include both sagittal and transverse components. It is generally accepted that an aortic measurement of greater than 3.0 cm in diameter is abnormal, with a significant risk of aortic rupture starting with measurements greater than 5.0 cm. This section illustrates the abdominal vasculature, which will aid in identification of the abdominal aorta and evaluation of AAAs.

Required Views for Emergency Department Abdominal Aorta Ultrasound

1. Transverse view
2. Sagittal view

The technique and common findings for each of these views are presented next.

Equipment: Recommended Transducers for Abdominal Aorta Ultrasound

- Convex array
- Microconvex
- Phased array
- Mechanical sector

Patient Preparation

- The patient is supine.

Techniques

Abdominal Aorta Window 1: Transverse View

- Place the transducer in the epigastrium with the transducer indicator oriented to the patient's right (Fig. 24.49).
- Identify the spinal stripe, the curvilinear hyperechoic reflection of the anterior vertebral body. The aorta is the circular anechoic structure anterior and slightly to the patient's left.
- Move down the abdominal aorta to the bifurcation (about the level of the umbilicus).
- Identify the liver, aorta, inferior vena cava (IVC), superior mesenteric artery (SMA), splenic vein (SV) (Fig. 24.50).
- Identify and measure the aorta at the mid- and distal aorta.

Abdominal Aorta Window 2: Sagittal View

- Place the transducer in the epigastrium with the transducer indicator oriented toward the patient's head. Move down the abdominal aorta to the bifurcation (about the region of the umbilicus) (Fig. 24.51).
- Identify the liver, aorta, inferior vena cava (IVC), celiac trunk, and superior mesenteric artery (SMA) (Fig. 24.52).

Abnormal Findings

- AAA: Anteroposterior measurements of more than 3.0 cm are suspicious for an aneurysm (Fig. 24.53).

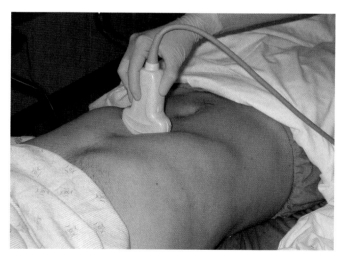

FIGURE 24.49 ■ Abdominal Aorta: Transverse Position. The transducer is placed in the epigastrium with the transducer indicator oriented to the patient's right; it is then moved down the abdominal aorta to the bifurcation. (Photo contributor: Stephen J. Leech, MD, RDMS.)

- Aortic dissection: An echogenic line (often moving with pulsations) of an aortic "flap" can be seen when present (Fig. 24.54).

Pearls

1. The EUS of the abdominal aorta should begin in the transverse view since this view provides the greatest amount of information and is essential for the diagnosis of a saccular aneurysm.
2. Measure the entire diameter (outer wall to outer wall) of the aorta or aneurysm and not just the lumen or false lumen. Include measurements of the proximal, mid-, and distal aorta.
3. If a significant amount of bowel gas is present, sit the patient at 45 degrees and apply constant gentle pressure.
4. The IVC will generally collapse when you have the patient abruptly sniff—a result of the negative pressure transmitted to the venous system by this maneuver.
5. If pulsed Doppler is available, it may be used to discriminate between the highly pulsatile flow of the aorta and the low-amplitude rumble of the IVC.

6. In patients with an aortic dissection, an intimal flap can be visible as a linear structure within the aorta. While this finding is highly specific, it is insensitive and its absence cannot be used to rule out a dissection.

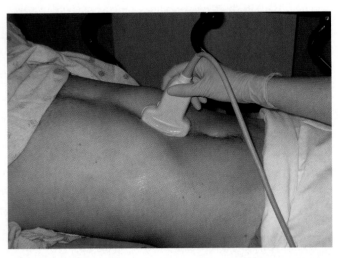

FIGURE 24.51 ■ Abdominal Aorta: Sagittal Position. The transducer is placed in the epigastrium with the transducer indicator oriented to the patient's head; it is then moved down the abdominal aorta to the bifurcation. (Photo contributor: Stephen J. Leech, MD, RDMS.)

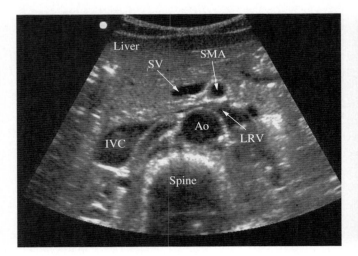

FIGURE 24.50 ■ Steve Abdominal Aorta: Transverse. Various structures are identified, including the liver, inferior vena cava (IVC), superior mesenteric artery (SMA), splenic vein (SV), aorta, and "spinal stripe." (Photo contributor: Stephen J. Leech, MD, RDMS.)

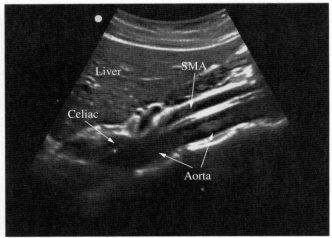

FIGURE 24.52 ■ Abdominal Aorta: Sagittal. The liver, aorta, celiac trunk, and superior mesenteric artery (SMA) are identified in this view. (Photo contributor: Stephen J. Leech, MD, RDMS.)

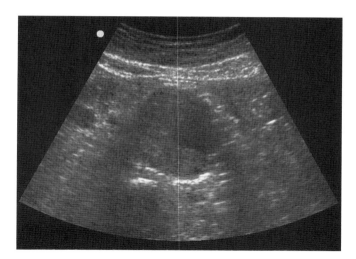

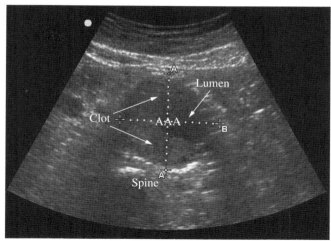

FIGURE 24.53 ■ Abdominal Aorta: Aneurysm. A large abdominal aortic aneurysm with clot in the vessel and small remaining lumen is seen in these views. (Photo contributor: Stephen J. Leech, MD, RDMS.)

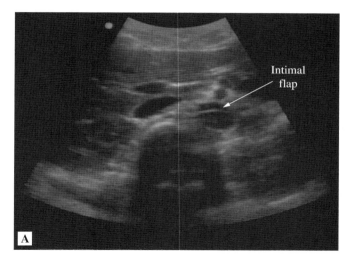

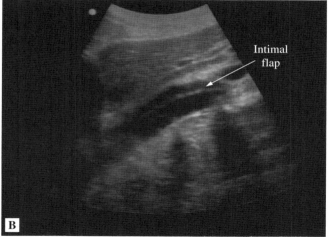

FIGURE 24.54 ■ Abdominal Aorta: Dissection. (A) An aortic dissection "flap" is seen in this transverse image of a 27-year-old female with undiagnosed Marfans syndrome. (B) The extent of the dissection is noted in this sagittal view. (Photo contributor: Paul R. Sierzenski, MD, RDMS.)

Clinical Summary

Renal ultrasound can yield helpful diagnostic information for the patient presenting with abdominal or flank pain consistent with renal colic. Obstructive uropathy due to kidney stones is the principal pathology identified with renal ultrasound. It is not standard practice for emergency physicians to perform renal ultrasound to identify renal or ureteral calculi, rather the kidneys are evaluated for hydronephrosis. The presence of hydronephrosis in the patient with renal colic is presumed to be a direct result of ureteral obstruction. There are no accurate means of determining the degree of obstruction by the presence of hydronephrosis.

Indications

- Flank pain
- Renal colic
- Abdominal pain in the elderly
- Hematuria
- Costovertebral angle (CVA) tenderness

The diagnostic dilemma for many emergency physicians is how to effectively utilize the renal EUS in the patient with suspected renal colic. Although hydronephrosis is the primary sonographic finding in renal EUS, renal cysts, calculi, and renal masses may also be identified.

The recommended sonographic approach to the kidney is identical to that for the RUQ and LUQ windows in the trauma/FAST examination previously discussed. The coronal view allows the sonographer to visualize the right or left kidney from the superior to inferior poles. The renal EUS is best interpreted when comparative images are obtained between the right and left kidneys. It is important to realize that many approaches to the renal system, described in other texts, may be useful at times; however, the coronal view is familiar to the emergency physician. For that reason it is our primary window for evaluating the kidneys on the renal EUS.

Required View for Emergency Department Renal Ultrasound

1. Coronal view

The technique and common findings for this view is presented next.

Equipment: Recommended Transducers for Renal Ultrasound

- Convex array
- Microconvex
- Phased array
- Mechanical sector

Patient Preparation

- The patient is supine.

Technique

Right and Left Coronal Views

- The transducer indicator is oriented toward the patient's head.
- The transducer is directed as a coronal section through the body in the midaxillary to posterior axillary lines (Fig. 24.55). Begin scanning between the 9th to 11th ribs on the right and the 8th to 11th ribs on the left.
- Identify the liver, right kidney, renal cortex (with pyramids), and central renal sinus (Fig. 24.56).
- Identify the spleen, left kidney, renal cortex (with pyramids), and central renal sinus (Fig. 24.57).

Abnormal Findings

- Hydronephrosis: Dilatation of the renal sinus with black, anechoic fluid within the bright renal sinus (Fig. 24.58)

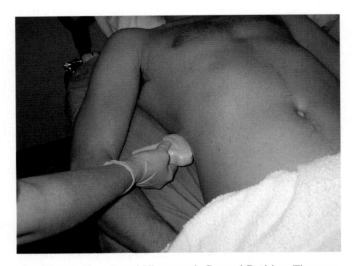

FIGURE 24.55 ■ Renal Ultrasound: Coronal Position. The transducer is directed in the midaxillary to posterior axillary lines for scanning between the 9th and 11th ribs on the right and the 8th and 11th ribs on the left. (Photo contributor: Stephen J. Leech, MD, RDMS.)

- Renal calculi: Bright hyperechoic oval/round structures within the cortex or renal sinus (posterior shadowing is often present)
- Renal cyst: Anechoic structure often at the periphery of the renal cortex with a thin wall, and posterior acoustic enhancement

Pearls

1. If your machine has "dual" or "multi-image" modes, selecting this feature will allow you to make an on-screen side-by-side comparison of both kidneys.

2. Rib shadows will be evident with this coronal view. Have the patient hold his or her breath in inspiration and move the transducer a rib space higher or lower to visualize the kidney from the superior to the inferior pole.

3. The presence of a "ureteral jet" confirms the passage of urine into the bladder from a specific side. Its absence is sensitive, but not specific for complete ureteral obstruction (Fig. 24.59).

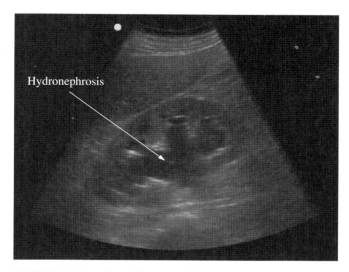

FIGURE 24.58 ■ Renal Ultrasound: Hydronephrosis. Dilatation of the renal sinus with dark black, anechoic fluid within the bright renal sinus is consistent with hydronephrosis. (Photo contributor: Stephen J. Leech, MD, RDMS.)

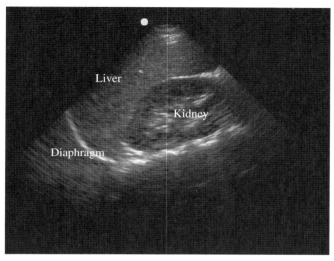

FIGURE 24.56 ■ Renal Ultrasound: Right Coronal. The liver, right kidney, and diaphragm are seen in this view. (Photo contributor: Stephen J. Leech, MD, RDMS.)

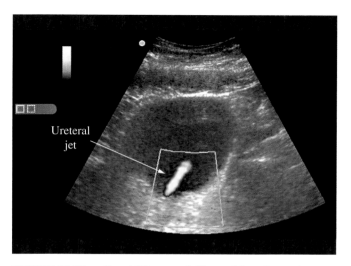

FIGURE 24.57 ■ Renal Ultrasound: Left Coronal. The spleen, left kidney, and diaphragm are seen in this view. (Photo contributor: Stephen J. Leech, MD, RDMS.)

FIGURE 24.59 ■ Renal Ultrasound: Ureteral Jets. Power Doppler imaging demonstrates a right ureteral jet as urine flows into the bladder. (Photo contributor: Stephen J. Leech, MD, RDMS.)

Clinical Summary

Pelvic ultrasound is frequently used to evaluate the patient presenting with pelvic pain and/or vaginal bleeding, who may have a host of underlying clinical conditions. Among these are ovarian cyst, tuboovarian abscess, ovarian torsion, fetal demise, urinary retention, incomplete or threatened abortion, molar pregnancy, appendicitis, urinary tract infection, ureteral calculi, or pelvic inflammatory disease. However, the primary goal of the pelvic EUS is to exclude an ectopic pregnancy. Pelvic ultrasound is accomplished with two different scanning techniques: transabdominal and endovaginal.

Pregnant patients presenting with abdominal pain or vaginal bleeding during the first trimester must have an ectopic pregnancy excluded. This is commonly accomplished in the emergency department setting by identifying an intrauterine pregnancy.

Indications

- Pelvic/abdominal pain
- Vaginal bleeding (pregnant or nonpregnant patient)
- Suspected pregnancy

Required Views for Emergency Department Pelvic Ultrasound

1. Sagittal view
2. Transverse view

The technique and common findings for each of these views are presented next.

Equipment: Recommended Transducers for Pelvic TAS

- Convex array
- Microconvex
- Phased array

Patient Preparation

- The patient is supine for transabdominal views.
- The patient is supine and preferably in the lithotomy position for endovaginal views.

Techniques

Pelvic Transabdominal Sonography (TAS) Window 1: Sagittal View

- Place transducer superior to symphysis pubis, with the transducer indicator directed toward the umbilicus (Fig. 24.60).
- Identify the bladder (triangular), uterus, rectum, ovaries, and the vesicouterine and rectouterine pouches (pouch of Douglas) (Fig. 24.61).

Pelvic Transabdominal Sonography (TAS) Window 2: Transverse View

- From the TAS sagittal view, rotate the transducer 90 degrees counterclockwise or place it superior to symphysis pubis, directed in a line connecting the anterior superior iliac crests (gradually angle caudally) (Fig. 24.62).
- Identify the bladder (rectangular), uterus (if present), rectum, ovaries, and the vesicouterine and rectouterine pouches (pouch of Douglas) (Fig. 24.63).

Endovaginal Sonography (EVS) Window 1: Sagittal View

- With a latex condom/shield covering the transducer, place it into the vagina, directed toward the anterior fornix in a line through the umbilicus (Fig. 24.64).
- The transducer indicator is directed upward.
- Identify the bladder (sliver), uterus, rectum, ovaries, and the vesicouterine (anterior) and rectouterine (posterior) cul-de-sacs (Fig. 24.65).

Endovaginal Sonography (EVS) Window 2: Coronal View

- From the EVS sagittal view, rotate the transducer counterclockwise 90 degrees and place into the vagina directed toward the posterior fornix in a line through the umbilicus (Fig. 24.66).
- Identify the bladder (sliver), uterus (ovoid) (Fig. 24.67), rectum, ovaries (Fig. 24.68), and the vesicouterine and rectouterine pouches (pouch of Douglas).
- Identify an intrauterine pregnancy if present (Fig. 24.69).

Abnormal Findings

- Free intraperitoneal fluid: Anechoic (black) bands of fluid located in the vesicouterine and/or rectouterine pouch.

- Intraperitoneal free fluid: Anechoic (black) bands of fluid located in the vesicouterine and/or rectouterine pouch.

- Ectopic pregnancy: Extrauterine gestation may have an accompanying pseudosac (an anechoic fluid collection within the endometrial echo of the uterus) in the uterus (Fig. 24.70).

- Free intraperitoneal fluid: Anechoic (black) bands of fluid located in the vesicouterine (anterior) or rectouterine (posterior) cul-de-sac.

- Live intrauterine pregnancy: Greater than 5-mm gestational sac with a thick, concentric echogenic ring within the endometrial echo of the uterus and both of the following: fetal pole with cardiac activity.

- Intrauterine pregnancy (IUP): Greater than 5-mm gestational sac with a thick, concentric echogenic ring within the endometrial echo of the uterus and one of the following: yolk sac, fetal pole, or double decidual sign (the decidua capsularis and decidua vera seen as two distinct hypoechoic layers surrounding the early gestational sac) (Fig. 24.71).

- Abnormal IUP: Gestational sac greater than 10 to 12 mm without yolk sac, gestational sac greater than 16 mm without fetal pole, or definitive fetal pole without cardiac pulsation.

- No definitive IUP: The uterus appears empty and no definitive ectopic pregnancy is visualized. Possible diagnosis includes early IUP, abortion, ectopic pregnancy.

- Ectopic pregnancy: Greater than 5-mm gestational sac and thick, concentric echogenic ring *outside* the endometrial echo of the uterus and one of the following: definitive yolk sac, obvious fetal pole, cardiac activity.

Pearls

1. A full bladder allows better visualization of structures posterior to the bladder in transabdominal ultrasound. An empty/minimally filled bladder is preferred for endovaginal ultrasound.

2. A *small* amount of free fluid found in the posterior cul-de-sac of the pelvis can be physiologic.

3. On insertion of the transducer, identify the bladder.

4. In the sagittal view, identify the endometrial stripe from the fundus of the uterus to the cervix. This is accomplished by tilting the probe (anteriorly to posteriorly) while maintaining a sagittal plane of the uterus.

5. Return to the fundus of the uterus in a sagittal view and slowly evaluate the right and then left borders of the uterus in the longitudinal axis.

6. Turn the transducer counterclockwise 90 degrees to enter the coronal plane. The uterus should appear oval in this view. Scan posteriorly to the cervix and then superiorly to the fundus of the uterus to exclude the presence of a bicornuate uterus.

7. If a pregnancy or intrauterine sac is identified, further evaluate with measurements and an assessment of fetal cardiac activity.

8. To evaluate the ovaries, begin with the patient's right ovary and scan initially in the longitudinal (sagittal) plane, then rotate the transducer counterclockwise 90 degrees and evaluate the ovary in the coronal plane. The ovaries ideally will be located anteromedially to the external iliac vessels. This is often only a guide to their location, and a methodical approach is often required to visualize both ovaries.

9. If the uterus is difficult to identify, withdraw the transducer slightly. A common error in EVS is inserting the transducer too far, thus bypassing the uterus and imaging only bowel.

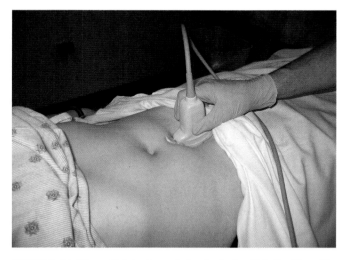

FIGURE 24.60 ■ Pelvic Transabdominal: Sagittal Position. The transducer is placed superior to symphysis pubis, with the transducer indicator directed in a line through the umbilicus. (Photo contributor: Stephen J. Leech, MD, RDMS.)

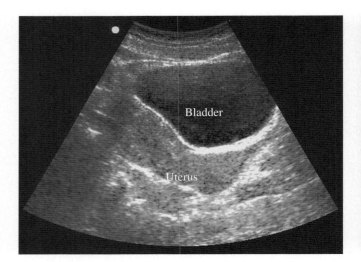

FIGURE 24.61 ■ Pelvic Transabdominal Ultrasound: Sagittal. The bladder (triangular in this view) and uterus are seen. The rectum, ovaries, vesicouterine, and rectouterine (pouch of Douglas) pouches may be seen with movement of the probe. (Photo contributor: Stephen J. Leech, MD, RDMS.)

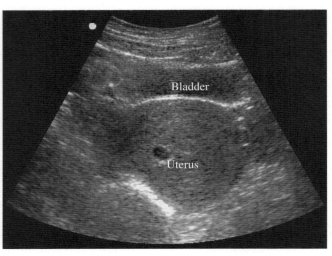

FIGURE 24.63 ■ Pelvic Transabdominal: Transverse. The bladder (rectangular in this view) uterus, and ovary are seen as well as a small gestational sac. The rectum and the vesicouterine and rectouterine pouches (pouch of Douglas) may be seen with movement of the probe. (Photo contributor: Stephen J. Leech, MD, RDMS.)

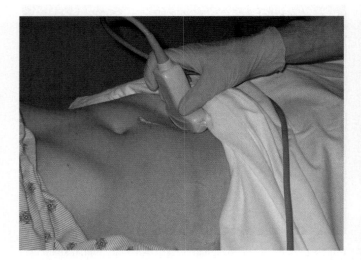

FIGURE 24.62 ■ Pelvic Transabdominal: Transverse Position. The transducer is rotated 90 degrees counterclockwise from the sagittal view and directed in a line connecting the anterior superior iliac crests. The transducer is angled caudally to complete the view. (Photo contributor: Stephen J. Leech, MD, RDMS.)

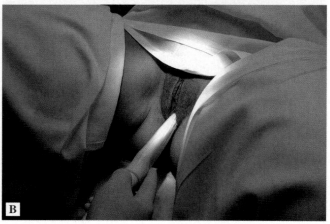

FIGURE 24.64 ■ Endovaginal: Sagittal Position. The transducer is directed toward the anterior fornix in a line through the umbilicus (**A**); it is placed into the vagina (**B**). The probe is advanced gradually. (Photo contributor: Windy City Ultrasound, Inc.)

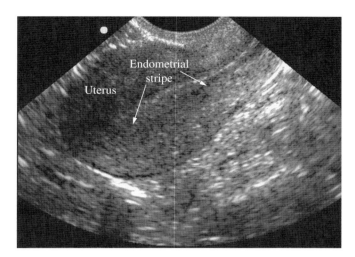

FIGURE 24.65 ■ Endovaginal: Sagittal. The uterus with an endometrial stripe is seen in this view. Other structures to be identified include the bladder, rectum, ovaries, and vesicouterine and rectouterine pouches. (Photo contributor: Stephen J. Leech, MD, RDMS.)

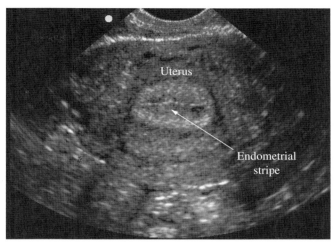

FIGURE 24.67 ■ Endovaginal: Coronal. The oval-shaped uterus with a hyperechoic endometrial stripe is seen in this view. Other structures to be identified include the bladder, rectum, ovaries, and the vesicouterine and rectouterine pouches. (Photo contributor: Stephen J. Leech, MD, RDMS.)

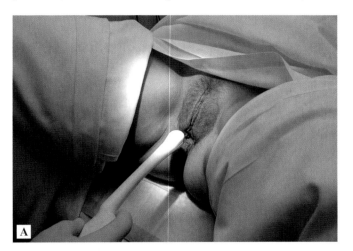

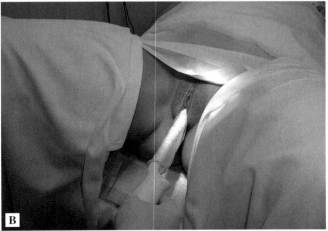

FIGURE 24.66 ■ Endovaginal: Coronal Position. From the sagittal view, the transducer is rotated counterclockwise 90 degrees (A) and directed toward the posterior fornix in a line through the umbilicus (B). (Photo contributor: Windy City Ultrasound, Inc.)

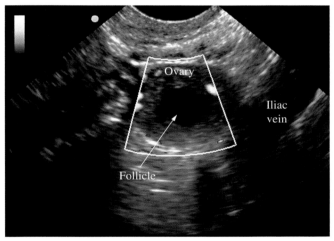

FIGURE 24.68 ■ Endovaginal: Ovary. An ovary with a small cyst and a follicle are seen in this view. Color-flow Doppler, if available, facilitates identification of vascular structures. The iliac vein is seen in this view. (Photo contributor: Stephen J. Leech, MD, RDMS.)

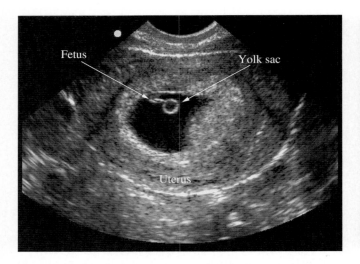

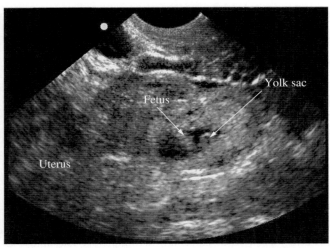

FIGURE 24.69 ■ Endovaginal: IUP. An intrauterine pregnancy of about 6 weeks' gestation is seen. (Photo contributor: Stephen J. Leech, MD, RDMS.)

FIGURE 24.70 ■ Endovaginal: Ectopic Pregnancy. An extrauterine gestation with echogenic ring, yolk sac, and fetal pole, is seen outside the uterus in the left adnexa. (Photo contributor: Stephen J. Leech, MD, RDMS.)

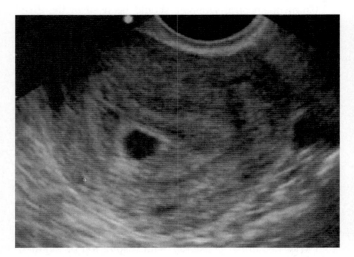

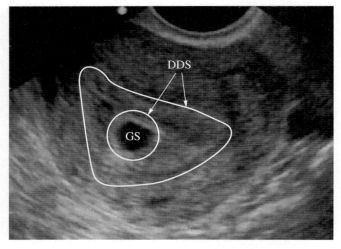

FIGURE 24.71 ■ Intrauterine Gestational Sac. Discrete ring of an intrauterine gestational sac seen on transvaginal ultrasound. No yolk sac is visualized. A double decidual sac sign is seen, however, lending evidence of a true gestational sac versus a pseudo gestational sac formed from a decidual cast in ectopic pregnancy. A thorough look in the adnexa is important in diagnosing ectopic pregnancy when a gestational sac in the only finding. (Photo contributor: Stephen J. Leech, MD, RDMS.)

Clinical Summary

The presence of a deep venous thrombosis (DVT) is a part of the differential diagnosis of a variety of signs and symptoms. Although clinical scoring algorithms have been developed to gauge risk, no clinical findings are conclusive of this condition and imaging is necessary to confirm the diagnosis. Ultrasonography is a sensitive, noninvasive imaging modality that can be performed rapidly essentially without contraindication. Unfortunately, it is not always readily available to the emergency physician and empiric treatment is used until the DVT is excluded.

Most DVTs occur in the lower extremity but upper extremity DVTs are increasing in frequency. The complete sonographic examination of the venous system of an extremity typically consists of Doppler and B-mode imaging of the entire extremity. A limited examination of the proximal venous system requires less time and complexity than the complete study and has been shown to be highly sensitive. The description of the DVT ultrasound in this section will refer only to the limited study of the proximal extremity.

Indications

- Extremity swelling
- Extremity pain
- Extremity erythema
- Dyspnea
- Chest pain

Required Views for DVT Ultrasound

Upper

1. Internal jugular vein (IJ)
2. Axillary vein (AxV)
3. Brachial vein (BV)

Lower

1. Common femoral vein (CFV)
2. Popliteal vein (PV)

Equipment: Recommended Transducers for DVT Ultrasound

- Linear
- Convex

Patient Preparation

- The patient is supine for upper extremity imaging.
- Ideally the patient is recumbent with the head of bed elevated 20 to 40 degree for lower extremity imaging.

Technique

Upper Extremity

- The transducer should be oriented in a transverse plane to the course of the vein (Fig. 24.72).
- Imaging typically begins at the distal IJ, moving proximally to the junction of the IJ and subclavian vein.
- Next, trace the proximal AxV from under the clavicle to the axilla, continuing to follow the brachial vein into the antecubital fossa (Fig. 24.74).
- The vein is gently compressed until the walls completely coapt, this process is repeated every few centimeters.
- Color or spectral Doppler should be used in the distal portion of each vein to document phasicity with respiration or augmentation (where applicable).

Lower Extremity

- The transducer should be oriented in a transverse plane to the course of the vein (Fig. 24.75).
- Imaging begins at the proximal CFV, moving distally to the PV.
- The vein is gently compressed until the walls completely collapse, this process is repeated every few centimeters (Fig. 24.76).
- Color or spectral Doppler should be used at the CFV and PV to document phasicitiy with respiration or augmentation (Fig. 24.76).

Abnormal Findings

- Inability to compress the vein: Suggests DVT. This may be acute or chronic, or due to technical limitations (unable to apply enough direct pressure [Fig. 24.77]).
- Poor or absent phasicity: Suggests occlusion at location proximal to transducer.
- Poor or absent augmentation: Suggests occlusion at location distal to transducer.

Pearls

- Ensure that the vascular structure is a deep vein. Deep veins are paired with arteries. Veins are easily compressible, arteries generally are not. Color or spectral Doppler should demonstrate characteristic arterial or venous waveforms.

- If unable to adequately compress vessels (especially in the adductor canal), apply pressure from under the extremity toward the transducer.
- Echogenic material within the vein may be an artifact and not a DVT. Visualize any abnormality in more than one plane and optimize settings to exclude artifacts.

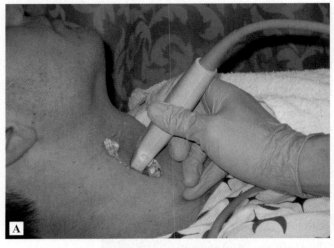

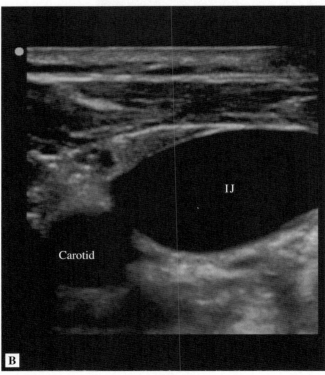

FIGURE 24.72 ■ Internal Jugular: Transverse. Transducer position (**A**) and anatomy (**B**) for transverse view of the internal jugular vein. (Photo contributor: Paul R. Sierzenski, MD, RDMS.)

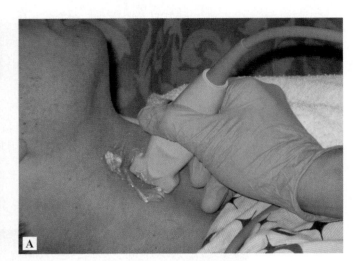

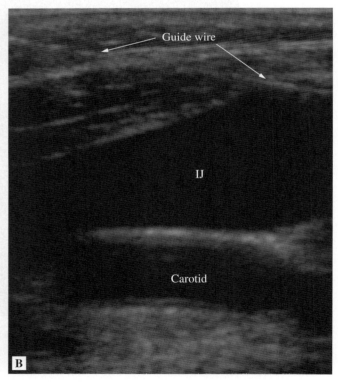

FIGURE 24.73 ■ Internal Jugular: Sagittal. Transducer position (**A**) and anatomy (**B**) for sagittal view of the internal jugular vein and carotid artery. A guidewire is noted entering the jugular to the right of this image. (Photo contributor: Paul R. Sierzenski, MD, RDMS.)

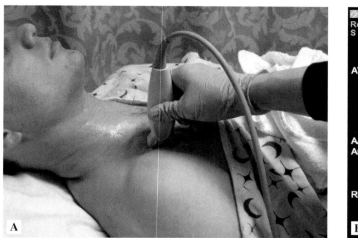
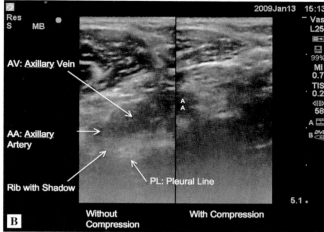

FIGURE 24.74 ▪ Venous: Upper Extremity. (**A**) Probe position is just inferior to the clavicle in the transverse plane. (**B**) Note the location of the axillary artery (AA), axillary vein (AV), and the pleura (PL). (Photo contributor: Paul R. Sierzenski, MD, RDMS.)

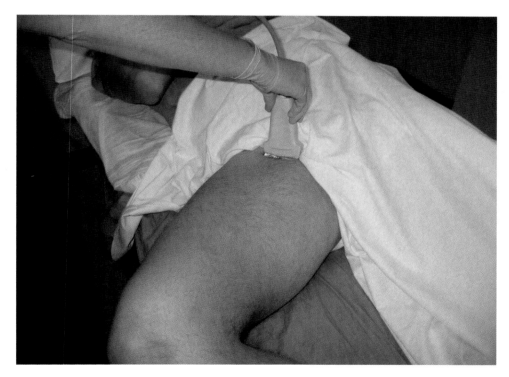

FIGURE 24.75 ▪ Venous: Lower Extremity. Transducer position with the probe in the transverse plane located over the femoral vessels. (Photo contributor: Stephen J. Leech, MD, RDMS.)

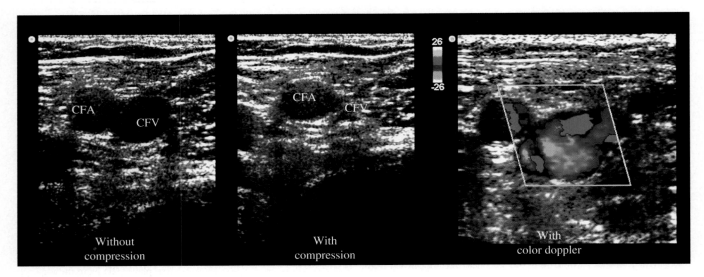

FIGURE 24.76 ■ Venous: Normal Compression, Doppler Lower Extremity. This is a side-by-side comparison of the common femoral vein (CFV) with and without compression and normal total collapsing of the CFV. Note the color Doppler filling of the CFV and the saphenous vein (SV) as it enters the CFV. This finding may be accentuated with venous augmentation. (Photo contributor: Stephen J. Leech, MD, RDMS.)

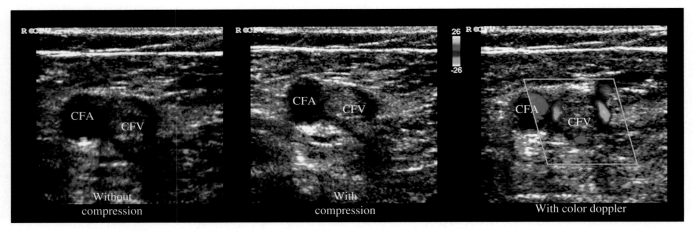

FIGURE 24.77 ■ Venous: DVT, Compression, Doppler Lower Extremity. This image shows a side by side, of the common femoral vein with and without compression. Since the vein does not fully collapse, this is an evidence of a DVT. Clot is also seen, as well as a filling defect in the vessel of the noncompressed vein with color Doppler. (Photo contributor: Stephen J. Leech, MD, RDMS.)

Clinical Summary

Vascular access is a necessity for evaluation and treatment of many patients in the emergency department. Traditionally, knowledge of common venous anatomy in experienced hands was the standard method of obtaining venous access. Factors such as obesity, prior access, and volume depletion increase the difficulty of the conventional approach. Increased difficulty not only leads to failure to obtain access, but also increases the risk of complications.

Ultrasound-guided vascular access reduces the variables associated with the traditional landmark-based approach. Other specialties have been using ultrasound for this purpose for some time and its use is increasing in emergency medicine. Many studies document the ease of use, accuracy and safety of this technique, and several national organizations have declared ultrasound-guided central venous access as the standard of care when available.

While much of the attention has focused on ultrasound guidance in central venous access, it has also proved beneficial in peripheral venous access. Likewise, it is also facilitates arterial access.

Indications

- Need for venous access
- Obscured landmarks (obesity, trauma, etc)
- Cardiac arrest

Equipment

- Linear
- Convex

Patient Preparation

- Position and prepare the patient as would be convention for access and use a sterile sheath for the transducer.
- For central venous access the patient is supine with the access site in a dependent position (Fig. 24.78).

Technique

Note: Ultrasound may either be used dynamically, where it is used throughout the entire procedure, or static, when only the anatomy is identified and the procedure is then carried out blindly. These descriptions refer to the dynamic technique.

Central Venous Access

Typical sites include the internal jugular as well as the femoral vein, but may also include the subclavian, axillary, and brachial veins.

- In a transverse view, identify the structures of interest:
  - Deep vein
  - Corresponding artery
  - Others (nerve, trachea, etc)
- Confirm the vein as the collapsible vascular structure as well as the orientation of the transducer
- Transverse technique (Fig. 24.78):
  - In a transverse view, position the vein in the center of the image, trace the course of the vein and estimate its depth.
  - Introduce the needle at a site distal to the transducer at a distance that would allow you to intersect the imaged vein using an approximate angle of 45 degree.
  - Direct the needle toward the middle of the transducer at an angle perpendicular to the long axis of the probe.
  - Maintaining the probes position on the skin, angle it distally to indentify the path of the advancing needle as indicated by:
    - Identifying the needle tip
    - Observing tissue movement
    - Observing ring-down artifact from the needle
  - Follow the tip of the needle until it contacts the anterior surface of the vein.
  - Continue to advance until a venous flash is seen or the needle has reached the intended depth.
  - If no flash is seen at an appropriate depth in the correct path, slowly withdraw the needle and observe for venous return.
  - Continue catheter placement as per common practice.
- Longitudinal technique (Fig. 24.79):
  - Position the transducer in-line with the long axis of the vein and estimate its depth.
  - Introduce the needle at the distal edge of the transducer.
  - Direct the needle along the long axis of the probe.
  - Identify the path of the advancing needle as indicated by:
    - Identifying the needle tip
    - Observing tissue movement
    - Observing ring-down artifact from the needle
  - Follow the tip of the needle until it contacts the anterior surface of the vein.
  - Continue to advance until a venous flash is seen or the needle has reached the intended depth.

- If no flash is seen at an appropriate depth in the correct path, slowly withdraw the needle and observe for venous return.
- Continue catheter placement as per common practice.

Peripheral Venous Access

Typical sites include the cephalic and basilic veins of the upper extremity and the external jugular (Fig. 24.80).

- Apply a tourniquet if indicated.
- In a transverse view, identify the peripheral vein.
- Confirm the vein as the collapsible vascular structure as well as the orientation of the transducer.
- Transverse technique:
    - In a transverse view, position the vein in the center of the image, trace the course of the vein, and estimate its depth.
    - Introduce the needle at a site distal to the transducer at a distance that would allow you to intersect the image the vein using an approximate angle of 45 degree.
    - Direct the needle toward the middle of the transducer at an angle perpendicular to the long axis of the probe.
    - Maintaining the probes position on the skin, angle it distally to indentify the path of the advancing needle as indicated by:
        - Identifying the needle tip
        - Observing tissue movement
        - Observing ring-down artifact from the needle
    - Follow the tip of the needle until it contacts the anterior surface of the vein.
    - Continue to advance until a venous flash is seen or the needle has reached the intended depth.
    - If no flash is seen at an appropriate depth in the correct path, slowly withdraw the needle and observe for venous return.
    - Continue catheter placement as per common practice.
- Longitudinal technique:
    - Position the transducer in-line with the long axis of the vein and estimate its depth.
    - Introduce the needle at the distal edge of the transducer.
    - Direct the needle along the long axis of the probe.
    - Identify the path of the advancing needle as indicated by:
        - Identifying the needle tip
        - Observing tissue movement
        - Observing ring-down artifact from the needle

- Follow the tip of the needle until it contacts the anterior surface of the vein.
    - Continue to advance until a venous flash is seen or the needle has reached the intended depth.
    - If no flash is seen at an appropriate depth in the correct path, slowly withdraw the needle and observe for venous return.
- Continue catheter placement as per common practice.

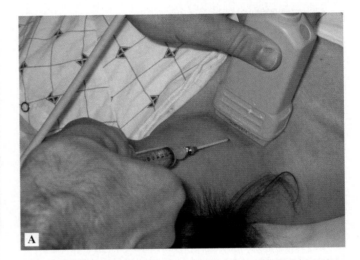

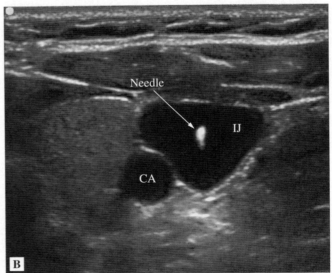

FIGURE 24.78 ■ Central Venous Access: Transverse IJ. (**A**) Probe position is transverse, patient is in Trendelenburg with needle in position. (**B**) The internal jugular (IJ) vein and carotid artery are seen. The hyperechoic area in the center of the IJ is the needle tip. (Photo contributor: Paul R. Sierzenski, MD, RDMS.)

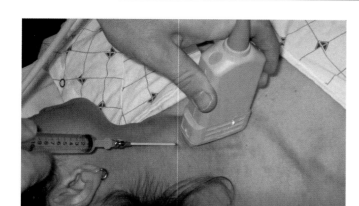

Pearls

1. Ultrasound identifies the relevant anatomy, but care must be used to follow the typical procedure of venous access.

2. When using a sterile sheath (or glove), use conductive media both inside (gel) and outside (gel or liquid antiseptic) the sheath.

3. Having the patient cough or performing the Valsalva maneuver may be used to further distend the IJ to facilitate placement.

4. Venous access may be performed by a single operator or with an assistant.

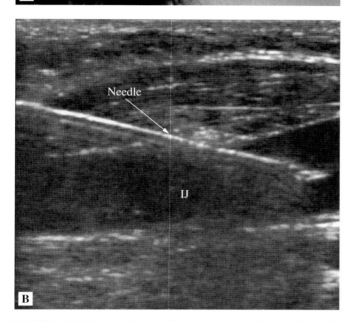

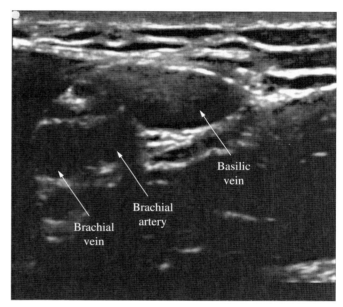

FIGURE 24.79 ■ Central Venous Access: Longitudinal IJ. (**A**) Longitudinal probe position with image (**B**) of needle entering into the internal jugular vein, needle tip within the lumen, and carotid artery deep to the IJ. (Photo contributor: Paul R. Sierzenski, MD, RDMS.)

FIGURE 24.80 ■ Peripheral Venous Access: Basilic Vein. A transverse view of the basilic vein in the upper arm. Note the humerus, brachial artery, and brachial vein. (Photo contributor: Paul R. Sierzenski, MD, RDMS.)

Clinical Summary

Ocular ultrasound may be used to identify serious intraocular disorders, particularly when a direct funduscopic examination is needed, but difficult or impossible to obtain.

Indications

- Visual loss/decrease
- Ocular pain
- Ocular trauma

Equipment: Recommended Transducers for Ocular Ultrasound

- Linear with high frequency (>10 MHz) is best.
- Confirm that the energy output levels of your ultrasound system are approved for ocular ultrasound.
- Ocular ultrasound often necessitates increasing gain settings to visualize detailed structures.

Patient Preparation

- The optic nerve should be oriented in plane with the ultrasound beam in a straightened position (eye looking slightly laterally).
- Identify the globe, lens, anterior chamber, retina, and optic nerve and sheath (Fig. 24.81).
- The patient's eyes remain closed, place ample gel over the eyelid and stabilize your fingers on the bridge of the nose and the zygomatic arch (Fig. 24.82).

Techniques

Transverse Technique

- In a transverse view, position the optic nerve in the middle of the screen with depth sufficient to view 1 cm beyond the optic nerve.

Abnormal Findings

- Retinal detachment: The retina is a dense neurovascular structure that is highly reflective of ultrasound. For this reason a detachment can be clearly identified when the sound beam strikes it (Fig. 24.83).
- Vitreous detachment: The normally anechoic vitreous will demonstrate various echoes that move with eye movement and can be consistently visualized in multiple planes. These small, filament-like threads of the vitreous

membrane can be missed if the image is not appropriately gained or over gained when needed (Fig. 24.84).

- Vitreous hemorrhage: Hyperechoic areas in the vitreous or anterior chamber may represent hemorrhage (Fig. 4.20B).
- Dilated optic nerve sheath: As intracranial pressure increases, this pressure is transmitted to spinal fluid and along the optic nerve sheath. When the ultrasound beam is directed in plane with the straightened optic nerve, a measurement of the width of the sheath can be taken at a point 3 mm deep to the retina. A diameter greater than 5 mm is considered abnormal and suggests elevated intracranial pressure (Fig. 24.85).
- Dislocated lens: The lens has an abnormal lie or position. A lens subluxation can be subtle and visualized as instability of the lens with eye movement.

Pearls

- Confirmation of an abnormality can often be made by using unaffected eye as the control. Using multiple planes to image a structure will also help to clarify artifacts from true pathology.

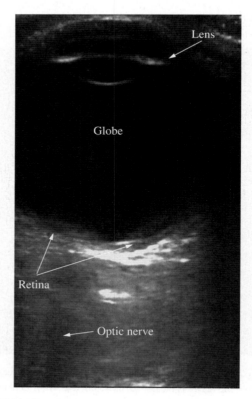

FIGURE 24.81 ■ Ocular: Transverse Anatomy. This image demonstrates the lens, globe, retina, and optic nerve. (Photo contributor: Jason Nomura, MD.)

- Over gain the image, then gradually decrease the gain. This will allow subtle clots such as in a small vitreous hemorrhage, or the lacy appearance of a vitreous detachment to be readily identified.

- Both retinal and vitreous detachments are tethered to their origin and can be seen moving when the eye is moved by the patient medial or lateral.

- The optic nerve sheath diameter can be falsely increased when measured if the optic bundle is imaged at an angle.

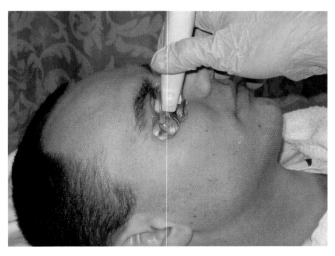

FIGURE 24.82 ■ Ocular: Transverse Position. The transducer is held and the fingers are stabilized on the zygomatic arch and the bridge of the nose to prevent applying pressure to the globe. It is essential to fill the area over closed eye with gel to allow the transducer to float and not apply pressure to the globe. (Photo contributor: Stephen J. Leech, MD, RDMS.)

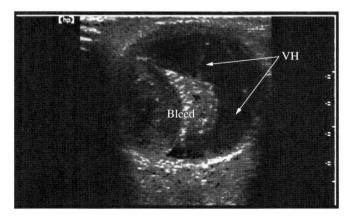

FIGURE 24.84 ■ Ocular: Vitreous Detachment with Hemorrhage. A large pre-retinal bleed along with vitreous hemorrhage is seen. The subtle findings of the vitreous detachment; lacy, spider-like lines are noted in this image. Detection of a small vitreous detachment or hemorrhage may require a high gain setting to be visualized. (Photo contributor: Paul R. Sierzenski, MD, RDMS.)

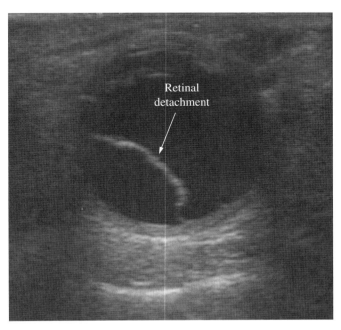

FIGURE 24.83 ■ Ocular: Retinal Detachment. The bright echogenic signal from the retina is clearly identifiable, due to the density of the retina, note how it separates from the posterior wall in the patient with a retinal detachment. (Photo contributor: Stephen J. Leech, MD, RDMS.)

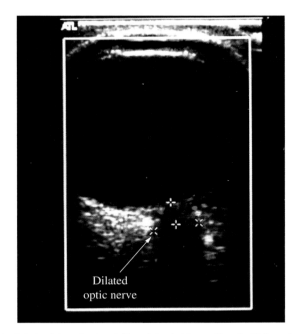

FIGURE 24.85 ■ Ocular: Dilated Optic Nerve Sheath. This patient's optic nerve sheath is dilated at 0.59 cm, larger than the top normal of 0.5 cm in an adult. This finding has been shown to correlate with increased intracranial pressure as in this patient with ventriculo-peritoneal shunt failure. The sheath diameter is measured 3 mm posterior to the retinal plateau. (Photo contributor: Paul R. Sierzenski, MD, RDMS.)

Clinical Summary

Superficial ultrasound has been shown to increase diagnostic accuracy, speed disposition, and reduce complications of procedures.

Indications

- Suspected fluid collection (abscess, hematoma, etc)
- Suspected tendon/ligament injury/pathology
- Localization of subcutaneous foreign body
- Guidance for procedures

Equipment

- Linear

Patient Preparation

- Expose the area of interest and position it to allow for maximal ultrasound visibility.
- Apply ultrasound gel to area.

Technique

- Image the area of interest by gently sweeping the probe across the skin. This should be done in two perpendicular planes. If possible, orient the planes along conventional axes (ie, transverse and longitudinal to a tendon).
- Identify normal subcutaneous tissue, tendon, muscle, ligament, and bone.
- Apply superficial marking to overlying skin if necessary.

Abnormal Findings

- Edema/cellulitis: Increased interstitial fluid appears similar on ultrasound regardless of cause. Initially, increased echogenicity and loss of definition of the tissue is noted with localized increased depth. As the condition progresses, fluid is noted to accumulate diffusely in a reticular pattern creating a cobblestone appearance (Fig. 24.86).
- Abscess: Focal fluid accumulation, often with significant cellulitic changes surrounding it. The fluid may appear anechoic or have complex echoes (Fig. 24.87). If drainage will be attempted, note should be made of the depth of the abscess as well as any associated tracts or other adjacent structures (vessels, nerves, etc).

- Tenosynovitis: Anechoic or heterogeneous echogenic fluid in flexor tendon sheath; may be associated with surrounding cellulitic changes (Fig. 24.88).
- Joint effusion: Ultrasound can readily identify fluid accumulation within joints. A distended joint capsule will be visualized with anechoic or heterogeneous echogenic fluid (Fig. 24.89). Thickened synovial lining may be noted as well. Drainage can be assisted either statically, locating and marking area of maximal effusion, or dynamically, using ultrasound throughout the entire procedure. Standard sterile precautions must be followed either way.
- Tendon/ligament injury: Ultrasound can be used to directly visualize tendon or ligament injury of almost any extremity. A defect will be noted in the structure of the tendon or ligament, often with a small fluid accumulation/hematoma (Fig. 24.90). Functional images can be obtained with active/passive use of the corresponding part of the limb while directly viewing the tendon/ligament with ultrasound.
- Subcutaneous foreign body: Most foreign bodies are visible using ultrasound. The foreign body's appearance depends on the shape, size, and composition of the object. Careful, slow passes should be made over the likely location, noting any abnormal object or defect in tissue (Fig. 24.91). EUS can assist in removal by either a static approach, marking the skin overlying the location, or dynamic technique guiding removal during real-time ultrasound. Care should be taken to identify any structures damaged by the foreign body or that may complicate removal.

Pearls

- Always scan the area in two planes. This will help to identify the exact location of the abnormality and exclude artifacts.
- Use surrounding, unaffected tissue or other extremity as a control.
- Optimize image: Reduce depth to appropriate level and increase frequency of probe. Structures that are extremely superficial (<0.5 cm) may not be well visualized due to artifact. Consider the use of a standoff pad or waterbath evaluation technique.
- Waterbath evaluation technique (WET): Distal extremities can be placed in a tub of water covering the area of interest and the water can be used as a conductive media

for the ultrasound (Fig. 24.92). Ultrasound waves travel well through water, permitting a standoff approach where the probe need not actually touch the skin. This is better tolerated by the patient as no contact with the painful area is necessary and this technique facilitates imaging of extremely superficial structures. WET technique for hand and flexor tendon evaluation was first described in emergency medicine by Dr Paul Sierzenski.

- Sterile technique for dynamic ultrasound procedure: For procedures requiring sterile precautions, a sterile sheath should be used to cover the transducer. Many sterile ultrasound sheaths are commercially available although, less preferably, a sterile glove or transparent adherent dressing (ie, Tegaderm) can be used. Sterile ultrasound gel or another sterile liquid (ie, Betadine or chlorhexidine) should be used as a conductive medium.

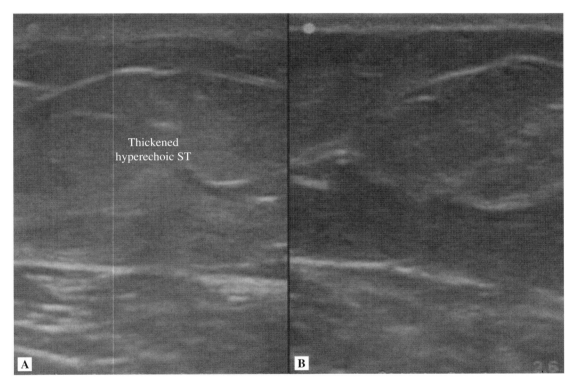

FIGURE 24.86 ■ Superficial: Cellulitis/Edema with Cobblestoning. (A) A side-by-side image shows the affected side left image with thickened dermis and increased echogenicity when compared to the matching portion of the upper arm in this patient with early cellulitis. (B) "Cobblestoning" is noted in this image which is sensitive for both advanced cellulitis and peripheral edema. (Photo contributor: Paul R. Sierzenski, MD, RDMS.)

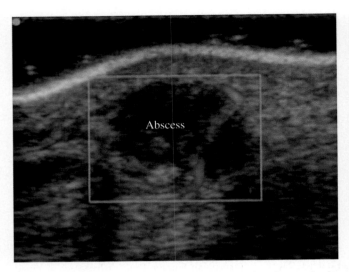

FIGURE 24.87 ■ Superficial: Hand Abscess. An abscess in the hand is noted using the water-bath technique. Power Doppler demonstrates the hyperemic "rim flow" seen around but not within the hypoechoic abscess. (Photo contributor: Paul R. Sierzenski, MD, RDMS.)

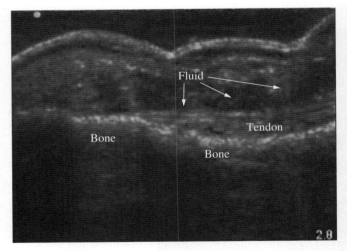

FIGURE 24.88 ■ Superficial: Tenosynovitis. A longitudinal image of the index finger using a water-bath technique shows fluid and debris surround the flexor tendon; diagnostic of tenosynovitis. (Photo contributor: Paul R. Sierzenski, MD, RDMS.)

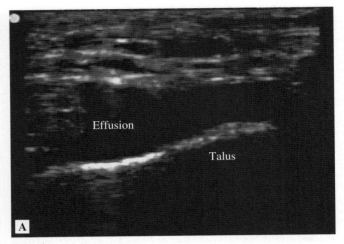

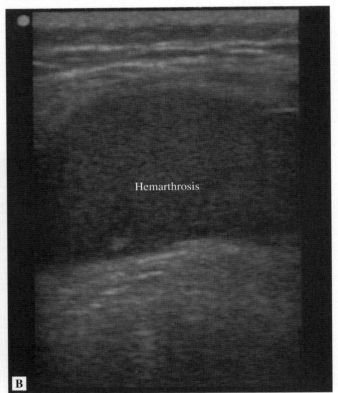

FIGURE 24.89 ■ Superficial: Joint Effusion/Hemarthrosis. (A) The anechoic wedge-shaped effusion is readily identified in this anterior sagittal image of the foot with the talus as the predominant land-mark. (B) The homogenous echogenicity of clotting blood is noted in this patient with a right knee hemarthrosis. (Photo contributor: Paul R. Sierzenski, MD, RDMS.)

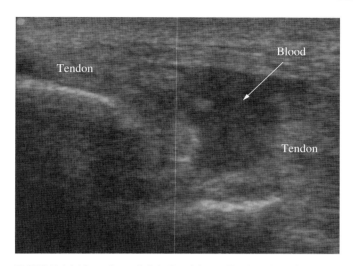

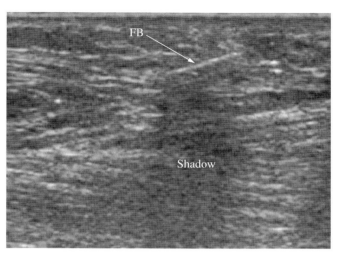

FIGURE 24.90 ■ Superficial: Quadriceps Tendon Tear. Complete rupture of the quadriceps tendon is noted in this sagittal image. The irregular boarders of the tendon partially retracted can be seen, as well as the anechoic blood that filled the defect after the rupture. This patient was diabetic and on fluoroquinolone antibiotics. (Photo contributor: Paul R. Sierzenski, MD, RDMS.)

FIGURE 24.91 ■ Superficial: Foreign Body. A hyperechoic small gage needle is seen in this plantar foot ultrasound. Note the edge artifact and shadowing that occurs for this metal foreign body. (Photo contributor: Paul R. Sierzenski, MD, RDMS.)

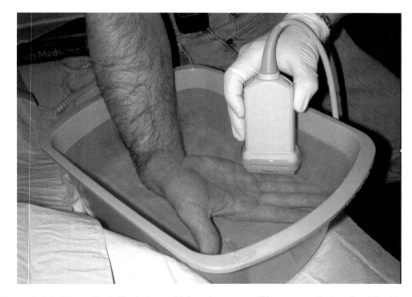

FIGURE 24.92 ■ Superficial: Water-Bath Technique. Using the water. (Photo contributor: Paul R. Sierzenski, MD, RDMS.)

Chapter 25

MICROSCOPIC FINDINGS

Diane M. Birnbaumer

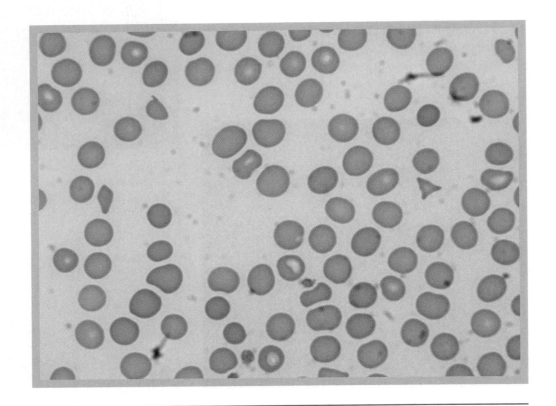

MICROSCOPIC URINALYSIS

Uses

To evaluate for the presence of cells, casts, and crystals.

Materials

Freshly collected urine specimen, centrifuge, graduated centrifuge tubes, glass microscope slide, and coverslip.

Method

1. Pour 10 mL of freshly collected urine into a graduated centrifuge tube.
2. Centrifuge at ×400 to ×450 gravity for 5 minutes.
3. Decant 9 mL of supernatant, leaving 1 mL in the tube.
4. Resuspend the centrifuged pellet in the remaining 1 mL of urine by stirring with a pipet.
5. Place one drop of resuspended urine on a glass microscope slide.
6. Overlay with a coverslip.
7. Examine initially using scanning ×10 power, emphasizing the periphery of the coverslip, since urinary elements tend to gather at the edges.
8. Switch to ×40 power to focus on specific urinary elements such as cells, casts, and crystals. Use ×100 power as needed for specific identification.

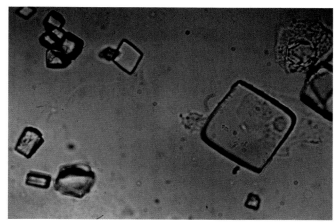

FIGURE 25.2 ■ Uric Acid Crystals. Uric acid crystals often have a yellow hue and a variety of sizes and shapes. They are found in acidic urine. (From Susan K. Strasinger. *Urinalysis and Body Fluids.* 3rd ed. Philadelphia, PA: Davis; 1994.)

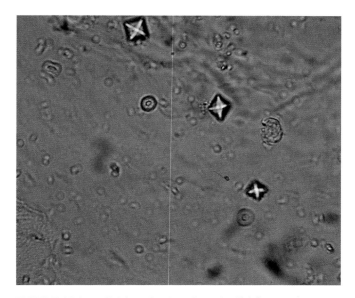

FIGURE 25.1 ■ Calcium Oxalate Crystals. Calcium oxalate crystals come in two shapes. The classically described octahedral, or envelope-shaped, crystals are made of calcium oxalate dihydrate. Calcium oxalate monohydrate crystals are needle-shaped. They are seen in acid or neutral urine. They may be found in the urine of patients with ethylene glycol ingestion. In addition, the urine of patients with ethylene glycol ingestion may also fluoresce under a Wood lamp. (From Susan K. Strasinger. *Urinalysis and Body Fluids.* 3rd ed. Philadelphia, PA: Davis; 1994.)

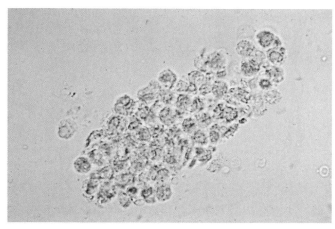

FIGURE 25.3 ■ White Blood Cell Casts. Usually two to three cells in width, white blood cell casts are indicative of upper urinary tract infection such as pyelonephritis. (Photo contributor: the American Society of Clinical Pathologists.)

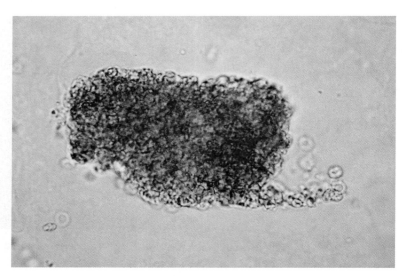

FIGURE 25.4 ■ Red Blood Cell Casts. Red blood cells casts range from 3 to 10 cells in width and are seen in glomerulonephritis. (Photo contributor: the American Society of Clinical Pathologists.)

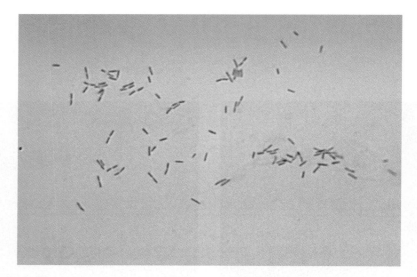

FIGURE 25.5 ■ Bacteria. Bacteria are often seen in urine specimens and either can be consistent with infection or may result from local contamination from surrounding skin during specimen collection. (Photo contributor: Roche Laboratories, Division of Hoffman-LaRoche Inc., Nutley, NJ.)

Uses

To determine the presence of uric acid crystals (in patients with gout) or calcium pyrophosphate crystals (in patients with pseudogout) in joint fluid.

Materials

Freshly collected joint fluid, glass microscope slide, coverslip, and polarizer.

Method

1. To prevent interference from polarizing artifacts, clean the slide and coverslip with alcohol prior to using them.
2. Using freshly collected unspun joint fluid, place a drop of joint fluid on the glass microscope slide.
3. Overlay coverslip.
4. View the slide using the polarizer.
5. Scan at ×10 power; ×100 power is needed to see intracellular crystals.

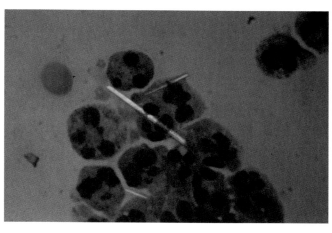

FIGURE 25.6B ■ Compensated Polarized Uric Acid Crystals (×500). Once crystals are found with a direct polarizing light, identification is made by using a compensated polarized light. The yellow crystal is aligned parallel to the slow vibration component of the compensator (negatively birefringent). The blue crystal is perpendicular (Crossed Urate Blue). (From Susan K. Strasinger. *Urinalysis and Body Fluids.* 3rd ed. Philadelphia, PA: Davis; 1994.)

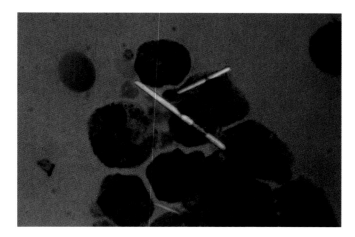

FIGURE 25.6A ■ Polarized Uric Acid Crystals (×500). Intracellular needle-like uric acid crystals are seen within the polymorphonuclear cells from the joint fluid in a patient with gout, using a direct polarizing light. (From Susan K. Strasinger. *Urinalysis and Body Fluids.* 3rd ed. Philadelphia, PA: Davis; 1994.)

FIGURE 25.6C ■ Extracellular Uric Acid Crystals (×100). Extracellular uric acid crystals are seen under compensated polarized light. Notice the change of color with crystal alignment. (From Susan K. Strasinger. *Urinalysis and Body Fluids.* 3rd ed. Philadelphia, PA: Davis; 1994.)

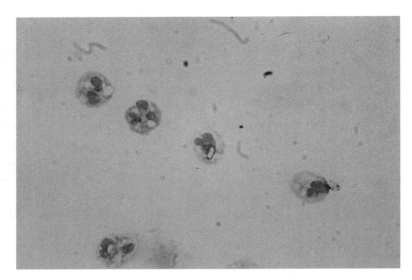

FIGURE 25.7A ■ Polarized Calcium Pyrophosphate Crystals (×1000). Intracellular rhomboid crystals in the joint of a patient with pseudogout. They may also appear as rods. (From Susan K. Strasinger. *Urinalysis and Body Fluids.* 3rd ed. Philadelphia, PA: Davis; 1994.)

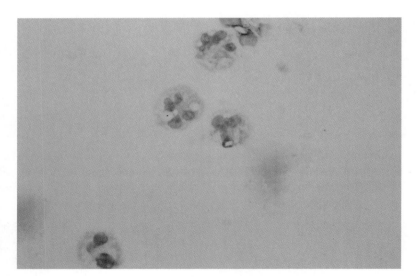

FIGURE 25.7B ■ Compensated Polarized Calcium Pyrophosphate Crystals (×1000). The blue calcium pyrophosphate crystal is aligned parallel to the slow vibration component of the compensator (positively birefringent). (From Susan K. Strasinger. *Urinalysis and Body Fluids.* 3rd ed. Philadelphia, PA: Davis; 1994.)

Uses

The first step in the identification of a predominant bacterial organism in a specimen. Classifies an organism by its cell wall's ability to retain crystal violet dye during solvent treatment. Morphology of the organism is also identified.

Materials

Freshly collected specimen to be examined, glass microscope slide, crystal violet, Gram iodine, acetone-alcohol (acetone, 30 mL, and 95% alcohol, 70 mL), safranin, and Bunsen burner.

Method

1. Put specimen on dry, clean glass microscope slide and allow to air dry.
2. Heat-fix specimen by gently passing over flame.
3. Cover specimen with crystal violet for 1 minute.
4. Rinse off completely with water; do not blot.
5. Cover specimen with Gram iodine for 1 minute.
6. Rinse off completely with water; do not blot.
7. Decolorize for 30 seconds with gentle agitation in acetone-alcohol.
8. Rinse off completely with water; do not blot.
9. Cover with safranin for 10 to 20 seconds.
10. Rinse off completely with water and let air-dry.

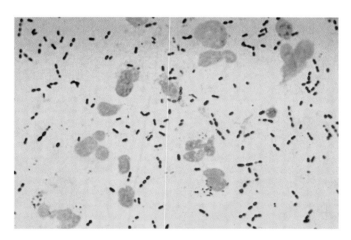

FIGURE 25.8 ■ Gram Stain—*Streptococcus pneumoniae.* Gram-positive, kidney-shaped diplococci of *S pneumoniae.* (Photo contributor: Roche Laboratories, Division of Hoffman-LaRoche Inc. Nutley, NJ.)

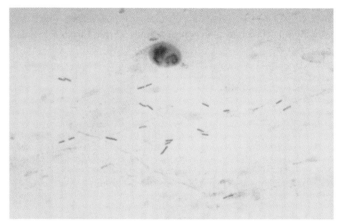

FIGURE 25.10 ■ Gram Stain—Gram-Negative Rods. Gram-negative rods of *Pseudomonas aeruginosa.* (Photo contributor: Roche Laboratories, Division of Hoffman-LaRoche Inc. Nutley, NJ.)

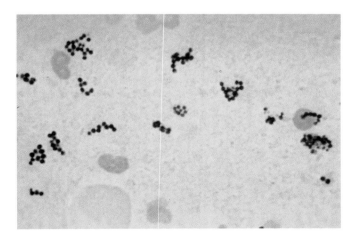

FIGURE 25.9 ■ Gram Stain—*Staphylococcus aureus.* Small clusters of gram-positive cocci seen in *S aureus* infection. (Photo contributor: Roche Laboratories, Division of Hoffman-LaRoche Inc. Nutley, NJ.)

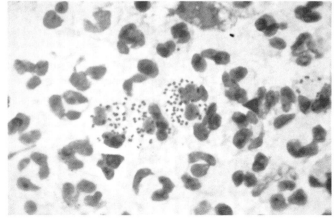

FIGURE 25.11 ■ Gram Stain—*Neisseria gonorrhoeae.* Multiple gram-negative, intracellular diplococci from a patient with *N gonorrhoeae.* (Reproduced with permission from Morse, Moreland, Thompson. *Atlas of Sexually Transmitted Diseases.* London: Mosby-Wolfe; 1990.)

Uses

To evaluate a lesion (chancre, mucous patch, condyloma lata, skin rash) for the presence of *Treponema pallidum*.

Materials

Compound microscope with dark-field condenser (dark-field microscope), glass microscope slide, coverslip, and physiologic saline.

Method

1. From chancre or condyloma lata:
   a. Gently abrade the lesion with dry gauze.
   b. Dab away any bleeding.
   c. Touch slide to exudative fluid in base of lesion.
   d. Overlay coverslip and view immediately under dark-field microscope using ×40 and ×100 objectives.
2. From mucous patch:
   a. Touch slide to mucous patch.
   b. Overlay coverslip and view immediately under dark-field microscope using ×40 and ×100 objectives.
3. From skin lesion:
   a. Gently scrape surface of skin lesion with edge of a number 15 scalpel blade.
   b. Dab away any bleeding.
   c. Touch slide to exudative fluid rising from skin lesion.
   d. Overlay coverslip and view immediately under dark-field microscope using ×40 and ×100 objectives.

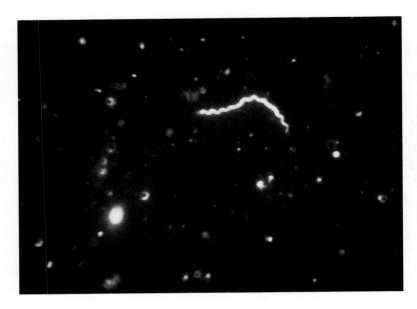

FIGURE 25.12 ■ Dark-Field Microscopy. Examined under a dark-field microscope at ×40 or ×100 power, spirochetes appear as motile, bright corkscrews against a black background. (Reproduced with permission from Morse, Moreland, Thompson: *Atlas of Sexually Transmitted Diseases*. London: Mosby-Wolfe; 1990.)

Uses

To examine for clue cells, *Trichomonas,* and sperm.

Materials

Aqueous sodium chloride, glass microscope slide, and coverslip.

Method

1. Place a drop of saline onto the middle of the glass slide. (Alternative method: Place several drops of saline in a small glass test tube and place the swab in the tube. The swab can then be wiped onto a slide at a later time.)
2. Mix a small amount of vaginal fluid to be examined into the saline drop.
3. Overlay a coverslip.
4. Examine directly through microscope at ×40 and ×100 (oil immersion).

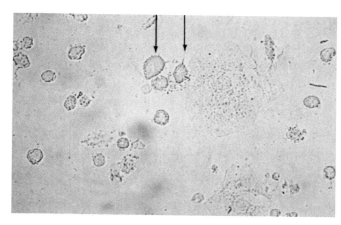

FIGURE 25.14 ■ *Trichomonas.* Saline wet mount demonstrating oval-bodied, flagellated trichomonads. They are similar in size to leukocytes and can be distinguished from them by their motility and presence of flagella. (Photo contributor: H. Hunter Hansfield. *Atlas of Sexually Transmitted Diseases.* New York, NY: McGraw-Hill; 1992.)

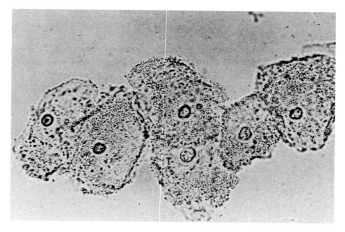

FIGURE 25.13 ■ Clue Cells. "Glitter cell" or "clue cell": Epithelial cell covered with adherent bacteria in a wet mount of a vaginal specimen from a patient with *Gardnerella vaginalis* (also known as nonspecific vaginitis or bacterial vaginosis). Note the refractile appearance, indistinct borders, and ragged edges of the epithelial clue cell. (Photo contributor: Curatek Pharmaceuticals.)

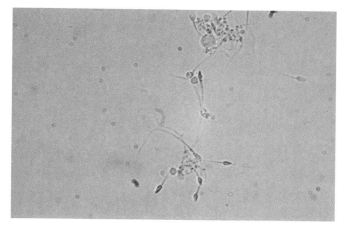

FIGURE 25.15 ■ Spermatozoa. Spermatozoa may be motile or immotile. (From Susan K. Strasinger. *Urinalysis and Body Fluids.* 3rd ed. Philadelphia, PA: Davis; 1994.)

Uses

To examine for yeast and fungus.

Materials

Aqueous potassium hydroxide (KOH) 10%, glass microscope slide, and coverslip.

Method

1. Place a drop of KOH onto the middle of the glass slide.

2. Suspend a small amount of vaginal fluid into the drop of KOH.

3. Overlay a coverslip.

4. Let sit at room temperature for 30 minutes; as an alternative, gently heat the slide over a Bunsen burner but do not boil.

5. Examine under microscope for hyphae and spores.

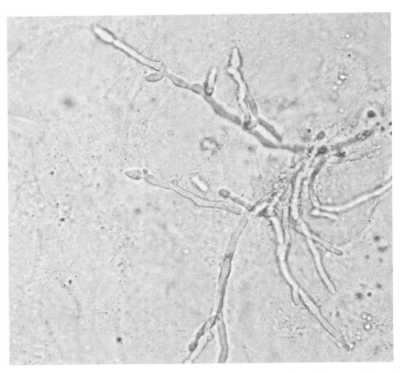

FIGURE 25.16 ■ *Candida albicans.* Potassium hydroxide preparation of vaginal secretions from a patient with vaginal candidiasis due to *C albicans.* Note the pseudohyphae characteristic of this organism. (Photo contributor: H. Hunter Handsfield. *Atlas of Sexually Transmitted Diseases.* New York, NY: McGraw-Hill; 1992.)

Uses

To evaluate a patient's stool sample for the presence of fecal leukocytes.

Materials

Freshly collected liquid stool specimen, glass microscope slide, coverslip, and methylene blue.

Method

1. Place a drop of liquid stool onto the glass slide.
2. Add two drops of methylene blue to the stool specimen.
3. Mix thoroughly.
4. Overlay with a coverslip.
5. Place the edge of a piece of filter paper adjacent to the coverslip to absorb any excess methylene blue.
6. Examine using ×10 objective to scan specimen and ×40 and ×100 to identify specific leukocytes.

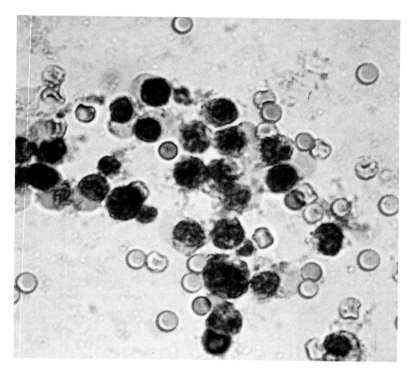

FIGURE 25.17 ■ Fecal Leukocytes. Multiple white cells in the stool specimen from a patient with bacterial diarrhea. (Photo contributor: Herbert L. DuPont, MD.)

Uses

To determine fungal dermatoses or skin infestations.

Materials

Fresh skin scraping, glass microscope slide, coverslip, 10% potassium hydroxide or mineral oil.

Method

1. Specimen collection:
   a. Gently scrape skin lesion with edge of a number 15 scalpel.
2. Slide preparation:
   a. Pediculosis may be seen grossly clinging to individual hairs or under low power. Live nits may fluoresce with a Wood lamp.
   b. For scabies, place a drop of KOH or mineral oil onto the slide.
   c. Suspend a small amount of the scraping onto the drop.
   d. Overlay a coverslip.
   e. Let sit at room temperature for 30 minutes; as an alternative, gently heat the slide over a Bunsen burner but do not boil.
   f. Examine under microscope for hyphae, spores, or infestations.

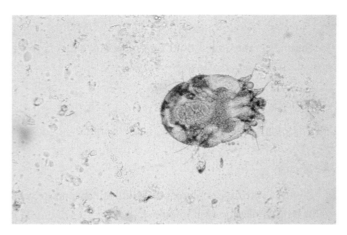

FIGURE 25.19 ■ Scabies. Adult female scabies mite. (Reproduced with permission from Morse, Moreland, Thompson. *Atlas of Sexually Transmitted Diseases*. London: Mosby-Wolfe; 1990.)

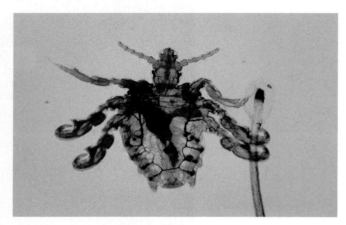

FIGURE 25.20 ■ Pediculosis. *Phthirus pubis,* the crab louse. Note the short body and claw-like legs, which are ideally suited for clinging to the hair shaft. (Photo contributor: the Department of Dermatology, Naval Medical Center, Portsmouth, VA.)

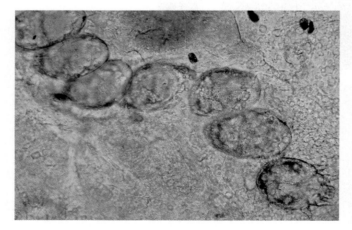

FIGURE 25.18 ■ Scabies. Skin scraping from a patient with scabies. Note the intact mite at the lower right of the photograph, and the ova and fecal pellets. (Photo contributor: the Department of Dermatology, Naval Medical Center, Portsmouth, VA.)

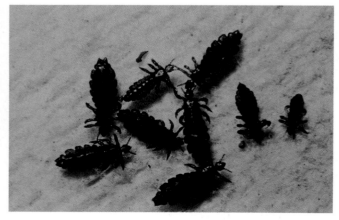

FIGURE 25.21 ■ Pediculosis. *Phthirus corporis,* the body louse. Note the elongated body. (Photo contributor: the Department of Dermatology, Naval Medical Center, Portsmouth, VA.)

Uses

To examine cerebrospinal fluid for organisms with capsules, particularly *Cryptococcus neoformans*.

Materials

India ink, glass microscope slide, and coverslip.

Method

1. Lightly centrifuge cerebrospinal fluid to concentrate cells at bottom of tube (1-2 minutes).

2. Pour off excess fluid (retain if further testing may be necessary).

3. Take a drop from the bottom of the centrifuge tube and place it in the middle of a glass microscope slide.

4. Place a drop of India ink into the specimen drop; gently mix.

5. Overlay a coverslip.

6. Examine at ×10 to screen specimen, use ×40 objective to confirm findings.

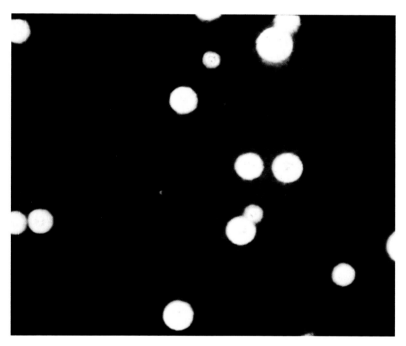

FIGURE 25.22 ■ India Ink Preparation. Budding yeast with prominent capsule on India ink preparation from a patient with *C neoformans* meningitis. (Reproduced with permission from Morse, Moreland, Thompson. *Atlas of Sexually Transmitted Diseases*. London: Mosby-Wolfe; 1990.)

Uses

To evaluate for the presence of ring trophozoites.

Materials

Air-dried blood smear, Coplin jar of Wright stain, slide rack, pH 7.2 buffer, and blotting paper.

Method

1. Place a drop of blood on the middle of a slide.

2. Hold another slide evenly on top of the slide at a 45-degree angle and drag the slide over the drop of blood to the opposite edge to spread the blood evenly.

3. Allow the blood to dry for 5 to 10 minutes.

4. Stain air-dried smears in a closed Coplin jar of Wright stain for 5 minutes.

5. Place the slide on a rack.

6. Rinse and treat with pH 7.2 buffer primed with 1 mL Wright stain per 400 mL for 3 minutes.

7. Rinse in pH 7.2 buffer for 20 seconds.

8. Blot dry and mount on microscope at ×100 (oil immersion).

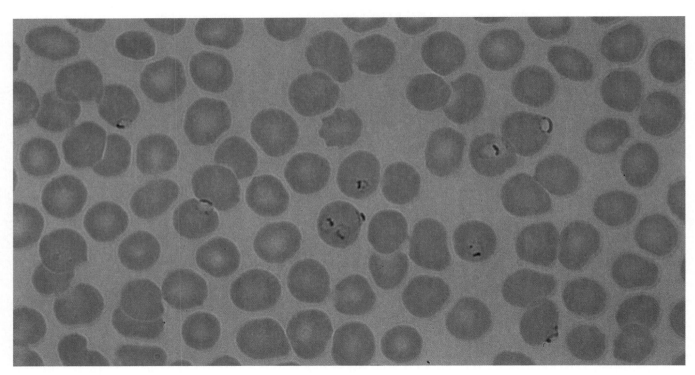

FIGURE 25.23 ■ *Plasmodium falciparum* Thin Film. Ring forms (trophozoites) of *P falciparum* are seen on the Wright stain thin film in a patient with intermittent fever who had recently traveled to Africa. (Photo contributor: James P. Elrod, MD, PhD.)

Uses

To distinguish between amniotic fluid due to membrane rupture and normal vaginal secretions in patients beyond the 20th week in preganacy who present with spontaneous vaginal fluid passage. Characteristic arborization, or typical ferning pattern, confirms amniotic fluid and spontaneous membrane rupture.

Materials

Sterile speculum, vaginal fluid, microscope slide, microscope, and serile swab or pipette.

Method

1. Place patient in dorsal lithotomy position.
2. Do not use lubricants or cleaning agents.
3. Place sterile speculum into vaginal vault.
4. Obtain sample of vaginal secretions from posterior vaginal pool using a pipette or sterile swab.
5. Place a drop of vaginal fluid on a microscope slide.
6. Spread the specimen evenly so that a thin smear is formed.
7. Allow the fluid to air-dry for 5 to 10 minutes. Do not apply heat.
8. Examine slide under low power (10×) for ferning pattern.

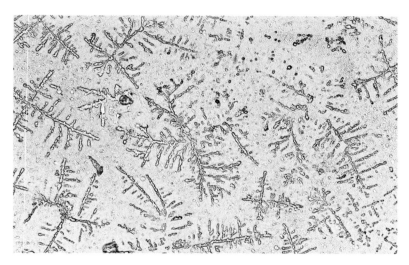

FIGURE 25.24 ■ Ferning Pattern. The arborization pattern found when a drop of amniotic fluid is allowed to air dry on a microscope slide, known as ferning. (Photo contributor: Robert Buckley, MD.)

Uses

To detect the presence of schistocytes in a peripheral blood smear. Shistocytes are fragmented red blood cells due to shearing forces in microarterioles lined or meshed with fibrin strands. They are found in patients with disseminated intravascular coagulation, throbotic thrombocytopenic purpura/haemolytic uremic syndrome, microangiopathic haemolytic anemia, uremia, and carcinoma. Turbulent blood flow due to congestive heart failure, artificial heart valves, or vavlular stenosis may cause schistocyte formation. Greater than 1% of forms or greater than 2 schistocytes per high-powered field suggest schistocytosis.

Materials

Two glass microscope slides, drop of blood, pipette, Wright stain, Giemsa stain, immersion oil, and microscope.

Method

Smear Preparation

1. Agitate sample well, by inversion of tube or mechanical rocker.
2. Place a 2- to 3-mm drop of whole blood $1/4$ in from the right edge of a 1×3 in slide using a wooden applicator stick.
3. Place the slide on a flat surface and hold securely.
4. Grasp a second slide (spreader slide) in the right hand between thumb and forefinger.
5. Place the spreader slide onto the lower slide in front of the blood drop, and pull the slide back until it touches the drop.
6. Allow the blood to spread by capillary action almost to the edges of the lower slide.
7. Push the spreader slide forward at a 30-degree angle, using a rapid even motion. The weight of the spreader slide should be the only weight applied. The drop of blood must be spread within seconds or the cell distribution will be uneven.
8. Allow to air dry.

Wright Stain of Peripheral Smear

1. Completely cover peripheral smear with Wright stain using a pipette. The stain layer should be $1/2$ in thick.
2. Wait for 2 minutes.
3. Cover with equal amount of Giemsa solution.
4. Blow gently on the slide to mix solutions.
5. Allow to stand for 4 minutes.
6. Wash slide for 30 seconds with distilled water.
7. Allow to air dry
8. View smear with oil emersion at high (100X) power.

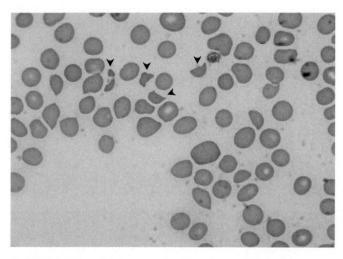

FIGURE 25.25 ■ Schistocytes. Mulitple fragmented red blood cells (black arrowheads) seen on this peripheral smear at 100X in a patient with microangiopathic hemolytic anemia. (Photo contributor: James P. Elrod, MD, PhD.)

Uses

To detect the presence of eggs of *Enterobias vermicularis* in patients who present with nocturnal perianal pruritis or concern for pinworm infestation.

Materials

Microscope slide, clear transparent tape, tongue blade, microscope, or a cellulose-tape slide preparation.

Method

1. Affix $^1/_2$ in of a 4-in piece of tape to the underside of a microscope slide.

2. Hold the slide against the tongue depressor 1 in from the end and lift the long end of the tape from the slide.
3. Loop tape over end of the depressor to expose gummed surface.
4. Hold tape and slide firmly against the tongue depressor.
5. Press gummed surfaces of the tape against several areas of the perianal area.
6. Affix long portion of the tape to the slide.
7. Smooth tape with cotton gauze.
8. View specimen under low (10×) power.

Note: Specimens are best obtained several hours after going to sleep or upon waking before a bowel movement or bath.

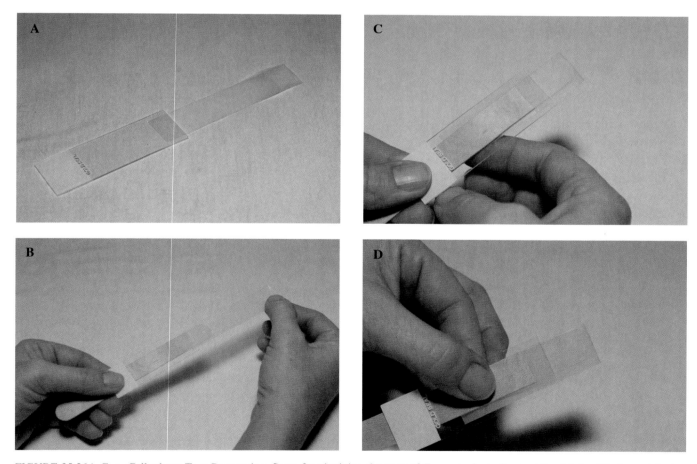

FIGURE 25.26A-G ■ Cellophane Tape Preparation. Steps for obtaining the eggs of *E vermicularis*. See text for details. (Photo contributor: Lawrence B. Stack, MD.)

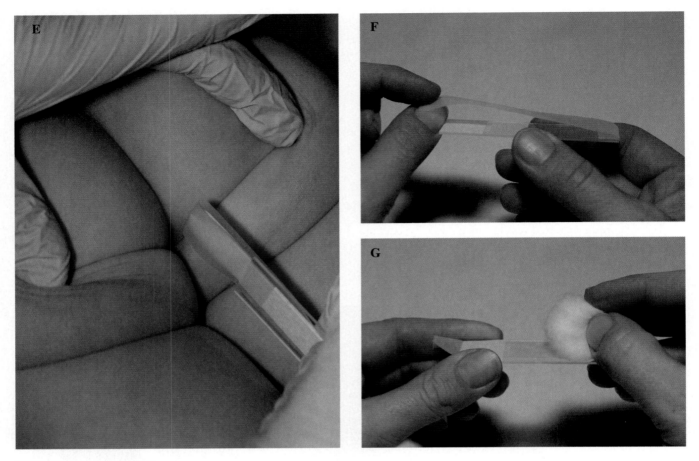

FIGURE 25.26 (*Continued*)

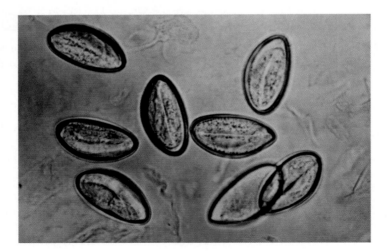

FIGURE 25.27 ■ *Enterobius vermicularis.* Characteristic appearance of the *E vermicularis* egg with contained larval form.

TZANCK PREPARATION

Uses

To detect the multinucleated giant cells confirming the presence of a herpes infection.

Materials

Microscope, Bunsen burner, glass microscope slide, 5% methylene blue or Wright stain, or Geimsa stain, immersion oil, and sterile scalpel or hypdermic needle.

Method

1. Unroof a fresh, uncrusted vesicle with a sterile hypodermic needle or scalpel.

2. Scrape the floor of the vescicle with the scalpel and smear scrapings of the lesion onto a glass microscope slide.
3. Let air dry.
4. Fix specimen with absolute alcohol or gentle heat.
5. Stain with blue stain (5% methylene blue, Wright stain, Geimsa stain) for 5 seconds, rinse and air dry.
6. View preparation through immersion oil at high power (40-50×).

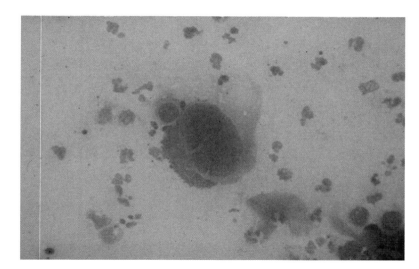

FIGURE 25.28 ■ Tzanck Preparation. A Tzanck preparation of both the roof and floor of a herpetic vesicle demonstrating a multinucleated giant cell. (Photo contributor: the Department of Dermatology, Wilford Hall USAF Medical Center and Brook Army Medical Center, San Antonio, TX.)

Note: Page numbers followed by "f" indicate figures; those followed by "t" indicate tables.

We have a passion for improving patient care. Our journey with *The Atlas of Emergency Medicine* began with an aggressive goal of producing the most comprehensive source of high-quality emergency department images available. The emergency department is, perhaps, the most diverse melting pot of patient conditions in the hospital. Diagnostic accuracy and prognostic prediction often rely heavily on visual clues. Our efforts are directed toward maximizing this skill. We also strongly believe the visual experience is critical to education in medicine, and that great images are the next best tool besides actual bedside exposure. Images often teach faster and with greater impact than many pages of text or hours of lecture.

We continue our pursuit of these goals with a substantially updated, expanded, and improved third edition of *The Atlas of Emergency Medicine*. Nearly all of our changes and additions come from reader suggestions and criticisms, all of which we receive with sincere gratitude. First, we have changed the format to reduce text and allow for more images. Hence the text is more concise, providing only essential information. Each chapter item is now organized into: "Clinical Summary," which includes pertinent differential diagnosis where appropriate, followed by "Emergency Department Treatment and Disposition" and, finally, "Pearls." We have endeavored to provide "Pearls" that are more relevant and represent tips for diagnosis or unique aspects of a condition that are difficult to find in a typical text. Second, after extensive review and critique, hundreds of new and replacement images have been added.

Third, four new chapters grace the pages of this new edition: Tropical Medicine, Toxicology, Airway, and Electrocardiography. Our increased emphasis on worldwide delivery of healthcare and easier patient travel is represented with Tropical Medicine. Toxicology is one of our core skills and a welcome addition as a separate chapter. We have made a decision to expand beyond our main emphasis on pictorial presentations with the addition of the Airway and ECG chapters. We included these topics, beautifully displayed in an atlas format, as they represent critical areas of emergency medicine expertise and are extremely visual. We believe they significantly contribute to the *Atlas*' ability to provide important visual information in a single source. These new chapters also complement our greatly expanded and updated Emergency Department Ultrasound chapter.

The primary audience for this text is emergency medicine clinicians, educators, residents, nurses, prehospital caregivers, and medical students who provide emergency and primary care. We hope it will aid them in making diagnoses and help take the student "to the bedside." Many have found it extremely useful as a review for the ABEM written examination. Other healthcare workers, such as internists, family physicians, pediatricians, nurse practitioners, and physician assistants will find the *Atlas* a useful guide in identifying and treating the many conditions for which visual cues significantly guide, improve, and expedite diagnosis and treatment.

We would also like to thank the many contributors and readers who have helped make this possible. Lastly, and most importantly, we express our gratitude to our patients who were willing to be a "great case" in the *Atlas*, thus ultimately paving the way for improved emergency care.

Kevin J. Knoop, MD, MS
Lawrence B. Stack, MD
Alan B. Storrow, MD
R. Jason Thurman, MD

The third edition of *The Atlas of Emergency Medicine* once again illustrates the breadth of emergency medicine. As emergency medicine has expanded, so too has this new edition with added chapters on the airway, electrocardiography, toxicology, and images related to tropical diseases. This newest edition improves upon the prior two generations of the *Atlas* by changing the format to reduce the text and more than doubling the number of images. It also has a newly formatted "Pearls" section to succinctly summarize key pictorial learning points. With these changes, the *Atlas* continues to be the book one can rely on to provide the single most authoritative collection of clinical images, illustrations, ultrasounds, radiographs, and now ECGs that are seen in the emergency department.

Reading this book is a comprehensive journey through emergency medicine. It can be used as a supplemental text for the study of emergency medicine, or as a reference and diagnostic tool when evaluating individual patients. Medical students, residents in training, new graduates preparing for their certification exam, the practicing physician, and those who teach will all find this authoritative and pictorial encyclopedia of images a valuable resource.

It is frustrating to view a physical finding, rash, or ECG and to have to say that "I don't know, I've never seen that before." *The Atlas of Emergency Medicine* compiles examples of common classic images along with the less common to create a reference encyclopedia for practitioners. This third edition of the *Atlas* is a substantial revision of the second edition and a reflection of the continuing scholarship of the editors and contributors.

Corey M. Slovis, MD